Adult and Family Nurse Practitioner Certification Examination: Review Questions and Strategies

Second Edition

Adult and Family Nurse Practitioner Certification Examination: Review Questions and Strategies

Second Edition

Jill E. Winland-Brown, EdD, MSN, APRN, BC
Professor and Director
Christine E. Lynn College of Nursing
Treasure Coast Campus
Florida Atlantic University
Vero Beach, Florida

Family Nurse Practitioner

Lynne M. Dunphy, PhD, APRN, BC
Professor and Assistant Dean, Graduate Studies
Christine E. Lynn College of Nursing
Florida Atlantic University
Boca Raton, Florida

Family Nurse Practitioner
Palmetto Park Medical Associates
Boca Raton, Florida

F. A. Davis Company • Philadelphia

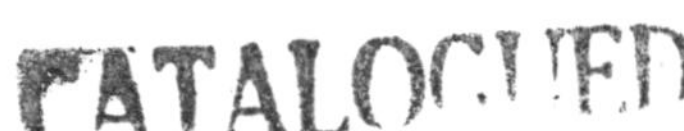

F. A. Davis Company
1915 Arch Street
Philadelphia, PA 19103

Printed in the United States of America

Last digit indicates print number: 10 9 8 7 6 5 4 3 2

Publisher, Nursing: Joanne P. DaCunha, RN, MSN
Developmental Editor: Kristin L. Kern
Production Editor: Jessica Howie Martin
Design Manager: Joan Wendt

ISBN 0-8036-1126-9

I would like to dedicate this book to my husband, Harvey, who is my "true north," and to my daughter, Cydney, who put up with me during the process.

Jill E. Winland-Brown

To my dear husband, Jim, with thanks for his steadfastness, good humor, loyalty, and affection, and to Bradley James Arthur Hektor, the best little boy in the world!

Lynne M. Dunphy

Preface

When we took the certification examination for adult and family nurse practitioners, the only resources available to assist us, other than review classes and associated materials, were review books for physician assistants and physicians. As nurse educators who have been preparing undergraduate students for the NCLEX exam for many years, we knew the importance of taking sample exams in the discipline that reflects the test content. Thus the idea for the book was born.

We believe that answering numerous sample test questions is the best way to prepare for taking a multiple-choice exam such as the current certification exam. We saw a tremendous need for a book that contained a large number of sample test questions with rationales as well as reinforcement in test-taking skills. In the second edition, we have updated information using new standards and guidelines. We have also increased the number of questions.

We suggest reading Chapters 1 and 2 first to get a feeling for both taking the exam and setting up an individualized study plan. Next, you might want to take one of the sample tests in the back of the book to assess your baseline score. This will help you design your individual study plan. We then suggest that you go to the chapter containing test questions for the content area in which you feel you are the weakest.

Because medicine is rapidly changing and is an art as well as a science, there are many conflicting viewpoints and practices regarding treatment options. Every effort was made to ensure that the content is current and relevant, and several sources were used for the rationales of each question. For further information regarding content, see the references that were used for the questions at the end of each chapter.

After you pass the certification exam, this text can be used as a study guide to continually refresh your knowledge base. We suggest writing comments next to each question that will assist you in remembering and noting ideas to be researched further.

We sincerely wish you success on certification and hope that this book contributed in a small way to that success. Best of luck.

Jill E. Winland-Brown
Lynne M. Dunphy

Acknowledgments

I would like to thank Bruce Wishnov, DO, for his continuing mentorship and his never being too busy or too irritable for any question!!! You are a caring physician and an all-around great guy.

LMD

We would both like to thank the entire F. A. Davis team, especially Joanne DaCunha, Publisher, F. A. Davis, for her enthusiasm, support, and friendship; and Kristin Kern, Developmental Editor, for her kind hand and guidance (as well as her culinary skills).

JW-B & LMD

Contributors

Priscilla Dunson Bartolone, RN, MSN
Director, Nursing Program
South University
West Palm Beach, Florida
Doctoral Student
Christine E. Lynn College of Nursing
Florida Atlantic University
Boca Raton, Florida

Karen Stuart Champion RN, MS
Department of Nursing
Indian River Community College
Fort Pierce, Florida

Janice S. Hayes, RN, PhD
Professor
Christine E. Lynn College of Nursing
Florida Atlantic University
Boca Raton, Florida

Gretchen Hope Miller Heery, APRN, BC
Occupational Health Nurse Practitioner
WorkForce Wellness Program
Gnaden Huetten Memorial Hospital
Lehighton, Pennsylvania

Deborah A. Raines, RNC, PhD
Associate Professor
Christine E. Lynn College of Nursing
Florida Atlantic University
Boca Raton, Florida

M. Christopher Saslo, MSN, APRN-C
Adult Nurse Practitioner, Infectious Diseases
VA Medical Center, Infectious Disease Clinic
West Palm Beach, Florida

Susan Elaine Sloan, RN, MS
Cardiovascular Nurse Clinician
The Cardiology Center
Delray Beach, Florida

Sharon A. Thrush, MSN, APRN, BC
Family Nurse Practitioner
Palm Beach Family Physicians
West Palm Beach, Florida
Adjunct Faculty
Christine E. Lynn College of Nursing
Florida Atlantic University
Boca Raton, Florida

Contents

UNIT ONE

INTRODUCTION

1 Achieving Success on a Certification Exam

LYNNE M. DUNPHY and PRISCILLA DUNSON BARTOLONE

Congratulations! With the purchase of this book, you have taken your first step along the road to becoming a certified advanced-practice nurse. The earlier in your educational process you begin preparing for the certification examination (we will be using the term *exam* from now on), the greater your chance of success. If you are a practitioner who has been "out there" for a number of years, this book will help you understand the certification process and the steps you need to take to be successful on the certification exam of your choice. Regardless of your situation, the important point is that you have begun! Remember that the longest journey begins with a single step.

Certification and Why It Is Important

There are basic differences between becoming licensed (something you achieved at the completion of your basic nursing program by sitting for the state boards or the National Council Licensure Examination for Registered Nurses [NCLEX-RN]) and becoming certified. A good understanding of these differences is important to your ultimate success on the certification exam. Becoming "test savvy" demands a thorough understanding of the underlying premises and purposes of the exam for which you are sitting.

LICENSURE

Licensure is a legal requirement. You must be licensed by a state in order to practice nursing in that state. The purpose of licensure is to protect the public from unsafe practitioners. Legal regulation of nursing practice is the joint responsibility of the state legislature and the state board of nursing. Minimum competency is assessed on a licensure exam. This exam asks: Have you met the basic criteria for safe and effective nursing practice? The test questions on the licensure exam are from frequently updated job analyses of entry-level nursing practice. They reflect the concepts and functions that a registered nurse (RN) needs to know and perform for safe entry-level practice.

Currently, the licensure exam is prepared and administered by the National Council of State Boards of Nursing. Composed of representatives from every nursing board in the United States and five of its territories, this body is responsible for setting a national standard for safe and effective entry-level nursing practice and assessing it through administration of a national licensing exam, the NCLEX-RN. Every state now mandates passage of this exam as a prerequisite for state licensure as a registered nurse.

CERTIFICATION

Certification is the process by which a nongovernmental agency or association grants recognition to an individual who has met predetermined standards for specialty practice. The purpose of certification (Table 1–1) is quite different from that of licensure. Certification is a voluntary process, although at present many states require passage of the appropriate certification exam as a prerequisite to licensure to perform advanced-practice nursing functions.

Certification validates superior knowledge of a nursing specialty; the process of recertification recognizes continued high achievement in that specialty. In 1974, the American Nurses Association (ANA) initiated a national voluntary certification process to recognize excellence in nursing practice. By 1978, the purpose had broadened to include the assurance of quality in advanced nursing practice. This was done partly to recognize professional achievement, but also to identify nurses who were potentially eligible for third-party reimbursement.

TABLE 1–1. PURPOSE OF CERTIFICATION

- Required for practice in some states
- Indicates specialized and advanced knowledge base
- Provides greater career opportunities
- Increasingly required for third-party reimbursement

By the 1990s, the regulation of advanced-practice nursing had become a topic of increasing concern within the nursing profession. Whether a secondary level of licensure, rather than certification, is the more appropriate regulatory mechanism has been debated for some time.

The current system for recognizing advanced-practice nursing through certification was established by, and has been operated by, various specialty nursing organizations since the 1990s. An umbrella board, the American Board of Nursing Specialties (ABNS), was established in 1991 (American Association of Colleges of Nursing, 2002, p. 3). Modeled after the American Board of Medical Specialties, this board recognizes advanced-practice nursing certifying bodies by establishing that these bodies have met certain uniform standards, such as education.

Debate remains heated on the continuation of voluntary certification administered through professional associations such as the ANA, its subsidiary, the American Nurses Credentialing Center (ANCC), and the American Academy of Nurse Practitioners (AANP), versus the institution of a mandatory second-level licensure exam specifically for advanced-practice nursing functions. At present, however, certification remains the only nationally recognized means available for validating advanced-practice nursing knowledge. Table 1–2 lists associations and organizations offering advanced-practice nursing certification.

National certification and specialty designation play an increasingly central role in state licensure at an advanced-practice level as well as in reimbursement for advanced nursing services. They are also linked to prescriptive authority in certain states. Some forms of reimbursement are contingent on national certification. Since 1998, certification has been a prerequisite to Medicare reimbursement. The Veterans Affairs Medical Systems now mandate national certification for advanced-practice nurses. Likewise, certain managed-care organizations, as well as hospitals, require national certification as a criterion for credentialing providers.

Certification of advanced-practice **registered** nurses (**APRNs**) ensures that individuals titled at an advanced-practice level have mastered a specific body of knowledge and acquired a particular set of specialized skills unique to their practice area. **APRNs** are expected to have expert competence, knowledge, and skills. Consensus has increasingly emerged regarding what these competencies and skills are. As outlined by the National Council of State Boards of Nursing in 1992, they include:

- Advanced assessment skills
- Advanced ability to synthesize and analyze data
- Advanced ability to apply nursing principles
- Ability to provide expert guidance and teaching
- Ability to work with clients, their families, and other healthcare workers
- Ability to manage clients' health or illness status
- Ability to recognize practice limits
- Ability to use abstract thinking and conceptualization
- Ability to make decisions independently
- Ability to diagnose and prescribe
- Ability to consult with or refer to other healthcare workers

YOUR ROLE

You are making an important, timely, and professionally astute decision by choosing to become certified. In 1998 Margretta Madden Styles, President of the ANCC, noted in *Credentialing News*, "(A)s the global tide turns from governmental regulation and public protectionism toward competitive quality improvement of services and informed consumer choice, voluntary credentialing is a movement whose time has come." We concur.

Certification Exams

This book is geared toward the nurse who is seeking certification as an adult nurse practitioner (ANP)

TABLE 1–2. ASSOCIATIONS AND ORGANIZATIONS OFFERING ADVANCED-PRACTICE NURSING CERTIFICATION

ASSOCIATION OR ORGANIZATION	*ADVANCED-PRACTICE NURSING CERTIFICATION*
American Academy of Nurse Practitioners	**Nurse Practitioner** • Adult • Family
American Nurses Credentialing Center	**Nurse Practitioner** • Acute care (jointly with American Association of Critical Care Nurses) • Adult • Family • Gerontological • Pediatric • Palliative Care • Psychiatric, Adult • Psychiatric, Family **Clinical Nurse Specialist** • Community health • Gerontological • Home health • Medical-surgical • Psychiatric and mental health (adult) • Psychiatric and mental health (child and adolescent)
American Association of Nurse Anesthetists	**Certified Registered Nurse Anesthetist**
American College of Nurse-Midwives	**Certified Nurse Midwife**
National Certification Board of Pediatric Nurse Practitioners and Nurses	**Nurse Practitioner** • Pediatric
National Certification Corporation for the Obstetric, Gynecologic, and Neonatal Nurse Practitioner Nursing Specialties	**Nurse Practitioner** • Neonatal • Women's health
Oncology Nursing Certification Corporation	**Advanced Oncology Nursing for Nurse Practitioners and Clinical Nurse Specialists**

and/or family nurse practitioner (FNP). The ANP certification exam is designed to assess your abilities as an **APRN** in the delivery of primary care services to an adult population, defined as adolescence through old age. The FNP certification exam is designed to assess your abilities as an APRN in the delivery of primary care services, including prepartum and postpartum care and pediatrics, to a population covering the entire family life span. Table 1–3 lists the requirements for nurse practitioner certification.

AMERICAN NURSES CREDENTIALING CENTER

In 1973, the ANA established a certification program to recognize professional achievement in a defined clinical or functional area of nursing. This was in response to the proliferation of specialties in nursing, as well as the increasing emphasis on clinical specialization in graduate nursing education. The exams were first offered in 1974. Certification was a voluntary process, and 691 nurses were initially certified, including psychiatric mental health clinical nurse specialists, the first group of APRNs to promote certification and use it for reimbursement. A master's degree was required to sit for this advanced-practice certification. In 1978, 10 generalist and specialty-level certification examinations were available; in 1997, the number of exams available had expanded to 28. Currently, more than 130,000 nurses have achieved certification at both the generalist and advanced-practice levels. Exams are available in **11** generalist categories, **13** advanced-practice categories (including clinical nurse specialist certifications and nurse practitioner certification), and **4** nursing systems and administration categories. There is also **1 modular** certification in case management.

In 1991, the ANCC was established as a separate subsidiary of the ANA. This is in compliance with nationally accepted standards for certification, which require that credentialing bodies be separate from their parent organizations to prevent conflicts of interest.

To qualify to take an examination and become certified at either the generalist or advanced level, a nurse must (1) meet requirements for clinical or functional

TABLE 1–3. REQUIREMENTS FOR NURSE PRACTITIONER CERTIFICATION

AMERICAN NURSES CREDENTIALING CENTER (ANCC)	*AMERICAN ACADEMY OF NURSE PRACTITIONERS (AANP)*
SPECIALTY AREAS	
• Acute Care Nurse Practitioner • Adult Nurse Practitioner • Family Nurse Practitioner • Gerontological Nurse Practitioner • Pediatric Nurse Practitioner • Palliative Care Nurse Practitioner • Psychiatric Nurse Practitioner, Adult • Psychiatric Nurse Practitioner, Family	• Adult Nurse Practitioner • Family Nurse Practitioner
REQUIREMENTS	
• Master's-level nurse practitioner program from an accredited institution of higher learning • Meet practice requirements specific to certification type	• Master's-level nurse practitioner program from an accredited institution of higher learning • Nurse practitioners without this degree may petition the certification board for permission to sit for the examination
EXAMINATIONS	
• Check ANCC Website	• Given in February, June, and September (Computerized/paper & pencil)
• Over 300 centers operated by Sylvan Technology Centers	• Check Website
• Check Website for current cost	• Check Website for current cost
CONTACT	
ANCC 600 Maryland Ave, SW Suite 100 West Washington, DC 20024-2571 800-284-2378 http://www.ana.org/ancc/index.htm	AANP Certification Program Capitol Station PO Box 12926 Austin, TX 78711 512-442-5202 http://www.aanpcertification.org email: *certification@aanp.org*

practice in a specialized field; and (2) show evidence of having pursued education beyond basic nursing preparation, and in the case of both the FNP and ANP exam, provide evidence of successful completion of an approved master's-level curriculum. In some specialties, the nurse must also receive the endorsement of his or her peers. After meeting these criteria as they relate to a given specialty, the nurse must take and pass the relevant certification exam. Only then will the nurse be certified in that specialty.

Once you have sent in your application for the ANCC exam, you will receive a copy of the *Candidate's Handbook*, a valuable source of help in preparing for the exam. The handbook contains a test content outline (TCO) that describes the practice and content areas, topics, and subtopics that will be covered on the exam. It also includes information about how that content is weighted; that is, the number of test questions in each of the major content areas.

The TCO for the Family Nurse Practitioner Certification Exam indicated that there would be 50 questions (33%) on assessment, 22 questions (14.7%) on diagnosis, 12 questions (8%) on client education, 43 questions (28.7%) on planning and intervention, 8 questions (5.3%) on evaluation of responses to care, 9 questions (6%) on health promotion strategies, and 6 questions (4%) on scope of practice and ethics.

Note the large number of questions in the area of *assessment*. This domain reflects health promotion applications across the life span and includes growth and development questions, as well as wellness/risk-factor identification, history taking, and physical examination in acute/episodic and chronic illness.

The domain of *planning and intervention*, which comprises about 29 % of the exam, contains questions on management of high-risk populations, including subtopics such as dependency behaviors (e.g., substance abuse), victims of violence, and crisis intervention. It also includes management, therapeutics (both pharmacological and nonpharmacological), and counseling.

The domain content of *diagnosis* reflects epidemiology and pathophysiology, including diagnostic data and laboratory test results.

Client education includes health promotion applications across the life span and acute/episodic and chronic illness.

Health promotion strategies includes questions on primary, secondary, and tertiary prevention; family, cultural, community, and environmental factors; lifestyle and health behaviors; and health and wellness research.

The domain content of *scope of practice and ethics* includes consultation and referral, client advocacy, ethical and legal considerations, access to care, and research-based practice.

Additionally, all questions are classified along a second dimension: *life span*. Classifications include non–age-specific content, aging adult, adult, adolescent, child, infant, and childbearing woman. Finally, a third dimension, *problem areas*, organizes question content by body systems such as respiratory and cardiovascular.

What this means is that each test question is characterized across three dimensions. For example, a test question that asks about the treatment of a 70-year-old man with a diagnosis of benign prostatic hypertrophy would be categorized as a planning and intervention test question, requesting content about the aging adult, specifically to do with the genitourinary system. Be aware that the TCO may change from exam to exam, so you need to examine your handbook carefully for the most current content breakdown.

As of 1999, the ANCC began giving its certification exams by computer. The number of items on the test may vary from 75 to 250, depending on your pattern of testing. As of 2003, the ANCC exam had 175 test questions. Of these, 150 were scored questions and 25 were nonscored sample questions under evaluation for future use on the exam. The nonscored questions could not be distinguished from the scored items. This is one reason to use good test-taking skills and not spend too much time on any one question: Any question might be one of the nonscored items!

In 2003 the passing score was based on 150 *scored* questions. The passing score for the 2003 FNP exam was 110 out of 150. Of 1692 persons who sat for the exam, 1271 (75.1%) passed. The passing score for the 2002 ANP exam was 91 out of 150. Of 750 persons who sat for the exam, 540 (72%) achieved a passing score.

A *criterion-referenced standard* is used to assess each examinee's level of specialty knowledge independent of the group taking the exam. In this approach, each examinee's score is compared to an absolute number determined by the content experts who develop the exam.

The test development committee determines the passing score after careful consideration of the content of the test questions. The passing score is always expressed in terms of the number of questions you must correctly answer on the total test, as well as statistical examinations of the reliability and validity of the "piloted" test questions. Additional statistical examination of the piloted questions is assessed for inclusion in the final graded pool of test questions on the next exam.

Your score report will provide you with detailed information regarding how many test questions you correctly answered in each of the major content domains. However, it is your performance on the total test that determines your success or failure. The report will be mailed to you 5 to 7 days after you take the test.

You will need to be recertified every 5 years. This may be accomplished by accumulating continuing education credits. Please check the ANCC Website; guidelines for recertification are subject to change.

AMERICAN ACADEMY OF NURSE PRACTITIONERS

The AANP offers competency-based national certification examinations for the ANP and FNP. Reflecting nurse practitioner knowledge and expertise, the content areas of these exams include health promotion, disease prevention, and diagnosis and management of acute and chronic diseases. The exams given by the AANP were developed in conjunction with the Professional Examination Service, a not-for-profit organization with over 50 years of experience in developing and administering national licensing and certification exams in health-related fields.

Historically, examinees were required to be graduates of approved master's-level ANP or FNP programs. As of this writing, non–master's-prepared practitioners may petition the certification board for permission to sit for the examinations. This certification program is fully accredited by the National Commission for Certifying Agencies (NCCA).

The Academy Certification Program, in conjunction with the Professional Examination Service, conducted a role delineation study to determine areas of clinical knowledge to be tested. Based on the study's results, the exam tests clinical knowledge in the following areas: assessment, diagnosis, formulation and implementation of treatment plans, evaluation, follow-up, and applicable professional issues. The FNP exam tests clinical knowledge of prenatal, pediatric, adolescent, adult, and geriatric primary care, whereas the ANP exam tests knowledge of late adolescence, adult, and geriatric primary care. Examinees must be able to integrate knowledge of pathophysiology, psychology, and sociology with the assessment, diagnosis, and treatment of patients in primary care. Knowledge of health promotion and disease prevention is tested as well as management of acute/episodic and chronic illness in the primary care setting.

These exams also consist of 150 test questions, with a minimum passing score of 91. **The June 1997**

FNP exam had 750 candidates; 540 candidates (72%) passed.

Certification is good for 5 years, after which you must recertify. This may be accomplished (1) by sitting for the exam again or (2) by keeping your practice current: working 1000 hours in your clinical area *and* pursuing 75 contact hours of continuing education in your relevant area of specialization.

Achieving Success

Practitioner programs generally focus on assessment, management, and evaluation of *disease*. Indeed, this is the role most of you perform in your respective work settings. The ability to diagnose and treat disease is paramount to your safe and effective functioning as an APN, and certification exams increasingly reflect this reality. However, it is important never to lose sight of the fact that these exams are certifying your abilities as an APN, and as such have an underlying bias toward *health, health promotion*, and *human responses to health and illness*.

As a nurse, your reaction to the various manifestations of health and illness phenomena is instinctively different than that of other primary care providers. This is manifested in different ways on each exam, but it is an important distinction to keep in mind as you sit and ponder various distractors and wonder what answer the examiner wants. Similarly, the test blueprints and type of questions asked reflect a continued commitment to concepts of health promotion and disease prevention, as well as the underlying principles of therapeutic communication skills that are so essential to the forging of meaningful nurse-client relationships. Nursing-based elements of growth and development, nutrition, and therapeutic communication, as well as questions about cultural differences and cross-cultural communication, will be integrated with content concerning specific aspects of diagnosis, pharmacology, and disease management.

Physical assessment and history-taking skills, as well as content from advanced physical assessment courses, remain prominent. Although a certain amount of basic pharmacologic content is included, the latest drugs and pharmacologic interventions may not always appear, because the exam questions are prepared and tested well in advance. (Note: Questions about your knowledge of safe prescribing for the pregnant woman almost always appear on the FNP exams.)

If you have been in active practice for some time, you must exercise care as you take the exam. Distractors (see Chap. 2) will not necessarily correlate with what you currently see and do. Remember, the exam reflects the *ideal* answer according to the certifying body, which may not always mirror the realities of your practice! Test answers draw on national guidelines and standards of practice promulgated by a variety of bodies. Your practice is likely to be focused on a specialty, and to reflect the practice patterns and priorities of your particular geographic region and site. The questions on the exam are looking for much more generalized responses and might well reflect phenomena that you very seldom experience. Allowing yourself to become frustrated with the distractors offered will not help you, but rather will hinder your ability to succeed. This is why it is essential that you study large numbers of sample test items (see Chap. 2).

Being test savvy and succeeding on a multiple-choice exam is a far different skill from the expert skills you bring to your practice. But these skills are not mutually exclusive. It is a matter of having the correct mindset. This mindset is predicated on an awareness of the *nursing base* of the certification exam coupled with an understanding of the *test blueprint*. Develop a determination not to select an anecdotal answer based on experience from your own practice, but rather to select an answer based on nationally recognized, clinically based guidelines and rooted in clinical literature.

You have taken the first and hardest step: you have purchased this book! Mentally review the important reasons to become nationally certified. Fix the end goal vividly in your mind. Imagine how you will feel opening the envelope telling you that you have succeeded, that you are a nationally certified APRN. It is a worthwhile goal.

Take the next step on the road to success. Turn to Chapter 2. It will assist you in the development of important test-taking skills, as well as providing guidelines for your individualized study plan.

You can succeed!

Bibliography

American Academy of Nurse Practitioners: National Competency-Based Certification Examinations for Adult and Family Nurse Practitioners. American Academy of Nurse Practitioners, Austin, TX, 2003.

American Association of Colleges of Nursing, Position Statement, 2002.

American Nurses Certification Corporation: 2003 Certification Catalog, American Nurses Certification Corporation, Washington, DC, 2003.

Henerson, T, et al.: Scope of Practice and Reimbursement for Advance Practice Registered Nurses: A State-by-State Analysis. Intergovernmental Health Policy Project, Washington, DC, 1995.

King, CS: Second licensure. Advanced Practice Nursing Quarterly 1(1):7, 1995.

National Certification Board of Pediatric Nurse Practitioners and Nurses: Pediatric Nurse Practitioner Certification and Certification Maintenance Programs. National Certification Board of Pediatric Nurse Practitioners, Cherry Hill, NJ, 2003.

National Council of State Boards of Nursing: Regulation of Advanced Practice Nursing—2002 National Council of State Boards of Nursing Position Paper. National Councils of State Boards of Nursing, Inc., 2002.

Oncology Nursing Certification Corporation: Oncology Nursing Certification Corporation Test Bulletin, Oncology Nursing Certification Corporation, Pittsburgh, PA, 2003.

Pearson, L: Annual update of how each state stands on legislative issues affecting advanced nursing practice. Nurse Pract 23:1, 2003.

Sheehy, CM, and McCarthy, M: Advance Practice Nursing: Emphasizing Common Goals, FA Davis, Philadelphia, 1998.

Resources

American Academy of Nurse Practitioners (AANP)
Capitol Station
P.O. Box 12926
Austin, TX 78711
512-442-5202
http://www.aanpcertification.org

American Nurses Credentialing Center (ANCC)
600 Maryland Ave, SW
Suite 100 West
Washington, DC 20024-2571
800-284-2378
http://www.ana.org/ancc/index.htm

2

Test-Taking Skills and Designing Your Study Plan

LYNNE M. DUNPHY and KAREN STUART CHAMPION

This chapter has several parts. The first part actively assists you in assessing your study and testing style. It prepares you to develop an individualized study plan that will enable you to achieve your goal: becoming a nationally certified advanced-practice nurse. The remaining parts deal with the specifics of answering multiple-choice test questions and the skills necessary to succeed on a multiple-choice examination (we will use the term exam *from this point on). We will specifically discuss the American Nurses Credentialing Center (ANCC) adult and/or family nurse practitioner exam and the American Academy of Nurse Practitioners (AANP) exam. Evaluating test taking skills and development of a formal study plan are also covered.*

Study Habits and Test-Taking Skills: Know Yourself

WHAT TEST-TAKING TYPE ARE YOU?

This fun exercise will allow you to diagnose your own studying and test-taking style. Are you a tortoise or a hare? Are you a peacock? Or are you more like a pig? Knowing your style can assist you in designing your study plan for the exam and answering test questions on exam day. For example, are you a *tortoise*, moving slowly and laboriously through each question, taking far too long, and then having to rush at the end, thereby increasing your chance of error? Or are you a *hare*, racing through the exam questions as fast as you can, often misreading information, and likely to make quick guesses rather than carefully thought-out responses?

Are you preoccupied with grades and personal achievement, viewing the certification exam as a threat? Do you procrastinate about studying rather than developing and sticking to a well-designed study plan, thus increasing your anxiety? Do you argue with some test questions, convinced that none of the options are right according to your practice! Then you may be a *peacock*. Remember, exam questions are **not** perfect, but still require that you choose the **best** available option. Do **not** waste time and energy arguing mentally with a test question. Select what you feel is the best option and **move on!**

Or are you a pig? *Pigs* frequently doubt their own knowledge and may waver from their correct initial responses. Most pigs are smart, but lack confidence. They are often academically successful, but experience anxiety when information is presented in an unfamiliar format.

Table 2–1 will assist you in identifying your test-taking personality.

TABLE 2–1. IDENTIFYING YOUR TEST-TAKING TYPE*

HARE	*TORTOISE*	*PEACOCK*	*PIG*
Study Style			
• Crams • Feels anxious during study sessions	• Obsessive • Focuses on details; misses the bigger picture	• Procrastinates • Puts off studying; does not think there is a need to study	• Diligent • Smart, has good study habits, but lacks self-confidence
Test-Taking Style			
• Often first to finish • Rushes, does not thoroughly read questions and answers • Makes quick guesses • Feels anxious when answer is not readily apparent	• Often last to finish • Spends too much time examining details and re-reading questions and answers • May have to rush at end to complete exam in allotted time	• Reads own ideas into questions • Changes initial responses often because expected answer is not present • Selects answer based on anecdotal experience	• Questions own knowledge • Changes initial responses • Feels anxious when faced with information that is presented differently from expected way • Voices self-doubt during testing
Test-Taking Strategies			
• Develop and stick to a study plan: avoid last-minute cramming. • Focus on decreasing test-taking speed. • Read questions as though speaking them aloud in your head to avoid scanning. • Read all options. • Time yourself in practice tests; allow no less than 1 minute per question.	• Focus on concepts and not details during study periods. • Use concept maps. • Focus on increasing testing speed. • Do not linger too long over one question. • Time yourself in practice tests; allow 45 to 60 seconds for each question. • Keep a watch in front of you while taking the test; determine the halfway point and mark it on the exam.	• Develop and stick to a study plan. • Practice with sample tests. • Maintain objectivity; avoid adding own interpretation. • Avoid changing answers.	• Continue usual study activities. • Work on self-confidence. • Develop a self-confidence mantra to recite if you find yourself doubting your knowledge. • Use practice tests to increase confidence. • Avoid changing answers.
Relaxation Techniques			
• Breathe deeply. • Practice positive visualization. • Avoid caffeine. • Develop a test-taking mantra to recite if you find yourself losing focus.	• Breathe deeply. • Practice positive visualization. • Avoid caffeine.	• Breathe deeply. • Practice positive visualization. • Avoid caffeine.	• Breathe deeply • Practice positive visualization. • Avoid caffeine.

**Source:* Adapted from Sides, MB and Korchek, N: Successful Test-Taking Strategies, ed. 3, Lippincott. Philadelphia, 1998, p. 77; and Dickenson-Hazard, N: Test-taking Strategies and Techniques, in Kopec, CA and Millonig, VL (eds.): Gerontological Nursing Certification Review Guide, revised ed., Health Leadership Associates, Potomac, MD, 1996, pp. 3–5.

WHAT IS YOUR PREFERRED LEARNING STYLE?

Awareness of your learning style will also guide you in selecting study strategies. Learning styles are related to the pathways or channels through which you prefer to absorb information. The three types of learners are commonly identified as *visual, auditory,* and *tactile* (sometimes called *kinesthetic*).

Visual Learners

Visual learners learn better from reading and writing than from hearing and talking about information. They usually find background noise, such as music and television, distracting rather than helpful. Strategies for visual learners include:

- Reading texts in a quiet place
- Watching appropriate videos
- Using visual study aids such as concept maps, flashcards, and charts
- Using highlighting markers or colored paper to take notes

Auditory Learners

Auditory learners grasp information most effectively by listening and talking. Combining information with music often works well for auditory learners. Strategies for auditory learners include:

- Reading texts aloud
- Listening to audiotapes of course material
- Making up a song about the content and singing it aloud (especially helpful for assimilating difficult content)
- Listening to background music or other noise
- Talking about the content with a study partner

Tactile or Kinesthetic Learners

Tactile or kinesthetic learners prefer to learn "hands on." They have difficulty sitting still for long periods. During study sessions, they should stand and move around or take frequent stretch breaks. Integrating physical activity with study works well for these learners. Strategies for tactile learners include:

- Moving around while studying
- Reading while exercising on a stationary bicycle
- Listening to tapes of learning material while walking or biking
- Rewriting or typing notes

Although almost everyone is capable of learning through all of their sensory pathways, most have a preferred channel. Think about which of the three learning styles discussed works best for you. Time is often at a premium for nurses studying for certification, and capitalizing on your preferred learning style will help you study in the most efficient way. Keep strategies for your preferred learning style in mind as you develop your study plan.

No matter what your personal style, your test-taking skills **can** be improved! Remember how you improve your other skills, such as playing an instrument or a sport: **practice.** The same holds true for test-taking skills. The best way to succeed on the exam is through practice, practice, and more practice. The more you practice answering sample test questions, the better you will become at it. That is why we have written this book for you. This book will provide you with 2000 sample test questions. Research has shown that two-thirds of study time should be spent taking sample tests, and only one-third of the time should be spent reviewing content. A number of exam preparation books are available to you; however, very few contain nearly the number of test questions you need to develop and flex your test-taking muscles. This book provides enough questions to enable you to do that.

GETTING STARTED

Studying, like regular exercise, is good for the brain. As a healthcare professional, you will find that it will always be your job to keep abreast of the professional literature and spend some time studying. To recertify, you are mandated to keep your practice current through a combination of a number of clinical hours and continuing education options. The earlier you begin to plan for certification or recertification, the better.

The principles of effective study are simple but often ignored. There is one central law about study: the law of mass effect. Any worthwhile studying takes time. And in today's world, time is a precious commodity. Therefore, if you want to study, you need to set aside adequate time and plan accordingly. There is no way around the hours involved. There are no shortcuts! But you need to make it easy to begin.

TIPS FOR STUDYING

Just as a cold engine will run a little rough, settling down to study when one is out of the habit can be difficult. The following suggestions should make it easier to begin studying, and to return to it on a regular and consistent basis:

- *Create a pleasurable personal environment.* This is a very basic but frequently overlooked requirement for successful study. Organize all your study materials in one area. Try to create a pleasant and regular workspace for yourself: perhaps just a part of a room, but an inviting part. Decorate it with flowers, pictures, or whatever makes the area appealing to you. For the kinesthetic learner, an open area that allows free movement may be better than a small office. Some literature suggests that playing classical music, especially from the baroque era, in the background increases concentration and retention. Decide whether background music is helpful for you or distracting to you. Background music may be helpful for an auditory learner, whereas a visual learner may find it a distraction. For the kinesthetic learner, an open area that allows free movement may be better than a small office.

- *Plan your activities in advance and be realistic.* Plan in advance what you are going to work on and do not be overly ambitious. Blocks of $1^1/_2$ hours at most are recommended, with a 10-minute break every 45 minutes. List the tasks beforehand; otherwise you might spend valuable time trying to decide what material to review. Set specific targets for the time available.
- *Keep focused on the goal: becoming certified!* Keep the benefits of the study clearly in mind, in this case the joy of receiving your passing score in the mail, followed by your embossed certificate. Visualize how the envelope feels when it comes in the mail. Feel your relief and joy when you open the envelope and read your passing score! Picture the certificate framed, hanging in your office. Write down a list of all the things that you stand to gain from passing the exam and reread it when you are ready to begin to study. Maybe they include a raise, an advanced level of licensure, a new job, or prescriptive privileges. Focus on these results and how they make you feel. Close your eyes and allow the feelings to flood through you!
- *Leave the environment in readiness for your next session.* Leave your work environment inviting for the next time. Put your materials away so that they are easily accessible. Do not leave the area cluttered; instead, make it more pleasing. Spend the last few minutes of your study time tidying up so that your environment is all set for your next session. This is also an excellent time to plan what you will do the next time you sit down to study. Believe it or not, these small, concrete habits can make a big dent in your natural tendency to procrastinate.
- *Reward yourself.* Last but not least, reward yourself! Reward yourself for each study period. You might decide that if you spend 3 hours studying on Saturday, you will see a movie on Saturday evening, or go to the mall, or treat yourself to a long, leisurely bubble bath! Be good to yourself.

There are a number of ways you can make studying more fun. Make use of your best time of day. For some, this might mean rising early while the rest of the household sleeps and stealing time alone, undisturbed, with a hot cup of tea or coffee. For others, evening is preferable. Study for short periods with frequent breaks. Remember to integrate whatever learning modalities work best for you. For example, if you are an auditory learner, use audiotapes. Listening to tapes while you are walking is especially good for tactile learners. Think in terms of "bite-size" pieces and structure your study plan accordingly. This will keep you from becoming overwhelmed and defeated before you begin. Variety is also essential. For example, divide your time between test question review and content review, or break up the study period into a variety of different tasks. Take notes part of the time and read for a part of the time. Do not keep at any one activity—even your practice exams—for longer than 45 minutes. Try studying with a study group part of the time. Discussing the materials with others is an especially good strategy for auditory learners.

Study with your purpose in mind: in this case, passing the certification exam. As stated earlier, research has shown that two-thirds of your study time will be most effectively spent taking sample test questions. Do not lose sight of this! Studying does not necessarily mean sitting and reading textbooks. Reading books in a linear fashion is often not the most effective way to master information. Always keep the end result in mind.

Use the "salami" principle: Cut large tasks into smaller ones and digest them one at a time. Also, be prepared to delay the start of new projects until this one is complete and you have successfully taken the exam.

Now that you understand yourself better, we will move on to understanding multiple-choice questions.

TEST-TAKING SKILLS: AN ACQUIRED ART

The ANCC and AANP certification exams consist of multiple-choice test questions. The ability to select the best response to each question is what determines your success on the exam. Knowledge of the content is, unfortunately, not enough to guarantee success. If you are not able to **communicate** your knowledge through the medium of a multiple-choice exam, you will not succeed in becoming certified. Achieving success on a multiple-choice test is a skill, and like any other skill, it can be learned. Think of it as like playing tennis. The more you practice, the stronger the muscles in your arm become and the better you get. The same is true for test taking. To begin strengthening your test-taking "muscles," we will discuss some specific strategies.

Strategy #1: Understanding and Analyzing the Anatomy of a Test Question

A multiple-choice test question consists of three parts:

- An *introductory statement*, which sets up the clinical scenario
- A *stem*, which poses a question
- *Options*, from which you must select the correct answer

The first step in analyzing a multiple-choice test question is to separate what the question **tells** you from what it **asks** you. The **introductory statement**, which may vary considerably in length, provides information about a clinical scenario, a disease process, or a nursing response. This statement includes a specific question, referred to as the **stem**, which you must answer on the basis of your advanced-practice nursing knowledge. Stems are worded in different ways. Some stems are in the form of a question; others are in the form of an incomplete statement. You must select the one **option** that best answers the question or completes the incomplete statement from a number of potential options, sometimes referred to as distractors.

Knowing these components will assist you in analyzing the information presented and focusing on the question's intent or issue. Let's look at an example that includes an introductory statement in the form of a clinical scenario. The stem is in bold print.

EXAMPLE 1

A 32-year-old woman comes to your office for a routine examination. Her blood pressure is 120/80. ***You should recommend that the client have her blood pressure checked again in:***
A. 6 months.
B. 1 year.
C. 2 years.
D. 5 years.

The introductory statement of Example 1 gives you information about the clinical situation (a 32-year-old female client came to your office for a routine exam and has a normal blood pressure), and the stem asks you for a clinical judgment (when should she have her blood pressure checked again?). You must select the option that provides the most accurate response (in this case, option C).

Understand what the question is asking. Test questions designed to assess nursing knowledge do so in two ways: (1) *recall* (memory-based questions) and (2) *comprehension* (application-based questions). This question is an example of a recall question. Nursing, however, is a practice-based discipline. Application of nursing knowledge is essential to safe, competency-based practice. Application frequently implies **analysis** of information. Review the following example.

EXAMPLE 2

Julie, age 18 months, is up to date with her immunizations and is due to receive her diphtheria, tetanus, and pertussis (DTP) and oral polio (OPV) vaccinations today. Her father is bedridden at home with AIDS. Which immunizations should Julie receive today?
A. DTP and OPV as scheduled
B. DTP and IPV
C. DTP, IPV, and measles, mumps, and rubella (MMR)
D. DTP, OPV, and MMR

You must synthesize several concepts regarding immunizations to select the correct answer (option B) for this question. You must integrate your recall knowledge regarding standard and current immunization schedules (e.g., that Julie should receive DTP and polio immunizations on this visit) with the specific clinical scenario of a family member, in this case her father, with AIDS. This calls for you to modify the regular regimen for immunizations, administering a dose of inactivated polio vaccine (IPV) rather than the standard OPV because of viral shedding and close proximity to her father, who might be susceptible to the live poliovirus present in OPV.

Additionally, a stem will request one of two types of responses: a **positive response** or a **negative response.** Remember, the stem asks you to answer a question, solve a problem, or select a response. To select the correct **option,** you need to determine the **type of stem.** Positive-response stems request an answer that is true, appropriate, or accurate, whereas negative-response stems request an option that is incorrect, false, inaccurate, or inappropriate. Negative-response stems frequently contain words such as **except**, **not**, **false**, or **least.** Consider this example.

EXAMPLE 3

Risk factors for osteoporosis include all of the following ***except:***
A. alcohol.
B. obesity.
C. age.
D. sedentary lifestyle.

Example 3 is a straight recall question testing your knowledge about osteoporosis and its risk factors. The key word in the stem, **except**, is a negative. In other words, to select the correct response for this question, which is B, you must select the answer that is wrong or is **not** a positively correlated risk factor for osteoporosis. It is necessary to determine whether the stem is a positive-response stem or a negative-response stem in order to select the correct answer.

Strategy #2: Identifying the Question's Critical Elements and Key Words

The ability to identify the **critical elements** and **key words** in a test question is crucial to correct interpretation of the question. Key words usually appear in the stem, whereas critical elements, such as the key concepts and conditions, tend to appear in the introductory statement.

Key words are important words or phrases that help focus your attention on what the question is specifically asking. For example, key words determine whether the stem is asking for a positive or negative response. Examples of key words include *most, first response, earliest, priority, on the first visit, on a subsequent visit, common, best, least, except, not, immediately,* and *initial.* Often, but not always, these words appear in bold or italicized print. Take a look at this example.

EXAMPLE 4

Which of the following is an example of a ***primary*** *preventive intervention?*
A. Tetanus prophylaxis
B. Screening sigmoidoscopy
C. Papanicolaou smear
D. Blood pressure screening

Example 4 is a recall question with a positive-response stem. Although all of the interventions are preventive, the key word is *primary,* allowing you to choose the correct answer, A.

You must also identify the **issue** the question is asking about. For example, the question might be requesting information about a disorder.

EXAMPLE 5

Mr. Williams, age 76, is seen in the ambulatory care clinic. He is complaining about incontinence, suprapubic pain, urgency, and dysuria. A urinalysis reveals the presence of white blood cells (WBCs), red blood cells (RBCs), and bacteria. Your ***assessment*** *is:*

A. prostatitis.
B. nephrotic syndrome.
C. benign prostatic hypertrophy (BPH).
D. cystitis.

By selecting the correct answer, D, you have demonstrated knowledge related to a disease process, the **issue** about which this question requested information. Other examples of issues include drugs, for example, antibiotics or immunizations; a diagnostic test, such as urinalysis or serum glucose; a toxic effect of a drug, such as rash or vomiting; a problem, for example, knowledge deficit or substance abuse; a procedure, such as bone marrow aspiration or cardiac catheterization; a behavior, for example, agitation or overeating; or, occasionally, a combination of the above. Consider this example.

EXAMPLE 6

Which drug is ***not*** *used in the treatment of acute gout?*

A. A nonsteroidal anti-inflammatory drug (NSAID)
B. Colchicine
C. An antibiotic
D. An analgesic

This is a **recall** question with a negative-response stem. The **key word** is **negative** (not) and the **issue** is knowledge of drugs. The correct answer is C.

Strategy #3: Using Therapeutic Communication

In communication-type questions, you are always looking for a **therapeutic response,** the cornerstone of the nurse-client relationship. To communicate therapeutically, you need to use communication tools and avoid communication blocks. Remember your basic therapeutic nursing role. The nurse, whether at a generalist or advanced-practice level, is **always** therapeutic. Your role is **not** that of an authority figure. This may cause some confusion for practitioners from other cultures in which healthcare providers are conceptualized as authority figures who give directions. Remember, this is a nursing-based exam. Your **initial response** is **always** the therapeutic response—the acknowledgment and validation of the client's feelings.

EXAMPLE 7

Ms. Doe, age 55, is very fearful because of a breast lump you have just identified. She begins to cry and states: "I'm afraid of having a mammogram." Your initial response is:

A. "You must have the mammogram."
B. "Don't worry; I'm sure it is nothing."
C. "Wonderful advances have been made in breast cancer research."
D. "You feel scared?"

The correct answer is D. Communication skills learned in Nursing 101 are important components of successful test-taking strategies. Table 2–2 reviews communication techniques that facilitate therapeutic communication and those that block therapeutic communication.

TABLE 2–2. COMMUNICATION TECHNIQUES

TECHNIQUES THAT FACILITATE THERAPEUTIC COMMUNICATION	
Techniques	***Examples***
Offering self	"I'll stay with you..."
Showing empathy	"I see you are upset."
Silence	Remaining present but silent
Giving information	"You need to take this drug two times a day."
Restatement	"You feel hurt?"
Clarification	"You are saying that..."
Reflection	"You seem to be anxious."
TECHNIQUES THAT BLOCK THERAPEUTIC COMMUNICATION	
False reassurance	"Everything will be okay."
Disapproval	"That was wrong."
Approval	"That was right."
Requesting an explanation	"Why did you do that?"
Giving advice	"I think you should..."
Deferring	"You need to talk with your doctor about that."
Defensiveness	"We are understaffed!"
Devaluing feelings	"That's silly, don't be upset!"

Another important component in selecting the correct answer to questions that address your ability to communicate therapeutically is prioritization of responses. More than one option may contain a therapeutic response. But which is the **first**, **best**, or **most therapeutic** response in that situation? Communication theory emphasizes that it is a priority to address the client's **feelings first.** Validate, validate, validate. "You seem to be very sad today, Mr. George." "I can see that you are upset." "You seem very anxious, Mrs. Smith." This should always be done **before** clarifying or presenting information. Is there a need to address the feelings? If so, this takes priority. Empathy, restatement, reflection, and being silent, as well as remaining with the client, are all excellent nursing strategies that can potentially validate clients' feelings. The only exception to this rule would be the presence of a pressing or interfering physical problem.

Identifying the Person Who Is the Focus of the Question

Another critical element is your ability to identify the person who is the focus of the question. This person might be the client or the person with the healthcare problem or a family member or neighbor of the person with the healthcare problem, or another member of the healthcare team. Take a look at this example.

EXAMPLE 8

Mr. Boyd, age 84, has dementia and is in a long-term care facility. His daughter and son-in-law are visiting. As they get ready to leave and begin to say good-bye, Mr. Boyd grabs his daughter's arm and begins to cry, saying "Don't leave me here. I will die in this place." As she leaves the room, his daughter is visibly upset and asks you if she should visit again soon because it has so upset her father. The ***best*** *reply for you to make is:*

A. "You might try telephoning next time instead of visiting. Your father will know that you are thinking of him then."
B. "I will give you the number of the social worker. She will be able to arrange a team conference and family meeting."
C. "This is a very upsetting time for all of you. However, it is important that you continue to visit regularly. For now, I will go in and sit with your father for a little while."
D. "He needs time to adjust to this new setting. Perhaps it might be easier on you all if you just didn't visit for a few days."

In this question, the person who is the focus of the question is Mr. Boyd's daughter, not Mr. Boyd. The **key word** in the stem is **best** response. It is also helpful to identify the **issue** the question is asking about. The issue in this question is one of therapeutic communication. The issue is Mr. Boyd's daughter's feelings of concern about her father. C is the correct response because it validates the daughter's feelings first.

Strategy #5: Determining the Best Response

There may be more than one option in a test question that is correct. But which is the **best**, **first**, or **most therapeutically sound** response to the question posed? Application-based test questions often involve decision making, which is based on prioritization. To assist you in the correct selection, follow a few tips:

- Assessment always comes before diagnosis and treatment.
- The key word **initial** usually implies the need to assess.
- Remember Maslow's Hierarchy of Needs.
- In communication-based questions, you must address the client's feelings **first.**
- In teaching and learning situations, learning is contingent upon **motivation.**

According to Maslow, physiological needs always come first. For example, you might recall the mnemonic "A, B, C" (referring to airway, breathing, circulation) from basic cardiopulmonary life support as a way of prioritizing treatment. This is handy to remember for questions that present a sudden emergency situation or any situation that is potentially life threatening for the client. Once basic physiological needs are met, **safety** is the next priority, followed by **psychosocial** needs. Therapeutic communication skills teach the acknowledgment of feelings first. Teaching and learning theory reminds us that unless the client is motivated to learn, no client teaching will be successful. If the client is not motivated, this issue must be addressed first.

Strategy #6: Avoiding Common Pitfalls

A very common cause of test-taking error is misreading the test question. To avoid common pitfalls, follow these tips:

- Ask yourself, "What is this question **really** asking?"
- Look for the key words.
- Restate the question in your own words. Eliminate any options that require you to make assumptions about information that was not presented in the case scenario and any options that contain information not presented in the scenario. **Do not read anything new into or overanalyze the test question!** Go with your first, most straightforward response. It is usually your best bet for answering the test question correctly.
- Carefully review the question using the systematic format and strategies suggested in this book.
- Make a decision about each option as you read it; this is an efficient approach to test taking. Do **not** go back to that option once you have eliminated it, do **not** overcomplicate the case scenario presented, and do **not** rely on anecdotal data from your own practice! These are national exams with testing content based on national standards of practice.

Strategy #7: Selecting the Best Answer When You Do Not Know the Answer

We now discuss some more specific strategies for selecting the best answer. Imagine that you are beginning your exam. You have answered a few questions easily, but now you have come to a test question to which you do not know the answer. You have identified the introductory statement and the stem, have determined whether it is a positive-response stem or a negative-response one, and have read through the distractors. You have identified the issue and the person who is the focus of the question. But you are still uncertain of the answer. If this happens, follow these tips:

- Eliminate incorrect options. This is very important. Frequently, you will be able to eliminate two choices easily. This gives you a 50% chance of guessing the correct answer, even on a test question that you do not know the answer to.
- Select the most global response option. The option that offers the most comprehensive or general statement is often a better answer than an option that is more specific and thus more limited.
- Eliminate similar options or those that contain words like "always" or "never." If two options say essentially the same thing, neither can be correct. If three of the four options sound similar, the "odd" one should win out.
- Eliminate options that contain words like "always" or "never." Absolute options containing the words "always or "never" are seldom correct.
- Look for words or phrases in the option that are similar to those in the introductory statement or stem. Try this strategy if you need to guess.
- Be alert to relevant information from earlier questions.
- Watch for grammatical inconsistencies between the stem and the options.
- Look for the longest option. It is often the correct response.

Key test-taking tips are given in Table 2–3.

TABLE 2–3. KEY TEST-TAKING TIPS

- Eliminate options you know are incorrect. If you can eliminate two options, even a guess has a 50% chance of being correct.
- Answer all questions as if the situations were **ideal.**
- Read the test question carefully.
- Separate what the question tells you from what it is asking.
- Identify all **false-response** stems.
- Select the most **global** response.
- Eliminate options that are incorrect or similar, or that contain words such as "always" or "never."
- Look for grammatical inconsistencies between the stem and the options, words in the options that have appeared in the stem, and the longest option.
- Be alert to information relevant to answering the question in the stem or in earlier questions.

Designing Your Study Plan

ASSESS

Review the phases of the nursing process in creating your study plan: *assess*, *plan*, *implement*, and *evaluate*. Begin by taking some sample exams. You might try an integrated content exam first and score yourself. This will give you an idea of your baseline and how intensive your study plan needs to be. Reflect, as part of your assessment, on your test-taking type, preferred learning style, and personality.

Use the analysis of scoring in Table 2–4 to help you make an accurate assessment of why you missed the questions you did. Did you miss the correct answer because you did not know or remember the content? Or did you miss a key word, read into the test question, or change the answer? If so, you need to continue to work on test-taking skills and building confidence. These objectives are best achieved through ongoing self-testing with sample exam questions, such as the ones provided for you in this book. Evaluate what percentage of questions you missed because of (1) content issues, (2) testing errors, and (3) confidence issues. Design your study plan accordingly. As you study, use the analysis of scoring to continue to track your progress.

TABLE 2–4. ANALYSIS OF SCORING

QUESTION NUMBER
TEST-TAKING ERROR
- Missed key word
- Did not read all of the distractors carefully
- Read into the question
- Misread or misunderstood the question
- Changed the answer

CONTENT WEAKNESS
- Forgot or did not recognize or understand the content
- Applied wrong concept or rationale

The ANCC and AANP exams are administered on computers but are not computer-adaptive testing at this time. (Computer-adaptive testing is the technique used for the NCLEX licensure exam. With computer adaptive tests each answer, correct or incorrect, determines the difficulty level of the next question a participant receives, and each participant may answer a different number of questions to meet a minimum passing level.) The ANCC and AANP certification exams consist of multiple-choice questions at a variety of difficulty levels, administered in no particular order. The benefit of giving the exams via computer testing centers is flexibility as to the locations where the test is offered (more than 300) and the number of days when testing is available. The ANCC and AANP exams consist of 150 questions and may include up to 25 additional pilot questions. The AANP exam is also given as a paper and pencil exam twice a year at a limited number of locations. Aim for an 85% grade on your practice exams to demonstrate a good level of mastery of each content area. Assess your passing score on an integrated content exam. Any test score below 80% indicates a need to initiate a more aggressive and intensive exam review. A score of 80% or above, however, does not mean that you shouldn't prepare! You should still aim to review approximately **2000** to **3000** sample test questions before sitting for the exam, as well as doing some basic content review.

An initial score below 80% means you should aim to review a minimum of **5000** sample test questions before the exam, as well as doing an intensive content review. Attending a certification review class is an additional way to shore up your knowledge base.

PLAN AND IMPLEMENT

The certification exam timeline and study calendar (Table 2–5) lays out a suggested 6-week timeline, providing a countdown to exam time from the day you register for your exam. Use the salami technique. Study a little every day. Improve your self-image! Believe you are a good student and behave like one! Stick to your study plan! Setting clear-cut goals and objectives is always helpful.

Answer approximately 100 test questions in a specific content area. Assess your score. If it is between 85 and 95%, move on. Feel confident—but continue to review sample test questions. If your score is lower than 85%, use the diagnostic grid.

As noted in chapter 1, both the ANCC and AANP

TABLE 2–5. CERTIFICATION EXAM TIMELINE AND STUDY CALENDAR*

	SUNDAY	*MONDAY*	*TUESDAY*	*WEDNESDAY*	*THURSDAY*	*FRIDAY*	*SATURDAY*
				Commitment			
			• **Register for the exam** • **Evaluate your test-taking type and preferred learning style** • **Take assessment exam** • **Evaluate exam with analysis of scoring** • **Develop study plan and gather study materials** • **Fill out study calendar and begin** • **Make arrangements for going to the exam**				
(Dates)							
WEEK 1	Content: Score:	Content: Score:	Content: Score:	Content: Score:	Content: Score:	Content: Score:	Content: Score:
(Dates)							
WEEK 2	Content: Score:	Content: Score:	Content: Score:	Content: Score:	Content: Score:	Content: Score:	Content: Score:
				Perseverance			
			• **Continue studying** • **Take a week off from studying**				
(Dates)							
WEEK 3	Content: Score:	Content: Score:	Content: Score:	Content: Score:	Content: Score:	Content: Score:	Content: Score:
(Dates)							
WEEK 4	Content: Score:	Content: Score:	Content: Score:	Content: Score:	Content: Score:	Content: Score:	Content: Score:
				Focus and Reward			
			• **Focus on content areas in which you scored less than 80% on sample questions** • **Make final arrangements for going to the exam**				
(Dates)							
WEEK 5	Content: Score:	Content: Score:	Content: Score:	Content: Score:	Content: Score:	Content: Score:	Content: Score:
(Dates)							
WEEK 6	Content: Score:	Content: Score:	Content: Score:	Content: Score:	Content: Score:	Content: Score:	Content: Score:

*Source: Adapted from Hoefler, P: Successful Problem Solving and Test-Taking for Nursing and NCLEX-RN Exams, ed. 4, MEDS, Silver Spring, MD, 1997, p. 111.

exams cover pathophysiological content organized by body system. This is how you should organize your study time: by body system as well as by associated content areas. We suggest following the table of contents of this book, which is modeled on the practice domains spelled out by both certifying bodies. After assessing your baseline knowledge through use of the integrated exams provided in this book, move on to the content areas in which you scored the lowest. For some people, this might be the neurological content; for others, it might be the endocrine or psychiatric content.

To review disorders and help you prioritize, use the following tips:

- Organize content by body system.
- Begin with the system you find the most difficult.
- Review the pathophysiology of that system, if necessary.
- List pertinent disorders of that system.
- Review incidence and contributing factors.
- Review early and late disease manifestations.
- Review the sequelae, prognoses, and life-threatening complications.
- Determine treatment; adjust for age.
- Review associated teaching and learning needs.
- Review coping techniques, prevention, and health promotion.

Using content maps is another approach to mastering content. Figure 2–1 is an example of a content map approach to reviewing disease processes. A content map is a picture or pattern of information. It also shows relationships between pieces of information. Developing content maps can help you to find content areas in which you are weak and avoid studying content you already know. People are drawn to study what they already know. They feel comfortable with that information, whereas new information can produce anxiety. In the long run, however, this is not a good strategy. Few people can read a book and visualize the exact page, word for word, in their minds. A content map helps you find the information in your memory, where it is usually stored in patterns related to other memories. Using this structure, you can find out what areas you may not completely understand. Content maps start with general information and move to specifics. They can be helpful for persons who spend so much time studying the details that they miss the bigger picture.

EVALUATE

To help you evaluate your progress, consider these tips:

- *Take a sample test and use the test-taking analysis of scoring.* Review one of your sample content area tests. Why did you answer the questions that you got wrong incorrectly?
- *If content is forgotten, use a content review.* Did you not recognize or remember the content? This would indicate a need to review content using a book of condensed information such as Hektor Dunphy's *Management Guidelines for Adult Nurse Practitioners* or an outline-review text, or attending a certification review. It does not mean that you should return to your textbook or class notes.
- *If a rationale is misunderstood, go back to textbooks.* Did you not comprehend the content? For example, perhaps your basic understanding of the cardiac cycle was not thorough enough to include the severity and implications of various murmurs (i.e., which ones are relatively normal physiological events and which ones are indicative of more severe pathology). This would indicate a need to go back to one of your textbooks, or perhaps obtain audio- and/or videotapes with more detailed content, and review basic pathophysiologic processes.
- *If the error is in test taking or you need to build confidence, continue to take the sample exams.* Did you answer a question incorrectly because you missed a key word? Did you not read all the distractors carefully enough? Did you read something into the question? Did you change an answer? All these are indications of test-taking error. This indicates a need to continue taking sample exams. If you are consistently scoring well on practice exams, it will make you feel more confident and comfortable with testing.
- *Practice, practice, practice sample test questions.*

Using the analysis of scoring as you score yourself on an integrated exam followed by exams for specific body-system content will enable you to design an individualized study plan that has specificity and relevance for you. For example, you may need to spend a week on neurological content but only a day on cardiac content. You **can** succeed in becoming certified!

Last-Minute Preparations: Relaxed and Ready

Well, you are finally there! The day of the exam has arrived. Several tried-and-true techniques can help you get through this day with success and confidence. The night before the exam, get a good night's sleep. Try relaxation techniques to assist you. Do **not** cram the night before, although you may want to review a few notes. It might be better to do something relaxing and enjoyable like going to a movie. Find the exam site the night before to ease your anxiety on the morning of the exam. Know where to park and how long it will take you to get there.

The morning of the exam, do a few exercises to get your blood pumping to your brain. Eat lightly, but **do** have breakfast. Bring identification, your registration for the exam, at least two sharpened pencils if you are taking a paper-and-pencil exam, and a watch. Dress in layers. Avoid stimulants and depressants. Go light on the caffeine. Find the restroom. Use it before the exam begins.

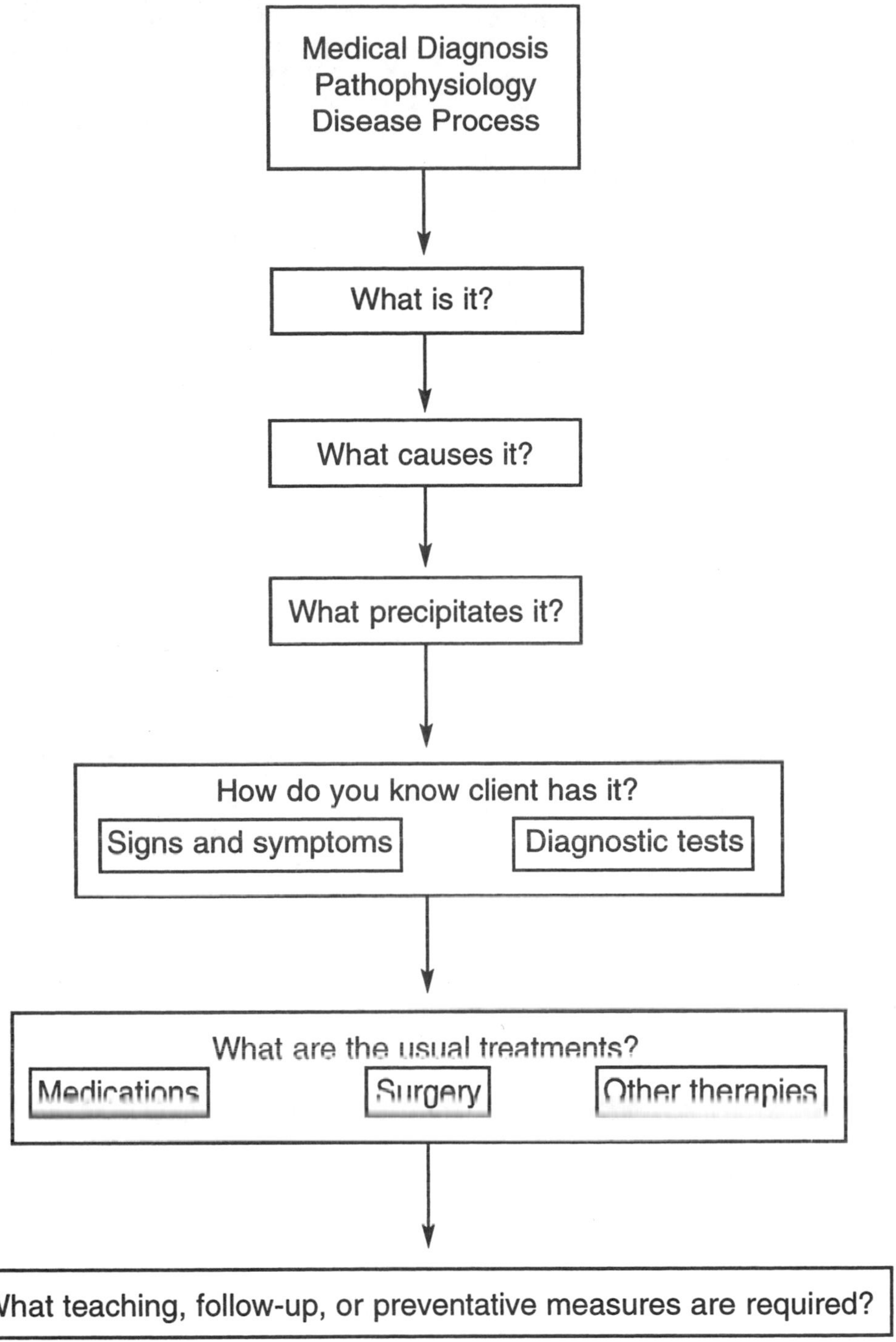

Fig. 2–1 Content map.

Pay careful attention to the instructions and tutorial for computer testing. Do deep breathing and positive relaxation exercises to calm yourself. Stay focused! Pace yourself—do not spend too long on any one test question. Go with your first choice. Move on. On a computerized exam, you will not be able to go back. Use test-taking strategies when you do not know the answer. Identify distractions, such as backache or neck ache, noise, reading the same questions over and over, feeling tired, or thinking of your vacation. If these occur, **stop,** take a a few deep breaths, refocus, then get back on track! In a testing center others will be taking different exams and will have started at different times, so do not panic if people come and go while you are testing. Stretch as necessary. Practice positive visualization if your mind begins to drift and you find it difficult to concentrate. Do not overcomplicate the test questions! Do not overanalyze the test questions! Move on! Think positively about your success. Stay focused on your goal: becoming a nationally certified advanced practice nurse.

Begin now by using this book as suggested. After all, the longest journey begins with a single step. Take that step now. Turn the page and begin.

Bibliography

American Nurses Credentialing Center: Credentialing News 1:1, 1998.

American Academy of Nurse Practitioners, *http://www.aanp.org/Certification/Certification.asp*, accessed March 25, 2003.

American Nurses Credentialing Center, *http://nursingworld.org/ancc/*, accessed March 25, 2003.

Dickenson-Hazard, N: Test-taking strategies and techniques. In Kopac, CA, and Millonig, VL (eds): Gerontological Nursing Certification Review Guide, revised ed. Health Leadership Associates, Potomac, MD, 1996.

Sides, MB, and Korchek, N: Successful Test-Taking, ed. 3. Lippincott Williams & Wilkins, Philadelphia, 1998.

Hoefler, P: Successful Problem Solving and Test-Taking for Beginning Nursing Students, ed. 3. MEDS, Silver Spring, MD, 2000.

Hoefler, P: Successful Problem Solving and Test-Taking for Nursing and NCLEX-RN Exams, ed. 5. MEDS, Silver Spring, MD, 1999.

Stein, A, and Mariano, D: Test Smart: How to Pass NCLEX-RN. In NCLEX Excel! Course. Allegheny University of Health Sciences, Philadelphia, 1997.

UNIT TWO

EVALUATION AND PROMOTION OF CLIENT WELLNESS

Health Promotion 3

SHARON A. THRUSH
and
JILL E. WINLAND-BROWN

3–1 *The best defense against colds, flu, and respiratory syncytial virus is:*

A. the flu shot.
B. prevention.
C. increased dosage of vitamin C.
D. rimantadine HCl (Flumadine).

3–2 *Susie, age 5, comes to the clinic for a well-child visit. She has not been in since she was 2. Her immunizations are up to date. What immunizations would you give her today?*

A. None. Wait until she is 6 years old to give her booster shots.
B. Diphtheria, tetanus, and pertussis (DTaP); *Haemophilus influenzae* type B (HiB); and measles, mumps, and rubella (MMR).
C. DTP, tetanus and diphtheria (Td), and polio.
D. DTP, polio, and MMR.

3–3 *Which of the following is a true contraindication to immunizations?*

A. Mild to moderate local reaction to a previous immunization
B. Mild acute illness with a low-grade fever
C. Moderate or severe illness with or without a fever
D. Recent exposure to an infectious disease

3–4 *Which immunization may prevent meningitis?*

A. Hepatitis B
B. *Haemophilus influenzae* type B (HiB)
C. Measles, mumps, and rubella (MMR)
D. Varicella

3–5 *Gerald, a 67-year-old male retired maintence worker, comes to your office for a physical. On reviewing Gerald's history, you discover that he has had pneumonia twice in the past 5 years. When you question Gerald about his immunization history, he reveals that his last tetanus and diptheria (Td) immunization was 6 years ago, and his last flu shot was 8 months ago during the last flu season. He denies ever having had a pneumonia vaccination. Which immunizations should you offer to Gerald today?*

A. Td
B. Pneumoccal vaccine
C. Influenza
D. Td and pneumoccal vaccine

3–6 *How much higher are healthcare costs for smokers than for nonsmokers?*

A. 20%
B. 40%
C. 60%
D. 80%

3–7 *The U.S. government report,* Healthy People 2010, National Health Promotion and Disease Prevention Objectives, *lists which of the following as leading health indicators?*

A. Obesity, substance abuse, and immunizations
B. Obesity, responsible sexual behavior, and driver education
C. Obesity, substance abuse, and driver education
D. Obesity, immunizations, and driver education

3–8 *Screening is considered a form of:*

A. health counseling.
B. primary prevention.
C. secondary prevention.
D. tertiary intervention.

3–9 *The broad-based initiative led by the United States Public Health Service (PHS) to improve the health of all Americans through emphasis on prevention, rather than just treatment, of health problems throughout the next decade is:*

A. the National Health Objectives Report.
B. Healthy People 2010.
C. the Surgeon General's Report.
D. the PHS Initiative.

3–10 *Performing range-of-motion exercises on a client who has had a cerebrovascular accident (CVA) is an example of which level of prevention?*

A. Primary prevention
B. Secondary prevention
C. Complications prevention
D. Rehabilitation prevention

3–11 *When performing a sports physical exam on Kevin, a 16-year-old healthy boy, which question in the history is important to ask Kevin or his guardian?*

A. Did anyone in your family ever have sudden cardiac death?
B. Does anyone in your family have elevated cholesterol levels?
C. Did you ever have any injury requiring stitches?
D. Does anyone in your family have a history of asthma?

3–12 *An example of an active strategy of health promotion is:*

A. maintaining clean water.
B. introducing fluoride into the water.
C. enacting a stress management program.
D. maintaining a sanitary sewage system.

3–13 *The best strategy to promote personal health is to:*

A. instill a sense of responsibility in persons for their own health.
B. provide complete health information in many languages.
C. encourage health-promoting habits.
D. teach clients about appropriate risk factors.

3–14 *Women tend to outlive men by an average of:*

A. 3–4 years.
B. 5–6 years.
C. 6–7 years.
D. 7 or more years.

3–15 *The goal of a sports physical is to:*

A. clear all athletes for full participation in their sport activity.
B. limit the number of athletes participating in a sport activity.
C. identify health risks that may be minimized or cured in order to allow participation.
D. identify students at risk for health problems and limit their sports participation.

3–16 *Harriet, a 76-year-old woman, comes to your office every 3 months for follow-up on her hypertension. Harriet's medications include one baby aspirin (ASA) daily, lisinopril 5 mg daily, and calcium 1500 mg daily. On today's visit Harriet's blood pressure is 168/88. According to the JNC VII guides, what should you do next to control Harriet's blood pressure?*

A. Increase her dose of lisinopril to 20 mg daily.
B. Add a thiazide diuretic to the lisinopril 5 mg daily.
C. Discontinue the lisinopril and start a combination of ACE inhibitor and calcium channel blocker.
D. Discontinue the lisinopril and start a diuretic.

3–17 *Marvin is a gay man who is ready to "come out." The last step in the process of coming out involves:*

A. testing and exploration.
B. identity acceptance.
C. identity integration and self-disclosure.
D. awareness of homosexual feelings.

3–18 *Ethnocentrism is:*

A. being concerned about the health needs of all Americans.
B. putting the group being studied at the center of dialogue.
C. thinking that ethnic groups other than one's own are inferior.
D. keeping a central focus on commonalities, not differences.

3–19 *The first step in alleviating the problem of homelessness is to:*

A. increase available housing for low-income individuals.
B. make public assistance more readily available.
C. correct the public's perception of homeless persons.
D. provide community support for deinstitutionalized persons.

3–20 *Which healthcare system delivers comprehensive health maintenance and treatment services to members of an enrolled group who pay a prenegotiated and fixed payment?*

A. Health maintenance organizations (HMOs)
B. Preferred provider organizations (PPOs)
C. Fee-for-service (FFS) independent practices
D. Exclusive provider organizations (EPOs)

3–21 *Utilization review refers to a system:*

A. of reviewing access to and utilization of healthcare services.
B. that uses retrospective review of client records to reveal problems that may be addressed in the future.
C. to monitor diagnosis, treatment, and billing practices to assist in lowering costs.
D. that has clients use an identification card to be able to use healthcare services.

3–22 *Which federal insurance program went into effect in 1966 to provide funds for medical costs for persons age 65 and older as well as disabled persons of any age?*

A. Medicare
B. Title XIX of the Social Security Act
C. Medicaid
D. Omnibus Reconciliation Act

3–23 *Which part of Medicare is basic hospital insurance?*

A. Medicare Part A
B. Medicare Part B
C. Medicare Part C
D. Medicare Part D

3–24 *A diagram that depicts each member of a family, shows connections between the generations, and includes genetically related diseases is referred to as a:*

A. family assessment diagram.
B. family generation illustration.
C. generations diagram.
D. genogram.

3–25 *Lewin's change theory involves fundamental shifts in persons' behaviors to evoke and successfully implement change. The final phase is referred to as:*

A. implementation.
B. refreezing.
C. finalizing.
D. change.

3–26 *The primary objective of screening is to:*

A. prevent a disease.
B. detect a disease.
C. determine the treatment options.
D. promote genetic testing to prevent passing on the disease.

3–27 *Which of the following questions does not provide a basis for designating a disease as screenable or not?*

A. Does the significance of the disorder ensure its consideration as a community problem?
B. Can the disease be screened?
C. Should the disease be screened?
D. What is the cost of treatment?

3–28 *To quantify the margin of error in a screening instrument, the measure of validity is divided into two components: sensitivity and specificity. Sensitivity refers to a screening test's ability to:*

A. recognize negative reactions or nondiseased individuals.
B. identify persons who actually have the disease.
C. predict populations at risk.
D. give the same result regardless of who performs the test.

3–29 *If a screening test used on 100 individuals known to be free of breast cancer identified 80 individuals who did not have breast cancer while missing 20 of the individuals, the specificity would be:*

A. 80%.
B. 60%.
C. 40%.
D. 20%.

3–30 *Mildred, a 92-year-old independent woman, is moving into her daughter's home. Her daughter comes to see you seeking information for helping to keep her mother from falling. Which of the following interventions would you suggest she do to help prevent Mildred from falling?*

A. Install an intercom system in Mildred's bedroom.
B. Limit the time Mildred is home alone.
C. Hire an aide to assist Mildred 24 hours a day.
D. Remove all loose rugs from floors and install hand grasps in bathtubs and near toilets.

3–31 *Mammography, as a method of screening for breast cancer, should be performed:*

A. every year after age 40.
B. only after a woman finds a lump when performing monthly breast self-examinations.
C. every 2 years from ages 40–80.
D. every 2 years from ages 40–50, then annually until age 65, then every 2 years until age 80.

3–32 *Which tumor marker is specifically elevated in prostate cancer?*

A. Prostate cancer tumor marker (PCTM)
B. Cancer antigen (CA) 125
C. Carcinoembryonic antigen (CEA)
D. Prostate-specific antigen (PSA)

3–33 *Sam, age 30, has a normal cholesterol level of 186 mg/dL. He should be screened for hypercholesterolemia:*

A. every 5 years.
B. every 2 years.
C. every year.
D. whenever blood work is done.

3–34 *Herbert, a 69-year-old man, comes to your office complaining of nocturia. On questioning Herbert you find that for the last 3 months he has been getting up at least five times a night to void. He came in to seek help today because of his wife's insistence that he be checked out. When you perform the digital rectal exam you find that his prostate protrudes 3–4 cm into the rectum. What grade would you assign to Herbert's prostate enlargement?*

A. Grade 1
B. Grade 2
C. Grade 3
D. Grade 4

3–35 *You are working with Iris, age 62, who has hypertension. Both of you are considering factors that contributed to her condition and will contribute to her probability of taking the appropriate plan of action. According to this information, you are formulating your plan using which of the following?*

A. Social learning theory
B. Precede-proceed model
C. Health belief model
D. Nursing process model

3–36 *The two leading causes of death in the United States for all ages are:*

A. cancer and stroke.
B. heart disease and cancer.
C. acquired immunodeficiency syndrome (AIDS) and heart disease.
D. accidents and heart disease.

3–37 *Sally, age 25, is of normal weight. She follows a diet of 70% carbohydrates, 10% fat, and 20% proteins. How do you respond when she asks you if this is a good diet?*

A. "Yes, this is a good diet."
B. "No, you should eat more proteins."
C. "You should be eating only about 55% carbohydrates."
D. "Make sure your fats are divided among saturated, polyunsaturated, and monounsaturated fats."

3–38 *The American Heart Association recommends that you eat a combination of how many fruits and vegetables per day?*

A. Two
B. Three
C. Four
D. Five

3–39 *A conservative, preventive health approach for healthy adults is to recommend limiting salt intake to how many grams per day?*

A. 2 g
B. 4 g
C. 6 g
D. 8 g

3–40 *Alcohol, especially when used with tobacco, is a dietary factor in which type of cancer?*

A. Liver
B. Esophagus
C. Bladder
D. Breast

3–41 *The National Cancer Institute recommends that adults eat how many grams of fiber a day?*

A. 10–20
B. 20–30
C. 30–40
D. 40–50

3–42 *Postmenopausal women who are not on hormone replacement therapy need how much calcium per day to help prevent osteoporosis?*

A. 1000 mg
B. 1200 mg
C. 1500 mg
D. 1800 mg

3–43 *Margaret, age 29, is of medium build and 5 feet 4 inches tall. You estimate that she should weigh about:*

A. 105 lb
B. 110 lb
C. 120 lb
D. 130 lb

3–44 *Max states that he cannot give up drinking beer, but will cut down. You suggest that his limit should be:*

A. one can of beer a day.
B. two cans of beer a day.
C. three cans of beer a day.
D. four cans of beer a day.

3–45 *Julia, age 18, asks you how many calories of fat she is eating when one serving has 3 g of fat. You tell her:*

A. 12 calories.
B. 18 calories.
C. 27 calories.
D. 30 calories.

3–46 *A high sodium intake contributes to the risk of:*

A. cancer.
B. heart disease.
C. osteoporosis.
D. hypertension.

3–47 *The ultimate goal of crisis intervention is to:*

A. assist persons to function at a higher level than in their precrisis state.
B. help persons eliminate the crisis and get back to where they were.
C. prevent further crises from happening.
D. eliminate stress altogether.

3–48 *Martin, an 83-year-old man, is at your office for his yearly physical exam. He has a history of* *hypertension, hyperlipidemia, cigarette smoking, and COPD. Martin states that he has been feeling increased fatigue with minimal activity, but denies any chest pain or shortness of breath. Martin's list of medications include the following: 1 baby ASA daily, 1 ACE inhibitor daily, diuretic daily, and statin medication daily. Martin's physical exam was normal. His blood pressure was 130/68, his heart rate was 88, and his respiratory rate was 22. Observing Martin during your examination, you detect that he utilizes pursed-lip breathing throughout the exam. What medication should he be started on for his COPD?*

A. Inhaled corticosteroid
B. Inhaled anticholinergic and inhaled beta-2 agonists
C. Oral steroids daily
D. Inhaled beta-2 agonists

3–49 *Eileen, a 42-year-old woman, comes to your office with the chief complaint of fatigue, weight loss, and blurred vision. Eileen has a negative past medical history for any chronic medical problems. You obtain a fasting chemistry panel, lipid profile, CBC, and a HgbA1c. The results of the blood work show Eileen's blood sugar to be elevated at 356 mg/dL, total cholesterol elevated at 255, HDL low at 28, LDL elevated at 167, triglycerides 333, and HgbA1c 12. On questioning Eileen further, you discover that both her grandmothers had adult-onset diabetes mellitus. You diagnose type 2 diabetes mellitus. Your treatment plan should include a cholesterol-lowering agent, a blood sugar-lowering agent, and which other class of medication?*

A. ACE inhibitor
B. Diuretic
C. Weight loss medication
D. Beta blocker

3–50 *You are sharing with your client the idea that he needs to get some counseling to deal with his severe stress because it is affecting his physiological condition. Which of the following hormonal changes occurs during severe stress?*

A. A decrease in catecholamines
B. An increase in cortisol
C. A decrease in antidiuretic hormone
D. A decrease in aldosterone

3–51 *Josephine, a 60-year-old woman, presents to your office with a history of elevated total cholesterol, triglycerides, and LDL. She was started on a statin medication 4 weeks ago and is concerned about some muscle pains she has been experiencing. On questioning Josephine, you discover that she has had pain in both her thighs for the past 2 weeks. What possible complication of statin therapy are you concerned that Josephine might be experiencing?*

A. Liver failure
B. Renal failure
C. Rhabdomyolysis
D. Rheumatoid arthritis

3–52 *Jan's mother has Alzheimer's disease (AD). She tells you that her mother's recent memory is poor and that she is easily disoriented, incorrectly identifies people, and is lethargic. Jan asks you, "Is this as bad as it gets?" You tell her that her mother is in which stage of the disease?*

A. Stage I
B. Stage II
C. Stage III
D. Stage IV

3–53 *Which of the following criteria is not diagnostic for a child with attention deficit hyperactivity disorder (ADHD)?*

A. The child frequently blurts out the answer to a question before the question is finished.
B. The child has difficulty following directions.
C. The child talks very little but is very restless.
D. The child often engages in physically dangerous activities.

3–54 *Carol, a nursing student, is at your office for her nursing school admittance physical exam and immunizations. On reviewing Carol's allergies, you find that she is allergic to baker's yeast. What would you tell Carol regarding the hepatitis B vaccine?*

A. You recommend that she receive the first hepatitis B vaccine today.
B. You advise her to wait until she is starting her clinical rotations to get the first hepatitis B injection.
C. You advise her that she cannot receive the hepatitis B vaccine because of her allergy to baker's yeast.
D. You instruct her to receive the first hepatitis B vaccine today, the second injection in 6 months, and the third injection in 1 year.

3–55 *Which statement is true regarding testicular cancer?*

A. White men are at a higher risk.
B. All races are equally susceptible.
C. Although testicular self-examination (TSE) alerts the person to the presence of a tumor, it has not been shown to decrease mortality.
D. TSE should be taught to all middle-aged men.

3–56 *An indicator of body fat measured by dividing weight in kilograms by height in meters is the:*

A. weight/height chart.
B. body mass index.
C. body fat measurement.
D. anthropometric measurement.

3–57 *A lab value that is commonly decreased in older adults is:*

A. creatinine clearance.
B. serum cholesterol.
C. serum triglyceride.
D. blood urea nitrogen.

3–58 *Anorexia nervosa is a steady, intentional loss of weight with maintenance of that weight at an extremely unhealthy low level. Which statement is true regarding anorexia nervosa?*

A. The poor eating habits result in diarrhea.
B. It may cause tachycardia.
C. It may occur from prepubescence into the early 30s.
D. It may cause excessive bleeding during menses.

3–59 *Mary, a 70-year-old woman with diabetes, is at your office for her 3-month diabetic checkup. Mary's list of medications includes Glucophage XR 1000 mg daily, ACE inhibitor daily, and 1 baby ASA daily. Mary's blood work showed a fasting blood sugar of 112 and HgbA1c of 6.5. You tell Mary that her blood work shows:*

A. that her diabetes is under good control and she should remain on the same medications.
B. that her diabetes is controlled and she needs to have her medications decreased.
C. that her diabetes is not controlled and her medications need to be increased.
D. that her diabetes has resolved and she no longer needs any medication.

3–60 *What is the term used to describe a disorder characterized by excessive sleep?*

A. Insomnia
B. Narcolepsy
C. Nocturnal myoclonus
D. Cataplexy

3–61 *Marie, a Russian Jew, married Endo, a Filipino, and is currently adapting to his culture. This is referred to as:*

A. acculturation.
B. biculturalism.
C. cultural relativity.
D. enculturation.

3–62 *Joseph, a 55-year-old man with diabetes, is at your office for his diabetic follow-up. On examining his feet with monofilament, you discover that he has developed decreased sensation in both feet. There are no open areas or signs of infection on his feet. What health teaching should Joseph receive today regarding the care of his feet?*

A. Wash your feet with cold water only.
B. See a podiatrist every 2 years, inspect your own feet monthly, and apply lotion to your feet daily.
C. Go to a spa and have a pedicure monthly.
D. See a podiatrist yearly; wash your feet daily with warm soapy water and towel dry between the toes; inspect your feet daily for any lesions; and apply lotion to any dry areas.

3–63 *Sandra, a 27-year-old nurse, states that she does not want to get the hepatitis B virus vaccine because of its adverse effects. You tell her that the most common adverse effect is:*

A. fatigue.
B. headache.
C. pain at the injection site.
D. elevated temperature.

3–64 *In discussing sexuality with the mother of a 4-year-old, you should be concerned if the mother gives a "yes" answer to which of the following questions?*

A. Has your child asked questions about anatomic differences between sexes?
B. Does your child touch his or her own genitals?
C. Does your child play "doctor" with children of the opposite sex?
D. A "yes" answer to any of these questions is of no concern.

3–65 *Mimi, age 52, asks why she should perform a monthly breast self-examination (BSE) when she has an annual exam by the physician as well as a yearly mammogram. You respond:*

A. "If you are faithful about your annual exams and mammograms, that is enough."
B. "More breast abnormalities are picked up by mammograms than by clinical exams or BSE."
C. "More than 90% of all breast abnormalities are first detected by self examination."
D. "Self-examinations need to be performed only every other month."

3–66 *When does the National Cholesterol Education Program recommend cholesterol screening for persons with no family history of coronary heart disease before age 55?*

A. Starting at age 20, then at least every 5 years thereafter if the cholesterol level was normal
B. Whenever any other blood test is ordered
C. At the annual routine physical
D. Starting at age 20, then annually thereafter

3–67 *A heart-healthy diet should be recommended to clients:*

A. with a low-density liproprotein (LDL) cholesterol level greater than 160 mg/dL.
B. with a total cholesterol level greater than 200 mg/dL.
C. with a high-density liproprotein (HDL) cholesterol level below 35 mg/dL.
D. regardless of age or risk.

3–68 *Harvey, age 55, comes to the office with a blood pressure of 144/96 mm Hg. He states that he did not know if it was ever elevated before. When you retake his blood pressure at the end of the examination, it remains at 144/96. Your next action would be to:*

A. start him on an angiotensin-converting enzyme (ACE) inhibitor.
B. start him on a diuretic.
C. have him monitor his blood pressure at home.
D. try nonpharmacologic methods and have him monitor his blood pressure at home.

3–69 *Martha, age 82, has an asymptomatic carotid bruit on the left side. You recommend:*

A. ASA therapy.
B. coumadin therapy.
C. surgery.
D. no treatment at this time.

3–70 *According to the JNC VII guidelines for hypertension, Jesse, who has stage 1 hypertension, should be placed on which treatment plan for control of his hypertension?*

A. Thiazide diuretic
B. Diet and exercise
C. One drug from one of the following classes: ACE inhibitor, calcium channel blocker, or ARB.
D. Thiazide diuretic, and either ACE inhibitor, calcium channel blocker, or ARB.

3–71 *The CAGE screening test for alcoholism is suggestive of the disease if two of the responses are positive. What does the E in CAGE stand for?*

A. Every day
B. Eye opener
C. Energy
D. Ego

3–72 *Twenty percent of colorectal cancers can be attributed to which dietary cause?*

A. High-fat diet
B. High-carbohydrate diet
C. Use of alcohol
D. Lack of fiber in the diet

3–73 *For primary prevention of skin cancer, you would recommend a sunscreen with how much ultraviolet (UV) wave protection?*

A. 15
B. 25
C. 30
D. 45

3–74 *Screening test recommendations for human immunodeficiency virus (HIV) infection include:*

A. all clients.
B. persons getting married.
C. teenagers who have been sexually active for 1 year.
D. intravenous drug users and clients with high-risk behaviors.

3–75 *When should glaucoma screening be instituted?*

A. When the client is age 65
B. When the client exhibits vision problems
C. At the client's annual exam
D. Starting at age 40

3–76 *When should an African-American man start to be screened for prostate enlargement by a digital rectal exam?*

A. Age 60 and then yearly
B. Age 40 and then yearly
C. Age 40 and then every 2 years
D. Age 55 and then yearly

3–77 *Who is the most important source of social support for an adult?*

A. Spouse (if applicable)
B. Parents
C. Close friends
D. Children

3–78 *Which of the following 4-year-olds should not receive an immunization today?*

A. Jerry, who has an upper respiratory tract infection (URI) with a mild fever
B. Timmy, who has otitis media
C. Joan, who needs several other immunizations
D. Joe, who had a previous reaction to egg protein

3–79 *Mark, a 50-year-old man, comes to your practice seeking help to quit smoking. You prescribe Zyban, a prescription medication, to aid with his attempt. What instructions do you give Mark regarding how to stop smoking with Zyban?*

A. Start the Zyban today and take it twice a day for one week, then stop smoking.
B. Start the Zyban today and take one a day in the morning for 3 days, then twice a day, then pick a date to stop smoking about 2 weeks after starting the Zyban.
C. Pick a date to stop smoking and start the Zyban that day. Take one a day for 3 days, then take one twice a day.
D. Start the Zyban today, take it twice a day for 2 weeks, then stop smoking.

3–80 *Andrea, a 20-year-old nursing student, never had her second MMR immunization. What test must you do before giving Andrea her second MMR?*

A. Complete blood count
B. Complete metabolic panel

C. Lipid profile
D. Urine pregnancy test

3–81 *Emily, a healthy 26-year-old woman, asks you how she can prevent bone loss as she ages. She is concerned because both her maternal grandmother and now her mother have severe osteoporosis. What guidance would you give to Emily?*

A. Drink all the soda you like—it has no effect on your bone density.
B. Smoking has not been proven to affect bone loss.
C. Replace estrogen when you reach menopause.
D. Perform aerobic exercise at least three times a week.

3–82 *Drugs causing the most adverse reactions are:*

A. chemotherapeutic agents.
B. anticonvulsants.
C. antibiotics.
D. antidepressants.

3–83 *One of the major criteria for diagnosing chronic fatigue syndrome is:*

A. generalized headaches.
B. unexplained generalized muscle weakness.
C. sleep disturbance.
D. fatigue for more than 6 months.

3–84 *One of the most common causes of involuntary weight loss is:*

A. malignancy.
B. pulmonary disease.
C. endocrine disturbances.
D. substance abuse.

3–85 *Which industry is responsible for the most injuries?*

A. Mining
B. Construction
C. Transportation and utilities
D. Manufacturing

3–86 *The most common type of occupational illness in the United States is:*

A. poisoning.
B. respiratory conditions caused by toxic agents.
C. disorders caused by physical agents.
D. skin disorders.

3–87 *Sandy, a 68-year-old woman, presents to your office for screening for osteoporosis. Sandy states that her grandmother and mother both lost inches in their old age. Sandy has been postmenopausal for the past 15 years and never took any hormone replacement medications. She is Caucasian, weighs 108 lb, and is 5 feet 1 inch tall on today's measurement. When do postmenopausal women lose the greatest amount of bone density?*

A. The first 7 years after menopause.
B. The first year of menopause.
C. The first 10 years after menopause.
D. Bone loss occurs continuously at the same rate from menopause to death.

3–88 *Margo, age 50, is perimenopausal. She tells you that she is taking dehydroepiandrosterone (DHEA) and wants to start on hormone replacement therapy (HRT). When she asks for your opinion, you tell her that:*

A. Taking both DHEA and HRT is not recommended because it is like "double dosing."
B. DHEA is safe and will not affect prescribed medications.
C. She will be safe as long as she takes the minimum dose of both therapies.
D. DHEA has the same pharmacotherapeutic effects as HRT.

3–89 *In women with human immunodeficiency virus (HIV) infection, there is a high prevalence of additional infection from:*

A. *chlamydia.*
B. syphilis.
C. human papillomavirus (HPV).
D. *Candida.*

3–90 *Most anal cancers are potentially preventable. Which of the following is a cause of anal cancer?*

A. Sexually transmitted diseases (STDs)
B. A low-fiber diet
C. Hemorrhoids
D. Foreign bodies used as sexual stimulants

3–91 *Marian's husband, Stu, age 72, has temporal arteritis. She tells you that his physician wants to perform a biopsy of the temporal artery. She asks if there is a less invasive diagnostic test. What test do you tell her is less invasive?*

A. Computed tomography (CT) scan
B. Magnetic resonance imaging (MRI)
C. Electroencephalogram (EEG)
D. Color duplex ultrasonography

3–92 *Dennis, age 62, has benign prostatic hyperplasia (BPH). He tells you that he voids at least four times per night, and that he has read about a preventive drug called terazosin hydrochloride (Hytrin) that might help him. What do you tell him?*

A. "It's not a preventive drug, but it relaxes smooth muscle in the prostate and bladder neck."
B. "It changes the pH of the urine and prevents infections caused by urinary stasis."
C. "It relaxes the urethra."
D. "It shrinks the prostate tissue."

3–93 *Molly, age 48, is healthy except for her well-controlled asthma. She asks if she should* *get an annual flu vaccination. You tell her that she should:*

A. get it only after she reaches age 65.
B. get it only during the fall season when her asthma is bothering her.
C. get it on an annual basis.
D. not get it because she has a respiratory problem (asthma).

3–94 *How do you respond when Mattie, who is taking levothyroxine (Levothroid, Synthroid), says she has read that she should not eat brussels sprouts?*

A. "Brussels sprouts contain a high amount of iodine, and therefore you should not eat them."
B. "Brussels sprouts interfere with the absorption of the medication."
C. "There is no reason why you should not eat brussels sprouts."
D. "It is safe if you take the medication in the morning and don't eat brussels sprouts until the evening."

3–95 *A child's head circumference should be measured until the child reaches what age?*

A. 6 months
B. 12 months
C. 18 months
D. 24 months

3–96 *When should children have their first visual acuity testing?*

A. When they are able to read.
B. When they enter kindergarten.
C. At age 2.
D. At age 3.

3–97 *When should children be screened for lead poisoning?*

A. Only if they are in high-risk groups
B. At age 12 months
C. At age 3 years
D. Only if they live in or regularly visit a house built before 1960

3–98 *How do you respond when Jill, age 42, asks you what constitutes a good cardiovascular workout?*

A. Exercising for at least 30 minutes every day
B. Exercising a total of 2 hours per week
C. Exercising for at least 20 minutes, 3 or more days per week
D. Exercising for at least 30 minutes, 5 days per week

3–99 *Bone density studies to screen for osteoporosis should be performed on which of the following?*

A. Perimenopausal women who used to smoke but no longer do
B. All women after menopause
C. All women who have had hysterectomies
D. Women with drinking problems

3–100 *When can Pap smears be safely discontinued?*

A. At age 80.
B. At age 65 if the previous 3 Pap smears have been normal.
C. Never; they should be continued throughout life.
D. After menopause or hysterectomy.

3–101 *Sal is traveling out of the country and asks for a prescription to prevent traveler's diarrhea. What do you give him?*

A. Trimethoprim with sulfamethoxazole (TMP-SMX) double strength daily.
B. Bismuth subsalicylate, 2 tabs q.i.d.
C. Nothing, but tell him to "cook it, boil it, peel it, or forget it."
D. Nothing, but tell him to use bottled drinking water.

3–102 *Harry is taking his entire family to Central America and is wondering about protection against mosquito bites causing malaria. You tell him to:*

A. Use an insect repellent with diethyltoluamide (DEET) for the entire family, applying it sparingly to small children.
B. Make sure the family is in well-screened or indoor areas from dusk to dawn.
C. Use an insect repellent with DEET for adults only; apply permethrin to children's clothing; and stay inside from dusk to dawn.
D. Stay inside from dusk to dawn and use an insect repellent with permethrin.

3–103 *Susan is traveling to South America and wonders if she should get a tetanus and diphtheria (Td) vaccination. You tell her that:*

A. She needs one if she has not had a Td shot within the past 10 years.
B. She should have tetanus immune globulin administered before departure.
C. She should receive a tetanus shot now.
D. Tetanus and diphtheria are no longer a serious problem in South America.

3–104 *When is routine screening for hypothyroidism performed?*

A. When a client reaches age 65.
B. Whenever a client exhibits symptoms.
C. Never; it is not routinely recommended.
D. When a client has a family history of thyroid problems.

3–105 *Tuberculin skin testing using the Mantoux test should be considered for:*

A. high-risk adolescents, recent immigrants, and homeless individuals.
B. all clients every 2 years.
C. all clients at their annual physical.
D. all children before entrance into first grade.

Answers

3–1 Answer B

The best weapon against infection such as colds, flu, and respiratory syncytial virus is prevention, although the flu shot has improved the basic preventive measures such as hand washing, good hygiene, and isolation of infected persons. Although many persons believe that taking extra vitamin C and echinacea will shorten the length of a cold, vitamin supplements have not been proven necessary in persons who follow balanced diets. Rimantadine HCl (Flumadine) is effective against influenza A only if given within 24–48 hours of symptom onset.

3–2 Answer D

Because Susie has not been in for several years, one cannot assume that she will come in next year to get the immunizations that are due between the ages of 4 and 6; therefore, this opportunity to give her her immunizations cannot be missed. Between the ages of 4 and 6, a child is due for diphtheria, tetanus, and pertussis (DTP); polio; and measles, mumps, and rubella (MMR) if all other immunizations are up to date.

3–3 Answer C

The only true contraindications to immunizations, according to the American Academy of Pediatrics, are a moderate or severe illness with or without a fever and an anaphylactic reaction to a vaccine or a vaccine constituent. Illnesses themselves are not true contraindications to vaccinations. Early symptoms may be a prodrome of something else; however, risks of the diseases are usually greater than the complications of vaccination. Even a fever of 104.5°F (40°C) with a previous diphtheria, tetanus, and pertussis (DTP) immunization is not a contraindication to a subsequent DTP shot.

3–4 Answer B

Meningitis is one of the most severe manifestations of *Haemophilus influenzae* infection, and the *H. influenzae* type B (HiB) immunization may help prevent its occurrence. The HiB vaccination is especially important for children age 5 years and younger. It should be given at ages 2 months, 4 months, and 6 months, with the fourth dose given between ages 12–18 months. Hepatitis B vaccination is important for all infants to help prevent liver disease as adults. A measles, mumps, and rubella (MMR) vaccination protects against measles, mumps, and rubella (German measles), and varicella vaccination protects against chickenpox.

3–5 Answer B

Prevention of pneumococcal disease in older people is one of the health initiatives of the United States government report, *Healthy People 2010, National Health Promotion and Disease Prevention Objectives.* The goal for healthcare providers is to have 90% of all clients over 65 years old immunized against pneumococcal disease by the year 2010. The pneumococcal vaccine is a one-time injection that may need to be repeated in 8 years. Gerald does not need a TD booster because his last injection was only 6 years ago. The CDC recommends a TD booster every 10 years. The influenza injection would not be appropriate at this time. Influenza vaccine is adjusted yearly to address the type of influenza that is thought to be prevalent in that year. Also, the influenza vaccine is given just before flu season.

3–6 Answer B

Healthcare costs for smokers at any given age are as much as 40% higher than for nonsmokers. Although smokers have more diseases than nonsmokers, nonsmokers live longer and can incur more health costs at advanced ages.

3–7 Answer A

The United States government report *Healthy People 2010, National Health Promotion and Disease Prevention Objectives* presents measurable objectives organized into 22 priority areas within four broad categories: health promotion, health protection, preventive services, and surveillance and data systems. Driver education is not considered a leading healthcare indicator.

3–8 Answer C

Screening is considered a form of secondary prevention because one aspect of it is identifying such diseases as high blood pressure, glaucoma, and diabetes.

3–9 Answer B

The broad-based initiative led by the United States Public Health Service to improve the health of all Americans through an emphasis on prevention and not just treatment of health problems throughout the next decade is called *Healthy People 2000, National Health Promotion and Disease Prevention Objectives*. It took its lead from the 1979 report, *Healthy People: The Surgeon General's Report on Health Promotion and Disease Prevention*. Although all the objectives in that report were not achieved, it had such a positive impact that *Healthy People 2000* was conceived. The major difference is in the 2000 report's primary emphasis on health promotion and individual responsibility.

3–10 Answer D

Performing range-of-motion exercises on a client who has had a cerebrovascular accident (CVA) is an example of rehabilitation prevention. Primary prevention would be eating a healthy diet as a young adult to prevent atherosclerosis, which might precipitate a

CVA. Secondary prevention would include taking lipid-lowering drugs to prevent a CVA after having already developed hyperlipidemia. Although it is desirable to prevent any complications from the CVA, there is no level of prevention called complications prevention.

3–11 Answer A

The risk of sudden death during sports activities from hypertrophic cardiomyopathy may be greatly reduced with a thorough cardiac history and examination. If a child has a relative who died of sudden cardiac disease before age 55, that child could possibly have hypertrophic cardiomyopathy. Family history of asthma is not relevant to this exam question.

3–12 Answer C

Enacting a stress management program is an active strategy of health promotion because it requires individuals to become personally involved. Maintaining clean water, introducing fluoride into the water, and maintaining a sanitary sewage system are all examples of passive strategies—those done for individuals and communities by others.

3–13 Answer A

The best strategy to promote personal health is to instill a sense of responsibility in persons for their own health. Until persons have made a commitment to assume personal responsibility for their own health, their health-promoting behaviors will not change. One of the nurse practitioner's functions is to effect changes in human behavior. Encouraging the adoption of personal responsibility is one way to do this.

3–14 Answer C

Since the late 1970s, the difference in life expectancy for men and women has narrowed, but women still outlive men by 6–7 years.

3–15 Answer C

The goal of the preparticipation sports exam is to protect the student from injury by identifing health risks and miniminzing or curing them so the student may participate in a sports activity. You might feel pressured by parents or coaches to pass the student regardless of your findings. Your responsibility is to further evaluate any abnormal findings on your exam before clearing the student to participate.

3–16 Answer B

The seventh report of the Joint National Committee on Prevention, Detection, and Treatment of Hypertension (JNC VII) recommends that stage 2 hypertension be treated with a combination of a thiazide diuretic and an ACE inhibitor, ARB, calcium channel blocker, or beta blocker.

3–17 Answer C

The last step in the process of a gay man or lesbian "coming out" is that of identity integration and self-disclosure. The process of discovering and revealing one's sexual orientation can occur at any age and is known as "coming out." Stage theories for coming out have been summarized as a four-step process: (1) awareness of homosexual feelings, (2) testing and exploration, (3) identity acceptance, and (4) identity integration and self-disclosure. If the ultimate costs of self-disclosure are felt to be too high, an individual may become socially isolated or deny gay or lesbian identity.

3–18 Answer C

Ethnocentrism is thinking that ethnic groups other than one's own are inferior. An ethnocentric perspective is a barrier to establishing and maintaining positive relationships with others.

3–19 Answer C

The first step in alleviating the problem of homelessness is to correct the public's perception of homeless persons. Current stereotypical opinions hinder effective delivery of healthcare as well as other resources that should be available. Lack of housing for low-income persons, restrictions on public assistance, and inadequate support for deinstitutionalized persons are all factors that have contributed to the problem of homelessness.

3–20 Answer A

Health maintenance organizations (HMOs) deliver comprehensive health maintenance and treatment services to members of an enrolled group who pay a prenegotiated and fixed price. Preferred provider organizations (PPOs) allow persons to go to any doctor in the network, whereas clients of HMOs must choose their doctor ahead of time. Fee-for-service (FFS) independent practices permit an individual to be treated in any facility, with the full fee paid by the client. Exclusive provider organizations (EPOs) limit clients to providers belonging to one organization. Some may be able to use outside providers at an additional out-of-pocket charge.

3–21 Answer C

Utilization review is a system to monitor diagnosis, treatment, and billing practices. It assists in lowering healthcare costs by discouraging unnecessary procedures.

3–22 Answer A

Medicare was established in 1966 by the U. S. government as a federal insurance program to provide funds for medical costs for persons age 65 and older as well as disabled persons of any age. Medicaid, an amendment to Title XIX of the Social Security Act, went into effect in 1967 to provide basic health services to low-income persons. The Omnibus Budget Reconciliation Act was implemented in 1982, when 20 programs were combined into four block grants.

3–23 Answer A

Medicare Part A is basic hospital insurance. Medicare Part B is supplementary voluntary medical insurance supported by tax revenues and by additional moneys paid by the insurer to cover physician services, laboratory services, home healthcare, and outpatient hospital treatments.

3–24 Answer D

A genogram is a diagram that depicts each member of a family and shows connections among the generations (including all members of the extended family for several generations). It includes the health status of each member (including any genetically related diseases).

3–25 Answer B

Lewin's change theory involves fundamental shifts in persons' behaviors that evoke and successfully implement change. It is a three-stage process. Stage 1 is unfreezing, in which there is recognition of the need to change and methods are suggested to minimize resistance to the change; stage 2 is the actual changing process, in which the tasks and structure are actually implemented; and stage 3 is refreezing, in which the outcomes are reinforced and results are evaluated.

3–26 Answer B

The primary objective of screening is to detect a disease in its early stages in order to be able to treat it and change its progression. Treating a disease at the early asymptomatic period can significantly alter the course of the disease.

3–27 Answer D

To designate a disease as screenable or not, several questions are taken into account: Does the significance of the disorder ensure its consideration as a community problem? Can the disease be screened? Should the disease be screened? Questions such as "What is the cost of treatment?" are not taken into account and therefore do not provide a basis for designating a disease as screenable or not.

3–28 Answer B

Sensitivity refers to a screening test's ability to identify persons who actually have a disease (true positives), whereas specificity measures a screening test's ability to recognize negative reactions or nondiseased individuals (true negatives). For example, if a screening tool were used on 100 individuals known to have prostate cancer and detected 90 persons with prostate cancer, missing 10 of the individuals, the sensitivity would be 90%.

3–29 Answer A

Specificity measures a screening test's ability to recognize individuals who are nondiseased or those with negative reactions (true negatives). It can be represented by a ratio of true negatives to the total number of known true negatives. In this case, the number of true negatives that the test recognized was 80, with the total number of known true negatives being 100. Therefore 80 out of 100 (80/100) equals a specificity of 80%.

3–30 Answer D

The correct answer is to allow Mildred her independence but provide a safe environment by removing loose rugs that she could easily trip over and installing hand rails by the toilet and in the bathtub. The rails will provide support for her as she goes from a sitting to a standing position. Hiring an aide 24 hours a day would decrease Mildred's independence. Leaving Mildred home, alone or not, will not change her chance of falling.

3–31 Answer D

The American Cancer Society recommends that mammograms, as a method of screening for breast cancer, be performed every 2 years from ages 40–50, then annually until age 65, then every 2 years until age 80.

3–32 Answer D

The tumor marker that is specifically elevated in prostate cancer is prostate-specific antigen (PSA). Determined by a simple blood test, PSA is a tumor marker whose level in the bloodstream becomes elevated with prostate cancer, although it may also become elevated with benign prostatic hypertrophy (BPH). There is no prostate cancer tumor marker (PCTM). Levels of cancer antigen (CA) 125 are increased in the following cancers: epithelial ovarian, fallopian tube, endometrial, endocervical, hepatic, and pancreatic. It is used to monitor for persistent or recurrent serous carcinoma of the ovary in the postoperative period or during chemotherapy. Measurement of the level of carcinoembryonic antigen (CEA) is used primarily for monitoring persistent, metastatic, or recurrent cancer of the colon after surgery and less frequently for breast or other cancers.

3–33 Answer A

The National Cholesterol Education Program (NCEP), launched by the National Heart, Lung and Blood Institute, recommends that persons with normal cholesterol levels be tested every 5 years.

3–34 Answer C

The degree of prostate enlargement is based on the

amount of projection of the prostate into the rectum. The normal prostate protrudes less than 1 cm into the rectum. Grade 1 enlargement is a protrusion of 1–2 cm, Grade 2 is 2–3 cm, Grade 3 is 3–4 cm, and Grade 4 is greater than 4 cm.

3–35 Answer C

The health belief model follows a paradigm that analyzes factors contributing to a client's perceived state of health or risk of disease and to the client's probability of taking the appropriate health plan of action. Social learning theory assists in explaining, predicting, and influencing behavior change. The precede-proceed model is a comprehensive planning guide to administering health education programs. The nursing process model is a series of activities that nurses perform as they provide care to clients. The steps include assessment, diagnosis, planning, implementation, and evaluation. Depending on the nursing diagnosis, the plan may be similar to that using the health belief model, but the assessment phase would have to incorporate data related to the client's perceived state of health, at which the health belief model excels.

3–36 Answer B

The two leading causes of death in the United States for all ages are heart disease and cancer. Almost two-thirds of the deaths in the United States every year are from these causes.

3–37 Answer C

The National Cholesterol Education Program recommends that total fat in a diet be no more than 30% total calories, carbohydrates about 55% of total calories, and proteins about 15–20% of total calories.

3–38 Answer D

The American Heart Association has a saying, "Five Alive," meaning that everyone should eat a combination of five fruits and vegetables per day. This recommendation is also supported by the American Cancer Society.

3–39 Answer C

A conservative, preventive health approach for healthy adults is to recommend limiting salt intake to 6 g or less per day. This includes salt added to food during cooking or at the table, salt added as an ingredient to processed foods, and salt that occurs naturally in foods. Table salt is approximately 40% sodium by weight; therefore a diet incorporating 6 g of salt contains about 2.4 g of sodium.

3–40 Answer B

Alcohol, especially when used with tobacco, is a dietary factor in cancer of the esophagus. Alcohol is also a factor in liver cancer. Dietary factors related to bladder cancer are unknown. A high-calorie diet (with high fat and low fiber) is a factor in breast cancer.

3–41 Answer B

The National Cancer Institute recommends that adults eat 20–30 g of fiber a day to prevent colon cancer. The plant kingdom is the only source of fiber-containing foods.

3–42 Answer C

Postmenopausal women who are not on hormone replacement therapy need 1500 mg of calcium a day to help prevent osteoporosis. Because treatment for osteoporosis is limited, prevention is necessary to reduce the occurrence.

3–43 Answer C

To estimate a client's ideal weight, use the following formula: For women over age 25, allow 100 lb for the first 5 ft, then add 5 lb for each inch thereafter. For men, allow 106 lb for the first 5 ft, then 6 lb for each inch thereafter. Multiply the number by 110% for a client with a large frame and 90% for a client with a small frame.

3–44 Answer B

The Committee on Diet and Health of the National Research Council recommends that alcohol consumption per day be limited to the equivalent of less than 1 oz of pure alcohol. This equates to two cans of beer, two small glasses of wine, or two average cocktails. This does not apply to pregnant women, who should avoid alcohol altogether.

3–45 Answer C

A gram of fat contains 9 calories, whereas a gram of either carbohydrates or proteins contains 4 calories. In this case, Julie was eating 3 g of fat; therefore 9 calories per gram of fat times 3 g of fat equals 27 calories.

3–46 Answer D

The Food and Drug Administration states that sodium may contribute to the risk of hypertension; fat and fiber in grains, fruits, and vegetables decrease the risk of cancer; and insufficient calcium contributes to the risk of osteoporosis. Sodium intake should be reduced if there is a family health history of hypertension, diabetes, or any form of cardiovascular disease. Sodium intake should also be reduced if a personal health history indicates hypertension or glucose intolerance. Although hypertension is certainly a factor in heart disease, the best answer is hypertension, because not all cardiovascular diseases are affected by the amount of sodium consumption.

3–47 Answer A

The ultimate goal of crisis intervention is to assist persons to function at a higher level than their precrisis state. Eliminating the current crisis and returning persons to the functional level where they were before the crisis will put them back in the same situation and make them susceptible to the crisis all over again.

3–48 Answer B

According to the Global Initiative for COPD guidelines, all symptomatic COPD clients should be started on an inhaled anticholinergic drug and a beta-2 agonist. Both are well tolerated by older adults and have few side effects.

3–49 Answer A

Studies have shown the use of ACE inhibitors in clients with diabetes with or without hypertension has slowed the progression of nephropathy. You must monitor the client's creatinine and potassium levels routinely. If the client's renal function does decrease, elevated potassium levels may occur.

3–50 Answer B

During severe stress, the cortisol level increases, allowing mobilization of free fatty acids. Also, glucose production from amino acids increases with the increased cortisol level. During severe stress, catecholamine levels increase as glucagon release increases. The insulin-to-glucagon ratio decreases, glycogen breakdown increases, and glucose production from amino acids increases. The antidiuretic hormone increases during stressful periods and retention of water increases. Aldosterone is also increased and retention of sodium increases.

3–51 Answer C

Rhabdomyolysis is a syndrome that results from destruction of skeletal muscle. It is usually diagnosed from laboratory findings that are characteristic of myonecrosis. Although there are no standard creatine kinase values that establish the diagnosis of rhabdomyolysis, elevations above 10,000 IU/L are usually indicative of clinically significant rhabdomyolysis. It usually affects muscles used in exercise, but may present as generalized muscle weakness. It usually resolves on stopping the statin medication, but severe cases may lead to renal failure and death.

3–52 Answer C

Families of persons with Alzheimer's disease (AD) need to know that AD is a progressive disorder of the brain affecting memory, thought, and language. Although the progression of the stages is individual and changes may occur rapidly or slowly over the course of several years, knowing what stage their family member is in helps family members in planning and knowing what to expect. Stage I is the onset, which is insidious. Spontaneity, energy, and initiative are decreased; slowness is increased; word finding is difficult; the person angers more easily; and familiarity is sought and preferred. In Stage II, supervision with detailed activities such as banking is needed; speech and understanding are much slower; and the train of thought is lost. In Stage III, personality change is marked and depression may occur. Directions must be specific and repeated for safety, recent memory is poor, disorientation is easy, people are incorrectly identified, and the person may be lethargic. In Stage IV, apathy is noticeable. Memory is poor or absent, urinary incontinence is present, individuals are not recognized, and the person should not be alone.

3–53 Answer C

Diagnostic criteria for the child with ADHD include frequently blurting out answers before a question is finished, difficulty following directions, engaging in physically dangerous activities (often without thinking of the consequences of actions), tending to talk excessively, and often interrupting others. Behavior in which the child talks very little, but is very restless, is not indicative of ADHD.

3–54 Answer C

An allergy to baker's yeast is a definite contraindication to receiving the hepatitis B vaccine. Yeast is used in making the vaccine and is still present in the vaccine.

3–55 Answer A

White men are at a higher risk for testicular cancer than nonwhite men. Testicular self-examination (TSE), along with early detection and treatment, has decreased the mortality rates appreciably. TSE should be taught to all men beginning at adolescence.

3–56 Answer B

The body mass index (BMI) is an indicator of body fat. It is derived by dividing weight in kilograms by height in meters. It shows a direct and continuous relationship to morbidity and mortality in studies of large populations. The weight/height chart gives a range of what the ideal weight is for each height, but does not reflect body fat. Anthropometric measurement is the measurement of the size, weight, and proportions of the human body.

3–57 Answer A

The creatinine clearance value is commonly decreased in older adults because of impaired renal function. Serum cholesterol, serum triglyceride, and blood urea nitrogen values are usually increased in older adults.

3–58 Answer C

Anorexia nervosa may occur from prepubescence into the early 30s, and occurs most commonly from early to late adolescence. It occurs more frequently in women and may cause bradycardia, arrhythmias, and amenorrhea. Constipation is common in clients with anorexia because of their poor eating habits.

3–59 Answer A

A person with diabetes mellitus type 2 should have a hgbA1c of 6.5 or less and fasting blood sugar (fbs) less than 120 for optimal control. Because the client's lab results fall in that category, she is under good control and her medications should stay the same.

3–60 Answer B

Narcolepsy is a disorder characterized by excessive sleep. Narcolepsy with involuntary daytime sleep attacks may begin in adolescence. The person may have symptoms of this problem years before it is diagnosed. Insomnia is the inability to fall asleep or to stay asleep for a sufficient amount of time. Nocturnal myoclonus is a condition characterized by stereotypic kicking movements of the legs during sleep. It is more common in older adults. Cataplexy is often associated with narcolepsy. It is marked by abrupt attacks of muscular weakness and hypotonia triggered by an emotional stimulus such as anger or fear.

3–61 Answer A

Acculturation is the process of adapting to a culture belonging to someone else. Biculturalism refers to taking components of both cultures and making them fit one's lifestyle. Cultural relativity refers to the attempt to view the behavior of culturally different individuals within one's own framework. Enculturation is the process of acquiring one's cultural identity as it is transferred down from the older generation.

3–62 Answer D

The ADA recommends careful inspection of a diabetic client's feet for corns, callouses, and open lesions in order to prevent further deterioration into diabetic foot ulcers. The client should wash his or her feet daily with warm soapy water and towel dry them, especially between the toes, to prevent fungal infections. Diabetic clients should see a podiatrist yearly.

3–63 Answer C

The most common adverse reaction to the hepatitis B virus vaccine is pain at the injection site (13–20% in adults, 3–9% in children). Other mild, transient systemic adverse effects are fatigue and headache (11–17% in adults, 8–18% in children), and temperature elevation (1–6% of all injections).

3–64 Answer D

A "yes" answer to any of these questions is of no concern. These are all normal behaviors for preschool children ages 3–6. These are the ways in which children express their concerns and explore their anatomy. Parents should honestly answer questions posed by their children regarding sexuality in terms the children can understand.

3–65 Answer C

More than 90% of all breast abnormalities are first detected by self-examination. All women over age 20 should examine their breasts monthly, a week after their period. After menopause, women should examine their breasts at the same time each month.

3–66 Answer A

The National Cholesterol Education Program recommends cholesterol screening for persons with no family history of coronary heart disease before age 55. This should start at age 20, then be done at least every 5 years thereafter. Earlier screening at ages 10–15 should be considered for children with a family history of coronary heart disease that developed before age 55.

3–67 Answer D

A heart-healthy diet should be recommended for all clients regardless of age or risk. It is especially important that children learn healthy eating habits early in life. A heart-healthy diet follows the Dietary Guidelines for Americans as developed by the U.S. Departments of Agriculture and Health and Human Services. It is designed for healthy people over age 2 to maintain their health. The guidelines include: Eat a variety of foods; balance the food you eat with physical activity; maintain or improve your weight; choose a diet with plenty of grain products, vegetables, and fruits; choose a diet low in fat, saturated fat, and cholesterol; choose a diet moderate in sugars; choose a diet moderate in salt and sodium; and, if you drink alcoholic beverages, do so in moderation.

3–68 Answer D

Before drug therapy is instituted for hypertension, nonpharmacologic methods such as salt restriction, weight reduction, biofeedback, and exercise should be considered. Aggressive treatment of all clients with a systolic pressure greater than 140 mm Hg and/or a diastolic pressure greater than 90 mm Hg is essential. The client should monitor his or her blood pressure at home and call the healthcare provider if it exceeds the parameters discussed. In this case, Harvey should try nonpharmacologic methods and monitor his blood pressure at home, then return in 1 to 2 weeks for follow-up. If his diastolic pressure is still 96 mm Hg after 2 weeks, a diuretic or an ACE inhibitor would be indicated.

3–69 Answer D

Clients with asymptomatic carotid bruits have a 2% incidence of cerebrovascular accident (CVA) per year. Although ASA, anticoagulants, and surgery are frequently ordered, there are not sufficient data to prove that these treatments reduce the risk of CVA in clients with asymptomatic carotid bruits. Starting an asymptomatic older woman on ASA therapy may produce more problems, such as skin bruising or gastrointestinal bleeding.

3–70 Answer A

The JNC VII guidelines for treatment of stage 1 hypertension recommend use of a thiazide diuretic as first choice for treatment of hypertension.

3–71 Answer B.

The E stands for eye opener. The C stands for cutting down, the A stands for annoyed by criticism of drinking, and the G stands for guilt feelings about drinking.

3–72 Answer D

Twenty percent of colorectal cancers can be attributed to a lack of fiber in the diet. A high-fat diet has also been secondarily implicated.

3–73 Answer A

For primary prevention of skin cancer, a sunscreen with an ultraviolet (UV) wave protection factor of 15 has been shown to be as effective as those with higher numbers. In addition, for primary prevention of skin cancer, all clients should be counseled to avoid UV waves from either the sun or tanning booths and to wear protective clothing.

3–74 Answer D

The Centers for Disease Control and Prevention recommend that all clients with high-risk behaviors be encouraged to be screened for HIV antibodies to identify those who are already infected so that interventions can be started to further halt the spread of the virus.

3–75 Answer D

Glaucoma screening should be instituted starting at age 40 and continue every 5 years until age 60, then every 2–3 years thereafter. Glaucoma is an elevated intraocular pressure that is measured with the use of a tonometer.

3–76 Answer B

With respect to African-American men, the American Cancer Society recommends that screening for prostate cancer with a digital rectal exam start at age 40 and be done yearly.

3–77 Answer A

The spouse has been shown to be the most important source of social support for an adult. If there is no spouse, family members are the next most important source. Research has shown that support from outside the family cannot compensate for what is missing within the family.

3–78 Answer D

Egg protein is a vaccine component and may cause an anaphylactic reaction; therefore Joe, who has had a previous reaction to egg protein, should not receive his immunization. To maximize opportunities to vaccinate, every client visit should be assessed for an appropriate vaccination. Clients may receive multiple vaccinations. Mild febrile illnesses, such as upper respiratory tract infection or otitis media, are not contraindications for vaccinations.

3–79 Answer B

Zyban works in the craving center of the brain. For the plan to be successful, the client needs to build up a steady blood level before stopping smoking. Target date to stop smoking should be set for 1–2 weeks after beginning the Zyban. The Zyban may cause insomnia—this is why it is slowly started with once-a-day dosing for 3 days, then increased to twice a day. Avoid bedtime dosing, but doses should be 8 hours apart. The client then continues on the medication for 2 weeks before picking a stop-smoking date. The Zyban helps the client not to crave the nicotine while going through withdrawal. The client then stays on the Zyban for approximately 10 more weeks before stopping it altogether.

3–80 Answer D

The MMR is a live attenuated vaccine, and therefore a female client must not be pregnant when she receives the vaccination. Female clients must also be informed that they need to refrain from becoming pregnant for the next 3 months or risk birth defects to the fetus.

3–81 Answer D

Emily is only 26 years old and has not reached her peak bone mass yet. Aerobic exercise has been proven to increase bone mass. Smoking and soda drinking both have been shown to decrease bone mass. Estrogen replacement therapy is no longer reccommended for bone health; it is recommended only for short-term use to alleviate vasomotor symptoms.

3–82 Answer C

Of all the drug classes, antibiotics cause the most adverse reactions. The other drug classes that cause a high number of adverse drug reactions, in order, are chemotherapeutic agents, cardiovascular agents, antihypertensive agents, anticonvulsants, and antidepressants.

3–83 Answer D

Fatigue for more than 6 months and absence of other clinical conditions that may explain such fatigue are the two major criteria the client must demonstrate to be diagnosed with chronic fatigue syndrome. Other minor criteria include generalized headaches, unexplained generalized muscle weakness, sleep disturbances, sore throat, mild fever or chills, and migratory arthralgias without swelling or redness.

3–84 Answer A

Malignancies (lung, lymphoma, gastrointestinal tract) are the most common causes of involuntary weight loss, along with gastrointestinal diseases and psychiatric disorders. Other less common causes include pulmonary disease, endocrine disturbances, and substance abuse.

3–85 Answer B

The construction industry is responsible for the most injuries (15 injuries per 100 full-time workers per year). Next in line are the agriculture, fishing, and forestry industries, followed by the manufacturing, transportation and utilities, and mining industries.

3–86 Answer D

Skin disorders are the most common type of occupational illness in the United States, accounting for 41,800 illnesses or 33% of the cases per year. This is followed by disorders associated with repeated trauma, respiratory conditions, disorders caused by physical agents, poisoning, and dust diseases of the lungs.

3–87 Answer A

Bone loss begins at a rate of 0.5% a year in a woman's mid- to late 40s. When menopause occurs, the rate increases to 3% a year. This increase in the rate of bone loss is directly related to the decrease in a woman's estrogen loss. This high rate of bone loss continues for up to the first 7 years of menopause and then decreases to 0.5–1% a year until death.

3–88 Answer A

Dehydroepiandrosterone (DHEA) is an abundant hormone in the body and is naturally produced from cholesterol by the adrenal glands, with smaller amounts manufactured by ovaries. Taking DHEA and hormonal replacement therapy (HRT) is not recommended because it is like "double dosing." It is not absolutely contraindicated, but because most clients do not adequately regulate the dosage of over-the-counter medications, the combination therapy may produce excessively high levels of estrogen. Additionally, because almost a third of clients today are taking some sort of herbal therapy, it is essential to ask in the history and physical what other therapies are being used.

3–89 Answer C

Women with human immunodeficiency virus (HIV) infection have a high prevalence of human papillomavirus (HPV) infections. They are associated with an increased incidence of squamous intraepithelial lesions in HIV-seropositive women.

3–90 Answer A.

Sexually transmitted diseases (STDs) are a cause of anal cancer. For women, other risk factors for anal cancer include an increased number (greater than 10) of sexual partners, having their first sexual experience before age 16, having 4 or more sexual partners before age 20, and anal intercourse. For men, other risk factors include having more than 10 sexual partners and being homosexual or bisexual.

3–91 Answer D

A biopsy of the temporal artery is usually required to confirm the diagnosis of temporal arteritis. Color duplex ultrasonography (a combination of ultrasonography and the flow velocity determinations of a Doppler system) has been shown to examine even small vessels, such as the superficial temporal artery, and show a halo around the inflamed arteries when temporal arteritis is present. Therefore it is a much less invasive procedure. A computed tomography (CT) scan and magnetic resonance imaging (MRI) are done to detect neurologic damage from hemorrhage, tumor, cyst, edema, or myocardial infarction. These tests may also identify displacement of the brain structures by expanding lesions. However, not all lesions can be detected by CT scan or MRI. An electroencephalogram is used to evaluate the electrical activity of the brain. It can identify seizure activity as well as certain infectious and metabolic conditions.

3–92 Answer A

Terazosin (Hytrin) is an alpha-1 adrenergic blocker. It is not a preventive drug, but it does relax smooth muscle in the prostate and bladder neck and allows complete emptying of the bladder, relieving frequent nocturnal urination. Terazosin is begun at 1 mg at bedtime initially, then titrated upward to 10 mg once a day. Doxazosin (Cardura) is also effective as an alpha-1 adrenergic blocker. It is begun initially at 1 mg at bedtime, with the dosage doubled every 1–2 weeks to a maximum of 8 mg per day. Finasteride (Proscar), a 5-alpha reductase inhibitor, decreases the volume of the prostate within about 3 months. At 12 months, it seems to have reached its peak effectiveness. Finasteride is given 5 mg daily for at least 6 months; then the client is re-evaluated.

3–93 Answer C

Molly should get an annual flu vaccination because she has a long-term pulmonary problem. Other persons who should be vaccinated include those over age 64; nursing home residents; persons with diabetes, blood dyscrasias, suppressed immune systems, and long-term cardiac, urinary, and respiratory problems; and persons who come in close contact with other persons who are vulnerable to influenza.

3–94 Answer A

Clients taking levothyroxine (Levothroid, Synthroid) should avoid foods high in iodine such as brussels sprouts, cabbage, cauliflower, rutabagas, soy, and turnips because these foods, when added to the medication, raise clients' iodine levels.

3–95 Answer D

Head circumference should be measured until a child reaches age 24 months. It should be measured at birth; at 2–4 weeks; and at ages 2, 3, 6, 9, 12, 15, 18, and 24 months. Measuring growth and following its progression over the course of time can help identify significant childhood conditions. In addition to head circumference, height and weight should be measured at ages 3, 4, 5, and 6, then every 2 years thereafter.

3–96 Answer D

Children should have their first visual acuity testing at age 3. They should have their visual acuity tested using a pictorial wall chart and be tested for strabismus using the cover-uncover test. Visual acuity testing should be repeated at age 5 or 6.

3–97 Answer B

The Centers for Disease Control and Prevention recommend that all children be screened for lead poisoning at age 12 months. If resources allow, children should then be screened again at age 24 months. Children ages 3–6 years should be tested for lead levels (using an assessment tool) every 6 months if they have a high risk of lead exposure. Those with normal lead levels should be retested once a year until age 6 years.

3–98 Answer C

A good cardiovascular workout consists of exercising large muscle groups for at least 20 minutes, 3 or more days per week, at an intensity of at least 60% of the maximum heart rate (220 beats per minute minus age).

3–99 Answer A

There is still debate as to the recommendations for screening for osteoporosis for women. Bone density studies to screen for osteoporosis are recommended for women at age 65. Prior to age 65, the literature only supports screening for perimenopausal women with risk factors that include: Caucasian or Asian race, have a history of bilateral oopherectomy before menopause, have a slender build, smoke or have smoked tobacco, have low calcium consumption patterns, have a sedentary lifestyle, and have a positive family history of the condition. Women who have had a hysterectomy but not an oopherectomy are not considered at particular risk. Alcohol use at present is not listed as a risk factor.

3–100 Answer B

Pap smears may be discontinued at age 65 if the previous 3 Pap smears have been normal. For women before age 65, Pap smears should start at age 18 or at the time of first sexual intercourse, then every 1 to 3 years depending on risk factors, up to age 65. If a woman has had a hysterectomy, there is only a need for a Pap smear if the cervix has been left intact.

3–101 Answer C

Although antibiotics and bismuth subsalicylate are effective in the prevention of traveler's diarrhea, they are not generally recommended because of the potential side effects. Instead, advise clients to "cook it, boil it, peel it, or forget it."

3–102 Answer A

Insect repellents with high concentrations (greater than 35%) of diethyltoluamide (DEET) are effective in preventing mosquito bites; however, DEET is not recommended to be applied to the hands or faces of young children. Permethrin is effective as a scabicide (at 5%) and as a pediculicide (at 1%). It is very effective at a low concentration against malaria-carrying mosquitoes and is safe for all ages. Other preventive measures include remaining in well-screened or indoor areas from dusk to dawn, using mosquito nets, and wearing clothing that covers most of the body.

3–103 Answer A

Because tetanus and diphtheria remain serious problems in South America, it is recommended that all travelers be current (within 10 years) on these vaccinations. Tetanus immune globulin should be administered to persons not previously immunized.

3–104 Answer C

Screening for hypothyroidism is not routinely recommended. Because of the subtle presentation of hypothyroidism, healthcare providers should order a thyroid-stimulating hormone level (TSH) test at their discretion. Most clinicians add a T4 level test to routine blood work and, depending on the results, then order a TSH test.

3–105 Answer A

Tuberculin skin testing using the Mantoux test should be considered in high-risk adolescents, as well as recent immigrants and homeless individuals. For high-risk individuals, an induration of 10 mm or greater when read at 48–72 hours is considered positive.

Bibliography

Doherty, DE: Management of the Symptomatic Patient. Clinical Cornerstone 5(1):17–27, 2003.

Dunphy, LM, and Winland-Brown, JE: Primary Care the Art and Science of Advanced Practice Nursing. F.A. Davis, Philadelphia, 2001.

Edelman, CL, and Mandle, CL: Health Promotion Throughout the Lifespan. Mosby, St. Louis, 1998.

Follin, SL, and Hansen, LB: Current Approaches to the Prevention and Treatment of Post-Menopausal Osteoporosis. American Journal of Health-System Pharmacy 60(9):883–901, 2003.

Influenza and Pneumococcal Vaccination Levels Among Persons Age Greater than 65. Morbidity and Mortality Weekly Report. MMWR 51(45):1019–1024, 2002.

Lombardo, JA, and Badolato, SK: The Preparticipation Physical Exam. Clinical Cornerstone 3(5):10–25, 2001.

National Heart, Lung, and Blood Institute: Seventh Report of the Joint National Committee on Prevention, Detection, Evaluation, and Treatment of Hypertension (JNC VII) Express Report. National Institutes of Health. 2003.

Rakel, RE: Textbook of Family Practice. WB Saunders, Philadelphia, 2001.

Ragucci, E, Zonszein, J, and Frishman, WH: Pharmacotherapy of Diabetes Mellitis Implications for the Prevention and Treatment of Cardiovascular Disease. Heart Disease 5(1):18–33, 2003.

Schuval, S: Avoiding Allergic Reactions to Childhood Vaccine (and What to Do When They Occur). Contemporary Pediatrics. 20(4):29–31, 2003.

HOW WELL DID YOU DO?

85% AND ABOVE CONGRATULATIONS! THIS SCORE SHOWS APPLICATION OF TEST-TAKING PRINCIPLES AND ADEQUATE CONTENT KNOWLEDGE.

75–85% KEEP WORKING! REVIEW TEST-TAKING PRINCIPLES AND TRY AGAIN.

65–75% HANG IN THERE! SPEND SOME TIME REVIEWING CONCEPTS AND TEST-TAKING PRINCIPLES AND THEN TRY THE TEST AGAIN.

4

Care of the Emerging Family

DEBORAH A. RAINES
and
JILL E. WINLAND-BROWN

4–1 *Sally, who is 18 weeks pregnant, had a maternal serum alpha-fetoprotein (MS-AFP) level done. The results are elevated. What is the meaning of an elevated MS-AFP level?*

A. The fetus has trisomy 21.
B. There is an increased risk that the fetus has an open neural tube defect.
C. The infant will be born with hydrocephalus.
D. The fetus has an increased risk of developing cerebral palsy.

4–2 *Danger signs in the first trimester of pregnancy include:*

A. absence of fetal movement and vaginal bleeding.
B. edema extending to the upper extremities and vomiting.
C. presence of proteinuria and elevated blood pressure.
D. vaginal bleeding and persistent vomiting.

4–3 *Samantha, who has genital herpes, just found out that she is pregnant. Although she has not had a recurrence in years, she states that she has heard that genital herpes might cause a spontaneous abortion. You know that genital herpes:*

A. might cause a spontaneous abortion at any time if the client has an active occurrence.
B. might cause a spontaneous abortion if the primary infection was early in the pregnancy.
C. might cause a spontaneous abortion if the recurrence is during the second trimester.
D. will not cause a spontaneous abortion.

4–4 *What is the rationale for anemia seen throughout gestation?*

A. Iron stores are depleted by the fetus.
B. It is difficult for the mother to consume as much iron as needed.
C. Mild dilutional anemia is seen as a result of an increased circulating blood volume.
D. Hepatic function is affected by the growing fetus.

4–5 *When can you hear fetal heart tones with a conventional fetoscope?*

A. At 7–8 weeks' gestation
B. At 10–12 weeks' gestation
C. At 18–20 weeks' gestation
D. At more than 20 weeks' gestation

4–6 *The recommended first-trimester weight gain for an underweight woman is:*

A. 2 lb.
B. 3.5 lb.
C. 5 lb.
D. 7 lb.

4–7 *Heather, who is 5 weeks pregnant, is nauseous. She asks you how long this will last. You tell her the nausea usually disappears by the:*

A. 12th week.
B. 16th week.
C. 20th week.
D. 24th week.

4–8 *Which of the following dietary changes would you recommend to Heather, who is experiencing nausea during her first trimester?*

A. A bland diet taken frequently and in small amounts
B. An increase in fat intake
C. A decrease in carbohydrate intake
D. Restriction of fluid intake after 7 pm

4–9 *Which of the following is the best description of the Lamaze method of childbirth education?*

A. It focuses on the birth event and requires a dimly lighted room and a warm water bath.
B. It uses no medical interventions such as fetal monitors, intravenous fluids, or medications
C. It uses the child's father as a birthing coach and relies on deep abdominal breathing to handle the contractions.
D. It uses a focal point for concentration while the woman does controlled breathing techniques.

4–10 *During the 6-week postpartum visit, the nurse practitioner asks Jane if she has any concerns about her son. Jane replies, "He just lies there and doesn't do anything." Which activities typical of an infant at this age can you point out to Jane?*

A. Sucking of fingers or fist, staring at objects, and recognizing the parent's voice
B. Smiling, gurgling, and swinging arms and feet at an object
C. Sitting with support and bringing an object to his or her mouth
D. Creeping and babbling

4–11 *Ginny, who is planning on getting pregnant, is taking phenytoin (Dilantin). She states that she knows that the drug is in category D and asks what that means. You know FDA category D indicates that:*

A. positive evidence of human fetal risk exists, but benefits may outweigh risks in certain situations.
B. animal studies have not demonstrated a fetal risk, but there are no human studies in pregnant women; or animal studies have shown an adverse effect that was not confirmed in human studies.
C. studies or experience have shown fetal risk that clearly outweighs any possible benefits.
D. controlled studies in women failed to demonstrate a risk to the fetus in the first trimester, and fetal harm appears remote.

4–12 *When should zidovudine (sometimes called azidothymidine or AZT) be given to a pregnant woman with a human immunodeficiency virus (HIV) infection?*

A. Never
B. Beginning at 14 weeks' gestation
C. Beginning with the second trimester
D. During labor

4–13 *Allie, who has asthma, just found out that she is pregnant. She is wondering whether or not she should continue taking her medications. Which of the following is true regarding asthma and pregnancy?*

A. Only inhaled (rather than oral) medications should be used.
B. In the event of an acute exacerbation, glucocorticoids should not be used.
C. Management differs little from management in nonpregnant women.
D. All medications may be used except for theophylline.

4–14 *The drug of choice for the pregnant woman with diabetes is:*

A. insulin.
B. glyburide (DiaBeta, Glynase, Micronase).
C. glipizide (Glucotrol).
D. metformin (Glucophage).

4–15 *Screening for gestational diabetes mellitus (GDM) should be done on which of the following clients?*

A. On all pregnant women at month 5
B. Age 40 or older
C. All women with threatened miscarriage
D. Women who report hypoglycemic symptoms

4–16 *Hegar's sign, a physiological sign of pregnancy, is:*

A. cervical blueness.
B. softness of the uterus and ballottement at the isthmus.
C. cervical softness.
D. quickening.

4–17 *Beth thinks that she may be pregnant, but she does not want a blood test done and does not think home pregnancy tests are accurate. She asks when a urine test performed at the clinic office would be accurate. How soon after conception will a urine human chorionic gonadotropin test be positive if Beth is pregnant?*

A. 1 week
B. 2 weeks
C. 3 weeks
D. 4 weeks

4–18 *The G in APGAR stands for:*

A. gross appearance.
B. grunting.
C. grimace.
D. gas exchange.

4–19 *At birth, the anterior fontanelle has what shape?*

A. Triangular
B. Oval
C. Round
D. Diamond

4–20 *When you flex the hips and knees at a 90-degree angle and attempt to slip the femur heads onto the posterior tips of the acetabulums by lateral pressure of the thumbs and by rocking the knees medially with the knuckles of the index fingers, you are testing for normal hip movement. This test or maneuver is known as:*

A. Ortolani's maneuver.
B. Barlow's test.
C. Spock's test.
D. Moro maneuver.

4–21 *When evaluating Marge during her first obstetric visit, you assess the shape of her pelvis. While drawing her a picture of her android-type pelvis, you explain that it has:*

A. a rounded, slightly ovoid, or elliptical inlet with a well-rounded forepelvis (anterior segment).
B. a wedge-shaped inlet, a narrow forepelvis, a flat posterior segment, and a narrow sacrosciatic notch with the sacrum inclining forward.
C. a long, narrow, oval inlet; an extended and narrow anterior and posterior segment; a wide sacrosciatic notch; and a long, narrow sacrum.
D. a distinct oval inlet with a very wide, rounded retropubic angle and a wider, flat posterior segment.

4–22 *An example of an X-linked-recessive condition or trait is:*

A. muscular dystrophy.
B. hemophilia.
C. sickle cell anemia.
D. cystic fibrosis.

4–23 *Spontaneous abortion refers to the loss of a fetus of less than:*

A. 12 weeks' gestation.
B. 18 weeks' gestation.
C. 22 weeks' gestation.
D. 26 weeks' gestation.

4–24 *The brain configuration of a fetus is roughly complete at:*

A. 4 weeks' gestation.
B. 12 weeks' gestation.
C. 20 weeks' gestation.
D. 24 weeks' gestation.

4–25 *The presumptive symptom of pregnancy that involves tingling or frank pain of the breasts is:*

A. Montgomery's tubercles.
B. colostrum secretion.
C. melasma.
D. mastodynia.

4–26 *According to Nagele's rule, if a woman's last normal menstrual period was September 23, what is her estimated date of delivery?*

A. June 30
B. June 16
C. June 1
D. May 30

4–27 *Minnie is experiencing Braxton Hicks contractions. What should she do?*

A. Take a cold shower.
B. Immediately call her healthcare provider.
C. Go for a walk.
D. Lie down with her feet elevated.

4–28 *What is a fetus's gestational age when its mother's uterus is palpable just at the pubic symphysis?*

A. 4 weeks
B. 8 weeks
C. 12 weeks
D. 16 weeks

4–29 *Mindy, age 42, is pregnant for the first time. She wants a chorionic villus sampling (CVS) performed for genetic testing. Which statement is true regarding CVS?*

A. CVS may be offered at 11–14 weeks gestation.
B. CVS detects only chromosomal anomalies and not anatomic aberrations such as open neural tube defects.
C. CVS is extremely safe.
D. CVS can be done in the physician's office.

4–30 *Sandra, who is 5 months pregnant and of average height and weight, asks you how many extra calories she should be adding to her diet per day. You tell her to add:*

A. 200 calories.
B. 300 calories.
C. 500 calories.
D. 700 calories.

4–31 *Kim states that she has heard many old wives' tales of harmful things during pregnancy. Which of the following is harmful late in pregnancy?*

A. Intercourse
B. Swimming
C. Douching
D. Dental visits

4–32 *Cervical mucus changes throughout the menstrual cycle. The appearance of the cervical mucus consistent with fertile-type mucus is best described as:*

A. copious, clear, and stretchable
B. scant, thick, and sticky
C. copious, thick, and clotted
D. scant, clear, and elastic

4–33 *Gloria just delivered her baby and wants to start a vigorous exercise program to get back in shape. You advise her that she can start strenuous exercises:*

A. in 1 week.
B. in 3 weeks.
C. in 6 weeks.
D. whenever she wants.

4–34 *Nelda is breast-feeding her 6-week-old daughter. She comes today with pain, a lump in her right breast, and flulike symptoms. You see that the breast is engorged, erythematous, and warm to the touch. Her temperature is 101.8℉ (38.4℃). Your diagnosis is:*

A. breast abscess.
B. breast engorgement.
C. mastitis.
D. viral syndrome.

4–35 *Margie, who has been breast-feeding for 4 weeks, has mastitis in her right breast and is taking dicloxacillin. She asks you what she needs to do about feeding the baby. You respond:*

A. "You need to stop breast-feeding and start with a bottle."
B. "You can still breast-feed on your left side and express the milk from your right side until the problem is resolved."
C. "There is no need to stop breast-feeding, but start with your left side."
D. "Stop for 2 weeks, then continue."

4–36 *What are the clinical characteristics consistent with a diagnosis of trisomy 21?*

A. Low birth weight, small jaw with recessed chin, muscle rigidity, and short sternum
B. Cleft lip and palate, polydactyly, malformed ears, and absence of the iris
C. Lymphedema of the hands and feet, webbed neck, coarctation of the aorta, and urinary tract abnormalities.
D. Hypotonia, simian creases, epicanthial folds, and Brushfield's spots.

4–37 *Betsy is breast-feeding and complains of tenderness of the nipples all the time. You recommend that she:*

A. apply ice to the nipples between feedings.
B. apply dry heat to the nipples between feedings.
C. use nipple shields.
D. stop breast-feeding.

4–38 *Which of the following is the diagnostic standard for gestational diabetes?*

A. The presence of glycosuria on 2 urine samples within a 24-hour interval
B. A 50-gram oral glucose challenge
C. An abnormal 3-hour glucose tolerance test after a 100-g glucose load
D. A postprandial glucose blood serum level greater than 140 mg/dL

4–39 *Which of the following is the best description of the relationship between the hemoglobin A1C (glycosylated hemoglobin) level and the glucose concentration of the blood?*

A. The higher the glycosylated hemoglobin level, the lower the glucose concentration
B. The higher the glucose concentration, the lower the glycosylated hemoglobin level
C. The higher the glucose concentration, the higher the glycosylated hemoglobin level
D. The higher the glycosylated hemoglobin level, the higher the fetal blood glucose level

4–40 *Mildred is 6 months pregnant and presents with symptoms of urinary frequency, urgency, dysuria, and suprapubic discomfort. Her urine is cloudy and malodorous. She has no chills, fever, nausea, or vomiting. Your diagnosis is:*

A. urinary calculi.
B. acute cystitis.
C. acute pyelonephritis.
D. interstitial cystitis.

4–41 *Which of the following antibiotics is the best choice for acute pyelonephritis when it occurs during the seventh month of pregnancy?*

A. Nitrofurantoin (Furadantin)
B. Trimethoprim and sulfamethoxazole (Bactrim, Septra)
C. Ampicillin (Principen, Polycillin)
D. Tetracycline (Panmycin, Achromycin V)

4–42 *Linda, age 32, has multiple sclerosis (MS). She is concerned about pregnancy. You respond:*

A. "Unfortunately, pregnancy may exacerbate the symptoms of MS. I wouldn't advise it."
B. "Pregnancy has no deleterious effect on MS."
C. "It may or may not affect your MS; it could go either way."
D. "Because you may not be able to care for the baby, you shouldn't get pregnant."

4–43 *Nettie, who is pregnant, is suffering from an exacerbation of peptic ulcer disorder. Which is the best medication to order for her?*

A. Cimetidine (Tagamet)
B. Ranitidine (Zantac)
C. Sucralfate (Carafate)
D. Bellergal-S

4–44 *When is a pregnant woman at risk for developing congenital rubella syndrome?*

A. During the first 4 weeks of pregnancy
B. During the first 16 weeks of pregnancy
C. During the last trimester
D. Any time during the pregnancy

4–45 *Which of the following should be avoided by the pregnant woman who is constipated?*

A. Bulk-forming laxatives
B. Mineral oil
C. Stool softeners such as docusate sodium (Colace)
D. Drinking warm fluids on arising

4–46 *Liza is 34 weeks pregnant and has mild hypertension. You are performing a nonstress test (NST). The criterion for a reactive NST is:*

A. a minimum of 2 fetal activity patterns in a 20-minute test period
B. the presence of 2 contractions with no fetal heart decelerations in a 20-minute test period
C. at least 2 fetal heart rate accelerations in response to fetal movement in a 20-minute test period
D. the absence of uterine contractions following fetal stimulation during a 20-minute test period

4–47 *Aida, who is 29 weeks pregnant, received a blunt trauma to the abdomen during an argument with her boyfriend. She has no obvious injuries and denies pain. Aida needs to be monitored for the occurrence of:*

A. abruptio placentae.
B. liver hemorrhage.
C. ruptured spleen.
D. placenta previa.

4–48 *The best description of Bishop's score is*

A. a series of four maneuvers to determine fetal position.
B. a multiparameter evaluation of fetal condition following a nonreactive nonstress test.
C. an assessment of the cervix's readiness for elective induction.
D. an evaluation of fetal lung maturity and readiness for birth.

4–49 *In evaluating a mother-and-infant breastfeeding situation, signs of an effective latch at the breast are:*

A. infant's cheeks sucked in and slow, shallow sucking.
B. infant's lips flanged out, cheeks full.
C. rapid, short, nonrhythmic sucking by infant.
D. maternal nipple discomfort throughout the feeding.

4–50 *After 28 weeks' gestation, all women should perform fetal movement counts (FMCs). Which of the following statements is true regarding FMCs?*

A. Counts should be done as the woman is going about her work.
B. Ten movements should be obtained in 1 hour.
C. Ten movements should be obtained in 2 hours.
D. If decreased activity is perceived, a nonstress test (NST) should be performed at the next obstetric visit.

4–51 *During nursery rounds, you examine a 12-hour-old newborn. The infant has a yellow tint to the skin and sclera. What lab test will you order to further evaluate this infant?*

A. Blood glucose
B. Direct Coombs'
C. Blood cultures
D. Arterial blood gas

4–52 *Sam and Mary are planning to adopt a baby girl. Because they have seen pictures of the biological parents, who resemble them, they plan on not telling the child that she is adopted. They ask for your opinion. You respond:*

A. "It's a personal decision you have to make."
B. "If the biological parents look like you, she will probably never find out she is adopted."
C. "You should tell her when she is 18."
D. "It's your decision, but I'd advise telling her right from the beginning."

4–53 *You see G5P4015 written on a client's history form. You surmise that:*

A. the woman has been pregnant 5 times and has 5 living children.
B. the woman has 5 living children, which includes a set of twins, and she has had 1 abortion.
C. the woman has 4 living children and had 1 abortion, for a total of 5 pregnancies.
D. the woman is pregnant now and has 5 living children, including a set of twins

4–54 *To obtain the daily calcium intake recommended during pregnancy, what should a woman consume per day?*

A. One quart of cow's milk
B. Two cups of yogurt
C. Four slices of cheddar cheese
D. One cup of cottage cheese

4–55 *The nurse knows that a male client with vas deferens blockage can expect which of the following problems?*

A. Frequent urination
B. Oligospermia
C. Impotence
D. Decreased libido

4–56 *Which of the following instructions should be included in the discharge teaching plan to assist the postpartal woman in recognizing early signs of complications?*

A. The passage of clots as large as an orange is expected.
B. Call the office to report any decrease in the amount of brownish-red lochia.
C. Palpate the fundus daily to make sure it is soft.
D. Notify your healthcare provider of a return to bright red vaginal bleeding.

4–57 *Which of the following signs of thrombophlebitis must the nurse educate the postpartal client to assess at home after discharge from the hospital?*

A. Muscle soreness in the leg after exercise
B. Varicose veins in the legs
C. Local tenderness, heat, and swelling
D. Bruising

4–58 *A woman with hyperemesis gravidarum would most likely benefit from a plan of care designed to address which of the following nursing diagnoses?*

A. Imbalanced nutrition, more than body requirements, related to pregnancy
B. Anxiety, related to effects of hyperemesis on fetal well-being
C. Anticipatory grieving, related to inevitable pregnancy loss
D. Ineffective coping, related to unwanted pregnancy

4–59 *Lynne comes to the clinic for her initial prenatal visit. Based on her menstrual history, the client is at 9 weeks' gestation and is scheduled to have an ultrasound for estimation of the gestational age of the fetus. Which fetal measurement would be the best indicator of gestational age at this time?*

A. Biparietal diameter
B. Femur length
C. Abdominal circumference
D. Crown-rump measurement

4–60 *Which of the following signs or symptoms would indicate a need for colposcopy and biopsy for human papillomavirus?*

A. Rash on the palms of the hands and soles of the feet
B. Chancre sore noted on the vulva
C. A crusted ulcer inside the vagina
D. A 2–3 cm soft papillary swelling on the genitalia

4–61 *Early in pregnancy, all pregnant women need which of the following tests?*

A. 3-hour glucose challenge test
B. Rh status
C. Direct Coombs' test
D. Pap smear

4–62 *Rh_o(D) immune globulin (RhoGAM) should be administered:*

A. when an infant is in distress at birth.
B. after a mother gives birth to a macrosomic infant.
C. when a D-negative mother has received a transfusion of D-positive blood.
D. when an infant with type-A blood is born to a mother with type-O blood.

4–63 *What components make up the biophysical profile?*

A. Nonstress test, amniotic fluid composition, fetal breathing. and fetal tone
B. Fetal tone, breathing, motion, and contraction stress test
C. Amniotic fluid composition, contraction challenge test, fetal breathing, and motion
D. Fetal tone, breathing, motion, amniotic fluid volume, and nonstress test

4–64 *Which of the following statements about lesbian relationships is true?*

A. Battering is a concern only in heterosexual relationships, but in lesbian relationships, instead of physical abuse, there may be emotional or financial abuse.
B. Support from family, friends, and coworkers may be lost.
C. HIV infection is not a concern with two women who are in a firm relationship.
D. Childbearing issues do not affect lesbian couples.

4–65 *Joyce, who experienced some transient emotional disturbances around her third postpartum day, is just now feeling like herself again after about 2 weeks. It is most likely that Joyce experienced:*

A. maternity blues.
B. postpartum depression.
C. postpartum psychosis.
D. postpartum anxiety disorder.

4–66 *Which of the following drugs should be used with extreme caution in breast-feeding mothers?*

A. Azithromycin (Zithromax)
B. Phenobarbital (Luminal, Solfoton)
C. Propranolol (Inderal)
D. Cisplatin (Platinol)

4–67 *A couple come to you for infertility treatment. They have been having unprotected intercourse for 18 months without achieving pregnancy. Which of the following tests will be ordered for this couple?*

A. Semen analysis and hystersalpingography
B. Hystersalpingogram and PAP smear
C. Colposcopy with endocervical biopsy and sperm count
D. Sexually transmitted infection testing and artificial insemination

4–68 *Marta asks you how pregnancy will affect her rheumatoid arthritis. You respond:*

A. "There is a one-third rule: one-third get better, one-third remain the same, and one-third get worse."
B. "Pregnancy will have no effect on your rheumatoid arthritis."
C. "Seventy-five percent of women experience remission of the disease during pregnancy."
D. "It is advised that you don't get pregnant with this condition."

4–69 *A poorly defined, flat, blue-black macule, present at birth and usually on the trunk and buttocks, is a:*

A. blue nevus.
B. drug-induced blue macule.
C. Mongolian spot.
D. malignant melanoma.

4–70 *What is the minimum number of café-au-lait spots that should be of concern?*

A. 1–3
B. 4–5
C. More than 5
D. Any number

4–71 *Carrie is due to deliver her second baby. During your workup, you note that she hemorrhaged after delivering her first baby 2 years ago, has always had menorrhagia, and bruises easily. Her lab work reveals a normal blood workup, including a normal prothrombin time and activated partial thromboplastin time. You suspect:*

A. Von Willebrand's disease.
B. Hemophilia.
C. Sickle cell anemia.
D. Unfortunate coincidences.

4–72 *The reason most often cited to explain why women who have had a usual length of stay and normal delivery discontinue breast-feeding before 8 weeks postpartum is:*

A. that the mother returned to work or school.
B. the perception that the infant is not receiving enough milk.
C. the ease of formula use.
D. maternal or infant illness.

4–73 *Marisa was born with a red- to blue-purple nodule on her thigh that blanches dramatically with pressure. Over the last few months it has increased in size. Her mother asks you what you think it is. You respond:*

A. "It may be a hemangioma."
B. "It may be a melanoma."
C. "It might be fibromatosis."
D. "It may be a dermatofibrosarcoma protuberans."

4–74 *Children react to their parents' divorce in different ways, depending on their age. If a child reacted with guilt, self-blame for the divorce, a sense of loss, feelings of betrayal and rejection, and confusion, what age would you suspect the child to be?*

A. Preschool age (3–4 years old)
B. Early school age (6–8 years old)
C. Older school age (9–11 years old)
D. Adolescent (12–18 years old)

4–75 *Rebecca is seeking to become pregnant through artificial insemination using donor sperm. In teaching Rebecca about this procedure, which information should the nurse include?*

A. The client will be able to find out who the father of her baby is from the sperm bank before conception.
B. The client's child will be able to find out who its father is from the sperm bank when the child turns 18.
C. The identity of the sperm donor who becomes the father of this child is confidential and will not be released to the client or her child.
D. The identity of the sperm donor who becomes the father of the child will be unknown because the sperm bank does not document donor identity on the medical record.

4–76 *Cydney, who is 30 weeks pregnant, is planning to travel outside of the United States. She asks you which immunizations she should or should not have. Which immunization do you recommend she not receive?*

A. Pooled gamma globulin
B. Chloroquine for malaria prophylaxis
C. Yellow fever
D. Inactivated polio vaccine (IPV)

4–77 *Susie, who is 16 weeks pregnant, is having mild cramps with persistent and excessive bleeding. On examination, you find that some portion of the products of conception (placental) remain in the uterus, but the fetus has been expelled. What type of abortion is Susie having?*

A. Incomplete
B. Threatened
C. Inevitable
D. Missed

4–78 *Marci has had several abortions in the past and has been unable to carry a pregnancy to full term because of an incompetent cervix. She states that the physician mentioned cerclage to her and asks you what that means. You tell her that cerclage is:*

A. a treatment of bedrest with frequent pelvic exams to make sure that the cervix is not dilated.
B. a method in which an apparatus resembling a diaphragm is placed over the cervix to help it stay "tight."

C. a purse-string type of stitch placed around the cervix.
D. a treatment using intravaginal medicated sponges.

4–79 *What is the simplest and safest method of suppressing lactation after it has started?*

A. Administering oral and long-acting injections of hormonal preparations
B. Using breast binders
C. Gradually weaning the baby to a bottle or cup over a 3-week period
D. Stopping "cold turkey" (stopping breast-feeding immediately)

4–80 *At what age should children first be screened for lead toxicity?*

A. 3 months
B. 6 months
C. 1 year
D. 3 years

4–81 *When asking a family member if the family generally gets the things they want out of life, if there are any "rules" in the family that everyone believes are important, and what role religion plays in the family, you are trying to assess which functional health pattern?*

A. Role-relationship pattern
B. Cognitive-perceptual pattern
C. Value-belief pattern
D. Health-perception/health-management pattern

4–82 *An asymmetric, softened enlargement of the uterine corner caused by placental development is a probable sign of pregnancy called:*

A. Hegar's sign.
B. Chadwick's sign.
C. Goodrich's sign.
D. Piskaçek's sign.

4–83 *Lois is complaining of leg cramps during her pregnancy. What would you suggest to relieve them?*

A. Take a calcium supplement daily.
B. Do several quick stretches to relieve the cramping.
C. Massage the cramping muscle.
D. Point your toes when exercising.

4–84 *Which of the following statements regarding gender differences in fetal growth is true?*

A. Female fetuses grow faster than male fetuses in the third trimester.
B. Female fetuses are larger after 26 weeks' gestation.
C. Male infants are slightly heavier and longer at birth.
D. Female infants have a larger head circumference at birth.

4–85 *Marissa is a long distance runner with 9% body fat. Which of the following findings is consistent with this situation?*

A. Regular menses and a basal body temperature that indicates ovulation
B. Irregular menses and a basal body temperature that indicates ovulation
C. Regular menses and a basal body temperature that indicates lack of ovulation
D. Irregular menses and a basal body temperature that indicates lack of ovulation

4–86 *Sabrina, who has a 4-month-old daughter, is trying to decide what to take with her on her vacation. She asks you when her daughter should be able to sit in a straight-backed high chair. You tell her:*

A. Any day now.
B. At age 6 months.
C. At age 8 months.
D. At age 1 year.

4–87 *Which one of the following behavior ratings is not included on the Denver Developmental Screening Test?*

A. Complies with examiner's requests
B. Alertness
C. Fearlessness
D. Attention span

4–88 *Purposes of the Denver Developmental Screening Test include:*

A. screening apparently healthy infants for developmental problems.
B. measuring a child's intelligence.
C. predicting the development potential of at-risk children.
D. confirming the normal development of young children

4–89 *When counseling a woman about the use of a diaphragm for fertility control, which of the following would be important assessment data to collect?*

A. Current lactation status
B. Frequency of sexual activity
C. Regularity of menses
D. Willingness to touch her genitals

4–90 *When an infant is around 6 months of age, solid foods are usually added to the diet, generally in a recommended sequence. The first solid food recommended is cereal. What is the second type of solid food recommended?*

A. Yellow vegetables
B. Strained meats
C. Green vegetables
D. Fruits

4–91 *Which of the following tips will facilitate the introduction of solid foods into an infant's diet?*

A. A rougher texture is more noticeable to the infant and thus is more palatable.
B. Introduce only foods in the same category together; for example, introduce two fruits rather than one fruit and one vegetable.
C. Add small amounts of food to the feeding bottle and make a larger hole to allow "drinking" of the food.
D. Feed the solid food to the infant before the milk feeding.

4–92 *Nancy is concerned that her new breast-fed baby is not getting enough fluid. What do you tell her so that she can assess for an adequate intake?*

A. Weigh the infant every other day to see the weight gain in ounces.
B. If the infant is drinking and sleeping normally, an adequate intake is assumed.
C. If there are 6–10 wet diapers a day, intake is adequate.
D. If the infant is not irritable, an intake problem does not exist.

4–93 *Robert comes to the clinic to discuss having a vasectomy. Which of the following statements indicates that Robert understands the teaching received about the procedure?*

A. "I will be able to return to my job as a construction worker immediately after the procedure."
B. "The procedure will be performed at the hospital under general anesthesia."
C. "It will be safe for me to have unprotected sex one week after the procedure."
D. "The procedure will not affect my sexual function."

4–94 *At what age can an infant listen to talking, respond to simple commands, and begin to differentiate among words?*

A. Age 3–5 months
B. Age 6–8 months
C. Age 9–12 months
D. Age 12–18 months

4–95 *Which behavior of a mother indicates that the mother has good bottle-feeding technique?*

A. Keeps the nipple full of formula throughout the feeding
B. Props the bottle on a rolled towel
C. Points the bottle at the infant's tongue
D. Enlarges the nipple hole to allow for a steady stream of formula to flow

4–96 *Which of the following major pollutants has a high incidence of causing upper respiratory infection, pneumonia, bronchitis, and asthma, and is also linked to cancer?*

A. Carbon monoxide
B. Nitrogen dioxide
C. Sulfur dioxide
D. Passive smoking (second-hand smoke)

4–97 *A new mother asks, "Is it true that breast milk will prevent my baby from catching colds and other infections?" You should give which of the following replies based on current research findings?*

A. "Your baby will have increased resistance to illness caused by bacteria and viruses, but he may still contract infections."
B. "You should not have to worry about your baby's exposure to contagious diseases until he stops breast-feeding."
C. "Breast milk offers no greater protection to your baby than formula feedings."
D. "Breast milk will give your baby protection from all illnesses to which you are immune."

4–98 *Care of the infant experiencing neonatal abstinence syndrome should include which of the following?*

A. Place stuffed animals and mobiles in the crib to provide visual stimulation.
B. Position the infant's crib in a quiet corner of the nursery.
C. Avoid the use of pacifiers.
D. Spend extra time holding and rocking the baby.

4–99 *During the 6-week visit after a stillbirth, Mary states, "Sometimes I feel like I left my baby somewhere, and I can't remember where she is. Then I remember that she isn't alive." This is an example of:*

A. Anticipatory grieving
B. Disorientation
C. Reorganization
D. Searching and yearning

4–100 *Ruth is toilet training her daughter and has many concerns. What do you tell her about the process?*

A. Girls are usually completely trained an average of $2^1/_2$ months earlier than boys.
B. The majority of children achieve bowel training before bladder training.
C. About 80% of children are completely trained after age 3.
D. Boys are usually completely trained an average of $2^1/_2$ months earlier than girls.

4–101 *At what age can a child understand up to 1200 words?*

A. 18 months
B. 24 months
C. 30 months
D. 36 months

4–102 *The primary site of drowning for children under age 3 is:*

A. the ocean.
B. a backyard pool.
C. a lake.
D. a bathtub.

4–103 *Which of the following statements is true regarding infant car seats?*

A. An infant car seat should be placed facing backward until the infant's toes touch the seat.
B. An infant car seat should be placed facing backward until the infant weighs 20 lb.
C. An infant car seat should be placed facing forward until the infant outgrows it.
D. An infant car seat should be placed facing forward until the infant weighs 20 lb.

4–104 *When should a child be moved from a car seat to a regular seat with a seatbelt?*

A. At age 4
B. At age 3
C. When the child weighs 40 lb
D. When the child weighs 30 lb

4–105 *Mandy, age 16, approaches her parents and states that she knows that she is adopted. How should the parents respond?*

A. "That's crazy! Where did you get such an idea?"
B. "Everyone at your age has doubts about their parents."
C. "Yes, I'm glad you know."
D. "Why do you think that?"

4–106 *Glenda gave birth to Jack 4 weeks ago. Her postpartum course was complicated by an intrauterine infection that was successfully treated with antibiotics. Today Glenda calls the office because Jack has white patches on his tongue and gums. She is concerned that her milk has become "sour" and is causing the white patches in Jack's mouth. Based on this data, you suspect a diagnosis of:*

A. oral chlamydia infection.
B. oral candidiasis.
C. mastitis.
D. Epstein's pearls.

4–107 *Given the above information and confirmation of the diagnosis, you would anticipate treating Jack with:*

A. Vinegar and water.
B. Nystantin.
C. Fluconazole.
D. Antibiotics.

4–108. *Jack and Jill present for a preconception health counseling session. Jack is 34; Jill is 33; and they have a 5-year-old son, Jake. Jake is the product of an uncomplicated pregnancy and labor. At birth, Jake had an open neural tube defect and now has spinal bifida with a loss of function of his lower extremities. Jack and Jill want another child and ask if there is anything they can do to prevent the recurrence of a neural tube defect in future pregnancies. Your best response to this couple is:*

A. "Take 60 mg a day of an iron supplement to enhance stores to support fetal development."
B. "It is a matter of genetics and there is nothing you can do."
C. "Have a CVS performed at 12–14 weeks gestation to determine the health of the fetus."
D. "Take 4 mg/d of folic acid, beginning before conception."

4–109. *Patricia presents for her regularly scheduled prenatal visit at 34 weeks gestation. During the interview, you determine that Patricia has not felt fetal movement for the past week. On examination, you are unable to auscultate the fetal heart tones. Which of the following would be useful in the diagnosis of an intrauterine fetal death?*

A. Chadwick's sign
B. Piskaçek's sign
C. Spalding's sign
D. Homans's sign

4–110. *During a woman's initial prenatal visit, you are reviewing her lab results. The urine contained an increased number of white blood cells, nitrites and greater than 10,000 bacteria/mL of urine. Based on these findings, you suspect which of the following?*

A. Renal failure
B. Contamination of the urine with amniotic fluid
C. Urinary tract infection
D. Nothing unusual; this is a normal finding in pregnancy

4–111 *A low-risk woman who is 16 weeks pregnant should be instructed to return to the prenatal clinic in:*

A. 1 week.
B. 2 weeks.
C. 3 weeks.
D. 4 weeks.

4–112 *Karen is taking oral contraceptive pills for fertility control. Karen calls the clinic and reports the presence of chest pain and shortness of breath. You instruct Karen to:*

A. Eat smaller meals more frequently to prevent gastric distention.
B. Stop taking the pills and use a nonhormonal contraceptive method.
C. Wait for the physician to return a telephone call to the client.
D. Go to the nearest emergency room immediately to be evaluated.

4–113. *Susan is keeping a basal body temperature (BBT) graph as part of her infertility treatment. Today she shares the BBT graph with you. The BBT graph shows a nearly straight line. Which of the following is the best interpretation of Susan's BBT graph?*

A. The client is not ovulating.
B. The client is not having intercourse.
C. The client is ovulating late in her menstrual cycle.
D. The client is not taking her temperature correctly.

4–114. *During Kim's first prenatal visit, she denies having had rubella or the rubella vaccine. Based on this information, which of the following is the most appropriate action?*

A. Administer the rubella vaccine.
B. Take a blood sample to assess the rubella titer.
C. Tell the client to avoid infection with rubella during her pregnancy because it will result in a preterm birth.
D. Tell the client that, because rubella has little effect on the fetus, she should not worry about exposure to the disease.

4–115. *Bea delivered vaginally 36 hours ago. You made rounds this morning and determined that she is ready to be discharged. You are at the nurses' station completing your documentation when Bea's husband comes up to you and states that his wife is very sick. Upon arrival at her room, you find Bea sitting up in bed. She states, "I cannot breathe! My chest hurts so much!" You suspect:*

A. Myocardial infarction
B. Panic attack
C. Bacterial pneumonia
D. Pulmonary embolism

Answers

4–1 Answer B

Maternal serum alpha-fetoprotein (MSAFP) testing is a screening procedure used to detect an increased risk for neural tube defects and ventral wall defects. MSAFP screening should be considered for all pregnant women at 16–18 weeks' gestation because 90% of neural tube defects occur in the absence of a positive history. MSAFP is elevated in 80–90%of women whose fetuses have open neural tube defects or other fetal anomalies such as omphalocele, congenital nephrosis, and fetal bowel obstruction, and in women with multiple fetuses. MSAFP levels are not elevated with closed neural tube defects such as hydrocephalus. Birth trauma is the most common cause of cerebral palsy, so there is no available screening test. It is diagnosed after birth. An MSAFP is part of a triple screening test, and low values on triple screening testing are indicative of an increased risk for trisomy 21.

4–2 Answer D

Vaginal bleeding may be a sign of impending pregnancy loss; persistent vomiting may result in dehydration and ketosis, which in turn can affect organogenesis during the first trimester. During the first trimester, fetal movement is not perceptible. Quickening (the perception of fetal movement) occurs at 18–20 weeks' gestation. Edema of the hands and face are signs of a constricted intravascular space and worsening pregnancy-induced hypertension (PIH), which occurs in the last trimester of pregnancy. Other signs of PIH are proteinuria and elevated blood pressure. In the first trimester there is no change in the maternal blood pressure.

4–3 Answer B

If a primary infection of genital herpes simplex occurs early in a pregnancy, a spontaneous abortion may result. Primary infection or a recurrence later in a pregnancy is not associated with an increase in pregnancy loss or malformation. Before the initiation of labor, if a woman has a history of genital herpes simplex, she should have a thorough inspection of the vulva and lower genital tract. If active lesions are found, a cesarean section should be performed.

4–4 Answer C

Mild dilutional anemia is seen throughout gestation as the result of an increased circulating blood volume. Plasma volume expansion, which begins at 6–8 weeks' gestation, precedes and exceeds red cell volume. The circulating blood volume of a pregnant woman increases by 45%. Iron stores are not depleted by the fetus and hepatic function is not affected during gestation.

4–5 Answer C

Fetal heart tones can be heard with a conventional fetoscope at 18–20 weeks' gestation. At 7–8 weeks' gestation, a transabdominal ultrasound will show fetal heart movement. At 10–12 weeks' gestation, fetal heart tones can be heard with a Doppler stethoscope. At 20 or more weeks' gestation, fetal movements can be felt by the examiner.

4–6 Answer C

An underweight woman (less than 90% of ideal body weight) should gain 5 lb during the first trimester, for a total recommended weight gain of 28–40 lb. A woman of normal weight should gain 3.5 lb during the first trimester, for a total recommended weight gain of 25–35 lb. An overweight woman (greater than 120% of desirable pregravid weight for height) should gain 2 lb during the first trimester, with a total recommended weight gain of 15–25 lb. A severely overweight (greater than 135% of desirable pregravid weight) woman should gain 2 lb during the first trimester, for a total recommended weight gain of at least 15 lb during the pregnancy. These recommendations are from the U.S. Institute of Medicine, Subcommittee on Nutritional Status and Weight Gain During Pregnancy.

4–7 Answer C

Nausea and vomiting affect 50–90% of all pregnant women. Nausea, ranging from mild to severe, typically begins at about the 4th–6th week of pregnancy, peaks around weeks 8–12, and disappears by the 20th week of pregnancy. Severe nausea, known as hyperemesis gravidarum, affects about 1–2% of all pregnant women.

4–8 Answer A

Nausea during pregnancy may be helped somewhat by dietary changes, such as eating a bland diet taken frequently and in small amounts, increasing carbohydrate intake, decreasing fat intake, and trying to stay away from food odors. Good hydration is important in pregnancy; therefore fluid restriction is never recommended.

4–9 Answer D

Lamaze uses patterned, controlled breathing with concentration on a visual focal point during labor. A focus on birth in a dimly lighted room and a warm water bath is the Leboyer method. Natural childbirth uses no medical interventions. The Bradley method is father-coached childbirth.

4–10 Answer A

The infant at age 6 weeks sucks on his or her fingers, stares at objects, and recognizes the parent's voice. Smiling, gurgling, and swinging the arms and legs is typical of the 3–4-month-old infant. Infants can sit with support and bring an object to the mouth at 5–6 months and begin creeping and babbling at 7–9 months.

4–11 Answer A

The Food and Drug Administration (FDA) has five pregnancy categories. Category D indicates that positive evidence of human fetal risk exists, but benefits may outweigh risks in certain situations, such as when the client is using phenytoin (Dilantin). The other four FDA pregnancy categories are as follows: Category A indicates that controlled studies in women failed to demonstrate a risk to the fetus in the first trimester and fetal harm appears remote. Category B indicates that animal studies have not demonstrated a fetal risk, but there are no human studies in pregnant women, or animal studies have shown an adverse effect that was not confirmed in human studies. Category C indicates that animal studies show adverse effects and there are no controlled studies in women. Category E indicates that studies or experience have shown fetal risk that clearly outweighs any possible benefits.

4–12 Answer B

Zidovudine (AZT) should be given to a pregnant woman with a human immunodeficiency virus (HIV) infection beginning at 14 weeks' gestation. The dosage is 100 mg by mouth (po) 5 times a day. During labor, IV administration is recommended. Administration of AZT beginning at 14 weeks' gestation and continuing through labor significantly decreases the risk of HIV transmission to the infant.

4–13 Answer C

The management of asthma in pregnant women differs little from management in nonpregnant women. Beta-2 agonists, theophylline, epinephrine, cromolyn, and glucocorticoids are all safe to use. Whenever possible, inhalation rather than oral medications should be used. During exacerbations, IV and oral glucocorticoids may be used in the usual manner. Typically, asthma during pregnancy follows the one-third rule: one-third of the women have improved symptoms; one-third have no change; and one-third have worse symptoms.

4–14 Answer A

If medication is needed, the drug of choice for pregnant women with diabetes is insulin. Oral hypoglycemics such as glyburide, glipizide, and metformin should be avoided because they are all teratogenic. Diet remains the cornerstone of treatment for pregnant women with diabetes.

4–15 Answer B

Universal screening for GDM is no longer recommended. Screen women at risk. Age 40 or older is considered a risk factor. Other risk factors include: obesity, history of miscarriage or fetal death, history of premature infant, family history of diabetes, polyhydramnios, history of infant with macrosomia (>4,000 g) or congenital malformation, preeclampsia, excessive weight gain, and glycosuria. A threatened miscarriage without a history of a previous miscarriage is not a risk factor; the term "hypoglycemic" could be interpreted a variety of ways. This complaint would have to be evaluated before a decision to screen or not could be made.

4–16 Answer B

Hegar's sign is softness of the uterus and ballottement at the isthmus. Other physiological signs of pregnancy are Chadwick's sign (cervical blueness), Goodell's sign (cervical softness); and quickening (feeling fetal movement, usually at 18–22 weeks' gestation).

4–17 Answer D

A urine human chorionic gonadotropin (hCG) test will be positive 4 weeks after conception; hCG is detectable in urine 26 days after conception. It is detectable in serum 8 days after conception. A home urine pregnancy test is 99% accurate and becomes negative after 18–20 weeks' gestation because the hCG levels begin to drop.

4–18 Answer C

The G in APGAR stands for grimace. The acronym APGAR helps in the assessment of the five components of a neonate's responses: appearance, pulse, grimace, activity, and respiration.

4–19 Answer D

At birth, the anterior fontanelle has a diamond shape, whereas the posterior fontanelle has a triangular shape. The fontanelles are soft and flat and may bulge when the infant cries.

4–20 Answer B

Barlow's test is when you flex the hips and knees at a 90-degree angle and attempt to slip the femur heads onto the posterior tip of the acetabulums by lateral pressure of the thumbs and by rocking the knees medially with the knuckles of the index fingers. A palpable or audible hip click is not normally heard. With Barlow's test, the action is up and back like a piston. You are testing for normal hip movement. With Ortolani's maneuver, you are also testing for normal hip movement, but the action is to abduct: up and out. You flex the knees and hips, placing fingers bilaterally on the greater trochanters, thumbs gripping the medial aspect of femurs, then adduct and abduct. There is a positive jerking motion as the femur passes over the acetabulum. Very frequently, hip "clicks" are an indication for radiographic or orthopedic consultations. As in adults, clicks are caused by the movement of articular and periarticular parts, but the "clunks" attending subluxation and rearticulation are easily felt and often even grossly visible. There is no Spock's test. The Moro (startle) reflex is elicited by physical shocks and sudden changes in support of the infant.

4–21 Answer B

An android-type pelvis has a wedge-shaped inlet, a narrow forepelvis, a flat posterior segment, and a narrow sacrosciatic notch with the sacrum inclining forward. A woman's pelvis may be one of four types or a combination of them. A gynecoid-type pelvis has a rounded, slightly ovoid, or elliptical inlet with a well-rounded forepelvis (anterior segment). An anthropoid-type pelvis has a long, narrow, oval inlet; an extended and narrow anterior and posterior segment; a wide sacrosciatic notch; and a long, narrow sacrum, often with six sacral segments. A platypelloid-type pelvis has a distinct oval inlet with a very wide, rounded retropubic angle and a wider, flat posterior segment.

4–22 Answer B

Hemophilia is an example of an X-linked recessive condition, occurring more commonly in men than in women. Muscular dystrophy is an example of an autosomal-dominant condition in which the trait appears with equal frequency in both sexes. For inheritance to take place, at least one parent must have the trait unless a new mutation has just occurred. Sickle cell anemia and cystic fibrosis are both examples of autosomal-recessive conditions in which the trait appears with equal frequency in both sexes. For inheritance to take place, both parents must be carriers of the recessive trait.

4–23 Answer C

Spontaneous abortion refers to the loss of a fetus of less than 22 weeks' gestation and a weight less than 500 g. A delivered fetus of about 22–28 weeks gestation and weighing 500–1000 g is called immature. A delivered fetus of about 28–36 weeks' gestation and weighing 500–2000 g is called premature. A full-term fetus is one that has attained 37 weeks' gestation and weighs at least 3500 g.

4–24 Answer B

The brain configuration of a fetus is roughly complete at 12 weeks' gestation. Therefore it is important to teach the pregnant client to avoid all drugs, alcohol, smoking, and other teratogenic agents that may cause neurological harm to the infant, unless the client checks first with her healthcare provider.

4–25 Answer D

The presumptive symptom of pregnancy that involves tingling or frank pain of the breasts is called mastodynia. Mastodynia (breast tenderness) may range from tingling to frank pain and is caused by hormonal responses of the mammary ducts and alveolar system. Similar symptoms may also occur just before menses. Other presumptive symptoms, or early manifestations of pregnancy, are as follows. Montgomery's tubercles (enlargement of the circumlacteal sebaceous glands of the areola) occur at 6–8 weeks' gestation and are caused by hormonal stimulation. Colostrum secretion is a symptom that may begin after 16 weeks' gestation. Melasma (the mask of pregnancy) is darkening of the skin over the forehead, bridge of the nose, or cheekbones and is most marked in women with dark complexions. It usually occurs after 16 weeks' gestation and is more prevalent in women who spend a lot of time in the sun.

4–26 Answer A

According to Nagele's rule, which assists in calculating the estimated date of delivery (EDD) by adding 7 days to the first day of the last normal menstrual period (LNMP), then subtracting 3 months, if a woman's LNMP was September 23, her EDD would be June 30 ($23 + 7 = 30$; $9 - 3 = 6$; $= 6/30$).

4–27 Answer C

When a client is experiencing Braxton Hicks contractions (painless uterine contractions felt as tightening or pressure that usually begin at about 28 weeks' gestation), they usually disappear with walking or exercise. If they were true labor contractions, they would become more intense.

4–28 Answer B

The gestational age when the uterus is palpable just at the pubic symphysis is 8 weeks. At 12 weeks, the uterus becomes an abdominal organ, and at 15 weeks it is usually at the midpoint between the pubic symphysis and umbilicus. The uterus is palpable at 20 weeks at the umbilicus, and after that, the fundal size correlates roughly with the gestational age up until about 36 weeks. At 36 weeks, the fundal height may decrease as the fetal head descends into the pelvis.

4–29 Answer B

Chorionic villus sampling (CVS) detects only chromosomal anomalies and not anatomic aberrations such as open neural tube defects. CVS may be performed at 10–12 weeks' gestation, whereas amniocentesis may be performed at 15–18 weeks' gestation. Although safe, CVS has a slightly higher risk of loss of the pregnancy as compared to amniocentesis and is performed only in large facilities that offer experienced practitioners and real-time ultrasound imaging.

4–30 Answer B

A woman of average height and weight needs an additional 300 calories a day during pregnancy and an additional 500 calories a day when breast-feeding to ensure an adequate intake of essential nutrients for the child.

4–31 Answer C

Douching, which is seldom necessary, may be harmful during pregnancy. Intercourse late in the pregnancy may initiate labor, possibly because an orgasm might cause a uterine contraction reflex. Intercourse is usually cautioned against only in women who have had a previous premature delivery or are currently experiencing uterine bleeding. Water does not enter the vagina; therefore swimming is not contraindicated. However, diving should be avoided because of the possibility of trauma. Good dental care is important during pregnancy; however, the dentist should be told that the woman is pregnant.

4–32 Answer A

Right before ovulation, as estrogen levels increase, the cervical mucus is copious, thin, and stretchable. It feels like a lubricant and can be stretched between the fingers. This is called spinnbarkheit. This is the time of maximum fertility. During most of the menstrual cycle, cervical mucus is scant in quantity and thick.

4–33 Answer B

After delivery, exercises to strengthen the muscles of the back, pelvic floor, and abdomen are advocated, but strenuous exercises should be postponed until about 3 weeks after delivery. This allows the abdominal muscles to partially regain their original length and tone and prevents undue client fatigue.

4–34 Answer C

With a history of 6 weeks of breast-feeding, pain and a lump in the breast, flulike symptoms, and physical examination revealing an engorged, erythematous, and warm-to-touch breast and temperature of 101.8°F (38.5°C), your diagnosis is mastitis, an infection of the breast. Mastitis, which occurs in about 5% of lactating women, may be caused by tight clothing, missed infant feedings, poor drainage of the duct and alveolus, or infection with *Staphylococcus aureus, Escherichia coli,* or *Streptococcus*. A clogged duct, simple breast engorgement, breast abscess, and viral syndrome are differential diagnoses. A clogged duct and simple breast engorgement may be painful, but not erythematous or warm to the touch. Also, flulike symptoms would not be present. A breast abscess should be suspected if there is no resolution of symptoms after several days of antibiotic therapy. If an abscess is present, pitting edema over the affected area is possible. An abscess is usually treated with both antibiotics and drainage.

4–35 Answer C

When a woman who is breast-feeding develops mastitis, there is no need to stop breast-feeding unless the mastitis is very severe. The woman should begin breast-feeding on the unaffected side because the infant's first sucking is the strongest and would be more painful on the affected side. This also allows the affected breast to "let down." Sulfa drugs should not be prescribed if the nursing infant is less than 1 month old. Dicloxacillin sodium (Dynapen, Dycill, Pathocil), cephalexin (Keflex), and acetaminophen (Tylenol) may be safely prescribed.

4–36 Answer D

Characteristics of trisomy 21 (Down syndrome) include hypotonia, simian creases, epicanthial folds, and Brushfield's spots. Findings of low birth weight, small jaw and recessed chin, muscle rigidity, and short sternum are consistent with a diagnosis of Edwards' syndrome (trisomy 18). Patau syndrome is indicated by the presence of a cleft lip and palate, polydactyly, malformed ears, and absence of the iris. Clinical findings of lymphedema of the hands and feet, webbed neck, coarctation of the aorta, and urinary tract abnormalities are indicative of Turner's syndrome.

4–37 Answer B

If a woman is breast-feeding and complains of tenderness of the nipples all the time, suggest that she apply dry heat to the nipples between feedings.
A common symptom during the first days of breast-feeding, tenderness of the nipples usually begins when the baby starts to suck and then subsides as

soon as the milk begins to flow. If maternal tissues are unusually tender, dry heat usually helps. Ice tends to increase nipple tenderness. Nipple shields should be used only as a last resort because they interfere with normal sucking. If it is necessary to wear nipple shields, suggest glass or plastic shields with rubber nursing nipples rather than all-rubber shields. This is a temporary problem that can be resolved. Stopping breast-feeding for a temporary problem is an irreversible solution.

4–38 Answer C

The diagnostic standard for the diagnosis of gestation is an abnormal 3-hour glucose tolerance test (GTT). A 50-g oral glucose challenge test is a screening test to identify women who are candidates for the 3-hour GTT. A postprandial glucose level greater than 140 mg/dL is not indicative of gestational diabetes. Because of changes in renal filtration rates during pregnancy, many women have evidence of glucose in voided urine.

4–39 Answer C

The higher the glucose concentration, the higher the glycosylated hemoglobin. Hemoglobin A_{1c} measures the average blood glucose fluctuations over the life span of a maternal RBC. The glycosylated hemoglobin level is not influenced by or related to the fetal blood glucose concentration.

4–40 Answer B

Symptoms of urinary frequency, urgency, dysuria, and suprapubic discomfort in the absence of chills, fever, nausea and vomiting, along with cloudy, malodorous urine, are clinically diagnostic of acute cystitis. Acute cystitis and acute pyelonephritis are common renal disorders in pregnancy. Renal calculi may cause intermittent flank pain or pain that radiates around to the abdomen. Maternal symptoms of pyelonephritis include fever, shaking chills, malaise, flank pain, nausea and vomiting, headache, increased urinary frequency, and dysuria. Interstitial cystitis is a chronic, painful bladder disorder in which the course is unpredictable. The symptoms include urinary frequency, urgency, nocturia, and suprapubic pain in the absence of urinary pathogens. Although the etiology of interstitial cystitis is unknown, most attribute it to an initial insult to the bladder wall by a toxin, allergen, or immunologic agent that causes an inflammatory response.

4–41 Answer C

The antibiotic of choice for acute pyelonephritis occurring during the seventh month of pregnancy is ampicillin (Principen, Polycillin) because the most common offending pathogen is *Escherichia coli*. Ampicillin is safe for the mother and fetus and has minimal side effects. Earlier in the pregnancy, sulfonamides, nitrofurantoin, and cephalosporins may be prescribed along with ampicillin. Nitrofurantoin should be avoided in the last trimester because it may induce hemolytic anemia in the newborn. Sulfa drugs must be avoided in mothers with glucose-6-phosphatase deficiency and are best avoided late in pregnancy because of the increased likelihood of neonatal hyperbilirubinemia. Trimethoprim is a folic acid antagonist, so trimethoprim-sulfamethoxazole should be avoided in pregnancy.

4–42 Answer B

Pregnancy does not appear to exert any deleterious effect on multiple sclerosis (MS), and the initial occurrence of MS is not increased during pregnancy. Because MS is a progressive neurologic disease, the client's participation in long-term childcare may be impossible, but becoming pregnant or not is the client's decision to make.

4–43 Answer A

H_2-receptor antagonists such as cimetidine can be prescribed for pregnant clients who have peptic ulcer disease. Newer drugs such as ranitidine should not be used during the first trimester of pregnancy because animal studies have revealed possible teratogenicity. Sucralfate should be avoided because it has not been adequately studied during pregnancy. Bellergal-S, an anticholinergic agent, contains phenobarbital and is contraindicated. Symptoms should be treated initially by avoidance of irritating foods and by antacids. Supportive advice may be given regarding cessation of smoking; small, bland meals; avoidance of stress; and so forth.

4–44 Answer B

A pregnant woman is at risk for developing congenital rubella syndrome during the first 16 weeks of pregnancy. The risk of congenital rubella syndrome is related to the gestational age of the fetus at the time the pregnant woman is exposed to the infection. The fetal infection rate is 90% before 11 weeks' gestation, 33% at 12 weeks gestation, 11% at 14 weeks' gestation, and 24% at 16 weeks' gestation. It then goes down to 0% after 16 weeks' gestation. Prenatal testing should be performed to determine if a woman is seronegative, in which case she should avoid anyone with a rash or viral illness.

4–45 Answer B

Mineral oil should be avoided by the pregnant woman who is constipated because it decreases the absorption of fat-soluble vitamins. Cathartics are also contraindicated because they may cause preterm labor. Bulk-forming laxatives and stool softeners can be used along with dietary interventions, such as drinking warm fluids on arising, eating foods high in bulk, and drinking 6–8 glasses of water per day to stimulate bowel motility.

4–46 Answer C

A nonstress test examines fetal heart reactivity in response to fetal movement. The criterion for a reactive test is the presence of at least 2 fetal heart rate accelerations of at least 15 beats in amplitude and lasting at least 15 seconds, in response to fetal movement during a 20-minute testing window. The relationship between uterine contraction and fetal heart response is the basis of a contraction stress test.

4–47 Answer A

Trauma to the pregnant abdomen can result in *abruptio placentae* (premature separation of the placenta). *Abruptio placentae* is a life-threatening event. The enlarged uterus and its contents actually provide some protection to the other abdominal organs from trauma.

4–48 Answer C

Bishop's score is an assessment of the cervix's readiness for elective induction. Leopold's maneuvers are used to determine fetal position. The multiparameter evaluation following a nonreactive nonstress test is a biophysical profile. An L/S (lethicin/sphignomyelin) ratio is used to evaluate fetal lung maturity.

4–49 Answer B

Signs of an effective latch-on are lips flanged out and cheeks full. Rapid, short, nonrhythmic sucking is consistent with non-nutritive sucking. With an effective latch-on, if maternal nipple discomfort is present, it subsides quickly because the pressure of the infant's sucking motion is on the areola, not the nipple.

4–50 Answer B

After 28 weeks' gestation, when the woman is performing fetal movement counts (FMCs), 10 movements should be obtained in 1 hour. Usually, 10 movements are felt within 30 minutes, but 10 movements in 1 hour are considered acceptable. FMCs should be performed at the same time every day, preferably after a meal or when the fetus is most active. The woman should be lying in the left lateral position. If the woman senses decreased activity, a nonstress test (NST), or, at the very least, fetal surveillance, should be initiated within 12 hours.

4–51 Answer B

The infant is showing signs of jaundice. Jaundice in an infant less than 24 hours of age is often caused by Rh or ABO incompatibility. A direct Coombs' test will determine the presence of maternal antibodies in the baby's blood. The other lab tests are not related to hyperbilirubinemia.

4–52 Answer D

Even though children may look like the adoptive parents, they usually find out one way or another that they are adopted. Studies have shown that the least traumatic way of let a child know that he or she is adopted is to tell them right from the beginning how special they are. For example, you can tell them that with biological children you had no choice, but with adoption, you "picked" them especially because they are unique and you wanted them in your family.

4–53 Answer B

G5P4015 written on the client's chart indicates that the woman has been pregnant five times (G for gravidity or total number of pregnancies), had four delivery experiences (P for parity or birth [alive or dead] of an infant or infants weighing more than 500 g; multiple gestation is counted as a single occurrence), and had one abortion. Because she has five living children, she must have had a set of twins because one of the pregnancies ended in an abortion. An abortion is a pregnancy that terminates before the 22nd gestational week or in which the fetus weighed less than 500 g. Another way to remember this is to think of FPAL (Florida Power and Light) as the four numbers following P. The first number (F) stands for full-term births (with multiple gestation counted as a single occurrence), P for premature births (preemies), A for abortions, and L for the number of living children.

4–54 Answer A

To obtain the daily calcium intake recommended during pregnancy, a woman should consume at least 1 quart of cow's milk per day. Calcium must be supplemented during pregnancy to meet fetal needs and preserve maternal calcium stores. Milk is relatively inexpensive and 1 quart of cow's milk contains 1 g of calcium, which is almost the 1.2 g recommended daily during pregnancy. The milk can be in forms other than liquid, such as in soups, custards, etc. However, caution your client that large quantities of milk, meat, cheese, and dicalcium phosphate (a supplement) may cause excessive phosphorus levels, which may result in leg cramps. If a woman is lactose intolerant, as in the case of many Native Americans, foreign-born African-Americans, and certain Asians, protein, calcium, and vitamins must be supplied in other forms.

4–55 Answer B

Vas deferens blockage prevents ejection of sperm (oligospermia). It has no effect on urination or sex drive.

4–56 Answer D

A return to bright red vaginal bleeding is a sign of a complication and potentially a late postpartum hemorrhage. The patient should not be passing clots. It is expected that the amount of lochia will decrease over time. The fundus should be firm. A soft uterine fundus would result in increased vaginal bleeding.

4–57 Answer C

Classic signs of thrombophlebitis are local tenderness, heat, and swelling. Varicose veins increase the woman's risk for clot formation but are not a sign of thrombophlebitis.

4–58 Answer B

The woman with hyperemesis gravidarum is anxious about the effect of her condition on the fetus. The etiology of hyperemesis is unknown, but the incidence is associated with conditions of elevated hCG levels, such as pregnancy. Although there may be an emotional component, there is no indication that the pregnancy is unwanted. With appropriate treatment and support, the fetal prognosis is favorable. Because of the excessive vomiting, a nursing diagnosis focused on nutrition would be Imbalanced Nutrition, Less Than Body Requirements.

4–59 Answer D

Before 12 weeks gestation, length as measured from crown to rump is the most accurate measure of gestational age. Biparietal diameter and femur length are used to monitor fetal growth in the second trimester of pregnancy. Abdominal circumference is useful in identifying some congenital anomalies.

4–60 Answer D

A small, soft papillary swelling is most likely human papillomavirus infection, which can be confirmed by colposcopy and direct biopsy. A rash on the palms of the hands and the soles of the feet, as well as chancre sores, are associated with syphilis. Crusted ulcers are characteristic of herpes.

4–61 Answer B

Early in pregnancy, all pregnant women need their blood type and Rh status determined and need an atypical antibody titer (indirect Coombs' test) done. Although there are more than 400 antigens of the Rh factor, 90% of cases of Rh isoimmunization are caused by the D antigen. Women lacking antigenic determinant D require two exposures to the Rh antigen to produce significant sensitization, unless the first exposure was massive. A direct Coombs' test is performed on a blood specimen from the fetus/neonate, usually obtained from the umbilical cord. The 3-hour glucose challenge is diagnostic of gestational diabetes and is done in the second half of pregnancy. A Pap smear is only performed if the woman has not recently had one. As a result of normal pregnancy-related changes to the pregnant cervix, the reliability of the Pap smear is changed during pregnancy.

4–62 Answer C

RhoGAM (Rho [D] immune globulin) should be administered when a D-negative mother has been given a transfusion of D-positive blood and whenever a potential for mixing Rh-positive fetal and Rh-negative maternal blood exists, such as with an abortion, ectopic pregnancy, amniocentesis, antepartum hemorrhage, fetal blood sampling, fetal death, or fetal surgery. If there is any doubt about whether or not to administer RhoGAM, it should be given.

4–63 Answer D

The biophysical profile (BPP) consists of the four parameters of fetal well-being—fetal tone, breathing, motion, and amniotic fluid volume—along with a nonstress test (NST). In high-risk pregnancies, the BPP is necessary for a comprehensive fetal assessment.

4–64 Answer B

Lesbian concerns include the loss of support from family, friends, and coworkers. Battering and physical, emotional, or financial abuses are possible in any relationship, and there are no boundaries regarding gender. However, a lesbian woman may not want others to be aware of her sexual preference because she may not be able to obtain needed help and counseling. HIV infection is possible in a casual lesbian relationship if one partner has used intravenous drugs or been in a relationship with an HIV-infected man or woman. In addition, women may exchange body fluids by using a dildo without a condom. If HIV infection is a concern, the healthcare provider should counsel the women about safe sex practices. Other concerns of lesbian women relate to childbearing issues such as in vitro fertilization, donor sperm, who is the "real" mother, adoption issues, and custody issues.

4–65 Answer A

Maternity blues, sometimes called "baby blues," which affect about 50–70% of postpartum women, are usually transient emotional disturbances that occur around the second to fourth postpartum day and may last from a few hours to several weeks. Postpartum depression, which affects about 10–15% of postpartum women, is characterized by a depressed mood, irritability, fatigue, feelings of worthlessness, sleeping and eating changes, and changes in personality. There is a slow, insidious onset over several weeks after delivery. It usually begins within 2–3 weeks after birth and may last up to a year. Postpartum psychosis, which affects about 1 or 2 of every 1000 new mothers, is severely impaired ability to perform activities of daily living. Its onset is within a few weeks up to 3 months postpartum, with primiparas being at greater risk.

4–66 Answer B

Drugs that have significant effects in nursing infants and should be used with extreme caution in breastfeeding mothers include phenobarbital, clemastine, primidone, and sulfasalazine. Drugs that do not have significant effects in nursing infants and which may be used in breast-feeding mothers include azithromycin, propranolol, cisplatin, amoxicillin, cefoxitin, minoxidil, procainamide, and verapamil.

4–67 Answer A

Semen analysis and hystersalpingogram are appropriate to determine the reason for the couple's difficulty conceiving. Neither a Pap smear, colposcopy with endocervical biopsy, nor sexually transmitted infection testing will identify the cause of the couple's infertility.

4–68 Answer C

For women with rheumatoid arthritis, 75% will experience remission of their disease during pregnancy. Activities of daily living are easier to perform because of decreased joint stiffness, swelling, and an increase in grip strength. However, women with rheumatoid arthritis usually do experience major fatigue, and during labor and delivery, joint contracture may limit their positioning. Pain needs to be carefully assessed, and 95% of these women will experience a flare-up of their condition during labor and delivery.

4–69 Answer C

Mongolian spots (congenital dermal melanocytosis) are poorly defined, flat, blue to blue-black lesions. They are usually found on the trunk and buttocks of the newborn, but may occur anywhere. Mongolian spots are common in Asians and blacks. A biopsy reveals dermal melanocytes. They are usually asymptomatic, may fade with age, and do not require treatment. Some blue or blue-black macules that are acquired and not present at birth include blue nevus, a drug-induced blue macule, and malignant melanoma. A blue nevus usually occurs in an adolescent or adult and is asymptomatic. A biopsy reveals dermal melanocytes and there is usually an excision of the macule for cosmesis or concern about melanoma. A drug-induced blue macule most commonly occurs on sun-exposed areas of the body when the person takes phenothiazines, chloroquine, hydroxychloroquine, gold, minocycline, or silver-containing medications, as well as some others. A biopsy reveals increased melanin and deposition of the drug. There is very slow fading with time, and usually the focal lesions are removed surgically. Malignant melanomas may be assessed using the ABCDs: A for asymmetry (melanomas tend to be asymmetrical), B for border irregularity (the border of a melanoma lesion tends to be irregular), C for color (a melanoma is usually multicolored, blue-black, or black-brown), and D for diameter (a melanoma is usually greater than 6 mm in diameter).

4–70 Answer C

The presence of more than five café-au-lait spots suggests neurofibromatosis. Café-au-lait spots are uniformly pigmented tan, nonscaly, oval or irregularly shaped macules. The lesions are usually less than 0.5 cm in diameter and most commonly occur on the trunk, but can occur anywhere, although they are not usually found on mucosal surfaces. Ten percent of normal individuals have one to three café-au-lait spots. No treatment is necessary for normal individuals, although the spots may be associated with pulmonary stenosis and mental retardation.

4–71 Answer A

Von Willebrand's disease is the most common hereditary bleeding disorder, occurring in about 1% of the population. It is inherited as an autosomal dominant trait, so it is equally prevalent in men and women. Hemophilia is usually diagnosed during the first few years of life, and sickle cell anemia, if not diagnosed then, is usually diagnosed in childhood. Von Willebrand's disease is usually not diagnosed until after a severe hemorrhagic episode following surgery, trauma, dental procedures, or childbirth. Clients with von Willebrand's disease should be referred to a hematologist for coagulation studies. The treatment goal is to prevent bleeding or achieve hemostasis. Treatment depends on the severity of the disease and may range from intranasal desmopressin acetate spray (DDAVP nasal spray) to replacement of Factor VIII or blood transfusions.

4–72 Answer B

The most often cited reason why women who have had a usual length of stay after normal delivery discontinue breast-feeding before 8 weeks postpartum is the perception that the infant is not receiving enough milk. The other reasons, in descending order, are the mother's return to work or school, ease of formula use, maternal or infant illness, infant liking the bottle better, and breast pain. This is important to know when teaching new mothers about the benefits of breast-feeding and what to expect.

4–73 Answer A

Hemangiomas are single or multiple red to blue-purple nodules that blanch dramatically with pressure. Diffuse redness, increased hair growth, and scaling might occur over the lesions. They may occur anywhere and may be in a dermatomal distribution. Although usually present at birth, they may also increase in size during the first few months of life. Laser treatment can be done in selected cases. A melanoma may be multicolored, but will not blanch. A fibromatosis is a firm, flesh-colored nodule with normal overlying epidermis that may occur anywhere. In infancy, these nodules are usually on the trunk and shoulder. Surgical excision is usually performed, but the lesions may recur. A dermatofibrosarcoma protuberans is an erythematous, firm nodule that occurs more frequently on the trunk and more commonly in boys than in girls. The treatment consists of a wide local excision.

4–74 Answer B

The early school-age child (6–8 years old) reacts to a divorce with guilt, self-blame for the divorce, a sense of loss, feelings of betrayal and rejection, and confusion. The preschool-age child (3–4 years old) reacts with fears of abandonment and loss of custodial parent and confusion. The older school-age child (9–11 years old) reacts with shame, rejection, resentment, and loneliness. The child can view the divorce as his or her parents' problem, but still needs to find blame or reason. An adolescent (12–18 years old) has concerns about the loss of family life and his or her own future, feelings of responsibility for family members, and anger and hostility.

4–75 Answer C

The identity of sperm donors is confidential. Donors are usually assigned numbers, and the lists of donors and numbers are kept separate and secured by physical or electronic means.

4–76 Answer C

Live-virus immunization products, such as yellow fever, measles, and rubella vaccines, are contraindicated in pregnant women. Pooled gamma globulin to prevent hepatitis A and chloroquine for malaria prophylaxis have been proven safe to administer to a pregnant woman. Inactivated polio vaccine (Salk) can be administered instead of the oral vaccine. If a woman has a normal, low-risk pregnancy, travel can be accomplished safely between the 18th and 32nd weeks. Commercial airlines have pressurized cabins that do not pose a threat to the fetus. It is not advisable to travel to endemic areas of yellow fever in Africa or Latin America or to areas of Africa or Asia where chloroquine-resistant falciparum malaria is a hazard because complications of malaria are more common in pregnancy.

4–77 Answer A

An incomplete abortion occurs when some portion of the products of conception (usually placental) remains in the uterus. Usually, only mild cramps are reported, but bleeding is persistent and often excessive. A threatened abortion occurs when there is bleeding or cramping but the pregnancy continues. The cervix is not dilated. An inevitable abortion occurs when the cervix is dilated. The membranes may be ruptured, but passage of the products of conception has not occurred. Bleeding and cramping persist and passage of the products of conception is considered inevitable. A missed abortion occurs when the pregnancy has ceased to develop, but the conceptus has not been expelled. There is no bleeding, but a brownish vaginal discharge is present. Usually no pain is involved. Symptoms of pregnancy disappear and the uterus becomes smaller and irregularly softened, with the adnexa being normal.

4–78 Answer C

Cerclage is a purse-string type of stitch placed around the cervix. A variety of suture materials can be used to create the stitch around an incompetent cervix. Cerclage is used in conjunction with restriction of activities and should be used cautiously when there is advanced cervical dilation or membranes are prolapsed into the vagina. Rupture of the membranes and infection are specific contraindications to cerclage.

4–79 Answer C

The simplest and safest method of suppressing lactation after it has started is to wean the baby to a bottle or cup gradually over a 3-week period. The milk supply will decrease with the decreased demand and with minimal discomfort. Oral and long-acting injections of hormonal preparations used to be the practice to suppress lactation. Because of their questionable efficacy and associated adverse effects such as thromboembolic episodes and hair growth, this practice has been abandoned. In addition, lactation suppression with bromocriptine is not used because of the potential for severe hypertension, seizures, strokes, and myocardial infarctions associated with its use. The use of a snug bra, along with ice packs and analgesics, might help. If for some reason the mother must stop breast-feeding immediately, nipple stimulation should be avoided and the expression of milk should be discouraged.

4–80 Answer B

Children should first be screened for lead toxicity at age 6 months. All children ages 6 months through 6 years are considered at risk for lead poisoning and must be screened. Beginning at 6 months of age, a verbal risk assessment must be performed at every visit. If the screening tool used results in all negative responses to all the questions, a child is considered at low risk for high doses of lead exposure but must receive a blood lead test at 12 months and 24 months of age. If any response to the screening test is positive, the child is considered at high risk of lead exposure and a blood lead test must be done immediately. A blood lead test must be used to screen Medicaid-eligible children for lead poisoning.

4–81 Answer C

The value-belief functional health pattern includes the following questions to be asked during the family assessment: Does the family generally get things it wants out of life? What are the important things for the future? Are there any "rules" in the family that everyone believes are important? What role does religion play in the family? There are 11 different functional health patterns that are applicable to the assessment of families as well as individuals: health perception/health management, nutritional-metabolic, elimination, activity-exercise, sleep-rest, cognitive-perceptual, self-perception-self-concept, role-relationship, sexuality-reproductive, coping-stress tolerance, and value-belief. These guidelines provide information on family functioning, and the information obtained in a family assessment will assist the provider in setting goals with the family.

4–82 Answer D

A probable sign of pregnancy, Piskaçek's sign is an asymmetric, softened enlargement of the uterine corner caused by placental development. Hegar's sign is softening of the uterine isthmus. Chadwick's sign is a bluish or cyanotic color to the cervix and upper vagina. There is no Goodrich's sign.

4–83 Answer A

If a pregnant woman complains of leg cramps, the use of a daily calcium supplement may help relieve them. Leg cramps are a normal discomfort experienced during pregnancy. They are caused by a lack of calcium, pressure of the enlarged uterus on the blood vessels, fatigue or chilling, sudden stretching or overextension of the foot, and/or excessive phosphorus in the diet. Some nursing suggestions that might relieve the leg cramps are using calcium supplements, practicing gentle steady stretching to relieve the cramp, avoiding massage of the cramping muscle, and avoiding toe pointing when exercising.

4–84 Answer C

Gender differences occur in fetal growth. Boys are slightly heavier and longer at birth and have a larger head circumference than girls. Male fetuses also grow faster than female fetuses in the third trimester and are larger after 26 weeks' gestation than female fetuses.

4–85 Answer D

Fourteen percent body fat is considered adequate if a woman is to have regular menses and regular ovulation. A woman with less than 10% body fat will ovulate and menstruate very irregularly or not at all.

4–86 Answer B

At 6 months of age, a baby should be able to sit in a straight-backed high chair. At 7 months of age, a baby can sit leaning forward on both hands. At 8 months of age, a baby can sit well alone. At 1 year of age, a baby will begin to walk (cruise) by holding onto furniture.

4–87 Answer C

The Denver Developmental Screening Test (DDST) does not include fearlessness as a behavior rating. The behavior ratings included on the DDST are fearfulness (on a rating of none, somewhat fearful, or very fearful), complies with examiner's requests (on a rating of complies, usually complies, rarely complies), alertness (on a rating of interest in surroundings: alert, somewhat alert, or seriously disinterested), and attention span (on a rating of attentive, somewhat distractible, and very distractible).

4–88 Answer A

The Denver Developmental Screening Test (DDST) screens healthy infants for developmental problems. It is a screening test of a child's developmental level. By adding the number of accomplished and unaccomplished items on the test form, the person giving the test estimates the child's developmental level. It does not measure a child's intelligence, predict the child's potential, or confirm normal development.

4–89 Answer D

The woman needs to touch her genitalia to insert the diaphragm. The frequency of sexual activity and regularity of the menses are unrelated to diaphragm use. A diaphragm can be safely used by lactating and non-lactating women.

4–90 Answer D

The recommended sequence for adding solid foods to an infant's diet at 6 months of age is as follows: (1) cereal, particularly rice because it is nonallergenic; (2) fruits, such as peaches, pears, and applesauce; (3) yellow vegetables, such as squash and carrots; (4) green vegetables, such as peas or beans; and (5) strained meats, such as nonallergenic lamb or veal.

4–91 Answer D

A tip that will assist parents in making the introduction of solid foods to their infant's diet a smooth process is to feed the solid food to the infant before the milk feeding. The infant will not be completely full and therefore will be more interested in trying the food. The first solid foods should be very smooth and runny. Gradually, the infant will be ready to accept a slightly rougher texture. Only one new food at a time should be introduced, and in small amounts. This allows determination that there is no allergy to the food. Foods should not be added to the milk bottle, nor should a hole be made in the nipple to allow "drinking" of the food.

4–92 Answer C

To help assess for an adequate intake in a breast-fed baby, tell the mother that if there are 6–10 wet diapers a day in the first few months of life, the baby's intake is adequate. During the first few weeks, the infant's weight fluctuates greatly and is not an adequate indicator of fluid intake. If an infant is drinking and sleeping normally, it might be assumed that he or she is getting sufficient intake, although these assumptions may lead to problems. The infant may not be getting enough nourishment and actually may be sleeping because of decreased energy levels. An infant who is not irritable may be flaccid because of numerous other problems, such as neuromuscular conditions. Again, an adequate intake cannot be assumed.

4–93 Answer D

A vasectomy is usually performed in an outpatient setting with local anesthesia. The client needs to rest for 48 hours with minimal activity. He needs to use protection during sex for an additional 4–6 weeks because sperm that was in the reproductive tract before the procedure will continue to mature and can be ejaculated, resulting in pregnancy. A vasectomy does not affect sexual function, only fertility. Persons who have had this procedure ejaculate in a normal manner, but the ejaculate does not contain sperm.

4–94 Answer C

An infant can listen to speech, respond to simple commands, and begin to differentiate among words at age 9–12 months. At age 3–5 months, he or she can search for a sound in the room, stop sucking to listen, and locate the sound below the ear. At age 6–8 months, an infant reacts to changes in music volume and recognizes familiar sounds. At age 12–18 months, he or she begins to show voluntary control over responses to sound and to develop gross discrimination by learning to distinguish among sounds.

4–95 Answer A

Keeping the nipple full of formula prevents the infant from sucking in air and is good technique. Propping the bottle or enlarging the nipple hole can cause aspiration. Directing the nipple at the infant's tongue can cause the child to gag and vomit.

4–96 Answer D

Passive smoking creates a high incidence of upper respiratory infection (URI), pneumonia, bronchitis, and asthma, and is linked to cancer. Carbon monoxide, found in vehicle exhaust, replaces oxygen in red blood cells and causes dizziness, coma, and eventually death. Nitrogen dioxide, found in industrial wastes and vehicle exhausts, causes structural and chemical changes in the lungs and lowers URI resistance. Sulfur dioxide, found in burning coal and oil and industrial processes, causes an increase in colds, coughs, and asthma and contributes to acid rain.

4–97 Answer A

Breast-feeding increases resistance but does not protect the infant from all illnesses. Passive immunity is acquired through antibodies passed across the placenta.

4–98 Answer B

Neonatal abstinence syndrome or drug withdrawal results in hyperstimulation of the infant's nervous system. Nursing care focuses on decreasing environmental and sensory stimulation during the period of withdrawal.

4–99 Answer D

This is characteristic of the searching and yearning phase. The parent yearns for the deceased infant, is preoccupied with thoughts of the lost child, and may have physical manifestations such as aching arms, hearing the infant's cry, or looking for the infant.

4–100 Answer A

When talking to a mother about toilet-training her daughter, tell her the following: girls are usually completely trained an average of $2^1/_2$ months earlier than boys; the majority of children achieve bowel and bladder training at the same time; and about 80% of children are completely trained before age 3.

4–101 Answer B

At age 24 months, a child can understand up to 1200 words. At age 18 months, a child can understand up to 50 words; at age 30 months, up to 2400 words; and at age 36 months, up to 3600 words.

4–102 Answer D

Drowning is a major cause of death in toddlers. For children under age 3 years, bathtubs are the primary site of drowning. Toddlers should not be left unattended in the tub. They should also not be permitted to lean over the tub to play with water toys because they may fall in, hit their head, and not be able to get out. All swimming pools should be fenced in and have high latches on the gates. Children should be taught to swim as early as possible.

4–103 Answer B

Infant car seats should be placed facing backward until the infant weighs 18–20 lb and is able to sit up well. Infant car seats should also be placed in the rear seat of the car, preferably in the middle of the seat.

4–104 Answer C

A child should be moved from a car seat to a regular seat with a seat belt when he or she weighs 40 lb. Until the child weighs 70 lb, ideally, he or she should be in a booster seat. If the shoulder belt crosses the child's face or neck when buckled, it should not be worn, but tucked behind the shoulders with just the lap belt in place. Children should not ride in the cargo area of a pickup truck, van, or station wagon. They should be in the rear seat of the vehicle, preferably in the middle of the seat.

4–105 Answer D

Almost all adolescents think at some time that they are adopted. Asking "Why do you think that?" and exploring their reasons for thinking so will open up avenues for further discussion. Mandy may be adopted, and have never been told, or she may not have been adopted and is just curious as to why she looks slightly different from her parents. Finding out all the facts before responding will let the parent collect himself or herself and be able to respond satisfactorily. Children at this age should not be lied to but should be given all the information they need in language they can understand.

4–106 Answer B

Patchy white areas in the mouth of a breast-fed infant are consistent with a diagnosis of oral candidiasis or thrush. The mother may also have a candidiasis infection of the breast nipple or areola, which if left untreated may progress to mastitis. Neonatal chlamydia infections manifest as conjunctivitis or pneumonitis.

4–107 Answer B

The treatment for oral candidiasis is Nystantin. A vinegar and water solution is used to rinse the breast nipples between feedings. Fluconazole is used for ductal candidiasis infection of the breast. Candidiasis is a fungal infection; therefore antibiotics are not effective as a treatment.

4–108 Answer D

Adequate levels of folic acid supplements before conception and during the early stages of pregnancy have been shown to decrease the incidence of neural tube defects. Iron stores and supplementation do not affect neural tube development. A CVS procedure can identify chromosomal alterations but not structural abnormalities.

4–109 Answer C

Spalding's sign is overriding of the fetal cranial bones, as seen on ultrasound. It is a result of the decreased tissue turgor that occurs after fetal death.

4–110 Answer C

The presence of nitrites, white blood cells, and bacteria are signs of a urinary tract infection.

4–111 Answer D

The low-risk client is seen every 4 weeks until the 28th week of pregnancy. Between 28 and 34 weeks, the woman is seen every 2 weeks. After 34 weeks, she is seen weekly until delivery.

4–112 Answer D

Shortness of breath and chest pains are potentially life-threatening complications associated with the use of oral contraceptives. This situation requires immediate attention. Waiting for the physician's return phone call will delay treatment. Changing contraceptive method and eating patterns does not address the immediate life-threatening problem.

4–113 Answer A

A flat BBT graph indicates lack of ovulation. If ovulation is occurring, the BBT will rise 0.5–1.0°F 24–48 hours after ovulation.

4–114 Answer B

You need to determine immune status. Rubella during pregnancy can cause miscarriage or congenital anomalies. The woman should not be vaccinated during pregnancy because the fetus can be affected by the live virus. Immunity is best determined by assessing the rubella titer.

4–115 Answer D

Pregnancy is a hypercoagulable state, which increases the risk of clot development and formation of an embolism. The sudden onset of chest pain and shortness of breath is consistent with a pulmonary embolism. Because of the life-threatening nature of a pulmonary embolism, it is the first entity that needs to be ruled out. A myocardial infarction and bacterial pneumonia would have a more gradual onset.

Bibliography

Benson, RC, and Pernoll, ML: Handbook of Obstetrics and Gynecology. (10th ed). McGraw-Hill, New York, 2001.

Crombleholme, WR: Obstetrics. In Tierney, LM, et al: Current Medical Diagnosis and Treatment. Appleton & Lange, Norwalk, CT, 1998.

Cronin, C. First-time mothers—Identifying their needs, perceptions and experiences. Journal of Clinical Nursing 12(2):260–267, 2003.

Edelman, CL, and Mandle, CL: Health Promotion Throughout the Lifespan. Mosby, St. Louis, 2002.

Gabbe, SG, Niebyl, JR, and Simpson, JL: Obstetrics: Normal and Problem Pregnancies (4th ed.). Churchill Livingstone, New York, 2002.

Levasseur, SM, and Raines, DA: Perinatal Nursing Secrets. Hanley & Belfus, Philadelphia, 2003.

Littleton, LY, and Engebretson, JC: Maternal, Neonatal and Women's Health Nursing. Delmar, Albany, 2002.

Kupecz, D: Glycated hemoglobin test hits OTC market. Nurse Practitioner 28(5):49, 2003.

Murphy, PA: New methods of hormonal contraception. Nurse Practitioner 28(2):11–21, 2003.

Rakel, RE: Textbook of Family Practice. (6th ed) WB Saunders, Philadelphia, 2002.

Scott, JR: Danforth's Obstetrics and Gynecology (8th ed). Philadelphia, Lippincott Williams & Wilkins, 1999.

Youngkin, EQ, and Davis, MS: Women's Health: A Primary Care Clinical Guide. (3rd ed.). Appleton & Lange, Norwalk, CT, 2003.

HOW WELL DID YOU DO?

85% AND ABOVE CONGRATULATIONS! THIS SCORE SHOW APPLICATION OF TEST-TAKING PRINCIPLES AND ADEQUATE CONTENT KNOWLEDGE.

75–85% KEEP WORKING! REVIEW TEST-TAKING PRINCIPLES AND TRY AGAIN.

65–75% HANG IN THERE! SPEND SOME TIME REVIEWING CONCEPTS AND TEST-TAKING PRINCIPLES AND TRY THE TEST AGAIN.

5

Growth and Development

JANICE S. HAYES
and
JILL E. WINLAND-BROWN

5–1 *At birth, a baby's head circumference should:*

A. range from 32–37 cm.
B. be about 2 cm greater than the chest circumference.
C. correlate to the length and weight percentiles.
D. all of the above.

5–2 *At what age should a normally developing child be able to use a pincer grasp and pick up raisins and finger foods?*

A. 3–4 months
B. 5–6 months
C. 9–10 months
D. 12–14 months

5–3 *A baby can usually say two to three words with meaning at age:*

A. 8 months.
B. 10 months.
C. 12 months.
D. 24 months.

5–4 *Infants can sit alone without support at age:*

A. 1 month.
B. 3 months.
C. 5 months.
D. 7 months.

5–5 *The Moro reflex usually disappears by age:*

A. 2 months.
B. 3 months.
C. 4 months.
D. 6 months.

5–6 *Babies can imitate speech sounds, shake their head for "no," and wave "bye-bye" at age:*

A. 6 months.
B. 8 months.
C. 10 months.
D. 12 months.

5–7 *Sue takes her young son Michael to day care every day, and he has never been afraid of her leaving until now. At what age does this separation anxiety usually occur?*

A. 5–6 months
B. 8–9 months
C. 10–12 months
D. 15–18 months

5–8 *Which tooth is the first to erupt in an infant?*

A. A lower central incisor
B. A lower lateral incisor
C. An upper central incisor
D. An upper lateral incisor

5–9 *Delayed development can be the result of malnutrition from a deficiency of protein, calories, or both. This is referred to as protein energy malnutrition, kwashiorkor, or:*

A. protein-wasting disease.
B. hypermetabolic disease.
C. cachexia.
D. marasmus.

5–10 *Donna is breast-feeding her 3-month-old infant exclusively. She expresses concern to you that the* *baby's growth seems to be slowing down and she wonders if she should supplement the diet with other foods. What would be your response?*

A. "You are probably not producing enough milk. Try adding some rice cereal."
B. "As long as you are well nourished, the baby will get what she needs. Her growth pattern is normal for an exclusively breast-fed baby."
C. "We should add vitamin supplements for the baby."
D. "It is time for you to wean her and start her on solid foods."

5–11 *David, a new father, expresses his concern that his newborn son does not smile at him when he talks to him. What do you tell him?*

A. "True social smiles usually do not emerge until 6–9 weeks of age."
B. "Continue to watch his response so we can be certain that he is seeing."
C. "Babies usually have a preference for the mother's face. That's probably why he doesn't smile at you."
D. "This may just be his personality."

5–12 *The first tooth usually appears at age:*

A. 3–5 months.
B. 5–7 months.
C. 7–9 months.
D. 12 months.

5–13 *Daisy, age 2, has a "blankie" that she carries with her at all times. Her mother is concerned that if she does not get rid of it, Daisy will remain attached to this blanket forever. You tell her:*

A. "Yes, it is important at age 2 to get rid of it. It probably also encourages her to suck her thumb."
B. "Children should be weaned from their favorite toy or blanket gradually so that going without it is not so traumatic."
C. "Not to worry. This normal attachment may last throughout the preschool years."
D. "Try to reason with the child that this habit needs to be broken."

5–14 *Amanda states that her baby will not go to bed without her bottle. You tell her that if she has to have a bottle at night, it should be a bottle containing:*

A. milk.
B. juice.
C. sweetened water.
D. plain water.

5–15 *Sally Ann is concerned that she cannot afford special walking shoes for her baby, who is beginning to pull himself up to his feet. You tell her:*

A. "High-top shoes are necessary to prevent any ankle injuries from happening when your baby falls."
B. "Don't worry; special shoes are not necessary."
C. "Try to keep him in the playpen until you can obtain shoes."
D. "The sock-type booties you have are fine."

5–16 *Susie is 18 months old and does not seem the least bit interested in being toilet trained. You tell her mother that:*

A. although some babies are toilet trained earlier, most are not ready until age 2.
B. Susie should have started showing an interest in toilet training before now.
C. she should punish Susie whenever she soils her diapers—this will give her feedback.
D. she should try to let Susie be around other toddlers who are toilet trained so that she can learn from them.

5–17 *Because children are sexually curious at different ages, sex education should begin during:*

A. the first year of life.
B. the preschool years.
C. the school-age years.
D. adolescence.

5–18 *Why are younger children more predisposed to acute otitis media than older children?*

A. They are more susceptible to the new bacteria that they encounter.
B. Their eustachian tubes are more flaccid and more horizontal than those of older children.
C. They have more viral infections, which precipitate otitis infections.
D. They have more allergies, which are a frequent cause of serous otitis media.

5–19 *While assessing the skin of an infant, you note café-au-lait spots. What disease do you want to rule out?*

A. Tuberous sclerosis
B. Neurofibromatosis
C. Sturge-Weber syndrome
D. Fetal alcohol syndrome

5–20 *While assessing the eyes of baby Thomas, you observe inner canthal folds and Brushfield spots. What do you suspect?*

A. Trisomies
B. Turner's syndrome
C. Down syndrome
D. Neurofibromatosis

5–21 *You suspect autism in the young child of a client of yours, but the client says the child is just shy. For a diagnosis of autism, you know the* Diagnostic and Statistical Manual of Mental

Disorders *requires that three criteria be present. These include all of the following* **except:**

A. impaired reciprocal social interactions.
B. abnormal verbal and nonverbal communication (e.g., eye-to-eye contact).
C. reliance on an imaginary friend for all interactions.
D. a diminished repertoire of activities and interests, with onset during infancy or childhood.

5–22 *The most common inherited cause of mental retardation in boys is:*

A. Down syndrome.
B. fragile X syndrome.
C. meningomyelocele.
D. hydrocephalus.

5–23 *The behavioral feature(s) of fragile X syndrome include:*

A. being easily overwhelmed by stimuli.
B. excessive chewing on clothes.
C. frequent tantrums.
D. all of the above.

5–24 *Fragile X syndrome is usually diagnosed when a child:*

A. is a newborn
B. begins to walk
C. is past the toddler stage
D. begins puberty

5–25 *Justin, age 18 months, crosses his legs when lifted from behind rather than pulling them up. His legs are also hard to separate, making diaper changing difficult, and he persistently uses only one hand. What condition do you suspect?*

A. Cerebral palsy
B. Mild hydrocephalus
C. Mild spinal cord defect (spina bifida occulta)
D. Fetal alcohol syndrome

5–26 *Victoria's mother brings her for her 1-year checkup. As you are weighing her, you remember that at 1 year, her weight should be:*

A. double her birth weight
B. triple her birth weight
C. four times her birth weight
D. at least 25 pounds

5–27 *Mrs. Groome calls you to say that she is distressed that her 3-month-old baby is still not sleeping through the night. Your best response to her would be:*

A. "She should be sleeping at least 10 hours at night without waking."
B. "Perhaps she should have some sedation."
C. "The length of sleep for young babies is variable, but most sleep through the night by the end of the first year."
D. "Babies never sleep through the night until they are at least 6 months old."

5–28 *You are watching a baby play with a toy in the examining room. You move the toy and cover it with a cloth. The baby removes the cloth and reclaims the toy. This is an indication that the baby has achieved which of the following?*

A. Object permanence
B. Conservation
C. Basic trust
D. Initiative

5–29 *When assessing growth and development from a cross-cultural perspective, health-care providers need to be aware that:*

A. there may be differences in normal growth curves.
B. there may be differences in achievement of developmental milestones.
C. there may be differences in the onset of menarche.
D. All of the above.

5–30 *Cross-cultural studies of Piaget's theory of cognitive development provide all the following conclusions* **except:**

A. The rate of cognitive development is universal.
B. The sequence of achieving developmental stages is universal.
C. Some cultural groups achieve the task of conservation earlier than American and European children.
D. Conservation may appear as long as 6 years later in some cultures than in American and European cultures.

5–31 *Decades of research on differences between men and women has produced evidence that there is a difference between the genders in which of the following characteristics?*

A. Aggression
B. Appetite
C. Fertility
D. Intelligence

5–32 *While examining a 12-month-old boy, you notice that his weight is in the 95th percentile and his height is in the 50th percentile. You begin to discuss the implications of maintaining a healthy weight, and the mother tells you that she is very proud of her son's size. Your response to her is guided by your understanding that:*

A. some cultures believe that a fat baby is a healthy baby.
B. she is probably overfeeding the baby to stop his crying.

C. she does not understand the nutritional value of foods.
D. she does not care about the risk to the child's later health.

5–33 *The stage of adolescence is culturally defined. Some of the differences in the cultural approaches to adolescence are evidenced in:*

A. rites of passage or rituals marking the coming of age.
B. whether it represents a transition from child to adult identity.
C. the age at which adolescence is considered to end.
D. all of the above.

5–34 *Cyndy is 5 years old and cannot understand how the half-cup of vegetables on her plate is the same amount as the half-cup of vegetables in the saucepan. She is at which stage of cognitive development according to Piaget?*

A. Preoperational
B. Sensorimotor
C. Formal operations
D. Concrete operations

5–35 *Debbie is developing self-assertion, spontaneity, self-sufficiency, direction, and purpose as her mother encourages, reassures, and cheers her on. Which of Erikson's stages of ego development best characterizes Debbie?*

A. Trust versus mistrust
B. Autonomy versus shame and doubt
C. Initiative versus guilt
D. Industry versus inferiority

5–36 *Susan cannot see anyone else's point of view and feels no need to elaborate on her own point of view because she thinks everyone else sees things as she does. Which characteristic of Piaget's cognitive development is Susan displaying?*

A. Egocentricity
B. Self-importance
C. Centration
D. Delayed imitation

5–37 *Davy, age 4, is here for a well-child visit. To assess his fine motor skills, what activity would you ask him to perform?*

A. Copy a circle.
B. Cut on a line with scissors.
C. String beads.
D. Copy a square.

5–38 *Negativism and ritualism occur at age:*

A. 2 years.
B. 3 years.
C. 4 years.
D. 5 years.

5–39 *The preschool-age child (ages 3–6 years) develops initiative by accomplishing all of the following tasks* ***except:***

A. completing tasks given by the preschool/school teacher.
B. doing age-appropriate chores at home.
C. interacting with others in socially acceptable ways.
D. being allowed to say "no" when asked to put toys away.

5–40 *At what age can children use scissors successfully and fasten and unfasten simple buttons?*

A. 2 years
B. 3 years
C. 4 years
D. 5 years

5–41 *Johnny, age 3, is at the clinic for his well-child visit. You ask him to take off his shirt and he has trouble doing so. His mother yanks off his shirt after smacking his wrist and saying, "You must do as you're told—quickly." What should you do?*

A. Ignore the behavior because both Johnny and his mother are probably nervous about being there.
B. Tell the mother that Johnny's behavior is perfectly normal.
C. Observe Johnny for signs of child abuse.
D. Report the mother to Child Protective Services.

5–42 *Most children display a clear tendency for right- or left-handedness by what age?*

A. 2 years
B. 4 years
C. 6 years
D. 12 years

5–43 *In a game of hide-and-seek, 3-year-old Michael hides his face and believes that no one else can see him. This behavior is an example of:*

A. conservation.
B. object permanence.
C. egocentric thought.
D. concrete operations.

5–44 *Four-year-old Jamie believes that there is more juice in a tall thin glass than in a shorter, wider one. Jamie has not yet achieved which of the principles of Piaget?*

A. Conservation
B. Object permanence
C. Formal operations
D. Abstract reasoning

5–45 *Children begin to develop real friendships at the age of:*

A. 18 months.
B. 3 years.
C. 6 years.
D. 10 years.

5–46 *The 3-year-old child who has learned to put on a coat without help demonstrates the accomplishment of which of Erikson's tasks?*

A. Basic trust
B. Autonomy
C. Initiative
D. Industry

5–47 *Mrs. Anderson expresses to you that she is concerned about her 3-year-old's tendency to have verbal outbursts and hit people when he does not get what he wants. Your response to her would be:*

A. "His behavior is his way of expressing frustration. Although he shouldn't be allowed to hurt anyone, his behavior is not unusual at this age. It will likely diminish as he gains more language skill."
B. "This is bad behavior and should be punished so that it does not get worse."
C. "Just ignore him when he does that."
D. "Give him what he wants. He is too young to ask for it."

5–48 *Josephine, age 6, is just learning to hop on one foot. You know that:*

A. she should have been able to do this at age 3.
B. she should have been able to do this at age 4.
C. she should have been able to do this at age 5.
D. this is a normal age-related activity for her.

5–49 *Tasks of middle childhood (ages 6–10) include all the following* ***except:***

A. mastering skills that will be needed later.
B. developing a sexual identity.
C. winning approval from other adults and peers.
D. adopting moral standards.

5–50 *Preferring peer group activity over adult activities, conforming to group rules, using secret codes, and desiring acceptance are significant at ages:*

A. 2 through 4.
B. 4 through 6.
C. 6 through 10.
D. 12 through 15.

5–51 *A child should be able to focus on concrete operations at age:*

A. 4–6.
B. 5–8.
C. 7–11.
D. 10–13.

5–52 *During the school-age years, children usually grow how many inches annually?*

A. $^1/_2$ inch
B. 3 inches
C. 5 inches
D. 6–8 inches

5–53 *What is the approximate annual weight gain of a school-age child?*

A. 1–3 lb
B. 3–5 lb
C. 5–7 lb
D. 7–9 lb

5–54 *Hattie, age 6, appears to be masturbating when she rubs herself back and forth against the rug. Her mother asks you for advice because she believes masturbation may cause blindness. You tell her:*

A. "Masturbation causes no physical, sexual, or mental problems."
B. "Stop her now because she may progress to other sexual behaviors."
C. "There is no research to show that masturbation causes blindness."
D. "Don't worry; Hattie will be fine."

5–55 *Suzanne's 8-year-old daughter Natasha has attention-deficit-hyperactivity disorder (ADHD). She asks you if Natasha will "outgrow" her ADHD. You respond:*

A. "Yes; when they become young adults, most children outgrow the problem."
B. "No; unfortunately, Natasha will have this for the rest of her life."
C. "No, but there are many treatments available that we need to start now."
D. "About 50% or more of affected children will continue to have some difficulty as adolescents and adults."

5–56 *Ten-year-old Bobby is worried because his 10-year-old cousin Susan has suddenly gotten taller than he is. Your best response to him would be:*

A. "You will probably always be shorter than she is."
B. "At this age, girls have an average height greater than boys. They begin their adolescent growth spurt earlier."
C. "Perhaps you need to take growth hormones."
D. "Don't worry about it. Height is not important. You should just worry about getting good grades."

5–57 *Fine motor coordination improves during the middle childhood years. A person's ability to manipulate objects reaches adult capacity by the age of:*

A. 6 years
B. 9 years
C. 12 years
D. 21 years

5–58 *Jennifer has just developed the ability to play hopscotch with her older sister, Megan. Jennifer is probably what age?*

A. 4 years
B. 7 years
C. 10 years
D. 12 years

5–59 *Nine-year-old Mark is a highly active child with limited self-control. He is easily distracted and has difficulty staying on task and working toward a goal. You believe he should be evaluated by a neurologist because he is showing signs of:*

A. ADHD.
B. dyslexia.
C. autism.
D. impaired hearing.

5–60 *Miranda is playing with clay and realizes that she can roll a lump of clay into a long snakelike shape and then return that snakelike shape to a lump. She is exhibiting cognitive development typical of which of Piaget's stage?*

A. Sensorimotor
B. Pre-operational
C. Concrete operations
D. Formal operations

5–61 *At what age would you expect a child to be able to remember a string of 6 numbers and repeat them backwards?*

A. 3 years
B. 6 years
C. 9 years
D. 12 years

5–62 *Jason is in first grade. His mother expresses concern because he pronounces the "th" sound as "f." For instance, he says "free" for "three." Your response to his mother is:*

A. "This is normal at his age."
B. "He may have a hearing problem and does not know how it should sound."
C. "You should correct him when he does this or he will not learn the proper way to say it."
D. "He should be referred to a speech therapist for evaluation."

5–63 *A child who is meeting the challenges presented to him or her in school and in extracurricular activities is accomplishing which of Erikson's developmental tasks?*

A. Basic trust
B. Autonomy
C. Industry
D. Identity

5–64 *A 6-year-old would most likely view a friend as:*

A. someone to share enjoyable activities with.
B. someone who has the traits that satisfy the child's needs and wants.
C. someone to share loyalty with.
D. someone to be intimate with.

5–65 *Bullying has been recognized as a common problem in schools today. Victims of bullies are more likely than other children to exhibit which of the following characteristics?*

A. They are fairly passive.
B. They tend to lack social skills.
C. They cry easily.
D. All of the above.

5–66 *Developmental tasks of adolescence include which of the following?*

A. Searching for one's identity
B. Appreciating one's achievements
C. Growing independent from parents
D. All of the above

5–67 *According to Piaget, the ability to develop abstract thinking occurs during:*

A. early childhood.
B. middle school age.
C. adolescence.
D. early adulthood.

5–68 *When does the onset of menses usually occur?*

A. Between ages 10 and 11
B. Between ages 12 and 13
C. Between ages 14 and 15
D. Between ages 16 and 17

5–69 *James confides in his friend Mark that he had a "wet dream" and asks him if he has had one. How old do you think James is?*

A. 12 years
B. 13 years
C. 14 years
D. 15 years

5–70 *The first change to occur in the secondary male sexual characteristics is:*

A. testicular enlargement.
B. growth of axillary and pubic hair.
C. growth of facial and chest hair.
D. deepening of the voice.

5–71 *Marta, age 16, is not happy with the size of her breasts. She asks if her breasts will continue to enlarge. How do you respond?*

A. "Full breast growth occurs around age 15."
B. "No, this is probably the size your breasts will remain."

C. "Your breasts will continue to develop until about age 18."
D. "Your breasts will continue to develop until about age 20."

5–72 *When an adolescent girl's breasts and areolae are enlarged and there is no contour separation, which Tanner stage is she in?*

A. I
B. II
C. III
D. IV

5–73 *Jon, age 13, has some enlargement of the scrotum and testes, a reddened scrotal sac, and some hair texture alteration, but his penis is not enlarged. He is in Tanner stage:*

A. I.
B. II.
C. III.
D. IV.

5–74 *Sally, age 12, asks you when you think her periods will start. You tell her:*

A. "They should have started by now."
B. "They will probably start any day now."
C. "They will probably start when you're close to 13."
D. "It might not happen until you're 15."

5–75 *Adolescent thinking is egocentric, and adolescents sometimes perceive that they are the focus of everyone else's attention. This has been called the:*

A. imaginary audience.
B. personal fable.
C. invulnerable self.
D. ego ideal.

5–76 *Jaime, age 20, has had multiple sexual relationships. She has also moved repeatedly from one job to another. Which stage of Erikson's psychosocial development best describes her?*

A. Ego identity versus role confusion
B. Generativity versus stagnation
C. Intimacy versus isolation
D. Integrity versus despair

5–77 *Physical development and maturation are generally at their peak at which stage?*

A. Adolescence
B. Early adulthood
C. Middle adulthood
D. Later adulthood

5–78 *Developmental tasks of early adulthood (ages 20–45) include all the following* ***except:***

A. psychological separation from parents.
B. developing a capacity for intimacy with a partner.
C. achieving desired performance in a career.
D. choosing a career.

5–79 *Erikson's stage of intimacy versus isolation occurs between ages:*

A. 12 and 16.
B. 16 and 20.
C. 20 and 30.
D. 50 and 60.

5–80 *The tasks of middle adulthood include all of the following* ***except:***

A. affiliating with one's age group.
B. accepting and adjusting to the physical changes of middle age.
C. reviewing and redirecting career goals.
D. achieving desired performance in a career.

5–81 *What is the term used when the last child leaves home, either for school or to move out on his or her own?*

A. Longed-for freedom
B. Silent guilt
C. Empty nest
D. Abandonment

5–82 *Tasks of late adulthood include all of the following* ***except:***

A. achieving desired performance in a career.
B. adjusting to changes in physical strength and health.
C. forming a new family role as an in-law and/or grandparent.
D. adjusting to retirement and reduced income.

5–83 *Erikson's final ego stage in older adults occurs when successful resolution results in these adults feeling comfortable with their life choices and the knowledge that they would have done everything the same way again. This ego stage is called:*

A. generativity versus stagnation.
B. workaholism versus retirement.
C. success versus failure.
D. integrity versus despair.

5–84 *Middle-aged persons who still have responsibilities toward their children and are now caring for their own aging parents are sometimes said to:*

A. have institutional guilt syndrome.
B. have the "full nest" syndrome.
C. be the "sandwich" generation.
D. be "Generation X."

5–85 *Beginning at about age 55, most people can expect which of the following changes?*

A. A 1- to 2-inch decline in height

B. Stable body weight
C. Sharper vision and hearing
D. Increased strength

5–86 *The benefits of exercise during middle adulthood include all **except:***

A. slower decline in muscle mass.
B. slower decline in CNS processing.
C. slower decline in bone minerals.
D. delay in development of vision problems.

5–87 *Jane, age 45, is having her annual physical. She wants to know when she can expect to go through menopause. Your response to her would be:*

A. "You should not have any more periods after the age of 50."
B. "Most women begin having irregular periods in their late 40s, but age can range from 40–60."
C. "I'm surprised you haven't gone through it yet."
D. "You should think about hormone replacement therapy now."

5–88 *The major determinant of sexual activity in older adults is:*

A. physical and mental health.
B. social sanctions.
C. religious beliefs.
D. age.

5–89 *To determine your client's emotional and cognitive level of functioning when performing a mental status examination, you assess several individual behaviors. What is the term used when one ponders a deeper meaning beyond the concrete and literal?*

A. Thought process
B. Abstract reasoning
C. Consciousness
D. Perception

5–90 *When performing a mental status examination, you should keep in mind the ABCTs. The "C" stands for:*

A. cognition.
B. consciousness.
C. capabilities.
D. conscience.

5–91 *Jake, 8 years old, is brought in by his mother for evaluation of school problems. When he was 4 years old, his preschool teacher had expressed concern that his activity level was so high that it interfered with play with other children. Now, in third grade, he is underachieving in both math and reading. His teacher says that he constantly fidgets and bothers the other children. The school counselor has recommended that he be evaluated for ADHD. Your response to his mother is:*

A. "He is just being a normal 8-year-old."
B. "I think his teacher does not like dealing with active children."
C. "ADHD is often diagnosed in children with behavioral problems who underachieve in school. I agree that he should be evaluated."
D. "ADHD rarely shows up at this age."

5–92 *Jake's mother (in the above question) asks if he will have the problem for his entire life. Your response is:*

A. "Children always outgrow a high activity level."
B. "No one can say for sure right now. Some children diagnosed with ADHD continue to have the problem into adolescence and even adulthood, but many do not."
C. "Once you have ADHD, it never goes away."
D. "The medications will cure him over time."

5–93 *The diagnostic criteria for ADHD include:*

A. the criteria established by DSM-IV.
B. elevated blood levels of lead.
C. abnormal EEG.
D. failure on developmental screening tests administered by a licensed clinical psychologist.

5–94 *Common medications for treating ADHD include:*

A. Aminophylline and antihistamines.
B. Ritalin and Dexedrine.
C. Accutane and amphetamines.
D. Valium and codeine.

5–95 Some psychologists have suggested that at the end of adolescence, a kind of thinking emerges that goes beyond logic to encompass interpretive and subjective thinking. This is called:

A. postformal thought.
B. mature thinking.
C. adult cognition.
D. ephemeral perception.

5–96 *The body and the senses typically reach their peak during which stage of life?*

A. Adolescence
B. Early adulthood
C. Middle adulthood
D. Late adulthood

5–97 *Byron is 30 months old. His mother asks you what toys she should have for him to play with at home. Your suggestions to her could include:*

A. blocks and simple shape puzzles with few pieces.
B. a tricycle and a Wiffle ball and bat.
C. pop beads and Matchbox cars.
D. a mobile and a cloth book

5–98 *Jonathan, 2 ½ years of age, has come to see you because his mother says he has been very fussy* *and irritable. When you examine his ears, you note that the tympanic membrane in opaque. You look at his record and notice he has had 3 episodes of acute otitis media within the past 6 months. You are concerned about this because:*

A. children under 3 years of age with recurrent otitis media with effusion are at increased risk for impaired speech and language development.
B. children with opaque tympanic membranes are probably deaf.
C. the infection is highly likely to spread to the meninges.
D. he will not be able to be immunized for at least 6 months.

5–99 *Germaine, aged 12 years, comes to see you for her checkup. After weighing her, you note that her BMI is at the 96th percentile on the National Center for Health Statistics graph. Your response to this will be guided by the knowledge that:*

A. Her size is acceptable for her age and you will continue to follow up weight during subsequent checkups.
B. She has been in a phase of rapid growth and it will slack off within a year.
C. She is healthy but may be at risk for an eating disorder
D. She is obese and at risk for hypertension and diabetes.

5–100 *Shannon, age 4 months, is waiting in the exam room with her mother. When you walk into the room, you expect Shannon to:*

A. begin crying.
B. turn her head toward the sound of the door or your voice.
C. not notice you.
D. smile at you.

Answers

5–1 Answer D

At birth a baby's head is about 1/3 the size of an adult's head. For accurate measurement, the tape is placed over the most prominent part of the occiput and brought to just above the eyebrows. The circumference of a newborn's head ranges from 32–37 cm and is about 2 cm greater than the circumference of the chest. It will maintain that proportion for the next few months. If the child's weight is at the 40th percentile on the growth charts, the head circumference should be at the same or nearly the same percentile.

5–2 Answer C

At age 9–10 months, a baby's index finger is in apposition to the thumb, enabling the baby to use a pincer grasp and pick up finger foods such as raisins effectively. At age 3–4 months, a baby can use his or her thumbs in grasping objects such as a rattle; at 11 months, a baby can hold a crayon adaptively; and at 14 months he or she can build a tower of two blocks.

5–3 Answer C

At age 12 months, a baby can usually say 2 or 3 words with meaning. At age 9–10 months, a baby can imitate the sounds of others, but probably doesn't understand them. At age 24 months, a child can say 2-word phrases.

5–4 Answer D

Most infants can sit with support at 4 months and by 6 or 7 months are able to sit without support.

5–5 Answer D

The Moro reflex should be gone at age 6 months, when infants can roll from side to side and back to front. The prolonged presence of this reflex is a cause for concern.

5–6 Answer C

At age 10 months, infants can imitate speech sounds, shake their heads for "no," wave "bye-bye," respond to their names, and vocalize in varied jargon patterns.

5–7 Answer B

Separation anxiety starts a little later than stranger anxiety, which is common after 6 months. Separation anxiety is the distress displayed when the usual caregiver leaves. It begins around 8 or 9 months and peaks at about 14 months.

5–8 Answer A

The lower central incisors are the first teeth to erupt in an infant, usually at around age 5–11 months. The lower lateral incisors erupt at age 6–15 months, the upper central incisors at age 6 to 12 months, and the upper lateral incisors at age 7–18 months.

5–9 Answer D

Delayed development can be the result of malnutrition from a deficiency of protein, calories, or both. This is referred to as protein energy malnutrition, kwashiorkor, or marasmus. Marasmus is related to kwashiorkor and is a form of protein calorie malnutrition, occurring chiefly in the first year of life. It may be partly by a hypermetabolic disease. Muscle wasting is one of the symptoms.

5–10 Answer B

Human milk is the ideal food for human infants because it has nutritional characteristics that are matched to the needs of human infants. A well-nourished mother can meet all her infant's nutritional requirements with breast milk alone for the first 4–6 months of life as long as the infant did not begin life with a deficit and has no other problems. The addition of complementary foods only displaces the amount of breast milk taken and thus does not supplement the diet. The typical pattern of weight gain in breast-fed babies is rapid gain for the first couple of months, followed by a downward trend that leads some to question whether the intake is adequate. New growth charts for breast-fed babies during the first year of life are currently being developed by WHO.

5–11 Answer A

By age 6–9 weeks, babies smile at the sight of things that please them. The earliest smiles are fairly indiscriminate, becoming more selective over time. A true social smile is given in response to particular individuals.

5–12 Answer B

The first tooth usually appears between ages 5 and 7 months. Primary dentition is usually complete by age 2. Dentists are not overly concerned as long as children get their first tooth by their first birthday.

5–13 Answer C

Infants and toddlers often become attached to a particular toy or blanket, and seem especially attached to it at night or when they are upset. This attachment may last through the preschool years and should not be interfered with because it does provide comfort during stressful situations.

5–14 Answer D

To prevent milk-bottle syndrome and dental caries, children should not go to bed with a bottle. If one is absolutely necessary on occasion, it should be a plain water bottle.

5–15 Answer B

When an infant begins to walk, special walking shoes are not necessary. Bare feet, sneakers, or other shoes are fine. A proper fit is much more important than hard soles or high tops. Sock-type booties should not be used because they are slippery.

5–16 Answer A

Although other babies are toilet trained earlier than age 2, most are not ready until then because bladder and bowel control requires a great deal of coordination and maturity of the nervous system. Starting toilet training too early is frustrating for both parents and children.

5–17 Answer A

Because children are sexually curious at different ages, sex education should begin during the first year of life and continue thereafter. Children need truthful and factual information and their questions should be answered with age-appropriate, honest answers. Studies have shown that children who have received sex education at home before schooling and during the school years are less likely to get pregnant or have casual sexual experiences in adolescence.

5–18 Answer B

Younger children are more predisposed to acute otitis media than older children, primarily because their eustachian tubes are more flaccid and more horizontal than that of older children. Although younger children are more susceptible to the new bacteria they are encountering, have more viral infections, and have more allergies, the central role is played by the horizontal eustachian tube, which is anatomically predisposed to acute otitis media.

5–19 Answer B

Café-au-lait spots and neurofibromas would indicate neurofibromatosis. Hypopigmented macules and adenoma sebaceum would indicate tuberous sclerosis, whereas facial port-wine hemangiomas would indicate Sturge-Weber syndrome, and nail hypoplasia or dysplasia would indicate fetal alcohol syndrome and trisomies.

5–20 Answer C

If you notice inner canthal folds and Brushfield spots, you should suspect Down syndrome. Slanted palpebral fissures are seen with other trisomies, blue sclera and osteogenesis imperfecta with Turner's syndrome, and Lisch nodules with neurofibromatosis.

5–21 Answer C

The *Diagnostic and Statistical Manual of Mental Disorders* requires three criteria on which to base a diagnosis of autism. These are impaired reciprocal social interactions, abnormal verbal and nonverbal communication, and a diminished repertoire of activities and interests, with the onset during infancy or childhood. Reliance on an imaginary friend for all interactions is not a diagnostic criterion of autism.

5–22 Answer B

The most common inherited cause of mental retardation in boys is fragile X syndrome. It was discovered in 1969 and is responsible for about 30% of all cases of X-linked retardation. Involvement may range from mild learning and behavior difficulties to severe mental retardation. Other causes of mental deficiency include metabolic causes, such as hypothyroidism (cretinism), hyperbilirubinemia, and hypoglycemia; inherited or genetic causes, such as chromosomal abnormalities, Down syndrome, Turner's syndrome, Klinefelter's syndrome, autosomal-dominant inheritance, and autosomal-recessive inheritance; and acquired causes, such as maternal infection (rubella, toxoplasmosis, syphilis, and cytomegalovirus), maternal illness or drugs, birth injury, hypoxia, and trauma.

5–23 Answer D

The behavioral features of fragile X syndrome include being easily overwhelmed by stimuli, excessive chewing on clothes, and frequent tantrums. Other features include hand biting, hand flapping, hyperactivity, mood instability, perseveration in speech, poor eye contact, short attention span, shyness, social anxiety, and tactile defensiveness.

5–24 Answer C

It is rare for a child to be diagnosed with fragile X syndrome during the first year of life. Although it is possible to detect it by amniocentesis, it is not routinely done without a family history. The child is usually past the toddler stage when a diagnosis is made.

5–25 Answer A

Cerebral palsy needs to be detected early for effective treatment. You should suspect cerebral palsy whenever an infant crosses his or her legs when lifted from behind rather than pulling them up or bicycling like a normal infant; has legs that are hard to separate, making diaper changing difficult; persistently uses only one hand or, as he or she gets older, uses the hands well but not the legs; has difficulty sucking or keeping a nipple or food in his or her mouth; seldom moves voluntarily; or has arm or leg tremors with voluntary movement. Mild hydrocephalus should be noticed at an infant's well-baby checkup when measuring the head circumference. Spina bifida occulta is characterized by a depression or raised area and a tuft of hair over the defect in the spinal cord. A port-wine nevus may also be present. In many cases, neurologic status is normal because spina bifida occulta does not always cause neurologic dysfunction. Fetal alcohol syndrome would probably have been diagnosed earlier.

5–26 Answer B

The average infant doubles his or her birth weight by 5 months and triples it by 1 year. Growth slows over the second year but is still continuous; the child should weigh about 4 times their birth weight at age 2 years.

5–27 Answer C

New parents are often very tired and distressed when their infant does not sleep for an extended period of time. There are wide variations in the amount of sleep during infancy, but most infants sleep through the night by the age of 1 year.

5–28 Answer A

In Piaget's theory of cognitive development, the child in the sensorimotor period achieves object permanence. Before this achievement, the child will not search for a toy that is hidden right before his eyes. Later he or she will search for it even though it is out of sight, indicating that he or she knows it exists even when it is not in sight.

5–29 Answer D

Cross-cultural studies of child development reflect differences in the achievement of growth and development milestones. Factors that may influence these differences include nutrition, preferred activities, and lifestyle differences.

5–30 Answer A

Cross-cultural studies strongly support that the sequence of stages in Piaget's theory is universal but that there can be differences in the rate at which these stages are mastered.

5–31 Answer A

Researchers have reported a convincing contrast between males and females on aggressiveness/dominance and nurturance/submissiveness.

5–32 Answer A

In some poorer countries, stoutness is associated with good health and prosperity. Malnutrition is endemic in some areas, so fat stores are associated with health.

5–33 Answer D

In many cultures the period of adolescence is very short. On achieving sexual maturity, an individual is considered an adult and soon takes a mate and reproduces. In other cultures, adolescence is extended while the person makes decisions about and prepares for his or her life's work.

5–34 Answer A

Cyndy is at the *preoperational* stage (ages 2 through 7) of cognitive development as formulated by Piaget. She cannot *conserve* (understand that things remain the same even if their material is rearranged). She is also *egocentric* (unable to take another person's viewpoint) and uses *transductive* reasoning (reasoning from one specific fact to another specific fact). The *sensorimotor* stage is from birth to age 24 months. At this stage, there is *object permanence* (things continue to exist even when out of sight) and the beginning of verbal language. The stage of *concrete operations* occurs from ages 7–11. It is typified by the belief in the here and now, the ability to recognize the importance of rules, and the idea of *conservation* (not being fooled by the rearrangement of matter). Formal operations (from ages 12–18) is the stage of having the capacity for abstract thought, the ability to use hypothetical and deductive reasoning, and the ability to generate many possible solutions to a given problem.

5–35 Answer C

Debbie, who is learning self-assertion, spontaneity, self-sufficiency, direction, and purpose, is in the stage of *initiative versus guilt* in Erikson's stages of ego development. Her mother is appropriately stimulating her and she is developing a sense of initiative. This stage usually occurs around age 3–5 years. Debbie has already progressed through the *trust versus mistrust* stage (birth through age 15 months) and the *autonomy versus shame and doubt* stage (age 1–3 years). After her current stage, Debbie will progress to *industry versus inferiority* (around age 6 through early adolescence).

5–36 Answer A

When a child cannot see another's point of view and feels no need to elaborate on her own point of view because she thinks that everyone else sees things as she does, the child is displaying the *egocentric* characteristic in Piaget's cognitive development theory. This characteristic usually occurs in preschool-age children, who think that everyone sees things as they do. Self-importance is not a term used by Piaget. *Centration* is when a preschool-age child focuses on only one aspect of a situation at a time and ignores all others. *Delayed imitation* is when a preschool-age child can conjure up thoughts of something that occurred previously.

5–37 Answer B

To assess fine motor skills in a child, it is important to know that at age 3, a child can copy a circle; at age 4, a child can cut on a line with scissors; and at age 5, a child can string beads and copy a square, letters, and numbers.

5–38 Answer A

Negativism, along with ritualism, usually occurs at age 2 when the toddler wants things done in the same way each time. They are normal stages of development in a child's journey toward autonomy.

5–39 Answer D

The preschool-age child (ages 3–6) develops initiative by learning to accomplish things successfully and feel satisfaction in activities. As the child oversteps limits, there is a feeling of guilt for not behaving appropriately. This is the beginning of conscience.

5–40 Answer C

At age 4, children can draw stick figures with 3 parts, successfully use scissors, and lace shoes.

5–41 Answer C

Although both Johnny and his mother are probably nervous about being in the clinic, this behavior is not normal. If the mother spanks a child in front of an authority figure for an inconsequential act, it is possible that her behavior is indicative of child abuse. Although reporting the mother to a child protective services agency is a little drastic after only one encounter, you should document the incident and be alert to any other subtle or overt cues of child abuse.

5–42 Answer C

During infancy, some children show a preference for the use of one hand over the other. However by the end of the preschool period, handedness is usually clear.

5–43 Answer C

Preschoolers are unable to take someone else's perspective, and believe that others must see things as they see them.

5–44 Answer A

Conservation is the realization that quantity is unrelated to arrangement. Even when they view equal amounts poured into glasses of different shapes, young children cannot understand that the amount remains the same even when the level in the glasses is not the same.

5–45 Answer B

At about age 3 years, children begin to enjoy interaction with other children. Before this, they may have played alongside other children but have not engaged in real social interaction.

5–46 Answer B

Preschoolers between the ages of 18 months and 3 years are learning independence and mastery over their physical environment.

5–47 Answer A

Aggression begins to emerge in the preschool years. As the child becomes better able to express himself or herself with language, aggressive behaviors typically decline in frequency and duration.

5–48 Answer B

Although a child should be able to learn to hop on one foot by age 4, the ability to perform one particular activity is not sufficient to determine if the child is developing normal motor skills or not. A more complete assessment is required. At age 5, a child should be able to skip on alternate feet and jump rope.

5–49 Answer B

Tasks of middle childhood (ages 6 through 10) include mastering skills that will be needed later, winning approval from other adults and peers, and adopting moral standards. Development of a sexual identity occurs during adolescence. Other tasks of middle childhood include building self-esteem and a positive self-concept, and taking a place in a peer group.

5–50 Answer C

Preferring peer group activity over adult activities, conforming to group rules, using secret codes, and desiring acceptance are significant for the school-age child (ages 6 through 10).

5–51 Answer C

A child can focus on concrete operations during middle childhood (ages 7–11). During the *concrete operations* stage, as defined by Piaget, a child begins to apply logical processes to concrete problems.

5–52 Answer B

During the school-age years, when physical growth is relatively slow and smooth, children usually grow about 3 inches annually in height.

5–53 Answer C

The approximate annual weight gain in the school-age child is 5–7 lb. During the school-age years, children become slimmer, with longer legs and a lower center of gravity. On the average, boys are taller and heavier than girls until the adolescent growth spurt, which occurs earlier in girls.

5–54 Answer A

Masturbation is a common activity and should be ignored. It does not cause any physical, sexual, or mental problems. Drawing attention to the matter may make a child act out in other ways. Comforting the mother by telling her "not to worry, Hattie will be fine" is not addressing the mother's concern.

5–55 Answer D

Long-term studies have shown that adolescents with attention deficit hyperactivity disorder (ADHD) experience school failure, aggression, antisocial behavior, poor social skills, emotional immaturity, low self-esteem, and interpersonal conflicts. The same studies revealed that more than 50% of adults who had ADHD as children continue to exhibit anxiety, low self-esteem, personality disorders, alcohol and substance abuse, and interpersonal difficulties.

5–56 Answer B

This is the only time in the life span when girls are, on average, taller than boys. Girls have a slightly faster start on the adolescent growth spurt at about the age of 10 years.

5–57 Answer C

By the age of 8, a child can use each hand independently. The ability to manipulate objects continues to be refined and reaches adult capability by 11 or 12 years of age.

5–58 Answer B

Gross motor skills continue to develop during the school years. By age 7 years, a child can hop and jump accurately into small squares.

5–59 Answer A

ADHD is marked by inattention, impulsiveness, a low tolerance for frustration, and a great deal of inappropriate behavior. This can be exhausting for parents and teachers. In some cases, it can be managed by medications, but their use is controversial. A specialist should evaluate a child suspected of having ADHD.

5–60 Answer C

When the child uses concrete operations, the concept of *reversibility* can be applied. This is the idea that the process that changed an object can be applied to reverse the process.

5–61 Answer D

Short-term memory improves significantly during middle childhood. By the beginning of the preschool period, children can remember and reverse a sequence of two numbers. By the beginning of adolescence, they can perform the task with as many as six numbers.

5–62 Answer A

By the time they reach first grade, most children pronounce words fairly accurately. However, phonemes such as *th*, *zw*, *j*, and *v* remain difficult for some time.

5–63 Answer C

Industry versus inferiority is characterized by a focus on attaining competencies in the challenges presented to the child by parents, teachers, and others. It brings feelings of mastery and accomplishment.

5–64 Answer A

The development of friendship abilities undergoes three stages during middle childhood. In the beginning, children see friends as people who like them and whom they can have fun with. The next stage begins to take other people's traits and qualities into consideration, and the third stage begins to view friendship as entailing more closeness and mutual disclosure.

5–65 Answer D

Some 90% of middle-school children report being bullied at some time. Children who have a difficult time coping with bullying tend to be loners who are fairly passive. They cry easily and lack social skills to deal more effectively with the situation.

5–66 Answer D

The developmental tasks of adolescence include searching for one's identity, appreciating one's achievements, and growing independent from one's parents. Other developmental tasks of adolescence include forming close relationships with peers, developing analytic thinking, evolving one's own value system, developing a sexual identity, and choosing a career.

5–67 Answer C

According to Piaget, the ability to develop abstract thinking occurs during adolescence, as do the abilities to focus on formal operations, analyze situations, and use scientific reasoning. In early childhood, children are in the *preoperational* period of cognitive development, when thinking is egocentric. The middle-school-age child attains the *concrete operational* period when he or she can understand logical operations and principles and apply them to help interpret specific experiences or perceptions. The young adult should be capable of abstract thinking because the formal operational period begins with adolescence.

5–68 Answer B

The onset of menses (menarche) usually occurs at age 12 or 13; however, it may begin before or after that age.

5–69 Answer C

Nocturnal emissions ("wet dreams") usually begin during sleep at about age 14. The first ejaculation of seminal fluid usually occurs about 1 year after the penis begins its adolescent growth.

5–70 Answer A

Secondary sex characteristics occur in boys before puberty and may take 2–5 years to complete. Testicular enlargement is the first change, followed by penis and scrotal enlargement, deepening of the voice, growth of axillary and pubic hair, and finally growth of facial and chest hair.

5–71 Answer B

The approximate average age for full breast growth in girls is age 16.

5–72 Answer C

The Sexual Maturity Rating scale developed by Tanner consists of five stages based on pubic hair and breast development for girls and pubic hair and genitalia development for boys. For girls, the middle stage, stage III, is when the breast and areola are enlarged with no contour separation. Pubic hair is also considerably darker, coarser, and more curled. Tanner stage I is preadolescent, with an elevation of papilla only and no pubic hair. In stage II, there is a breast bud; elevation of the breast and papilla as a small mound with enlargement of the areolar diameter; and a sparse growth of long, slightly pigmented downy hair, straight or only slightly curled, along the labia. In stage IV, there is projection of the areola and papilla to form a secondary mound above the level of the breast, and the pubic hair resembles an adult's in type, but with the distribution considerably smaller. In stage V, the breasts are at the mature stage and the pubic hair is adult in quantity, with distribution of the horizontal pattern.

5–73 Answer B

Enlargement of the scrotum and testes, a reddened scrotal sac, some hair texture alteration, and a penis that is not enlarged are all characteristics of Tanner stage II. For boys, the Sexual Maturity Rating scale developed by Tanner consists of five stages based on pubic hair and genitalia. Stage I is when the penis, testes, and scrotum are preadolescent in development. Stage III is when there is further growth of the testes and scrotum and the penis enlarges and becomes longer. In stage IV there is an increase in the size of the penis with a growth in breadth and development of the glans, further enlargement of the testes and scrotum, and increased darkening of the scrotal skin. The pubic hair resembles that of an adult in type, but with the distribution considerably smaller than in the adult. In stage V, the genitalia are adult in size and shape and the pubic hair is adult in quantity.

5–74 Answer C

Most girls experience menarche at around the same age as their mothers did; however, the average age for American adolescents today is 13.3 years, with a standard deviation of 1.3 years.

5–75 Answer A

Adolescent egocentrism is a state of self-absorption in which the world is viewed from one's own point of view. This leads adolescents to believe that everyone else is watching them and is concerned about them. This is called *imaginary audience*.

5–76 Answer C

Intimacy versus isolation is the crisis of young adulthood (ages 18 through 25) that Erikson identified as occurring when there is an unsuccessful resolution of the bipolar crisis in intimacy versus isolation. It occurs frequently in this age group and is successfully resolved when the young adult develops the capacity to make commitments to work and relationships. Ego identity versus role confusion usually occurs during adolescence, with uncertainty implying unsuccessful resolution of that stage. Generativity versus stagnation is the stage of middle adulthood, and integrity versus despair is the stage of late adulthood.

5–77 Answer B

In most respects, physical development and maturation are complete at early adulthood. Most people are at their peak physical capabilities. They tend to be healthy and vigorous.

5–78 Answer C

Developmental tasks of early adulthood (ages 20 through 45) include growing independent from the parent's home and care, learning to cooperate in a marriage relationship, and forming a meaningful philosophy of life. Achieving desired performance in a career comes later (in middle adulthood). Other developmental tasks of early adulthood include establishing a career or vocation, forming an intimate bond with another and choosing a mate, setting up and managing one's own household, making friends and establishing a social group, assuming civic responsibility and becoming a citizen in the community, and beginning a parenting role.

5–79 Answer C

Erikson's stage of intimacy versus isolation occurs during early adulthood, and for some individuals lasts into the 30s. The adult is seeking a mature relationship involving mutual trust, cooperation, sharing, and complete acceptance. Without this relationship, the person is withdrawn and lonely.

5–80 Answer A

The tasks of middle adulthood include accepting and adjusting to the physical changes of middle age, reviewing and redirecting career goals, and achieving desired performance in one's career. Affiliating with one's age group occurs later in late adulthood when individuals retire and have more time to socialize. Other tasks of middle adulthood include developing hobby and leisure activities, adjusting to aging parents, helping adolescent children in their search for identity, accepting and relating to the spouse as a person, and coping with an empty nest at home.

5–81 Answer C

Empty nest is the term used when the last child leaves home, either for school or to move out on his or her own. It is a time when parents are alone as a couple once again.

5–82 Answer A

Tasks of late adulthood include adjusting to changes in physical strength and health, forming a new family role as an in-law and/or grandparent, and adjusting to retirement and reduced income. Achieving desired performance in a career is a task of middle adulthood. Other tasks of late adulthood include affiliating with one's age group; developing retirement activities that enhance self-worth and usefulness; arranging satisfactory physical living quarters; adjusting to the death of a spouse, family members, and friends; conducting a life review; and preparing for the inevitability of one's own death.

5–83 Answer D

Erikson's last ego stage in older adults is *integrity versus despair*. It is the stage when successful resolution results in adults feeling comfortable with their life choices and the knowledge that they would have done everything the same way again. Older adults who have successfully completed this phase in their life are in Erikson's *integrity phase*. When reviewing their life events, experiences, and relationships, they realize that these have been mostly good, and they have cherished memories. Failure to reach this point results in the *despair phase*, when older adults feel resentment, futility, hopelessness, and a fear of death.

5–84 Answer C

Middle-aged persons who still have responsibility toward their children and are now caring for their aging parents are considered (as a group) to be the "sandwich" generation because they are caught between the demands of their children and their parents. Although many individuals are hoping for the "empty nest" when children leave home, many, in reality, have a full house because their parents move in with them.

5–85 Answer A

Maximum height is reached in the 20s and remains stable until about age 55. Bones becomes less dense at that point and a slow loss of height begins, averaging 1 inch for men and 2 inches for women. "Middle-aged spread" continues, visual and hearing acuity drop, and strength diminishes.

5–86 Answer D

Visual acuity declines are related to changes in the shape and elasticity of the lens, which are not related to exercise. However, exercise can assist in maintenance of muscle strength and procession of CNS impulses, lower LDL, decrease cardiovascular risk factors, and decrease the risk of osteoporosis and fractures.

5–87 Answer B

The age of menopause can vary widely. There is usually a 2-year period of irregular periods beginning in the late 40s, but it occurs earlier for some and may be as late as age 60 for others. After a year goes by without a menstrual period, menopause is considered complete.

5–88 Answer A

Evidence suggests that people are sexually active well into their 80s and 90s. The two major factors are good physical and mental health and previous regular sexual activity. The phrase "use it or lose it" seems to be relevant.

5–89 Answer B

Abstract reasoning is the term used to describe the activity of pondering a deeper meaning beyond the concrete and literal. *Thought process* is the way a person thinks—the logical train of thought. *Consciousness* is being aware of one's own existence, feelings, and thoughts and environment. This is the most elementary of mental status functions. *Perception* is an awareness of objects through any of the five senses.

5–90 Answer A

The ABCTs are the four main headings of a mental status assessment. The "A" stands for appearance, the "B" for behavior, the "C" for cognition, and the "T" for thought processes.

5–91 Answer C

ADHD is among the most common neurodevelopmental disorders in children. Its hallmarks are hyperactivity, impulsiveness, and inattention beyond the norm for the child's age. The diagnosis is reliable if made by a standardized approach.

5–92 Answer B

Symptoms of ADHD may abate over time, but studies report anywhere from 22%–85% of adolescents and 4%–50% of adults who had ADHD as children continue to meet the criteria for diagnosis.

5–93 Answer A

The Diagnostic and Statistical Manual of Mental Disorders, 4th edition publishes the criteria for diagnosis of ADHD. There are five criteria that must be met.

5–94 Answer B

Dexedrine and Ritalin are preferred drugs for pediatric ADHD. Ritalin is a CNS stimulant that blocks the reuptake of norepinephrine and dopamine into the presynaptic neurons and increases the release of these monoamines into the extraneuronal space. Dexedrine probably causes the nerve endings to produce more norepinephrine at the synapse.

5–95 Answer A

Post-formal thought goes beyond logic and encompasses interpretive and subjective thinking. Developmental psychologist Giesela Labouvie-Vief has suggested that thinking changes qualitatively during the early adult years. She asserts that the complexity of society and the increasing challenges of getting through that complexity require more than logical thought. Thinking becomes more flexible and interpretive.

5–96 Answer B

In most respects, physical development and maturation are complete in early adulthood. Most people are at their peak in physical capabilities. The senses are as sharp as they ever will be. Even though there are changes in the elasticity of the eye, their effects at this point are usually minor.

5–97 Answer A

By 2–2 ½ years, the child has enough fine motor development to be able to assemble simple shape puzzles and build a tower with blocks or line up blocks to form a train.

5–98 Answer A

Acute otitis media is characterized by middle ear effusion in the presence of symptoms such as fever, ear pain, and irritability. When there is effusion, the tympanic membrane is opaque and has limited mobility. The time a child spends having middle ear effusion correlates with various cognitive delays and hearing deficits, which lead to speech and language delays.

5–99 Answer D

Obesity is the condition of having excess body fat and is defined as having a 95th percentile BMI. Childhood obesity is an increasingly prevalent problem and places children at risk for many health problems, including hypertension and type II diabetes. It is a problem that needs to be addressed immediately because research strongly suggests that the earlier a child is obese, the more obese the child will become; furthermore, a child who is obese is likely to become an obese adult.

5–100 Answer B

By 4 months, the infant shows attention to sights and sounds by turning the head toward the source of the sound.

References

De Onis, M, and Onyango, AW: The Centers for Disease Control and Prevention 2000 growth charts and the growth of breastfed babies. Acta Pediatric 92:413–419, 2003.

Dewey, KG: Nutrition, growth, and complementary feeding of the breastfed infant. Pediatric Clinics of North America 48(1):87–104, 2001.

Feldman, RS: Development Across the Life Span, 2nd edition. Prentice Hall, Upper Saddle River, NJ, 2000.

Gardiner, HW, Mutter, JD, and Kosmitzki, C: Lives Across Cultures: Cross-cultural Human Development. Allyn and Bacon, Boston, 1998.

Greenspan, SI: Clinical assessment of emotional milestones in infancy and early childhood. Pediatric Clinics of North America 38: 1371–1385, 1991.

Guevara, JP, and Stein, MT: Evidence-based management of attention deficit hyperactivity disorder. British Medical Journal 24: 1232–1235, 2001.

Lloyd, BT: A conceptual framework for examining adolescent identity, media influence, and social development. Review of General Psychology 6(1):73–91, 2002.

Olds, SB, London, ML, and Ladewig, PAW: Maternal-Newborn Nursing. A Family and Community-Based Approach. Prentice Hall, Upper Saddle River, NJ, 2000.

Potts, NL, and Mandleco, BL: Pediatric Nursing: Caring for Children and Their Families. Delmar Thomson Learning, Clifton Park, NY, 2002.

Sangare, J: ADHD: Making the appropriate pediatric assessment. Lippincott's Primary Care Practice 4(2):193–206, 2000.

Styne, DM: Childhood and adolescent obesity: Prevalence and significance. Pediatric Clinics of North America 48:823–854, 2001.

Valente, S: Treating attention deficit hyperactivity disorder. The Nurse Practitioner 26(9):1415, 19–20, 23–27, 2001.

Weber, SM, and Grundfast, KM: Modern management of acute otitis media. Pediatric Clinics of North America 50:399–411, 2003.

HOW WELL DID YOU DO?

85% AND ABOVE CONGRATULATIONS! THIS SCORE SHOWS APPLICATION OF TEST-TAKING PRINCIPLES AND ADEQUATE CONTENT KNOWLEDGE.

75–85% KEEP WORKING! REVIEW TEST-TAKING PRINCIPLES AND TRY AGAIN.

65–75% HANG IN THERE! SPEND SOME TIME REVIEWING CONCEPTS AND TEST-TAKING PRINCIPLES AND THEN TRY THE TEST AGAIN.

Health Counseling

6

LYNNE M. DUNPHY
and
JILL E. WINLAND-BROWN

6–1 *Having routine mammograms after age 50 is an example of:*

A. health promotion.
B. disease-prevention.
C. screening.
D. tertiary prevention.

6–2 *A smoking cessation program should be initiated when:*

A. the client states a readiness to quit.
B. the client is in the hospital.
C. an initial history and physical examination are performed.
D. the client's family convinces the client of the necessity to quit.

6–3 *Which of the following is the primary reason given by healthcare professionals as to why inadequate attention is paid to preventive services in the primary care setting?*

A. Lack of motivation because preventing problems is not as exciting as "curing" problems
B. Skepticism about the effectiveness of health promotion and counseling
C. Uncertainty about which and how much information to provide
D. The fact that counseling is not "billable" and is therefore not cost effective

6–4 *The most effective interventions available to healthcare providers for reducing the incidence and severity of the leading causes of disease and disability in the United States are:*

A. screening tests.
B. immunizations.
C. counseling interventions that address the personal health practices of clients.
D. chemoprophylaxes such as the use of drugs and nutritional and mineral supplements.

6–5 *The best way to promote a personal behavior change in a client is to:*

A. write an order for a treatment plan.
B. stress compliance with your treatment plan.
C. prescribe a health promotion regime.
D. discuss choices with the client and let him or her decide what will work best.

6–6 *The U.S. Preventive Services Task Force recommends screening which of the following groups for evidence of alcohol dependence, problem drinking, or excessive alcohol consumption?*

A. Individuals whom the provider thinks are abusing alcohol
B. Individuals with altered liver function studies
C. Individuals who have had several recent automobile accidents, regardless of precipitating cause
D. All adult and adolescent clients

6–7 *Which of the following is a four item screening tool useful in identifying a client who may have a problem with alcohol abuse?*

A. The AUDIT test
B. The CAGE questionnaire
C. The Michigan Alcoholism Screening Test
D. The Problem Drinker/Abuser Test

6–8 *As the nurse practitioner in an outpatient clinic, you will be performing a history and physical on Maria, age 15, whose mother comes to the clinic with her. How would you approach the topic of sexuality with Maria?*

A. Ask Maria's mother if you can discuss this issue with Maria.
B. Ask Maria, with her mother present, if it is OK for you to discuss this issue with them both.
C. Ask Maria's mother to leave the room.
D. When you are alone with Maria, tell her that you want to talk to her about this issue and ask her if she wants her mother to be present.

6–9 *You suspect that Ginger, age 6, has parents who smoke. Ginger is being seen in the office for an acute asthma attack. Her mother is present. How do you approach Ginger's mother about this risk factor?*

A. "You know that smoking is detrimental to Ginger's health."
B. "I hope that you don't smoke in front of Ginger."
C. "Is Ginger ever exposed to cigarette smoke?"
D. "I can smell smoke on your clothes. How many packs do you smoke per day?"

6–10 *Who should have a screening test for skin cancer?*

A. All individuals, starting at adolescence, then every 5 years thereafter
B. All individuals every 2 years
C. Individuals with risk factors for skin cancer
D. All individuals during every health examination

6–11 *Which of the following conditions, which may be detected by a complete blood count, has sufficient prevalence to make early detection beneficial?*

A. Anemia
B. Leukocytosis
C. Thrombocytopenia
D. Leukemia

6–12 *At what stage of life is it most important to target obesity prevention programs?*

A. Infancy, with interventions aimed at parents' understanding of adequate diet
B. Childhood
C. Adolescence
D. Middle adulthood, if there is onset of actual health problems such as diabetes mellitus

6–13 *It is important to counsel your clients of all ages regarding prevention strategies for cancers of the colon and rectum. These include:*

A. fecal occult blood testing on an annual basis after age 50.
B. the importance of regular physical exercise and colonoscopy after age 50.
C. stressing the importance of regular physical exercise; a diet rich in vegetables, fruit and fiber; and regular use of aspirin.
D. weight loss, smoking cessation, and a diet rich in fiber.

6–14 *Henry, age 57, is married and the father of three children. He is overweight and hypertensive, and has a sedentary lifestyle. His father died of a myocardial infarction at age 42. Which factor will provide the strongest motivation for Henry to change his lifestyle?*

A. The fear that he will not live to see his daughter get married.
B. Feeling "ownership" of the need to change.
C. Feeling guilty that his wife might be left alone to raise the children.
D. The desire to enjoy his retirement when the time comes.

6–15 *Joy wants to stop smoking but is afraid that she will gain weight like all of her friends did when they stopped. What might you say to her that will encourage her to stop?*

A. "Forget the weight gain; at least you'll live longer."
B. "The average weight gain is 5 pounds; it's worth it."
C. "Let's talk about several strategies you might use to prevent weight gain."
D. "Eat what you want and just exercise more."

6–16 *Alison asks you whether she should do anaerobic or aerobic exercise, and what the difference is between them. You tell her that a simple measure of whether or not an exercise activity is aerobic or not is:*

A. her heart rate.
B. whether or not she is sweating.
C. her degree of fatigue.
D. whether or not her muscles ache.

6–17 *When counseling a client about low-fat food choices, you recommend the following food as a good choice:*

A. Bluefish.
B. dark-meat chicken.
C. hot dogs.
D. swordfish.

6–18 *How do you respond to Trisha, who thinks that skipping breakfast is a way of banking calories for later in the day?*

A. "I do the same thing; that way I feel like I can have a bigger lunch."
B. "That's terrible. Didn't your mother always tell you that breakfast is the most important meal of the day?"

C. "Eating breakfast actually wakes up your system and gets your metabolism going."
D. "We all need some essential fatty acids that are obtained only from food."

6–19 *Coconut oil and cocoa butter are examples of which type of fatty acids?*

A. Saturated fats
B. Monounsaturated fats
C. Polyunsaturated fats
D. Both mono- and polyunsaturated fats

6–20 *What is the most common cause of injuries, the leading cause of hospital admissions for trauma, and the second leading cause of injury-related deaths for all age groups?*

A. Motor vehicle accidents
B. Falls
C. Bicycle or motorcycle accidents
D. Rollerblading and roller-skating accidents

6–21 *The most common agent(s) that cause(s) poisoning deaths in adults is (are):*

A. heroin and cocaine.
B. antidepressants and tranquilizers.
C. motor vehicle exhaust.
D. barbiturates.

6–22 *You are counseling the parents of a 2-year-old about accidental poisoning. What do you instruct them to administer if their child should accidentally ingest something poisonous?*

A. Burnt toast
B. Tea
C. Ipecac syrup
D. Milk of magnesia

6–23 *Your neighbors are building a swimming pool and have two children, ages 2 and 8. What is the best recommendation you could make to them to prevent an accidental drowning of the 2-year-old?*

A. Install a fence around the pool.
B. Have the 8-year-old learn cardiopulmonary resuscitation.
C. Never let the children out of your sight.
D. Keep the entrances to the backyard locked at all times.

6–24 *You suspect that a client is being physically abused by her husband because, in her last two visits to the office, she has had unexplainable ecchymotic areas on her face and upper arms. You would like to raise the issue of abuse. Which of the following statements might prompt the best response from the client?*

A. "These bruises are very unusual. Is your husband hurting you?"
B. "How did you get these bruises?"
C. "Would you like to talk about what's going on?"
D. "Do you frequently get a lot of bruises?"

6–25 *Melanie wants to start working on a tan before her Caribbean cruise. You warn her about the hazards of sun exposure, but she is still insistent about getting a tan. What do you recommend?*

A. Brief tanning periods using a sunscreen
B. Use of a tanning salon for several weeks before the cruise
C. Use of a self-tanning lotion or cream
D. Intervals of 1/2 hour in the sun and 1/2 hour out of the sun at intervals

6–26 *When performing a history and physical examination on Jason, age 16, he tells you that although he does not smoke, he uses snuff (smokeless tobacco). He says that he wants the nicotine "high" but does not want it to become a habit like cigarette smoking. What should you tell him about smokeless tobacco?*

A. It may lead to mouth or throat cancer.
B. Smokeless tobacco has no effect on teeth and gums.
C. Smokeless tobacco will increase his appetite.
D. It is less dangerous than cigarette smoking.

6–27 *While examining Marcia, age 12 months, you notice that her teeth are in very poor condition. What is the most appropriate question to ask the parents?*

A. "Does Marcia go to bed with a bottle at night?"
B. "Have you been cleaning Marcia's teeth with a piece of gauze around your finger every day?"
C. "What kinds of foods does Marcia eat?"
D. "Does Marcia chew on her toys?"

6–28 *Jenny is bringing in her 2-year-old daughter for her routine immunizations. She states that her daughter is up to date with all of her immunizations, but notes that at her previous physician's office, she was told her daughter did not need the* Haemophilus influenzae *type B (HiB) vaccine because she had HiB disease at age 15 months. You respond:*

A. "Having had the disease at that age is not a contraindication for receiving it. She needs only a single dose—we'll give it today."
B. "She definitely needs to be scheduled for all four doses. We'll do the first one today."
C. "Because she had the disease, she is immune."
D. "I have to check with the doctor."

6–29 *Tim, age 66, has chronic obstructive pulmonary disease. He comes in for counseling regarding a flu shot. He states that he thinks he needs one, but* *has heard some horror stories about the shot related to Guillain-Barré syndrome. What do you tell him?*

A. "You have to weigh the advantages against the disadvantages."
B. "Your chances of getting the flu are 10 to 1 and your chances of getting Guillain-Barré are 1,000,000 to 1."
C. "If you are worried, you shouldn't receive the flu shot."
D. "There is no relationship between the flu shot and neurologic complications."

6–30 *Dimitri, age 56, asks you about a prostate-specific antigen (PSA) screening test. He states that he has heard many arguments for and against having it done. Which of the following do you tell him?*

A. "Up to 70% of men over age 70 and up to 100% of men over age 90 have prostate cancer that is not clinically evident."
B. "Although the PSA test will increase case finding, it can't discriminate between clinically relevant and incidental cancer."
C. "There are no data showing that PSA screening leads to decreased mortality from prostate cancer."
D. All of the above.

6–31 *Jamie, age 7, is most likely to react to her parents' divorce with:*

A. sadness, crying, and depression.
B. whining, clinging, and fearful behavior.
C. conflicting loyalties toward her parents.
D. denial and perfect behavior.

6–32 *When planning health programs, a number of factors are important to take into consideration. Which factor is the* ***most*** *critical to achievement of success of a health program?*

A. Convenience
B. Content
C. Using visual images
D. Language

6–33 *You see a 3-year-old child in the office for a mild upper respiratory infection without fever. She is behind on her immunizations. What should you do?*

A. Tell the mother to bring her back when her infection is resolved.
B. Give her the killed-virus vaccines and wait to give the live-virus attenuated vaccines.
C. Give her the appropriate immunizations today.
D. Wait until her next scheduled visit.

6–34 *Marta states that her husband seems depressed lately and she is concerned that he will attempt suicide. In counseling her, you tell her that the risk factors for suicide include all of the following* ***except:***

A. a family history of suicide.
B. access to hypnotic medications.
C. a plan for the method of suicide.
D. self-imposed isolation.

6–35 *Gary, a gay male client of yours, age 45, arrives in your office with facial bruises. He states that he injured himself opening a door, but seems nervous. You suspect:*

A. that he is manifesting early signs of dementia.
B. domestic violence.
C. self-mutilation.
D. that he injured himself as stated.

6–36 *Mary, age 56, has been on antihypertensive medication. You have switched her regimen more than once. On some occasions when you see her for blood pressure checks, her blood pressure is fine; on other occasions, her blood pressure is out of control. She frequently complains about having to take antihypertensives. She feels she doesn't need them. You suspect that she is not taking her medication as ordered. You say:*

A. "Mary, you must take your medication as instructed."
B. "Mary, are you taking your blood pressure medication as prescribed?"
C. "Many people find it difficult to remember to take their medication. During the past week, have you missed **any** of your pills?"
D. "Mary, let's talk about the side effects of your medication."

6–37 *A recently HIV-diagnosed, asymptomatic male in his twenties has a CD4 T-cell count of less than 55/mm^3 and his plasma HIV RNA is less than 10,000. He comes to your office to discuss the pros and cons of early initiation of antiretroviral therapy. You tell him that:*

A. there could be a delayed progression to full-blown AIDS.
B. this is not a good idea because of potential side effects.
C. there is no documented potential maintenance of normal immune function.
D. there is extended duration of current antiviral therapy.

6–38 *Nathan, a long-distance runner, says he heard that a high-protein diet would increase his endurance. In counseling him, which type of diet do you tell him will increase an athlete's endurance?*

A. A fat-and-protein diet
B. A normal mixed diet with fat, protein, and carbohydrates
C. A high-carbohydrate diet
D. A fruit-and-vegetable diet

6–39 *Sam, age 26, likes to enter long-distance bicycle races. He asks you about carbohydrate loading to trick his muscles into storing energy before a competition. You advise him to:*

A. eat a high-carbohydrate diet for the first 4 days of the week before the competition, then a moderate-carbohydrate diet for the remaining 3 days.
B. increase his training time for 3 days before the competition to assist in releasing the stored energy.
C. avoid the practice of carbohydrate loading because it is very dangerous to his health.
D. cut back on activity and eat a very high-carbohydrate diet for the 3 days before the competition.

6–40 *In counseling an obese client to lose weight, which of the following is the best recommendation you could make?*

A. "Keep a diet history."
B. "Increase your activity."
C. "Cut down on the foods you eat."
D. "There is nothing to recommend because your obesity is hereditary and you will always be overweight."

6–41 *Sydney, age 15, has anorexia nervosa. Her mother is seeking nutrition counseling. You refer her to a specialist, but in the meantime you recommend:*

A. linking rewards to every pound gained.
B. that Sydney drink caffeinated sodas after meals to avoid filling her up before meals.
C. using liquid supplements in addition to solid foods.
D. eating three meals a day plus a bedtime snack.

6–42 *Nelda wants some counseling regarding her stepdaughter, age 18, whom she suspects has bulimia nervosa. You ask her if her stepdaughter exhibits:*

A. frequent urinary tract infections (UTIs), dental caries, and bruised or cut hands.
B. dental caries, dizziness, and dry, sparse hair.
C. amenorrhea, weakness, and sleep disturbances.
D. hyperactivity and bizarre behaviors around food

6–43 *Which of the following foods would be the best choice for a client recovering from bulimia nervosa?*

A. Rice
B. Baked potato
C. Pasta
D. French fries

6–44 *A folate deficiency can cause all of the following* ***except:***

A. depression.
B. fatigue.
C. diarrhea or constipation.
D. rough, red tongue.

6–45 *Chloe is chronically tired. During a telephone conversation, she asks you for advice. You recommend that she:*

A. not nap during the day and establish a routine for sleep at night.
B. add iron to her diet.
C. take a vitamin supplement with iron.
D. make an appointment.

6–46 *Raymond presents with bleeding gums and broken capillaries under his skin. What vitamin deficiency do you suspect he has?*

A. Vitamin A
B. Vitamin B_{12}
C. Vitamin C
D. Vitamin D

6–47 *Marvin has just been given a diagnosis of diabetes. To increase his adherence to a healthful lifestyle, you:*

A. initially have him come in every week for a urinalysis and fingerstick blood glucose test to see how he's doing.
B. tell him you will do a glycohemoglobin test every 3 months to assess his control of his blood sugar.
C. instruct him on self-monitoring of blood sugar.
D. tell him to call a nutritionist.

6–48 *George, age 52, is taking a diuretic to control his blood pressure. What foods should he also be eating that might help?*

A. Bananas and milk
B. Ribs and coleslaw
C. Avocados and soda
D. Popcorn and peaches

6–49 *Sam asks about saturated fats or "bad" fats, as he calls them. Which of the following is not a saturated fat?*

A. Soybean oil
B. Coconut oil
C. Palm oil
D. Cocoa butter

6–50 *Sally asks you if she is at risk for developing osteoporosis. You tell her that women at greater risk of developing osteoporosis include all of the following* ***except:***

A. white women.
B. Asian women.
C. petite women.
D. overweight women.

6–51 *Mary, who is obese, has started a walking program and wonders how much walking is too much. You tell her she has done too much walking when:*

A. her pulse rate increases by 30 beats per minute during the walk.
B. she starts sweating.
C. she still feels fatigued hours after walking.
D. she becomes slightly short of breath.

6–52 *Elyssa, age 69, lives alone. When talking about personal safety activities, you tell her:*

A. "Wear your slippers at all times and don't walk barefoot."
B. "Wear your reading glasses when walking around so you'll have them when you need them."
C. "When smoking in bed, be sure to turn on the light to keep you awake."
D. "Wear wide-base, low-heel shoes with corrugated soles to help prevent slips and falls."

6–53 *Smoking is a risk factor for the top three causes of death. What is your best course of action for dealing with your clients who smoke?*

A. Make your clients aware of the sequelae of smoking.
B. Ask, advise, assist, arrange.
C. Do not bring this topic up unless the client does.
D. Only bring this up if the client has symptoms related to smoking behavior; otherwise mentioning it is pointless.

6–54 *Sidney has diabetes and asks you why exercise is so essential for him. You tell him that:*

A. all persons with diabetes are overweight, and therefore exercise is the one tried-and-true method for weight loss.
B. going for a walk or exercising takes the mind off food, so he will not eat as much.
C. after exercising, people tend to be less hungry, and thus do not consume as much.
D. exercising lowers blood sugar and helps the body make better use of its food supply.

6–55 *Gene, who has insulin-dependent diabetes mellitus, is an avid tennis player. When counseling him about insulin and exercise, you tell him:*

A. "When your blood sugar is consistently high, you need to exercise more to try to lower it."
B. "After injection with regular insulin, the peak time to exercise is 2–4 hours later."
C. "Inject the insulin into your arms so that it will be absorbed well while you are playing tennis."
D. "Eat within an hour of exercising."

6–56 *Martha has many foot problems and asks you for some good general principles to help prevent them. You tell her:*

A. "Go barefoot outdoors."
B. "Do not massage your feet to improve circulation."
C. "Do not use cornstarch powder on your feet or sprinkle some in your shoes."
D. "Walk regularly."

6–57 *Sarah recently lost her husband and states that she thinks she is responding inappropriately at times. You tell her that the grief response:*

A. follows a predictable timetable.
B. follows progressive stages in all situations.
C. is effective when the pain of loss can be faced.
D. is all of the above.

6–58 *Jill states that she cannot tell when her grandmother is dehydrated and that she never seems to drink much fluid. What do you tell her about fluid and electrolyte changes associated with aging?*

A. Skin turgor is a reliable measure of body fluid levels.
B. Thirst sensation is the best indicator of body fluid balance.
C. Body weight is the best indicator of body fluid balance.
D. Peripheral edema is a reliable indicator of fluid and electrolyte balance in the older adult.

6–59 *Darlene, age 55, is shocked when she is weighed during her visit to your office. "I can't believe that I have gained so much weight! What should I do?" What stage in health behavior change is Darlene in?*

A. Contemplation
B. Preparation
C. Action
D. Maintenance

6–60 *Susan asks you about her husband, who was just told that he has degenerative joint disease (DJD). You know that the most likely joint to be affected by DJD is the:*

A. jaw.
B. elbow.
C. hip.
D. ankle.

6–61 *Susan asks why her husband developed degenerative joint disease (DJD) when there was no family history. You tell her that a cause of primary DJD is:*

A. trauma.
B. obesity.
C. sepsis.
D. a blood dyscrasia.

6–62 *Maury asks for advice on interventions that he can try to alleviate the discomfort of his arthritis. You tell him to:*

A. apply an ice pack to his stiff joints before exercising to reduce the discomfort.
B. place a rolled towel under his knees when he lies on his back.
C. rest frequently throughout the day.
D. eat more dairy products to increase the amount of calcium in his diet.

6–63 *You are teaching a client about his gout. You should include the following information:*

A. Once gout is treated, there is no danger of permanent damage.
B. Diet and alcohol may remain the same.
C. He should drink at least 1 quart of fluid per day.
D. Kidney stones and kidney damage may result if gout is not adequately managed.

6–64 *Sylvia has scleroderma and asks for counseling related to measures to help manage its effects. You tell Sylvia to:*

A. avoid becoming chilled.
B. cut down on smoking.
C. wear tightly layered clothing to keep the skin warm in winter.
D. begin physical therapy at the first signs of joint stiffness.

6–65 *Martin is marrying Laura, who has a seizure disorder. He asks for advice regarding her seizures. Which of the following is most important?*

A. Encourage Laura to begin jogging with him.
B. Remind Laura to take her anticonvulsant medication when she is experiencing seizures.
C. Do not let Laura drive for several weeks after she has a seizure.
D. Make sure that Laura wears a medical identification bracelet or necklace stating that she has a seizure disorder.

6–66 *Laura, age 26, has recently been diagnosed with multiple sclerosis. When advising her and her family you say the following:*

A. "You should avoid flying in airplanes because the altitude could trigger an exacerbation of your symptoms."
B. "You should initiate a vigorous exercise schedule to maintain function."
C. "You need to avoid all spicy foods, caffeine, and peppermints."
D. "You need to avoid hot showers."

6–67 *Jill, who is 8 months pregnant, calls you because her father has told her that her mother is gravely ill. Her parents live on the opposite coast of the continental United States from Jill and she would have to take a 4–5 hour flight to see her mother. How would you advise Jill?*

A. Tell her that she should **not** travel at this point in her pregnancy.
B. Evaluate her risk and make your recommendation on the basis of her risk factors and hemoglobin level.
C. Tell her that it is OK for her to make this flight.
D. Evaluate her risk and make your recommendation on the basis of an electrocardiogram.

6–68 *Helen is 24 weeks pregnant and needs to take a trans-Atlantic flight to attend to a sick parent. You make the following recommendations regarding her plane flight:*

A. Tell her to be sure to eat enough while traveling to avoid any drop in blood sugar.
B. Encourage her to decrease her fluid intake as it may be difficult to use the bathroom facilities and her bladder is over-distended related to her pregnancy.
C. Tell her to request an aisle seat so that she can ambulate frequently and advise her to do isometric exercises.
D. She should monitor her blood pressure before and after the flight.

6–69 *Nina has trigeminal neuralgia. She asks you what measures she can take to alleviate some of the nagging problems related to it. You advise her to:*

A. chew on the affected side of the mouth to strengthen those muscles.
B. eat and drink hot foods and fluids to help relax the oral mucosa.
C. avoid going to the dentist until the condition is in remission.
D. wear protective sunglasses or goggles when outside.

6–70 *You should advise any client who has received the following immunizations to use contraception for the next 3 months to avoid pregnancy:*

A. MMR, yellow fever, or varicella vaccines.
B. rabies postexposure prophylaxis.
C. tetanus-diphtheria.
D. hepatitis B.

6–71 *Olive has gastroesophageal reflux disease. She asks for advice as to what she can do to help her condition. You tell her to:*

A. take nonsteroidal anti-inflammatory drugs for the discomfort.
B. cut down on smoking.
C. monitor stools for steatorrhea.
D. avoid caffeine and chocolate.

6–72 *You are counseling a couple during pregnancy. To promote coping during pregnancy, which of the following interventions is* **not** *recommended?*

A. Discussing the normality of anxiety, fear, and tension during the client's pregnancy.
B. Encouraging the woman to share all her concerns and build a plan around these specific concerns.
C. Supporting the woman in her self-initiated coping strategies unless they are harmful to her or the fetus.
D. Referring the woman who is not developing adequate coping strategies for psychological care.

6–73 *Mandy is pregnant with her first baby. She asks you what the safest drug to use in pregnancy is. You suggest:*

A. acetylsalicylic acid (aspirin).
B. acetaminophen (Tylenol).
C. erythromycin (E-mycin, Eryc).
D. tetracycline (Achromycin, Sumycin).

6–74 *Martha is concerned because her 6-year-old daughter wets the bed almost every night. All of the following are appropriate counseling statements* ***except:***

A. "Enuresis is a common problem."
B. "A serious physical problem may be present."
C. "Nighttime enuresis is often inherited."
D. "Have the child strip the bed and put the sheets in the appropriate place."

6–75 *You suspect that Tania, age 16, is depressed. Her mother states that she exhibits many behaviors that suggest this. Which of the following would* ***not*** *be of concern?*

A. A change in weight or eating habits
B. Refusal to talk about death
C. Insomnia or hypersomnia
D. A drop in school performance

6–76 *Smoking cessation strategies are more effective when the healthcare educator:*

A. stresses the importance of not smoking and disease sequelae.
B. encourages persons to stop immediately.
C. conducts follow-up reinforcement sessions.
D. involves the entire family in the process.

6–77 *Primary prevention measures for sexually transmitted diseases and unwanted pregnancies should be based on an understanding of the following psychosocial determinants:*

A. Informing adolescents of disease risk is an essential component of primary prevention.
B. There must be multiple approaches and these should begin in middle childhood.
C. Working for personality change encourages adolescents to give up destructive behaviors.
D. Handing out latex condoms and showing people how to use them is the best defense against sexually transmitted diseases and unwanted pregnancies.

6–78 *Your client, whom you recently treated for a sexually transmitted disease, has returned with a reinfection. At this point, you:*

A. re-educate.
B. stress the importance of "safe sex" in more emphatic terms.
C. instruct the client that they must avoid all sexual contacts.
D. expect that the client will need to come back for more than one visit.

6–79 *It is appropriate to discuss smoking cessation techniques with a client who smokes:*

A. when the client presents with a smoking-related disease.
B. at every visit.
C. when the client indicates a readiness to stop smoking.
D. only when the client asks about them.

6–80 *James, a 32-year-old medical student, received 2 of 3 hepatitis B vaccinations last year. He is wondering if he needs to start the schedule all over again. You tell him:*

A. "We'll give the third dose now because it's been at least 4 months since the first dose."
B. "Yes, all 3 vaccinations need to be repeated if it's been longer than 1 year."
C. "No, but we'll need to repeat the second injection."
D. "If the third injection wasn't given within 6 months after the first one, all 3 will have to be repeated."

6–81 *Susan, who has systemic lupus erythematosus (SLE), asks for advice about getting pregnant. She states that she was told once that she should never get pregnant. You tell her that all of the following conditions result in a poor pregnancy outcome* ***except:***

A. uncontrolled hypertension.
B. deep venous thrombosis.
C. kidney disease.
D. a malar rash

6–82 *Mike was given three stool cards at the lab and told how to do a fecal occult blood test at home, but he was not counseled as to what foods or drugs to eat or avoid. You tell him to do all the following* ***except:***

A. do not take aspirin for 7 days before and during the collection period.
B. avoid red or processed meat for 3 days before and during the collection period.
C. do not take vitamin C or multivitamins containing more than 250 mg of vitamin C per day during the collection period.
D. avoid fruit juices.

6–83 *Your client, Casey, a 69-year-old chronic smoker, has called you to find out the result of his recent chest x ray, which you ordered because of his increasingly troublesome chronic cough. You have seen a large shadow on the chest x ray that you suspect is a carcinoma. You should say the following to Casey:*

A. "I need you to come to the office to discuss your chest x-ray results."
B. "I have seen an area on your chest x ray that concerns me."
C. "Please let me speak to your wife."
D. "I saw something on your chest x ray that we need to follow up on, but I am sure it will be all right."

6–84 *Asthma is increasing in all ages of the population. Primary prevention strategies include which of the following?*

A. Screen workers for hypersensitivity to lung irritants and counsel them to avoid jobs where they are exposed to irritants that affect them.
B. Provide masks for all industrial workers.
C. Provide pulmonary function tests for all industrial workers.
D. Provide yearly chest x rays for all industrial workers.

6–85 *Marcie is very depressed because she has fibromyalgia. She states that her husband thinks that she is just lazy. How can you help her deal with this?*

A. Tell her husband that fibromyalgia is a real syndrome and, although it cannot be cured, it can be managed.
B. Have her husband come in with her during her next visit and talk with them together.
C. Have him see a therapist, because most husbands do not understand the condition.
D. Tell Marcie that she just has to understand that her husband has made up his mind and will never change.

6–86 *Susan is a 32-year-old woman with chronic headaches. She has come to you specifically for a referral to a neurologist. She has already seen four neurologists but is not satisfied with the answer that any of them has provided. You do the following:*

A. Explain in an empathic way that there is no need to see another neurologist and that you cannot support another referral.
B. Agree to refer her to another neurologist and spend as little time with her as possible so that you can focus on clients who have more immediate concerns.
C. Do a complete history and physical and attempt to find out why the client was dissatisfied with the advice she received from the previous neurological consultations.
D. Rule out any immediate life-threatening problem and tell the client to return in a few weeks. If at that point she still wants the referral, you will provide it.

6–87 *Jane, age 72, is very upset about her stress incontinence. She asks you for advice. You tell her the following:*

A. "Unfortunately, stress incontinence is part of the normal aging process."
B. "There are many new pads on the market that provide an efficacious approach to this common problem, thus preventing social isolation."
C. "A diet that incorporates cranberry juice may be effective in curbing this problem."
D. "Kegel exercises may help."

6–88 *Sandra had a radical mastectomy 20 years ago and asks you why she still cannot have her blood pressure taken on the affected arm. You tell her that:*

A. after 20 years with no problem, she can have her blood pressure taken on that arm.
B. she no longer has to worry about injury or infection to that arm.
C. lymphedema can occur for up to 30 years after a mastectomy; therefore, precautions still need to be taken.
D. although she should not have blood drawn from that arm, she may have her blood pressure taken on that arm.

6–89 *Joanne is a second-grade teacher and is frustrated that her students do not seem to be getting any physical exercise at home. She asks you for advice. What do you recommend?*

A. "Advise parents to play outside with their children after dinner."
B. "Tell parents to let their children play outside after school."
C. "Assign homework to students that must be done with their parents and involves physical activity."
D. "Advise parents to turn the TV off for a week to get the children used to doing something else."

6–90 *Janice is recovering from osteomyelitis of her leg. She asks you for advice as to what she can do to promote healing. You tell her to:*

A. put weight on the affected leg more frequently to promote increased circulation, oxygenation, and nutrition to the tissues of the wound area.
B. eat foods high in vitamins and calcium and increase her calorie and protein intake.
C. spend time in the fresh air and expose the wound to fresh air and sunlight.
D. be sure to use strict aseptic technique when changing the dressing, which should be kept wet at all times to improve wound healing.

6–91 *Sam has lumbar spinal stenosis and asks which exercises he should do to help. You advise him to:*

A. do any exercise that results in hyperextension of the lumbar spine.
B. do exercises that encourage lumbar flexion and flattening of the lumbar lordotic curve.
C. refrain from exercising.
D. see a surgeon because surgery is the best treatment option.

6–92 *Elizabeth has juvenile psoriasis and asks for advice regarding conservative treatment. You advise her to use any of the following* ***except:***

A. ultraviolet light radiation.
B. tar preparations.
C. alcohol.
D. vitamin D_3 ointment.

6–93 *You must tell Casey that the biopsy results from his lung tumor were positive for lung cancer and that his prognosis is poor. This message should be delivered as follows:*

A. "Whatever I tell you in a moment, I want you to remember that the situation is serious, but there is plenty that we can do. It is important that we work closely together over the next several months. I am sorry, but your tests were positive for lung cancer."
B. "I am sorry, but your test confirmed that you have lung cancer. Although the situation is very serious, there is still plenty that we can do. It is important that we work closely together."
C. "Casey, can I ask that you have a family member or close friend with you when we talk?"
D. "Casey, we need to work together. I am sure that we can provide help for you."

6–94 *Jan states that his ears get plugged up frequently from ear wax and asks what he can do. You advise him to:*

A. use a cotton-tipped applicator to loosen the wax.
B. flush his ears regularly with water using a bulb syringe.
C. use several drops of mineral oil.
D. irrigate his ears with a commercial preparation and leave it in for 48 hours, using cotton wicks.

6–95 *Bob, age 46, has insulin-dependent diabetes mellitus. He asks your advice about foot care. You tell him to:*

A. use alcohol daily to keep his feet dry.
B. soak his feet in warm water daily to keep them from cracking and drying.
C. inspect the bottoms of his feet frequently with a mirror.
D. use emollients to prevent drying and cracking.

6–96 *Mark, age 26, has AIDS. He wants to know why you drew a viral load instead of a CD4 count at his last visit. You tell him that:*

A. a viral load is a more accurate measure of the progression of the disease.
B. CD4 counts do not contribute any information regarding diagnosis and treatment.
C. a viral load and a CD4 count are similar, but a viral load test is less expensive.
D. once a person has been given a diagnosis of AIDS, the CD4 count does not change.

6–97 *Cynthia brings her 15-year-old son David into the office. She wants some counseling regarding his behavior problems. David seems "laid back," quiet, and aloof. All of the information is volunteered by Cynthia. The first thing you do is:*

A. a urine test for drugs.
B. prescribe an antidepressant medication.
C. refer David to a psychiatrist.
D. talk to David about what is concerning him.

6–98 *Melinda brings in her daughter Shirley, age 2, with an ear infection. She asks why Shirley gets such frequent infections. You respond that:*

A. Shirley must be putting something in her ear.
B. a high-fat diet results in higher cerumen production; the cerumen traps bacteria, causing the infection.
C. her eustachian tubes are horizontal, which does not allow drainage.
D. Melinda must dry Shirley's ears more thoroughly after bathing.

6–99 *Ilene brings in her 14-year-old daughter Tracie because she fears that Tracie may be sexually active. What do you do?*

A. Start her on medroxyprogesterone acetate (Depo-Provera) immediately.
B. Perform a vaginal exam.
C. Ascertain in private from Tracie if she is contemplating becoming or is sexually active.
D. Call Child Protective Services.

6–100 *Phil, 14 years old, reluctantly tells you that he thinks he has something seriously wrong with him because he has awakened in the morning with a wet sheet around his penis. What do you do?*

A. Perform a test to rule out a sexually transmitted disease.
B. Tell him that this is a normal part of his sexual development.
C. Ask him if he is emptying his bladder before he goes to bed.
D. Tell him that this is abnormal and you want to refer him to a urologist.

6–101 *Ralph, age 66, comes to your office with concerns regarding declining sexual function. He states that it takes him much longer to get an erection and sometimes he cannot get or maintain an erection. He has also noticed a diminshed desire for sexual activity. He denies any change in his relationship with his wife of 35 years, with whom he has always enjoyed a satisfying sexual relationship. You do the following:*

A. Explain that you must investigate underlying causes, some of which are reversible and some of which are not.
B. Explain that diminished sexual desire and function are natural sequelae of aging.
C. Advise sexual counseling and prescribe Viagra.
D. Suggest that Ralph may be suffering from a low-grade depression and prescribe an antidepressant.

6–102 *Thomas, age 10, is sent home from school with pediculosis. You tell his mother that the cheapest and easiest remedy is to:*

A. use regular shampoo on his hair three times a day.
B. apply petroleum jelly (Vaseline) to the scalp and hair.

C. apply mayonnaise to the scalp and hair.
D. cut the hair very short or shave the head.

6–103 *Wes, age 60, wants advice regarding what to look for as signs of skin cancer. You tell him to observe lesions for all of the following and counsel him:*

A. to alert you if he observes a lesion with asymmetrical borders, a multicolored lesion, a lesion greater than 6 mm in diameter, or a change in the appearance of a nevus or mole.
B. to alert you if he observes a new papule that is 2 mm in size.
C. that any crusty-appearing lesion needs to be evaluated immediately.
D. that if there is no change in any lesion, he need not be concerned and does not need any formal screening.

6–104 *Betty brings her 2-year-old in for a routine visit and mentions that her husband has a gun at home for protection. In counseling her, which is most appropriate?*

A. Tell her that you are obliged to report this to the police.
B. Recommend that the bullets and gun be kept separately, discuss other home protection devices, and suggest a combination lock on the trigger.
C. Ask her, "Why on earth would you keep a gun in the house with a 2-year-old?"
D. Tell Betty that you must speak to her and her husband together about this situation.

6–105 *Mary is caring for her 83-year-old father at home. He has dementia and is unsteady on his feet. You recommend that Mary:*

A. put her father in a nursing home so that she can have a life of her own.
B. take in another elderly person so that her father can have company.
C. get information on home safety and community resources.
D. lock her father's bedroom door at night so that he will not wander into the street.

6–106 *Shelley, 55 years old, sees you for the first time. She has demonstrated osteopenia on a bone density test and you have prescribed the appropriate medication for her. What additional lifestyle changes should you counsel for this client?*

A. She should begin a rigorous swimming program to actively build bone.
B. She should cut down on coffee, but tea is OK.
C. She needs to take a multivitamin every day.
D. She should begin weight training.

6–107 *Mr. Green is a vigorous 70-year-old who comes for early assessment of dementia. He wants to "work" to keep up his mental capacities. You counsel that he should:*

A. make sure he gets enough rest because cells need time to regenerate because of the stress of the aging process.
B. begin taking a calcium supplement.
C. consider a hobby that challenges his mental capacity, like building model ships or airplanes.
D. play bridge (or any group card game) several times a week.

6–108 *You see a 19-year-old college student, Melissa, who is listless and speaks in monosyllabic language. Her affect is flat. Her mother has brought her to your primary care office because she is concerned about her. You know that risk factors for depression include the following:*

A. being a college student.
B. believing oneself to be incapable, helpless, a victim, or hopeless
C. having the summer free from school.
D. not having a car or transportation available.

6–109 *As you speak with Melissa and her mother, you ascertain more signs and symptoms that contribute to a clinical picture of depression. These include:*

A. sad, discouraged, irritable mood and feelings of loneliness.
B. going on a spending spree.
C. obsessively exercising.
D. constant handwashing.

6–110 *In counseling Melissa on dealing with her depression, you are aware of the successful strategies in managing a depressive illness. Apart from pharmacological interventions, some suggested strategies include:*

A. more exposure to daylight; rethinking one's situation
B. stressing the importance of rest.
C. doing complete blood work on Melissa and recommending a multivitamin and vitamin E.
D. recommending St. John's wort, an herbal remedy, because Melissa does not want to take antidepressants.

6–111 *Mr. Kent is a 60-year-old man who has a variety of cardiac risk factors. When you evaluate his risk profile, which of the following should be taken into consideration?*

A. Past surgeries
B. Number of children
C. Temperament
D. Economic advantage

6–112 *One specific intervention that might help Mr. Kent deal with his underlying CAD might be:*

A. frequent rest periods.
B. drinking at least one glass of red wine a day.
C. having a pet.
D. practicing relaxation exercises daily.

Answers

6–1 Answer C

Epidemiologists have identified three stages of the disease process at which preventive actions can be effective: primary prevention, secondary prevention, and tertiary prevention. Health promotion programs usually begin at the primary prevention level, which aims at keeping a disease from ever beginning or a trauma from ever occurring.

Immunization is an example of primary prevention. Primary prevention programs aim to reach the widest possible population group who is or might be at risk of a given health problem. Health promotion programs aimed at increasing exercise are another example of primary prevention of problems; their goal is to avert problems such as coronary artery disease and diabetes mellitus.

Secondary prevention involves early detection and early intervention against disease before it fully develops. Screening for potential disorders are considered secondary preventions. Mammography is an example of a strategy to detect breast cancer in its early stages. Pap smears are another example of secondary prevention, aimed at detecting cervical cancer in its early stages.

Tertiary prevention takes place after a disease or injury has occurred. Cardiac rehabilitation programs are an example of tertiary prevention.

6–2 Answer A

A smoking cessation program should be initiated when the client states a readiness to quit. Any smoking cessation program will have limited success when used to treat a highly dependent smoker who is not interested in smoking cessation. Therefore, the first crucial step is to assess a client's readiness to quit before initiating a smoking cessation program.

6–3 Answer A

There are many reasons why healthcare professionals give inadequate attention to preventive services in the primary care setting. The primary reason is a lack of motivation because preventing problems is not as exciting as "curing" problems. Another reason is that healthcare providers are skeptical about the benefits of counseling: Do clients really listen, or are they only present to receive treatment of their chief complaint? The fact that providers are not used to discussing risk factors and health promotion behaviors and counseling regarding self-care activities is another reason why information is withheld. The U.S. Preventive Services Task Force examined over 200 clinical preventive services and suggested health counseling and self-care activities that providers can recommend to their clients.

6–4 Answer C

The most effective interventions available to healthcare providers for reducing the incidence and severity of the leading causes of disease and disability in the United States are those counseling interventions that address the personal health practices of clients. This is the first type of clinical preventive service that providers should use, according to the U.S. Preventive Services Task Force. These counseling interventions address use of tobacco, diet, physical activity, sexual practices, and injury prevention. Other interventions that should be used include screening tests, immunizations, and chemoprophylaxis.

6–5 Answer D

The best way to promote a personal behavior change in a client is to discuss choices with the client and let him or her decide what will work best. Because medicine is moving away from the paternalistic model, healthcare providers are changing their way of thinking and are involving clients in a shared decision-making model that results in a discourse between providers and clients. Under this shared decision-making model, clients—because of a vested interest in their health and the way information is expressed—tend to listen to the information, make informed choices, and actually practice improved health promotion activities. Providers should use the words "choices" rather than "orders," "client initiative" rather than "compliance," and "partnership" rather than "prescription."

6–6 Answer D

The U.S. Preventive Services Task Force recommends screening all adult and adolescent clients for evidence of alcohol dependence, problem drinking, or excessive alcohol consumption. A client's self-report of the quantity and frequency of alcohol use does not usually provide accurate information. Responses such as "I only drink socially" need to be explored. By screening all adult and adolescent clients, you will screen the other individuals mentioned in answers A–C as well.

6–7 Answer B

The CAGE questionnaire is a four-item screening tool that is useful in identifying a client who may have a problem with alcohol abuse. C stands for "Have you ever felt you ought to *cut* down on your drinking?"; A for "Have people *annoyed* you by criticizing your drinking?"; G for "Have you ever felt *guilty* or bad about your drinking?"; and E for "Have you ever had a drink first thing in the morning *(eye opener)* to steady your nerves or get rid of a hangover?" The AUDIT Test and the Michigan Alcoholism Screening Test are also useful in identifying a client who may have a problem with alcohol abuse, but are not quite as short and easy to remember or administer. There is no Problem Drinker/Abuser Test.

6–8 Answer D

The U.S. Preventive Services Task Force and other groups advise healthcare providers to take a complete sexual history on all adolescent and adult clients.

Because of the sensitive nature of the topic, the provider needs to emphasize its importance to the client and state the relevance to a total history and physical. The client who is present with another in the room needs to be asked in private if he or she would be more comfortable addressing this topic alone or with the other person present.

6–9 Answer C

Asking "Is Ginger ever exposed to cigarette smoke?" is less threatening to a parent who may interpret the other questions as indictments of his or her parenting skills. Most parents know that they should not smoke around a person with a respiratory problem, and making them feel guilty does not address the problem of how they can stop smoking or how the risk factor can be eliminated from their child's environment.

6–10 Answer C

Individuals with risk factors for skin cancer should have a screening test for skin cancer. Although the U.S. Preventive Services Task Force has not found sufficient evidence to recommend for or against routine screening by primary care providers, other groups, such as the Canadian Task Force on the Periodic Health Examination and the American Academy of Family Physicians, recommend complete skin examinations of adolescents and adults who have risk factors for skin cancer. These risk factors include a personal or family history of skin cancer; clinical evidence of precursor lesions, such as dysplastic nevi, actinic keratoses, or certain congenital nevi; and increased occupational or recreational exposure to sunlight.

6–11 Answer A

Anemia, which may be detected by a complete blood count (CBC), has sufficient prevalence to justify screening and is a condition for which early detection may be beneficial. Although the CBC is often ordered as a routine screening test, it can detect anemia, leukocytosis, thrombocytopenia, and leukemia, as well as other hematologic disorders. Anemia is the only condition with sufficient prevalence for which early detection may be beneficial. Anemia is present in nearly 4 million Americans. Iron-deficiency anemia is easily treated and may be harmful in certain populations, such as young children and pregnant women.

6–12 Answer C

Adolescence may be the best time to mount primary and secondary prevention programs against obesity. It is at this age that adolescents become more independent in their food choices. It may also be the time when chronic overeating begins. Athough children may develop a taste for foods rich in sugar, fats, and salt, and some prevention aimed at parental education may be effective, the formative stage of adolescence is the time for preventive measures aimed at the individual.

6–13 Answer C

Colonoscopy is not a preventive strategy, but rather a form of secondary prevention, as is routine annual testing for fecal occult blood after age 50. Obesity is a weak risk factor for colon and rectal cancer, so weight loss is not the most valuable preventive strategy. No correlation between cigarette smoking and colon and rectal cancer has been discovered. However, the preventive power of regular physical exercise has been established as a protective factor against colon cancer, and also has some, but a lesser, effect on rectal cancer. Likewise, a healthy diet rich in vegetables, fruits, and fiber has been shown to have protective effects against colon and rectal cancer. The effect of regular aspirin use as a protector against colon cancers has been replicated in several nations. Aspirin also inhibits the growth of colonic and rectal polyps, perhaps by means of inhibiting prostaglandin synthesis.

6–14 Answer B

To change behaviors successfully, clients need to feel "ownership" of the need for change. Internal motivation has been shown to be predictive of successful treatment programs. To recognize that a change needs to take place and actually make the move to initiate a change, most clients need to feel that there is more to gain than to lose. The pleasure, comfort, or other gains the client receives from overeating, smoking, and other undesirable behaviors need to be outweighed by the gains the client values and believes are attainable. Although Henry wants to attend his daughter's wedding in the future and be able to enjoy his retirement when the time comes, they are temporary motivators that may not give him the needed impetus because they are far in the future. He needs to take ownership of the problem and start today to make changes that will enable him to enjoy his future.

6–15 Answer C

The appropriate response to a client who is concerned about gaining weight after smoking cessation is to suggest several strategies that the client might use to prevent a weight gain. Many clients who have stopped smoking and gain weight resume smoking. Therefore, this is an important area to address when the client is considering smoking cessation so that it can be dealt with before the weight is gained. The average amount of weight gained after smoking cessation is about 5 lb. Two strategies to be used are avoiding high-calorie foods (while keeping low-calorie foods available to satisfy the urge to eat), and increasing exercise.

6–16 Answer A

A simple measure of whether or not an exercise activity is aerobic or not is the client's heart rate. If the pulse reaches or exceeds a level of 60% of the maximum normal pulse, the exercise is considered aerobic. This only roughly measures the true degree of increased oxygen uptake by the muscles and is more accurate for measuring the intensity of exercise in beginners than in conditioned athletes. The formula to use is 220 minus the person's age times 0.6 (or 60% of the theoretical maximum normal pulse). One can usually assume that exercise is aerobic if breathing is deep and sweating occurs in mild to cold temperatures. For exercise to be beneficial in reducing the long-term risk for coronary artery disease, it must be aerobic, although any exercise is beneficial for weight loss.

6–17 Answer A

Low-fat varieties of fish include Dover sole, bass, bluefish, tuna, cod, haddock, northern pike, flounder, grouper, halibut, and red snapper. Of the many varieties of high-fat fish, swordfish is preferred over other high-fat fishes such as salmon, mackerel, pompano, or sardines. High-fat meats include sausages, hot dogs, luncheon meats (unless made from low-fat poultry), hamburger, and steak. Better choices of meat include flank steak, pork tenderloin, and loin lamb chops. All visible fat should be trimmed off meat before cooking. Poultry choices should include white meat rather than dark meat, and the skin should be removed, preferably before cooking.

6–18 Answer C

Eating breakfast and eating at regular intervals are elements of a successful weight-loss program that can be as important as the content of the meals. Eating breakfast actually wakes up the system and gets the metabolism going so that one will be able to digest all the essential nutrients. Saying, "We all need some essential fatty acids that are obtained only from food" is unrelated to the fact that Trisha skips breakfast. The other responses are inappropriate and critical.

6–19 Answer A

Coconut oil, cocoa butter, and palm and palm kernel oils are all examples of saturated fat, a type of fatty acid. Olive oil is an example of a monounsaturated fatty acid. Corn, cottonseed, soybean, and safflower oils are all types of polyunsaturated fatty acids. They are not combinations of mono- and polyunsaturated fats.

6–20 Answer B

Falls are the most common cause of injuries, the leading cause of hospital admissions for trauma, and the second most common cause of injury-related deaths for all age groups (about 12,000 annually). About 1 out of 20 persons receives emergency room care for injuries sustained in falls. Children typically fall from buildings or other elevated structures, whereas older adults are more likely to fall during normal household activities. Adult falls are usually a result of gait instability, decreased proprioception and muscle strength, or vision problems. Falls cause nearly 90% of all fractures among older adults. Motor vehicle and bicycle accidents are a cause of death in 1 out of 6 school-age children.

6–21 Answer C

The most common agent that causes poisoning deaths in adults is motor vehicle exhaust (25%), followed by cocaine and heroin (11%), antidepressants and tranquilizers (10%), and barbiturates (2%).

6–22 Answer C

When counseling parents about accidental poisonings in children, instruct the parents to administer ipecac syrup to induce vomiting if their child should accidentally ingest something poisonous. In some instances, however, inducing vomiting is harmful because the chemical ingested may be irritating to the gastrointestinal mucosa as it ascends. When in doubt about inducing vomiting, advise the parents to contact their local emergency room, which will put them in contact with the poison control hotline. If the parent is unable to get to a telephone, less damage will be done by administering ipecac syrup and inducing vomiting than by waiting. Of all poisoning cases, 85% involve children, and 70% of those are under 5 years of age. Families should have a bottle of ipecac syrup available to induce vomiting on the way to the hospital because many toxins are absorbed rapidly. Burnt toast, tea, and milk of magnesia are old-fashioned home remedies that should be replaced with ipecac syrup.

6–23 Answer B

Studies have shown that siblings are usually present when a brother or sister becomes a drowning victim. To help prevent an accidental drowning, young children (even as young as 8 years old) can learn cardiopulmonary resuscitation (CPR). A large number of swimming pool drowning deaths could have been prevented by immediate CPR. Children are very creative and can unlock doors and climb or go around fences. It is impractical to keep the backyard entrances locked at all times because the 8-year-old could certainly unlock them. It is almost impossible for a parent to keep a child in view 24 hours a day. Parents should also learn CPR.

6–24 Answer A

Although coming right out and stating, "These bruises are very unusual. Is your husband hurting you?" sounds very forthright, studies have shown that such a statement is what the client needs and is usually willing to respond to. Most clients who have been abused have been waiting to be confronted in a matter-of-fact manner, rather than an accusatory one or one that makes the client seem like the victim. If asked, "How did you get these bruises?" or "Would you like to talk about what's going on?", a client will usually continue the silence, denial, and victimization. Another common approach is to link the question to information that the client has already provided in the encounter, such as, "You said that one bad thing about working opposite shifts is that you frequently argue about child-rearing. Does your husband ever hurt you during these arguments?" Another approach is to normalize the problem, such as, "Many of my clients have told me that their husbands hit them; they complain of being abused. Is this how it is for you?"

6–25 Answer C

Self-tanning lotions or creams are a safe alternative to tanning from natural sunlight, tanning beds, or lamps. These substances contain dihydroxyacetone, a substance approved by the Food and Drug Administration (FDA), which binds to the epidermis and chemically produces a skin color resembling a sunlight-induced tan. Self-tanning does not affect melanocytes or melanogenesis, does not increase melanin levels, and does not depend on ultraviolet light. However, it is unrealistic to think that young women will always take your advice and stay completely away from the sun. While recommending a self-tanning lotion to Melanie, you should also stress that if she insists on getting a tan naturally, she should have brief tanning periods using a sunscreen with a skin protection factor (SPF) of 15 or higher.

6–26 Answer D

Almost 20% of teenage boys in the United States use smokeless tobacco. It is more common in rural areas than in urban settings. Long-term use is addictive, may lead to mouth or throat cancer, and can cause gum recession, which can lead to the loss of teeth. Smokeless tobacco does not affect appetite. All clients who use tobacco in any form should be counseled to stop because of the risks to oral and general health.

6–27 Answer A

Baby bottle tooth decay (BBTD) can occur when a child goes to bed with a bottle containing anything but water. Some parents use milk sweetened with sugar, sugared water, fruit juices, or carbonated or noncarbonated beverages. Even milk-based baby formula, because of its lactose content, is a potential promoter of BBTD. Some parents may use a sweetened pacifier at night, and this is also a contributing factor in BBTD. The child should be switched to a plain water bottle or weaned from the practice altogether.

6–28 Answer A

Children who have had *Haemophilus influenzae* type B (HiB) disease at less than 24 months of age still need to receive the vaccine because most fail to mount an immune response to the disease. Children over 2 years who have had a diagnosed invasive disease do not need vaccination. A single dose is indicated in children age 5 months to 5 years. It is not given after the age of 5 years. Under age 15 months, the routine schedule needs to be followed: a series of either three or four treatments, depending on the type of vaccine. There are currently four types of conjugate vaccines licensed for use in the United States by different companies. Each has a different schedule for administration.

6–29 Answer D

Although Guillain-Barré syndrome was associated with the use of the "swine flu" vaccine in 1976, studies done every year since then have not shown a clear association between influenza vaccination and neurologic complications. Sam is a definite candidate for a flu shot because he is over age 65 and has pulmonary disease. A flu shot is also recommended for residents and employees of nursing homes and other chronic care facilities; for clients with diabetes mellitus, renal dysfunction, hemoglobinopathy, and immunosuppression; and for healthcare personnel.

6–30 Answer D

The U.S. Preventive Services Task Force and the Group Health Committee on Prevention do not advocate prostate-specific antigen (PSA) screening, although most healthcare providers routinely perform it annually on men over age 50. Autopsy studies have shown that 30% of men over age 50, 70% of men over age 70, and 100% of men over age 90 have foci of prostate cancer that are not clinically evident. PSA as a screening test has very poor specificity (59%). Although the PSA test increases case finding, it cannot discriminate between clinically relevant and incidental cancer. There are also no data to show that PSA screening leads to decreased mortality from prostate cancer. If a client has an elevated PSA level, a prostate biopsy is often performed. If the biopsy is positive, the client may choose between a radical prostatectomy and radiation therapy, both of which have significant risks.

6–31 Answer A

Early school-age children (age 6–8) usually react to their parent's divorce with sadness, crying, and depression. They also have guilt and often blame themselves for the divorce. They long for the absent parent and have increased behavior problems. The preschool-age child (age 3–5) has a fear of abandonment and reacts with whining, clinging, and fearful behavior, or is in denial with perfect behavior. The older school-age child (age 9–11) sees the divorce as the parents' problem but needs to find blame or a reason and reacts with conflicting loyalties toward the parents.

6–32 Answer A

Health programs, to be effective, must be convenient. This includes convenience in location—someplace easily accessible, for example—convenience in times, and convenience and comfort in participating in the program. A friendly, culturally appropriate, "user-friendly" style is critical. Although the content, language, and visual images of the health information presented is important, nothing is more important than getting the participants to the program. No matter how excellent the content, if no one is there to participate, it is meaningless.

6–33 Answer C

Even though a child has a mild upper respiratory infection, if the child does not have a fever, immunizations should be administered. Missed opportunities for immunizations are lost forever. The contraindications for administering immunizations include anaphylactic reactions to egg ingestion (for live vaccines) and a moderate to severe infection with a fever.

6–34 Answer D

Self-imposed isolation is not a risk factor for suicide. In fact, most depressed persons isolate themselves. Risk factors for suicide include a family history of suicide; access to hypnotic medications or other means of self-destruction, such as a handgun; and a plan for the method of committing suicide.

6–35 Answer B

There is no reason to suspect dementia related to the amount of data presented in the question. Self-mutilation is not likely; this behavior usually manifests itself at a younger age and there would be a pattern of this behavior and usually concurrent behavioral problems. It is possible that the injuries are a result of the stated injury but Gary's "nervousness" should cause you to consider domestic violence, alcohol or drug abuse, and Gary being the victim of a "hate crime." Contrary to some popular beliefs, battery of lesbians and gay men by their partners exists, although the prevalence is not known. Gay men may find it more difficult to find services related to battery. All gay and lesbian clients should be screened for domestic violence, and just as with heterosexuals, this should be openly discussed. When clients present with nervousness and anxiety or symptoms of depression, you should consider violence, including hate crimes, as possible correlates. Perpetrators of hate crimes may include family members and community authorities. The incidence of alcohol and drug abuse among homosexuals is reported to be slightly higher than among their heterosexual counterparts. Substance abuse should therefore also be explored in a client presenting with Gary's symptoms.

6–36 Answer C

When asked, approximately 50% of noncompliant clients will admit to not taking their medication as ordered. Clients who admit to missing medication generally overestimate the amount of medication they do take. Although the direct approach may be effective, it is often more productive to inquire in such a way as to allow the patient to save face. Any questioning should be done in a nonthreatening and nonjudgmental manner.

6–37 Answer A

There may be a delay in the progression to full-blown AIDS so this is an important statement. Extended duration of antiviral therapies is a doubtful benefit. This consideration outweighs the potential for side effects. Thus, this option should be considered, not discouraged, as Answer C states.

6–38 Answer C

A high-carbohydrate diet will increase an athlete's endurance. A fat-and-protein diet provides 95% of total calories from fat and 5% from protein; a normal mixed diet with fat, protein, and carbohydrates provides 55% of total calories from carbohydrates; and a high-carbohydrate diet provides 83% of total calories from carbohydrates. Although fruits and vegetables should be a component of all diets, they should not make up the entire diet. A fruit-and-vegetable diet would not maximize an athlete's endurance time. In a study related to these diets and an athlete's maximum endurance time, a fat-and-protein diet gave 57 minutes of maximum endurance, a normal mixed diet gave 114 minutes, and a high-carbohydrate diet gave 167 minutes.

6–39 Answer D

Carbohydrate loading tricks muscles into storing extra glycogen before a competition. In training, a high-carbohydrate diet should be eaten regularly. During the first 4 days of the week before the competition, the individual should train moderately hard (1–2 hours per day) and eat a diet moderate in carbohydrates. During the 3 days before the competition, the individual should cut back on activity and eat a very high-carbohydrate diet. This practice can benefit an athlete who must keep going for 90 minutes or longer.

6–40 Answer B

The best recommendation when counseling an obese client to lose weight is to advise the client to increase activity. Because obese persons usually eat more and exercise less than nonobese persons, simply increasing energy expenditure may result in weight loss. Diet histories from obese persons have shown that their intakes are similar to, or even less than, those of nonobese persons. Although a diet history may not be totally accurate, it will show the types of food the person is eating. Heredity does play a major factor; if both parents are obese, there is an 80% chance that the children will be obese. Most experts conclude that overweight persons simply eat more and exercise less than nonobese persons.

6–41 Answer C

Principles of nutrition intervention in anorexia nervosa include using liquid supplements in addition to solid food when the client cannot achieve the desired intake with solid food; linking rewards to food energy intake, not to weight gain; reducing excessive caffeine intake; increasing food energy intake slowly by adding 200 kcal/week; giving multiple vitamin and mineral supplements at recommended daily allowance levels; enhancing elimination with dietary fiber from grain sources; and reducing sensations of bloating with small, frequent feedings.

6–42 Answer A

Signs and symptoms of bulimia nervosa include frequent urinary tract infections, which usually result from fluid and electrolyte imbalance; more than the average number of dental caries for the person's age and erosion of the teeth, usually as a result of vomiting, which can also cause irritation and infection of the pharynx, esophagus, and salivary glands; bruised or cut hands, which usually result from contact with the teeth when inducing vomiting; and injury to the lower intestinal tract from frequent use of strong laxatives. Bizarre behavior around food, hyperactivity, amenorrhea, and dry, sparse hair are all more typical of anorexia nervosa than bulimia.

6–43 Answer B

For the person with bulimia nervosa, foods that can be naturally divided into portions, such as a baked potato, should be given rather than rice, pasta, or French fries.

6–44 Answer D

A folate deficiency can cause a smooth tongue (because of atrophy of the tissues) rather than a rough, red tongue. Other signs and symptoms of a folate deficiency include depression, fatigue, diarrhea or constipation, anemia, heartburn, frequent infections, mental confusion, and fainting.

6–45 Answer D

A person who is chronically tired should see a healthcare provider rather than self-prescribe. Many self-diagnose iron-deficiency anemia and self-prescribe an iron supplement, which will relieve tiredness only if the cause is iron-deficiency anemia. If the cause is a folate deficiency, taking iron will prolong the tiredness. Taking a vitamin supplement with iron may cure the vitamin deficiency.

The symptoms of fatigue may have a non-nutritional cause. If the cause of the tiredness is actually a hidden blood loss because of cancer, the diagnosis may not be picked up as early as it could be. When tiredness is caused by a lack of sleep, no nutrient or combination of nutrients can replace a good night's sleep. If these possible causes of Chloe's fatigue are ruled out, a nursing measure that may be beneficial is a discussion of sleep-promoting behaviors.

6–46 Answer C

Two of the most notable signs of a vitamin C deficiency are bleeding gums and broken capillaries under the skin that occur spontaneously and produce pinpoint hemorrhages. Other signs of vitamin C deficiency include failure to promote normal collagen synthesis, which causes further hemorrhaging; degeneration of muscles, including the heart muscle; rough, brown, scaly, and dry skin; and wounds that fail to heal because scar tissue will not form.

Signs of vitamin A deficiency do not appear until after stores are depleted, which takes 1 to 2 years or less in a growing child. A deficiency of vitamin A affects the bones and teeth, with cessation of bone growth and painful joints; affects the blood with anemia; affects the eyes with night blindness; and affects the skin by plugging hair follicles with keratin, which forms white lumps (hyperkeratosis). Most vitamin B_{12} deficiencies reflect inadequate absorption, not poor intake. Inadequate absorption typically occurs for one of two reasons: a lack of hydrochloric acid or a lack of intrinsic factor. Many people over age 60 develop atrophic gastritis, a condition characterized by inadequate hydrochloric acid.

In vitamin D deficiency, production of the calcium-binding protein in the intestinal cells slows so that even when calcium is adequate in the diet, it passes through the gastrointestinal tract unabsorbed, leaving the bones undersupplied. The symptoms of a vitamin D deficiency are those of calcium deficiency: rickets and osteomalacia.

6–47 Answer C

Instructing Marvin on self-monitoring of his blood sugar makes him an active participant in his own healthcare, which in turn will improve his adherence to the plan of care. Although you may want him to call a nutritionist, he may never get around to this or may be in denial. Initially you will have Marvin come in frequently for a urinalysis and monitor glycohemoglobin levels every 3 months, but making him a participant in his care is one way to encourage ownership of the problem, which leads to an active approach.

6–48 Answer A

Foods high in potassium and calcium, such as bananas and milk, help to lower blood pressure. Also, a low-sodium diet is recommended to help reduce the amount of retained water, which in turn helps to lower blood pressure. In addition, some diuretics deplete serum potassium, which bananas will help to replace.

6–49 Answer A

Polyunsaturated fats ("good fats"), such as soybean oil, are liquid at room temperature and come from vegetables. Saturated fats ("bad fats"), such as coconut and palm oils and cocoa butter, harden at room temperature and are found in meat and dairy products made from whole milk or cream, as well as in solid and hydrogenated shortening.

6–50 Answer D

Women are at greater risk of developing osteoporosis if they are white, Asian, or petite. Osteoporosis affects 1 out of 4 women and 50% of women over age 65. The majority of women with osteoporosis are white and postmenopausal. Also prone to osteoporosis are individuals with small bones and thin bodies, because they have very small bone masses. Blacks have greater bone mass than whites, and men have greater bone mass than women; therefore, they are less prone to developing osteoporosis.

6–51 Answer C

Fatigue for hours after exercising or feeling sore and stiff means the exercise has either been done for too long or incorrectly. A person should never feel exhausted after the cool-down period of exercising. If that happens, the person should slow down and take it easier next time.

6–52 Answer D

For the promotion of personal safety, advise clients to wear wide-base, low-heel shoes with corrugated soles to help prevent slips and falls. Slippers or flimsy or slippery-soled shoes should not be worn. No one should walk around with glasses that are meant only for reading; they should be taken off before moving. Smoking should never take place in bed.

6–53 Answer B

Although the development of physiological symptoms related to smoking behavior may provide a "teachable moment," and although the client indeed will **not** stop smoking until ready, it is your job to assist that process. Simply informing your client of the dangers of smoking and the health-related consequences is not enough. The Agency for Health Care Policy and Research recommends the four "A's." (1) **Ask:** At every visit, ask "do you smoke?" and "are you interested in not smoking?" (2) **Advise** every smoker to stop smoking **now** at every visit. (3) **Assist:** If a client is ready to quit, ask him or her to set a "quit date" and provide self-help materials and possibly pharmacologic intervention. If a client is not ready to quit, provide motivational readings, discuss the dangers of exposing others to secondhand smoke, and indicate willingness to help when he or she is ready to quit. (4) **Arrange** follow-up visits. Make a follow-up appointment for one week after the quit date and assess smoking status; explore reasons for not stopping if the client has not been successful. Congratulate those that are successful, identify high-risk situations that they may encounter in the future, and provide coping strategies for those situations.

6–54 Answer D

Exercise provides several benefits for persons with diabetes. The most significant benefit is that exercise usually lowers blood sugar and helps the body to use its food supply better. Exercise also helps insulin work better; lowers cholesterol and triglyceride levels; improves blood flow through small vessels; increases the heart's ability to pump; helps burn excess calories; and relieves tension, anxiety, and depression.

6–55 Answer D

When counseling clients about insulin and exercise, advise them that, regardless of their blood sugar level, they should eat within an hour of exercising. If they are not able to eat a full meal, they should have a high-carbohydrate snack, such as 6 oz of fruit juice or half a bagel. If more intensive exercise is planned, they should consume a little more, such as half a meat sandwich and a cup of low-fat milk. Advise clients to avoid exercise when their blood sugar is consistently high and ketones are present in the urine. Exercise should also be avoided at the peak action time of insulin, for example, 2–4 hours for short-acting insulin or 12 hours for intermediate-acting insulin. In addition, insulin should never be injected into parts of the body that are being used during exercise, such as the arms for tennis players or the legs for joggers, because it will be absorbed into the bloodstream too quickly.

6–56 Answer C

When talking to clients about general guidelines for preventing foot problems, advise them not to use cornstarch powder on their feet or sprinkle it in their shoes because this practice may lead to a fungal infection. Instead, advise them to do the following: If feet perspire a lot, dust them with talc or a hygienic foot powder and sprinkle some in their shoes; do not go barefoot outdoors because a foreign body may cut or puncture feet; massage feet to improve circulation and promote relaxation daily; and walk regularly to improve circulation, increase flexibility, and encourage bone and muscle development. Walking is very important for maintaining overall foot health.

6–57 Answer C

The grief response is effective when the pain of loss can be faced. This may not occur for some time. Persons do not go through all the stages in the same order, nor does the passage through the stages follow a predictable timetable. There are many theories related to grief and loss, and most state that the response may be felt in many situations, not just in response to the death of a loved one. Grief may occur in many different life situations, such as loss of a breast, loss of a limb, loss of a parent through divorce, or loss of a job. Probably the best-recognized theory is by Elisabeth Kübler-Ross, who stated that there are five stages that define the response to loss and grief: denial, anger, bargaining, depression, and acceptance. These stages are not necessarily sequential.

6–58 Answer C

In older adults, there is a decline in all parameters of renal function, including decreased renal concentrating capacity, impaired sodium conservation, decreased glomerular filtration rate, altered acid-base regulation (decreased ammonia production), and a reduced response to antidiuretic hormone. Skin turgor is poor in older adults, so it is not a reliable measure of body fluids. Older adults are usually not thirsty; the best indicator of body fluid balance is body weight. In older adults, there is a decrease in the amount of total body water. This is attributable to an increase in body fat relative to a decline in lean body mass as intracellular water decreases. Edema in an older adult does not necessarily indicate pathology or fluid and electrolyte imbalance.

6–59 Answer B

A frequently cited model describes five stages in health behavior change: precontemplation, contemplation, preparation, action, and maintenance. Precontemplation is described as the stage in which the individual is not even considering the idea of change; contemplation is the stage when people begin to actively think about the health risk but no action is planned; preparation is when the individual begins to actively plan and move into early action such as developing a plan or joining a self-help group; action is marked by observable changes in health related behavior, where there may be relapses but this is part of the process; and maintenance, when the new health action is firmly consolidated as a permanent lifestyle. Prevention of relapse at this point is critical.

6–60 Answer C

Degenerative joint disease (DJD), also called osteoarthritis, is characterized by the degeneration and loss of articular cartilage in synovial joints. The joint most likely to be affected is the hip. DJD is the leading cause of disability in the older adult, affecting 20–40 million adults in the United States. By age 40, almost 90% of adults show changes characteristic of DJD in the weight-bearing joints, particularly the hips. Other joints affected include the knees, lumbar and cervical vertebrae, proximal and distal interphalangeal joints of the fingers, first carpometacarpal joint of the wrist, and first metatarsophalangeal (big toe) joint of the foot.

6–61 Answer B

A primary cause of degenerative joint disease (DJD) is obesity. Repetitive mechanical joint overuse is also a risk factor for DJD and can be seen in athletes such as tennis players and baseball pitchers. Arthritis also occurs in joints that have previously been injured or operated on. The etiology of the primary form of the disease is unknown, although genetic and immunologic factors appear to play a role in its development.

6–62 Answer C

Encourage the client with arthritis to rest frequently throughout the day to help alleviate discomfort and pain. Other interventions include applying heat to painful joints, usually in the form of warm packs or sitz baths or while in the shower or tub; applying splints to the affected joint to help maintain the joint in correct alignment; using good body mechanics and proper posture to reduce the stress on the affected joints; and losing weight (if overweight) to take the stress off the affected joint.

6–63 Answer D

When teaching clients about gout, include the following information: Although the initial attack of gout causes no permanent damage, recurrent attacks may lead to permanent damage and joint destruction. Kidney stones and kidney damage may result if the gout is not managed adequately. Clients should drink at least 3 quarts of fluid per day to help prevent kidney stones and damage to the kidneys from hyperuricemia, and should avoid alcohol. Other potential effects of continued hyperuricemia include tophaceous deposits in subcutaneous and other connective tissues.

6–64 Answer A

To help manage the effects of scleroderma, advise clients to avoid becoming chilled, which could trigger episodes of Raynaud's phenomenon; maintain good skin care; perform physical therapy, particularly of the hands and face, to help maintain mobility; wear loose, warm clothing, gloves, and warm stockings in the winter; and stop smoking altogether (because of the vasoconstrictive effect of nicotine as well as the respiratory effects of the disease).

6–65 Answer D

Martin should make sure that Laura is wearing a medical identification bracelet or necklace, such as those made by MedicAlert, stating that she has a seizure disorder. This will alert others in case she is not responsive. If a person has a seizure disorder, alcoholic beverages should be avoided completely and caffeine intake should be limited. The importance of continuing to take anticonvulsant medications should be stressed even when no seizures are experienced. State and local laws differ regarding persons with seizure disorders. Usually, driving a motor vehicle is prohibited for 6 months to 2 years after a seizure episode.

6–66 Answer D

Hot showers may transiently exacerbate symptoms. There is no evidence that flying exacerbates multiple sclerosis. Exercise is important to maintain function and flexibility but it needs to be balanced with rest to avoid excessive fatigue. There is no need to avoid spicy foods, caffeine and peppermint because of multiple sclerosis.

6–67 Answer B

Most airlines do not allow pregnant women to travel if they are at more than 35 to 36 weeks' gestation without a letter from their physician or healthcare provider. Commercial aircraft cruising at high altitude are able to pressurize only up to 5000 to 8000 ft above sea level. Women with moderate anemia (hemoglobin <8.5 g/dL) or with compromised oxygen saturation may need oxygen supplementation. Women with sickle cell disease may experience a crisis during the desaturation. Other medical risk factors include congenital or acquired heart disease, history of thromboembolic disease, hemoglobin <8.5 g/dL, and chronic lung disease such as asthma, and medical disease requiring ongoing assessment and medication.

Obstetric risk factors include history of miscarriage, threatened abortion or vaginal bleeding during the present pregnancy, history of ectopic pregnancy (rule out with ultrasound before flying), primigravia later than 35 or before 15 years of age, history of diabetes with pregnancy, hypertension, toxemia, multiple gestation in present pregnancy, incompetent cervix, history of infertility, or difficulty becoming pregnant. An electrocardiogram would only be indicated related to a specific risk factor, whereas it would be essential to check the hemoglobin level in making your decision. Even those with sickle cell trait may experience hematuria or renal microthrombosis during desaturation. The fetal circulation and fetal hemoglobin protect the fetus against desaturation during flight.

6–68 Answer C

An alteration in clotting factors and venous dilation during pregnancy may predispose pregnant women to superficial and deep venous thrombosis, or "economy class syndrome." Pregnant women have a rate of acute iliofemoral venous thrombosis that is six times more frequent. The pregnant traveler should request an aisle seat and should walk in the aisles at least once an hour during long airplane flights whenever it is safe to do so. General stretching and isometric leg exercises should be encouraged on long flights. Pregnant women should also be encouraged to drink nonalcoholic beverages to maintain hydration, and to wear seatbelts low around the pelvis throughout the entire flight. They should avoid heavy eating as intestinal gas expansion can be particularly uncomfortable for the pregnant traveler. Monitoring of blood pressure is not essential unless there is an identified underlying risk factor.

6–69 Answer D

Clients with trigeminal neuralgia should always wear protective sunglasses or goggles when outside, working in dusty areas, mowing the lawn, or using any type of spray material. They should also use artificial tears and an eye patch at night. Clients should be counseled to chew on the unaffected side of the mouth and avoid eating or drinking hot foods or fluids. They should also have regular dental examinations because they will not be able to feel pain associated with gum infection or tooth decay.

6–70 Answer A

Delay pregnancy for 3 months following measles, mumps and rubella (MMR), yellow fever, or varicella vaccines. These are all live attenuated vaccines. The others are not.

6–71 Answer D

Clients with gastroesophageal reflux disease should avoid caffeine and chocolate, as well as mints, citrus products, alcohol, aspirin, and other nonsteroidal anti-inflammatory drugs. They should also discontinue smoking altogether because it interferes with the action and effectiveness of H_2-receptor antagonists; and be advised to report worsening of symptoms, such as tarry stools, fever, sore throat, or hallucinations.

6–72 Answer B

When counseling, avoid making a decision and acting on a client's negative thoughts and ideas. Rather, encourage clients to open up and share their thoughts and feelings and assist them in recognizing and coping with the stresses in their lives.

6–73 Answer C

Erythromycin (E-Mycin, Eryc) has been found to be the safest drug to use in pregnancy because it has no teratogenic effects on the fetus. Acetylsalicylic acid (aspirin) alters platelet function and can cause maternal and newborn bleeding; acetaminophen (Tylenol) can be toxic to the liver; and tetracycline (Achromycin, Sumycin), if given to a pregnant mother between the fourth month of pregnancy and delivery, will cause abnormalities in tooth development, including brown spotting and unusual shape.

6–74 Answer B

Usually no serious physical problem is present with nighttime enuresis, although the child may have a small or immature bladder. When counseling the parents of a child with nighttime enuresis, tell them that it is a common problem that is often inherited. Stress the idea that the parents are not at fault. A family plan for dealing with the wet bed may include deciding who strips the bed and where the sheets should go. The child needs to play a major role in this plan, and positive reinforcement should be given when the child remains dry through the night.

6–75 Answer B

Adolescents who are depressed may have a preoccupation with death. They also exhibit the following behaviors: a change in weight or eating habits; insomnia or hypersomnia; a drop in school performance; fatigue; a change in motor activity, presenting as either inactivity or hyperactivity; loss of interest in usual activities; and strong feelings of self-reproach or guilt.

6–76 Answer C

The health counselor must work with the client because smoking cessation will not be effective unless the smoker is ready to quit. Follow-up reinforcement sessions are essential. The client should be followed first weekly, then monthly, then quarterly for a year. Treatment for smoking cessation is most effective when the healthcare counselor is perceived as being understanding, and when the expression of feelings and concerns is encouraged. If a client is smoking more than 20–30 cigarettes per day, he or she should be encouraged to start a tapering-off program; persons who smoke fewer than 20 cigarettes per day should be encouraged to set a "quit date." The client should announce the quit date to family and friends and all should provide additional support during this time. It is not necessary for the health counselor to meet with family, although strategies may be shared if the family requests.

6–77 Answer B

Although many sources do cite the condom as the most essential form of primary prevention against sexually transmitted diseases and unwanted pregnancies, in reality the best prevention tool is the brain. For this reason, an adequate understanding of psychosocial and cultural determinants underlying sexual behaviors is essential to individualize your counseling approaches depending on the client. Teaching should begin before puberty. Middle childhood is a "rationale period" for children. Sex education has vocal opposition in many subcultures. However, preventive teaching and participatory discussion need not focus on sex specifically. Teaching can be centered on making positive future choices and impulse control. This teaching should address girls in particular because of the lifelong consequences of unintended pregnancy and sexually transmitted diseases in women. Although sharing disease-specific information may help, it is only one prong of what should be a multi-pronged approach to prevention. Likewise, your job as a health counselor is not to change your client's personality or world view, nor to solve their deep conflicts; rather, you should offer better and healthier ways for patients to get what they want.

6–78 Answer D

When counseling clients, practice the "art of the possible." Your goal is not to increase the client's knowledge, but rather to effect behavioral change. Be realistic. For example, a client should not be asked to stop all intercourse. Clients who are not adequately helped the first time will be back again and again. It is practically impossible to counsel adequately clients in this area in one session. Personal connection, repeated messages, praise of progress, and negotiation are the name of the game. Even commercial sex workers, for example, might learn to be more restrictive by insisting on practicing only safe sex, or by avoiding high-risk situations such as working with belligerent or drugged clients.

6–79 Answer B

With a client who smokes, it is appropriate to discuss smoking cessation techniques at every visit. Because family practitioners see about 70% of the smokers in the United States during the course of each year, these encounters present excellent opportunities for providers to deliver smoking cessation advice to clients who smoke. This should be done at each visit, regardless of the reason why the client is being seen. Healthy People 2000 includes an objective to increase to at least 75% the proportion of healthcare providers who routinely advise their clients who smoke to quit.

6–80 Answer A

If the hepatitis B vaccine schedule is interrupted, it should be continued. If interrupted after the first dose, the second dose should be given as soon as possible; the third dose can be given 2 months after the second dose and at least 4 months after the first dose. This client's normal schedule would have been a series of 3 immunizations, with the second and third doses administered 1 month and 6 months, respectively, after the first dose.

6–81 Answer D

A malar rash (the "butterfly rash") is a classic initial symptom of systemic lupus erythematosus (SLE) and does not affect the outcome of pregnancy. SLE in general is not a reason to avoid pregnancy; however, the client with profound kidney disease, a low creatinine clearance, and a high blood urea nitrogen level has a high risk of miscarriage or preterm delivery. Other high-risk groups in which poor pregnancy outcomes may occur include clients with SLE who have uncontrolled hypertension, deep venous thrombosis, antiphospholipid antibodies, myocarditis, and a history of pulmonary infarction.

6–82 Answer D

To get an accurate result when collecting fecal occult blood samples, the following should be avoided: aspirin or aspirin-containing drugs for 7 days before and during the collection period; red or processed meat and raw fruits and vegetables for 3 days before and during the collection period; and vitamin C or multivitamins containing more than 250 mg of vitamin C per day during the collection period. Clients may have fruit juices and other beverages they normally drink, cooked vegetables or fruits, breads, cereal, fish, chicken, pork, and popcorn.

6–83 Answer B

Although it is always best to give bad news in person, if the client asks for the news over the telephone, it is best not to lie. Instead, begin a dialogue that provides basic information. News should always be conveyed directly to the client and not through a family member. False reassurance, even if bad news is still premature, never builds trust in the long run.

6–84 Answer A

Screening for hypersensitivity is correct because you are screening individuals before the development of disease and the commencement of counseling for it. Primary prevention for asthma includes cessation of tobacco smoking and the removal of environmental tobacco smoke left by smokers. The use of newer technologies to precipitate industrial air pollutants before they reach human airspace is another emerging strategy. The use of masks has not been shown to be effective as a primary preventive strategy. Screening yearly with pulmonary function tests is secondary prevention, as are chest x-rays; this question asked you about primary prevention strategies.

6–85 Answer B

Understanding that the pain and fatigue of fibromyalgia are real will enable the client, family, and friends to work with the healthcare provider to offer support and education that might assist the couple in dealing with this chronic condition. The couple should be seen together so that they may be counseled about the chronicity of the syndrome and how it may be managed. Support groups and educational classes are also a source of help for clients with fibromyalgia.

6–86 Answer C

The correct course of action is to do a complete history and physical exam and try to determine the cause of the client's discontent with the neurology consults. It may be that what this client needs is someone to listen to her and help her deal with her chronic headaches in a different manner. Conversely, there may still be some other underlying, undiscovered cause of her chronic headaches. Requests for repeated referrals are not uncommon.

6–87 Answer D

Stress urinary incontinence is not a normal part of the aging process. It may be controlled or alleviated in many women. The diagnosis must be confirmed first to rule out other causes of incontinence. Nonsurgical treatment options include drug therapy with estrogen vaginal cream, pelvic floor electrical stimulation, imipramine, Kegel exercises with biofeedback, pessaries, and occlusive devices. Very often, a combination of several of these will benefit the client. Surgery may be indicated, depending on which structure needs repairing. For example, if a cystocele is producing the symptoms, repair of the anterior vaginal wall prolapse is indicated. Pads may prove helpful, but underlying causes must first be investigated. There is no evidence that cranberry juice helps curb stress incontinence.

6–88 Answer C

Lymphedema is a lifelong potential complication of breast and axillary node surgery and radiation, and has been documented up to 30 years after surgery. Practicing good limb care is essential for managing and preventing lymphedema. You should advise the client of the following preventive measures: protecting the affected arm from extreme heat and burns (including sunburn); avoiding constriction of the affected arm (including by blood pressure cuffs); carrying heavy purses on the unaffected side; avoiding injury and infection of affected arm (venipunctures are contraindicated); wearing gloves when gardening and cleaning; caring for minor injuries on the affected arm promptly; and keeping regular appointments for follow-up care.

6–89 Answer C

To encourage physical activity along with parental involvement, advise teachers to assign homework to the students that must be done with their parents and involves physical activity, such as having the parents count how many times in 2 minutes the child can hop on 1 foot. Recommending play outside may not be safe, depending on the neighborhood. Turning off the TV is a good idea, but children may then substitute some other sedentary method of play, such as computer games or playing with dolls.

6–90 Answer B

To help Janice recover from osteomyelitis and promote healing, advise her to do the following: do range-of-motion and strengthening exercises; eat foods high in vitamins and calcium; and increase caloric and protein intake as well as fluid intake, which helps minimize the risks of kidney damage, yeast infections, and adverse gastrointestinal effects. You do not have enough history in the stem of the question to determine if the client should bear weight; likewise, it is unclear if exposing the wound to open air would be helpful, or if wet dressings should be applied.

6–91 Answer B

For the client with lumbar spinal stenosis, exercises that encourage lumbar flexion and flattening of the lumbar lordotic curve are particularly helpful. Also, exercises that strengthen the abdominal muscles and promote mobility of the lumbar paraspinal muscles can help minimize lordosis of the lumbar spine. Lumbar extension worsens the radiculopathy by increasing the laxity of the ligamentum. Any exercise that results in hyperextension of the lumbar spine should be avoided. Swimming and walking against the resistance of the water in a swimming pool also promote healthful cardiovascular function while maintaining lumbar flexion. Surgery may be necessary for clients who have severe neurologic dysfunction and pain.

6–92 Answer C

Alcohol should not be used for psoriasis because it is very drying. A conservative plan for managing juvenile psoriasis includes ultraviolet light radiation, tar preparations, vitamin D_3 ointment, sun baths, emollients, low-potency corticosteroids, and anthralin preparations. For a crisis, psoralen plus ultraviolet A, methotrexate, and retinoids may be tried.

6–93 Answer A

When delivering bad news, the following framework may prove helpful: (1) preparation (forecast possibility of bad news); (2) setting (give news in person if possible with privacy and adequate time); (3) delivery (give the news clearly but present the hopeful message first and then identify important feelings and concerns); (4) emotional support (remain with client and use empathic statements); (5) information (use clear words and summarize; use handouts as necessary); and (6) closure (make a plan for the immediate future and schedule a follow-up appointment). Do not provide false reassurance. Allow time for silence thoughout. The specific rationale for providing the hopeful message first is that typically clients remember very little after hearing the distressing news.

6–94 Answer C

Several drops of mineral oil can be used to soften ear wax. The old adage of "never insert anything smaller than your elbow in your ear" still applies, even with cotton-tipped applicators. Flushing the ears using a bulb syringe should be avoided, because the vacuum pressure may be excessive and rupture the tympanic membrane. Commercial preparations can be used to irrigate, but should never be left in longer than directed because they can cause local irritation.

6–95 Answer C

Clients with diabetes mellitus should be taught proper foot care, especially the use of a mirror to help them inspect the bottoms (soles) of their feet, because peripheral neuropathy may prevent them from feeling any foreign bodies or cuts. Preparations such as alcohol should be avoided because they tend to dry and crack the feet, allowing microorganisms to enter. Soaking the feet in water and use of emollients should also be avoided because they help to keep the feet moist and thus become a good medium for the growth of bacteria.

6–96 Answer A

For clients with AIDS, a viral load test is a more accurate measure of the progression of the disease than a CD4 count. The CD4 count is a surrogate marker that provides important, but indirect, measures of the state of a client's HIV disease and immunosuppression. The prognostic information it provides is useful, but incomplete, because the CD4 count can fluctuate depending on the status of the immune system, such as when the client has a cold, or as a result of dietary intake. A CD4 count is still recommended every 6 months.

6–97 Answer D

When an adolescent appears "laid back," quiet, and aloof, measures must be taken to ascertain from the client himself or herself as to what is concerning him or her. It may be appropriate to do a drug test, but first you should share that information with the client and ask if a urine test is necessary—is he or she in fact taking recreational drugs, or is there something else going on? You may still want to do a urine test if you do not think the client is credible, but certainly give the client the opportunity to talk. Eventually, the client may need to be referred to a counselor or psychiatrist or started on antidepressant medication, but this should not be the initial action.

6–98 Answer C

A viral infection enables pathogenic bacteria in the nasopharynx to ascend a child's horizontal eustachian tube into the middle ear by impairing local host defenses or by eustachian tube dysfunction. Thirty-five percent of children experience 6 or more episodes of acute otitis media by age 7. As the child grows, the eustachian tube angles more and is no longer horizontal. If Shirley inserted a foreign body into her ear and it remained in place, occluding the canal, she could develop an infection. But the mother is asking about frequent infections, which are more common than foreign-body-induced infections. A high-fat diet will not affect cerumen production. The mother cannot be expected to dry her daughter's ears completely after bathing. She should be drying the external canal with a cloth or tissue, nothing smaller.

6–99 Answer C

If a mother brings in her daughter because she thinks her daughter is sexually active, you should not take as fact the mother's perceptions of her daughter's sexual activity. You should find out directly from the daughter. If the daughter admits to being sexually active, you may want do to do a vaginal exam and discuss contraception methods or counseling. Notification of a child protective services agency may be warranted if the daughter admits to, or if you suspect, sexual abuse or an incestuous relationship with her father, stepfather, or other male relative.

6–100 Answer B

If an adolescent boy tells you that he thinks he has something seriously wrong with him because he has awakened in the morning with a wet sheet around his penis, tell him that this a normal progression in his sexual development. In this case, Phil may be embarrassed to ask his friends about this and not realize that "wet dreams" are a normal progression in sexual development. Ejaculation occurs in the early morning hours during an erection while sleeping and is referred to as a nocturnal emission. Phil should be assured that this is perfectly normal.

6–101 Answer A

You must investigate the underlying causes of this new change in sexual function and desire. Although testosterone deficiency is a common cause of low desire, and is more common in older adults, this change in sexual function is not a natural consequence of aging and should not be treated as such. It is too soon to send this client for sexual counseling as you must first attempt to ascertain the underlying reason behind the problem. You do not have enough data to presume depression, although depression is a common component of low sexual desire. Also, prescribing SSRIs may create other forms of sexual dysfunction, typically delayed or absent orgasm.

6–102 Answer C

The cheapest and easiest remedy for pediculosis (head lice) is to apply mayonnaise or White Rain conditioner to the scalp and hair. The solution smothers the live lice and loosens nits to facilitate their removal from the hair shaft. Although petroleum jelly (Vaseline) also works, it is extremely difficult to remove from the hair. Cutting the hair very short or shaving it should not be necessary.

6–103 Answer A

When advising clients what to look for in skin cancer and melanoma, tell them to look for the ABCDs: A for asymmetrical border, B for border irregularity, C for color variations, and D for diameter greater than 6 mm. A papule that is 2 mm in size sounds harmless, depending on the border and color. A crusty-appearing lesion may be an actinic keratosis and is not a medical emergency that needs to be seen immediately. It is overbroad to say that the absence of change in any lesion will negate the need for follow-up.

6–104 Answer B

Although you might like to report a gun in the house to the police, especially a gun in a house with a young child, this is not required; the gun may in fact be registered. What you do want to stress is the need to keep the gun in a locked place, where the child has no access to it, with a combination lock on the trigger, and to keep the ammunition and gun in separate places. You might also want to talk about other home safety devices, such as alarms, if the client feels that his or her home is not safe. Unfortunately, your personal bias and views on this situation, as expressed in distractors C and D, are not pertinent. You should not pass judgment; it is an ineffective strategy for behavioral change. Additionally, you cannot require a meeting with both parents regarding this issue.

6–105 Answer C

If a client is caring for an elderly parent with dementia, recommend that the client get information on home safety and community resources. In this case, Mary should be put in touch with support services for herself and given information about respite care. She should also receive information about resources regarding home safety that can be implemented so that she will not have to worry constantly about her father injuring himself. Mary should be encouraged to keep her father at home as long as possible because changing his environment may tend to worsen his dementia. However, she should not be made to feel guilty if she reaches the decision that she can no longer care for him at home. An elderly person's door should never be locked at night to keep him or her from wandering because there would be no way of escaping in case of a fire.

6–106 Answer D

Swimming greatly benefits the heart and lungs but does not help osteoporosis. All caffeine is a risk factor for osteoporosis. Cutting down on coffee is a good first step but black (regular) tea also contains caffeine. Herbal tea or decaffeinated coffee are better recommendations. Shelley needs an adequate calcium intake, not just a multivitamin. Regular exercise, especially weight-bearing exercise that includes walking and running, is recommended. This is because these types of exercise put the body's weight on the bones, pressing calcium into the bone matrix. Additionally, strengthening the leg muscles helps prevent falls; therefore, simply standing is more beneficial than sitting.

6–107 Answer D

Regular interaction with others exercises social and language skills, and playing a card game like bridge reinforces memory, providing a form of cognitive "exercise." Along those same lines, doing crossword puzzles and jigsaw puzzles helps exercise the mind. The benefits of video games and simulations are being researched at present. Although working on model ships or airplanes may provide some stimulation, the solitary nature of these hobbies over time makes them not as beneficial as an activity like card playing that demands social interaction in addition to mental effort. Engaging in rigorous physical activity, not resting, is considered protective of mental abilities. An older adult would do better to take a daily multivitamin, not just calcium, as a mental protective strategy. Research has also shown that a longer education as a youth is a protective factor. Maintaining a sense of self-efficacy—the belief, faith, and action that "I can do it"—and a "use it or lose it" approach are keys to effective mental functioning in older age.

6–108 Answer B

Although being a college student and lacking structure and transportation over a summer break might contribute to an ongoing depression, they are not risk factors in and of themselves. Believing oneself to be incapable, however, is a risk factor for depression. Other risk factors include being female, living in poverty or a powerless social position, having a severe physical illness, experiencing a severe stressor such as death or loss of a close person, and having a first-degree biological relative with a depressive mood disorder.

6–109 Answer A

Going on a spending spree is more indicative of a manic-depressive mood disorder; obsessively exercising is more consistent with anorexia nervosa; and obsessive hand-washing is more typical of an obsessive-compulsive disorder. Signs and symptoms of depression include sad mood, crying spells, loss of interest in activities and people, slowed movements, disturbed sleep cycle, trouble concentrating, and thinking about death. There may be an increase in alcohol or drug use. Co-morbidity is common, with anxiety symptoms accompanying depression in perhaps 70% of episodes (this figure differs in different cultural groups). This may bring on restlessness, fidgeting, worrying, and the inability to relax.

6–110 Answer A

Physical exercise, more daylight, and rethinking one's situation ("cognitive restructuring") are all important interventions for depression. Rest will not help, and although having a nutritionally sound diet is recommended, it is not as important as the other suggested strategies. St. John's wort, initially heralded as an important adjuvant treatment of depression, has in later studies proved to be virtually ineffective for depression.

6–111 Answer C

Past surgeries and number of children are not documented risk factors for coronary artery disease (CAD). Economic disadvantage, rather than economic advantage, is a risk factor. Temperament, however, is a risk factor. Studies from several industrialized nations suggest that people experiencing stressful situations who show their emotions are less likely to develop sustained high blood pressure, although their blood pressure may temporarily rise during the stressor. Social disadvantage, such as race, is another often-overlooked documented risk factor. Those who are discriminated against or who are poor face uncertain life situations and must constantly be vigilant. Both of these are risk factors for CAD. There are five documented risk factors: uncertain life situation, lack of experience to learn which behavioral response will solve a given problem, the possibility of serious harm, the fact that flight or fight are unlikely to help, and the need for sustained mental vigilance. Air traffic controllers, for example, experience all of the above except for lack of experience. These risk factors, as well as temperament, are often overlooked.

6–112 Answer D

The correct answer is D. Various relaxation exercises and yoga practices have been shown to lower blood pressure both acutely and chronically. Those on antihypertensive drugs may be able to lower their dose and experience fewer side effects. Although rest may be important, physical activity is even more important, and rest, if not of a relaxed nature, may create a more sedentary lifestyle, which is counterproductive. Although some studies have shown a glass of red wine every day to be cardioprotective, the evidence is not unequivocal, and in the case of a client who has a tendency to drink more alcohol than recommended, this practice is not advisable. Likewise, some studies have shown that a pet can reduce blood pressure, but the evidence is less conclusive than the evidence supporting relaxation practices.

Bibliography

Dunphy, LM, and Winland-Brown, JE: Primary Care: The Art and Science of Advanced Practice Nursing. FA Davis, Philadelphia, 2001.

Feldman, MD, and Christensen, J: Behavioral Medicine in Primary Care, ed. 2. Appleton & Lange, Stamford, CT, 2002.

Goodheart, JP: Identifying and managing common nail problems. Women's Health in Primary Care 1:3, 1998.

Goolsey, MJ: Nurse Practitioner Secrets. Hanley & Belfus, Philadelphia, 2002.

Horan, D, and McMullen, M: Assessment and management of the woman with lymphedema after breast cancer. J Am Acad Nurse Pract 10:4, 1998.

Jenkins, CD: Building Better Health: A Handbook of Behavioral Change. Pan American Health Organization Scientific and Technical Publication No. 590, Washington, DC, 2003.

Jong, EC, & McMullen, R: The Travel and Tropical Medicine Manual, ed. 3. WB Saunders, Philadelphia, 2003.

Lahita, RG, et al: Lupus: High stakes diagnosis, broad treatment options. Patient Care–Nurse Pract 1:2, 1998.

Nagler, W, and Hausen, HS: Conservative management of lumbar spinal stenosis. Postgrad Med 103:4, 1998.

National Center for Chronic Disease Prevention and Health Promotion, Centers for Disease Control and Prevention: Guidelines for school and community programs to promote lifelong physical activity among young people. J School Health 67:6, 1997.

Roodman, GD: Paget's disease of bone: Which patients need treatment? Women's Health in Primary Care 1:3, 1998.

Tallia, AF, et al: Swanson's Family Practice Review, ed. 4. Mosby, St. Louis, 2001.

Weg, JG, and Haas, CF: Long-term oxygen therapy for COPD. Postgrad Med 103:4, 1998.

Whitney, EN, et al: Understanding Normal and Clinical Nutrition. West/Wadsworth, Belmont, CA, 1998.

Winkler, HA, and Sand, PK: Stress incontinence: Options for conservative treatment. Women's Health in Primary Care 1:3, 1998.

Woolf, SH, et al: Health Promotion and Disease Prevention in Clinical Practice, ed. 2. Lippincott Williams & Wilkins, Baltimore, 2002.

Zimmerman, RK, et al: Hepatitis B virus infection, hepatitis B vaccine, and hepatitis B immune globulin. J Fam Pract 45:4, 1997.

HOW WELL DID YOU DO?

85% AND ABOVE CONGRATULATIONS! THIS SCORE SHOWS APPLICATION OF TEST-TAKING PRINCIPLES AND ADEQUATE CONTENT KNOWLEDGE.

75–85% KEEP WORKING! REVIEW TEST-TAKING PRINCIPLES AND TRY AGAIN.

65–75% HANG IN THERE! SPEND SOME TIME REVIEWING CONCEPTS AND TEST-TAKING PRINCIPLES AND THEN TRY THE TEST AGAIN.

UNIT THREE

ASSESSMENT AND MANAGEMENT OF CLIENT ILLNESS

Neurological Problems

7

JILL E. WINLAND-BROWN
and
LYNNE M. DUNPHY

7–1 *A carotid bruit heard on auscultation indicates:*

A. a normal finding in adults recovering from a carotid endarterectomy.
B. an evolving embolus.
C. a narrowing of the carotid artery because of atherosclerosis of the vessel.
D. a complete occlusion of the carotid artery.

7–2 *The typical perpetrator in a domestic violence situation is one who:*

A. has a history of being a victim of abuse.
B. has a criminal record.
C. is involved in a new relationship.
D. is on a lower socioeconomic scale.

7–3 *Karen Ann, age 52, has four children and a very stressful job. After you have performed her physical, which was normal, she tells you she has insomnia. You make several suggestions for lifestyle changes that might assist in promoting helpful sleep. Which one do you not suggest?*

A. "Wind down before bedtime by taking a warm bath or by reading for 10 minutes."
B. "Try some valerian extract from the health food store."
C. "Try exercising in the evening to tire yourself out before bed."
D. "Don't read or watch television while in bed."

7–4 *June, age 79, comes to your office with a recent onset of depression. She is taking several medications. All of the following medications have depression as a possible side effect* ***except:***

A. antiparkinsonian agents.
B. hormones.
C. cholesterol-lowering agents.
D. antihypertensive agents.

7–5 *Which of the following symptoms related to memory indicates depression rather than delirium or dementia in the older adult?*

A. Inability to concentrate, with psychomotor agitation or retardation
B. Impaired memory, especially of recent events
C. Inability to learn new material
D. Difficulty with long-term memory

7–6 *The older adult with delirium would present with which of the following behaviors?*

A. Fatigue, apathy, and occasional agitation
B. Agitation, apathy, and wandering behavior
C. Agitation and restlessness
D. Slowness and absence of purpose

7–7 *Dave, age 76, is brought in by his wife, who states that within the past 2 days Dave has become agitated and restless, has had few lucid moments, slept very poorly last night, and can remember only recent events. Of the following differential diagnoses, which seems the most logical from this brief history?*

A. Depression
B. Dementia
C. Delirium
D. Schizophrenia

7–8 *Which of the following is* ***not*** *characteristic of a major depressive episode?*

A. Weight loss or gain
B. Insomnia or hypersomnia

C. Diminished ability to think or concentrate
D. Grandiose delusions

7–9 *Bob, age 49, is complaining of recurrent, intrusive dreams since returning from his Marine combat training. You suspect:*

A. depersonalization.
B. schizophrenia.
C. post-traumatic stress disorder.
D. anxiety.

7–10 *Ed, age 50, has a chronic, episodic headache. He states that it can wake him up at night, lasts 15 minutes to 3 hours, and has occurred daily over a period of 4–8 weeks. You suspect a:*

A. tension headache.
B. migraine headache.
C. cluster headache.
D. potential brain tumor.

7–11 *Sigrid, age 83, has postherpetic neuralgia from a bout of herpes zoster last year. She has been having daily painful episodes and would like to start some kind of therapy. What do you recommend?*

A. A tricyclic antidepressant
B. A beta blocker
C. A systemic steroid
D. A nonsteroidal anti-inflammatory drug

7–12 *Persistent, excessive, or unreasonable fear of a specific object or situation, such as dogs or injections, is a description of which major anxiety disorder?*

A. Panic disorder
B. Agoraphobia
C. Phobia
D. Obsessive-compulsive disorder

7–13 *Which of the following statements about Parkinson's disease is false?*

A. It affects nearly 1% of the population over age 65.
B. The incidence is greater in women than in men.
C. The treatment is primarily pharmacological.
D. The average age of onset is 55–60 years.

7–14 *The first symptom seen in the majority of clients with Parkinson's disease is:*

A. rigidity.
B. bradykinesia.
C. rest tremor.
D. flexed posture.

7–15 *The goal of therapy for the client with Parkinson's disease is to:*

A. halt the progression of the disease.
B. keep the client functioning independently as long as possible.
C. control the symptoms of the disease.
D. ease the depression associated with the disease so that the client will be compliant with other therapies.

7–16 *Decreased facial strength indicates a lesion of:*

A. cranial nerve III.
B. cranial nerve V.
C. cranial nerve VII.
D. cranial nerve VIII.

7–17 *With which of the following movements might a client with a cerebellar problem have difficulty?*

A. Inserting a key into the narrow slot of a lock
B. Driving a car with a standard shift
C. Walking up stairs
D. Eating

7–18 Sophie is 82 and scores 25 on the Mini-Mental State Examination (MMSE). What is your initial thought?

A. Normal for age
B. Depression
C. Early Alzheimer's disease
D. Late Alzheimer's disease

7–19 *In which syndrome does the client often undergo multiple invasive procedures with negative findings?*

A. Masochist syndrome
B. Malingering syndrome
C. Munchausen syndrome by proxy
D. Munchausen syndrome

7–20 *Naloxone (Narcan) is the antidote for an overdose of:*

A. acetaminophen.
B. benzodiazepines.
C. narcotics.
D. phenothiazines.

7–21 *Bell's palsy affects which cranial nerve?*

A. Cranial nerve V
B. Cranial nerve VI
C. Cranial nerve VII
D. Cranial nerve VIII

7–22 *Sally, age 52, presents with a rapidly progressive weakness of her legs that is moving up the trunk. She also has absent reflexes and no sensory change. You suspect:*

A. peripheral neuropathy.
B. Guillain-Barré syndrome.
C. myasthenia gravis.
D. radiculopathy.

7–23 *The most common cause of cerebellar disease is:*

A. hypothyroidism.
B. use of drugs such as 5-fluorouracil or phenytoin.
C. cerebellar neoplasm.
D. alcoholism.

7–24 *Of the four types of strokes, which one is the most common and has a gradual onset?*

A. Thrombotic
B. Embolic
C. Lacunar
D. Hemorrhagic

7–25 *Which of the following is not a cause of death shortly after a stroke?*

A. Septicemia
B. Pneumonia
C. Pulmonary embolus
D. Ischemic heart disease

7–26 *Generalized absence seizures usually occur in which age group?*

A. Children
B. Adolescents
C. Middle-aged adults
D. Older adults

7–27 *When you ask a client to walk a straight line placing heel to toe, you are assessing:*

A. sensory function.
B. cerebellar function.
C. cranial nerve function.
D. the proprioceptive system.

7–28 *When you place a key in the hand of a client whose eyes are closed and ask him to identify the object, you are assessing:*

A. stereognosis.
B. graphesthesia.
C. two-point discrimination.
D. position sense.

7–29 *When assessing a client's deep tendon reflexes, you note they are more brisk than normal. You document them as:*

A. 3+.
B. 2+.
C. 1+.
D. 0.

7–30 *Jonas, age 62, experienced a temporary loss of consciousness that was associated with an increased rate of respiration, tachycardia, pallor, perspiration, and coolness of the skin. You would describe this as:*

A. lethargy.
B. delirium.
C. syncope.
D. a fugue state.

7–31 *Which cranial nerve do you test when you apply a small amount of sugar or salt to the anterior two-thirds of the tongue?*

A. Facial
B. Trigeminal
C. Abducens
D. Glossopharyngeal

7–32 *How is cranial nerve XI tested?*

A. Ask the client to say "ah."
B. Have the client shrug his or her shoulders while you resist the movement.
C. Have the client stick out his or her tongue and move it from side to side.
D. Touch the pharynx with a cotton applicator.

7–33 *Alternately touching the nose with the index finger of each hand and repeating the motion faster and faster with the eyes closed tests:*

A. cranial nerve X.
B. cranial nerve XI.
C. cranial nerve XII.
D. cerebellar function.

7–34 *When conducting a mental status exam, which question might you ask to assess remote memory?*

A. "How long have you been here?"
B. "What time did you get here today?"
C. "What did you eat for breakfast?"
D. "What was your mother's maiden name?"

7–35 *During a mental status exam, which question might you ask to assess abstraction ability?*

A. "What does 'a rolling stone gathers no moss' mean?"
B. "Start with 100 and keep subtracting 7."
C. "What do you think is the best treatment for your problem?"
D. "What would you do if you were in a restaurant and a fire broke out?"

7–36 *Which assessment tool rates the level of consciousness by assigning a numerical score to the behavioral components of eye opening, verbal response, and motor response?*

A. Mini-Mental State Examination
B. Brudzinski's sign
C. Glasgow coma scale
D. CAGE questionnaire

7–37 *Sam, age 29, has lost his sense of smell. You would document this as:*

A. hyposmia.
B. anosmia.
C. ageusia.
D. agnosia.

7–38 *Jim, age 45, has two small children. He states that his wife made him come to this appointment because she thinks he has been impossible to live with lately. He admits to being stressed and depressed because he is working two jobs, and sometimes takes his stress out on his family. About twice a week he complains of palpitations along with nervous energy. The most important question at this time to ask him is:*

A. "How is your wife handling stress?"
B. "Have you thought about committing suicide?"
C. "Do you and your wife spend time alone together?"
D. "Tell me more about what you think is causing this."

7–39 *Obsessive-compulsive disorder symptoms usually occur:*

A. before age 15.
B. during midlife crises.
C. during late adolescence and early adulthood.
D. in later life.

7–40 *The medication of choice for obsessive-compulsive disorders is:*

A. alpraxolam (Xanax).
B. carbamazepine (Tegretol).
C. clomipramine (Anafranil).
D. buspirone (Buspar).

7–41 *Extrapyramidal side effects of antipsychotic medications include all the following* ***except:***

A. akathisia.
B. dystonia.
C. parkinsonism.
D. hallucinations.

7–42 *All of the following drugs may be used to treat extrapyramidal side effects* ***except:***

A. benztopine (Cogentin).
B. trihexyphenidyl (Artane).
C. methylphenidate (Ritalin).
D. amantadine (Symmetrel).

7–43 *The most sensitive indicator of increased intracranial pressure and the first symptom to change as the pressure rises is:*

A. dilation of the pupil.
B. hyperventilation.
C. altered mental status.
D. development of focal neurological signs, such as hemiparesis.

7–44 *Mary, age 82, appears without an appointment. She is complaining of a new, moderately diffuse headache; fever; and muscle aches. She denies any precipitating event. On further examination, you note that her erythrocyte sedimentation rate is over 100 mm/min. What do you suspect?*

A. Temporal arteritis
B. Meningitis
C. Subarachnoid hemorrhage
D. Intracerebral hemorrhage

7–45 *George, age 52, has a recurring headache every Monday morning. Your plan is to order:*

A. an EEG.
B. a CT scan.
C. an MRI.
D. an NSAID.

7–46 *Which of the following may immediately follow a stroke in the older adult and be the body's attempt to maintain perfusion?*

A. Bradycardia
B. Tachycardia
C. Hypotension
D. Hypertension

7–47 *Gary, age 5, has a diagnosis of encopresis. After the diagnosis, your next action would be to:*

A. order extensive lab work.
B. send Gary to a psychologist.
C. rule out a neurological disorder.
D. bring Gary's parents in for counseling.

7–48 *James, age 58, has had several transient ischemic attacks. After a diagnostic evaluation, what medication would you start him on?*

A. Ticlopidine (Ticlid)
B. Aspirin
C. Warfarin (Coumadin)
D. Nitroglycerin (Nitro-Dur)

7–49 *Jessie, age 29, sees flashing lights 20 minutes before experiencing severe headaches. How would you describe her headache?*

A. Migraine without aura
B. Classic migraine
C. Tension headache
D. Cluster headache

7–50 *Which headache preparation has gastrointestinal distress as a side effect?*

A. Sumatriptan (Imitrex)
B. Nadolol (Corgard)
C. Naproxen sodium (Anaprox DS)
D. Ergot preparations (Cafergot)

7–51 *Which of the following tests is highly specific and fairly sensitive for myasthenia gravis?*

A. Electromyography nerve conduction tests
B. Magnetic resonance imaging scan of the brain and brainstem
C. Serum acetylcholine receptor antibody level
D. Lumbar puncture

7–52 *Current pharmacologic therapy for multiple sclerosis involves:*

A. high-dose steroids.
B. baclofen (Lioresal) or diazepam (Valium).
C. interferon B (Betaseron).
D. benzodiazepines.

7–53 *Which of the following is not an extra-axial brain tumor?*

A. Astrocytoma
B. Pituitary adenoma
C. Meningioma
D. Acoustic neuroma

7–54 *Deficiency of which nutritional source usually presents with an insidious onset of paresthesias of the hands and feet that are usually painful?*

A. Thiamine
B. Vitamin B_{12}
C. Folic acid
D. Vitamin K

7–55 *Jim, a 45-year-old postal worker, presents with a history of a sudden onset of intense apprehension, fear, dyspnea, palpitations, and a choking sensation. Your initial diagnosis is:*

A. anxiety.
B. panic attack.
C. depression.
D. agoraphobia.

7–56 *The persistent and irrational fear of a specific object, activity, or situation that results in a compelling desire to avoid the dreaded object, activity, or situation, is defined as:*

A. depression.
B. obsession-compulsion.
C. agoraphobia.
D. phobia.

7–57 *Marie, age 17, was raped when she was 13. She is now experiencing sleeping problems, flashbacks, and depression. Your initial diagnosis is:*

A. depression.
B. panic disorder.
C. anxiety.
D. post-traumatic stress disorder.

7–58 *Mark, age 29, tells you that he has thought about suicide. Which question should you ask next?*

A. "How long have you felt this way?"
B. "Tell me more about it."
C. "Do you have a plan?"
D. "Have you told anyone else?"

7–59 *In the depressed client, antidepressants are most effective in alleviating:*

A. suicidal feelings.
B. interpersonal problems.
C. sleep disturbances.
D. anxiety disorders.

7–60 *The two most common causes of dementia in older adults are:*

A. polypharmacy and nutritional disorders.
B. Alzheimer's disease and vascular disorders.
C. metabolic disorders and space-occupying lesions.
D. infections affecting the brain and polypharmacy.

7–61 *What is the most sensitive diagnostic test for identifying an alcoholic client?*

A. Aspartate transaminase (SGOT)
B. Mean corpuscular volume
C. Alkaline phosphatase
D. γ-glutamyltransferase (GGT)

7–62 *If you suspect that your client abuses alcohol, the most appropriate action would be to:*

A. confront the client.
B. obtain further confirmatory information.
C. consult with family members.
D. suggest Alcoholics Anonymous (AA).

7–63 *When a client is in the precontemplation stage of smoking cessation, which question should the healthcare provider ask?*

A. "What would it take for you to consider quitting?"
B. "What would it take for you to quit now?"
C. "What technique do you think will work best for you?"
D. "What do you think will be your biggest challenge to quitting?"

7–64 *The Agency for Health Care Policy and Research recommends that providers ask clients about their tobacco use status:*

A. at every visit.
B. at least every 6 months.
C. once a year.
D. at the initial history and physical examination.

7–65 *Which drug has been shown to be an effective aid to smoking cessation?*

A. Oxazepam (Serax)
B. Clorazepate dipotassium (Tranxene)
C. Bupropion (Zyban)
D. Alprazolam (Xanax)

7–66 *Drug screening tests of urine, often performed in the workplace, are frequently effective in finding a* *person who smokes marijuana because a urine test will be positive for marijuana for up to how long after a person stops smoking the drug?*

A. 24 hours
B. 1 week
C. 2 weeks
D. 30 days

7–67 *Susan has a slipped lumbar disk. When assessing her Achilles tendon, what would you expect her reflex score to be?*

A. 1+
B. 2+
C. 3+
D. 4+

7–68 *The position with the client supine, flexing the head to the chest, is referred to as:*

A. Brudzinski's sign.
B. Kernig's sign.
C. decorticate posturing.
D. decerebrate posturing.

7–69 *When you move a client's head to the left and the eyes move to the right in relation to the head, this is referred to as:*

A. extraocular eye movements.
B. oculomotor degeneration.
C. doll's eyes.
D. decerebrate posturing.

7–70 *Which type of intracranial hematoma is the most common and has the clinical manifestations of headache, drowsiness, agitation, slowed thinking, and confusion?*

A. Epidural
B. Subdural
C. Intracerebral
D. Meningeal

7–71 *Jeff, age 12, injured his spinal cord by diving into a shallow lake. He is in a wheelchair but can self-transfer. He can use his shoulder and extend his wrist, but has no finger control. At what level of the spinal cord was the damage?*

A. C4
B. C5
C. C6
D. C7

7–72 *Diane, age 35, presents with weakness and numbness of the left arm, diplopia, and some bowel and bladder changes for the past week. She states that the same thing happened last year and lasted for several weeks. What diagnosis is a strong possibility?*

A. Multiple sclerosis
B. Subdural hematoma
C. Pituitary tumor
D. Myasthenia gravis

7–73 *You assess for cogwheel rigidity in Sophia, aged 76. What is this a manifestation of?*

A. Alzheimer's disease
B. Parkinson's disease
C. Brain attack
D. Degenerative joint disease

7–74 *Which of the following conditions is most responsible for developmental delays in children?*

A. Cerebral palsy
B. Fetal alcohol syndrome
C. Down syndrome
D. Meningomyelocele

7–75 *Which of the following drugs used for parkinsonism mimics dopamine?*

A. Anticholinergics
B. Levodopa (l-dopa)
C. Bromocriptine
D. Tolcapone

7–76 *Mattie, age 52, has a ruptured vertebral disk with the following symptoms: pain in the midgluteal region as well as the posterior thigh and calf-to-heel area; paresthesias in the posterior calf and lateral heel, foot, and toes; and difficulty walking on her toes. Which intervertebral disks are involved?*

A. L4–5
B. L5–S1
C. C5–6
D. C7-T1

7–77 *Sandra has a ruptured intervertebral disk and is not responding to conservative management. She is requesting surgery for relief of her pain. She is going to have an enlargement of the opening between the disk and the facet joint to remove the bony overgrowth compressing the nerve. This describes which surgical procedure?*

A. Laminectomy
B. Diskectomy
C. Foraminotomy
D. Chemonucleolysis

7–78 *Grace, age 82, has Alzheimer's disease. Her daughter states that she is agitated, has time disorientation, and wanders during the afternoon and evening hours. How do you describe this behavior?*

A. Alzheimer's dementia
B. Sundowning
C. Deficits of the Alzheimer's type
D. Senile dementia

7–79 *Marian, age 39, has multiple sclerosis (MS). She tells you that she heard that the majority of peo-*

ple with MS have the chronic-relapsing type of disease and that she has nothing to live for. How do you respond?

A. "The majority of people have this response to MS."
B. "There are many different clinical courses of MS and the chronic-relapsing type is only one of them."
C. "The chronic-relapsing type of MS is in the minority."
D. "There is an even chance that you have this type."

7–80 *Some providers have successfully induced remission in clients with multiple sclerosis by using adrenocorticotropic hormone therapy or other pharmacological therapy along with:*

A. chelation therapy.
B. plasmapheresis.
C. bone marrow transplantation.
D. intravenous lipids

7–81 *A thymectomy is usually recommended in the early treatment of:*

A. Parkinson's disease.
B. multiple sclerosis.
C. myasthenia gravis.
D. Huntington's chorea.

7–82 *Which peripheral nervous system disorder usually follows a viral respiratory or gastrointestinal infection?*

A. Cytomegalovirus
B. Herpes zoster
C. Guillain Barré syndrome
D. Trigeminal neuralgia

7–83 *Lynne, age 72, presents for the first time with her daughter. Her daughter describes some recent disturbing facts. How can you differentiate between depression and dementia?*

A. You might be able to pinpoint the onset of dementia, but the onset of depression is difficult to identify.
B. A depressed person has wide mood swings, whereas a person with dementia demonstrates apathetic behavior.
C. The person with dementia tries to hide problems concerning his or her memory, whereas the person with depression complains about memory.
D. The person with dementia has a poor self-image, whereas the person with depression does not have a change in self-image.

7–84 *Clients with senile dementia of the Alzheimer's type often die of:*

A. pneumonia.
B. suicide.
C. pressure sores.
D. malnutrition.

7–85 *Clients with spinal cord injuries often have bowel incontinence and need to have a bowel program instituted. With the quadriplegic client, the most effective way to stimulate the rectum to evacuate is to:*

A. administer stool softeners every night.
B. insert a rectal suppository, then eventually perform digital stimulation.
C. administer laxatives every other night.
D. administer enemas on a regular basis.

7–86 *Which of the following lab results would indicate a specific infection in the central nervous system?*

A. Cerebrospinal fluid (CSF) glucose of 35 mg/dL
B. A CSF pressure of 250 mm of water
C. A CSF red blood cell count of 25/mm^3
D. A serum white blood cell count of 12,000/mm^3

7–87 *A rhizotomy may be performed for the client with:*

A. Bell's palsy.
B. tic douloureux.
C. Parkinson's disease.
D. myasthenia gravis.

7–88 *What is the first line of protection against an increase in anxiety?*

A. Mental defense mechanisms
B. An increase in the level of serotonin
C. A panic attack
D. Denial

7–89 *Barbara, age 36, presents with episodic attacks of severe vertigo, usually with associated ear fullness. Her attacks usually last several hours and she feels well before and after the attacks. You might attribute this to:*

A. Ménière's disease.
B. vestibular neuronitis.
C. benign paroxysmal positional vertigo.
D. otosclerosis.

7–90 *Janice, age 14, is markedly obese and has a poor self-image. How do you differentiate between compulsive eating and bulimia?*

A. Bulimia results in irregular menstruation.
B. A compulsive eater does not induce vomiting.
C. A compulsive eater has tooth and gum erosion.
D. A compulsive eater does compulsive exercising.

7–91 *Which statement is inaccurate regarding a client who is at highest risk for an eating disorder?*

A. The client is female.
B. The client is usually 12–24 years of age.
C. The client has high self-esteem.
D. The client has a perfectionist personality.

7–92 *Julie, age 15, is 5 feet tall and weighs 85 lb. You suspect anorexia and know that the best initial approach is to:*

A. discuss proper nutrition.
B. tell Julie what she should weigh for her height and suggest a balanced diet.
C. speak to her parents before going any further.
D. confront Julie with the fact that you suspect an eating disorder.

7–93 *Don, age 62, calls to complain of a severe headache. With which of his following statements are you most concerned?*

A. "It hurts whenever I turn my head a specific way."
B. "It's the worst headache I've ever had."
C. "Nothing I do seems to help this constant ache."
D. "I'm so worried, can you do a CT scan?"

7–94 *The Hallpike maneuver is performed to elicit:*

A. a seizure.
B. vertigo.
C. syncope.
D. a headache.

7–95 *In the stages of Elisabeth Kübler-Ross's anticipatory grieving, which stage follows that of anger?*

A. Denial
B. Bargaining
C. Depression
D. Acceptance

7–96 *Which of the following screening instruments is quick and easy to use and has a high level of diagnostic accuracy to detect alcohol abuse?*

A. The CAGE questionnaire
B. The HEAT instrument
C. The DRINK tool
D. MMSE

7–97 *How do you respond when Mavis, age 32, who is taking ergotamine tartrate (Ergostat), asks you about rebound headaches?*

A. "It's a headache that comes back if you don't take a sufficient dose of the medication."
B. "A daily or 'rebound' headache may occur if you take medication for a headache more than three times per week."
C. "A 'rebound' headache is another symptom indicating central nervous system involvement."
D. "Rebound headaches don't occur with ergotamine."

7–98 *Which of the following cardiac drugs is used to treat migraine headaches?*

A. Beta blockers
B. Nitrates
C. Angiotensin-converting enzyme inhibitors
D. Alpha-adrenergic blockers

7–99 *In teaching a client with multiple sclerosis, the provider should emphasize all of the following points* ***except:***

A. taking a daily hot shower to relax.
B. exercising to maintain mobility.
C. getting plenty of rest.
D. seeking psychological and emotional support.

7–100 *Which appropriate test for the initial assessment of Alzheimer's disease provides performance ratings on 10 complex higher-order activities?*

A. MMSE
B. CAGE questionnaire
C. FAQ
D. Holmes and Rahe Readjustment Scale

7–101 *Major depression occurs most often in which of the following conditions:*

A. Parkinson's disease
B. Alzheimer's disease
C. Myocardial infarction
D. Stroke

7–102 *Dan, age 82, recently lost his wife to breast cancer. He presents with weight loss, fatigue, and difficulty sleeping. What should your first response be?*

A. "Do you have a history of thyroid problems in your family?"
B. "Do you think a sleeping pill might help you sleep at night?"
C. "Things might look up if you added nutritional supplements to your diet."
D. "Have you thought of suicide?"

7–103 *Which of the following gaits in older adults includes brusqueness of the movements of the leg and stamping of the feet?*

A. Gait of sensory ataxia
B. Parkinsonian gait
C. Antalgic gait
D. Cerebellar gait

7–104 *Ivy, age 73, presents with limb paralysis, nystagmus, vertigo, nausea, slurred speech, and cerebellar ataxia. You suspect an occlusion of which part of the brain?*

A. Occipital and temporal lobes, dorsal surface of thalamus, upper part of cerebellum, midbrain
B. Anterior cerebral surfaces

C. Posterior cerebral surfaces
D. Parts of medulla

7–105 *Which type of encephalitis is the most common type?*

A. Microbial
B. Herpes simplex virus
C. Viral
D. Pneumococcal

7–106 *Herbert, age 58, has just been diagnosed with Bell's palsy. He is understandably upset and has questions about the prognosis. Your response should be:*

A. "Although most of the symptoms will disappear, some will remain but can usually be camouflaged by altering your hairstyle or growing a beard or mustache."
B. "Unfortunately, there is no cure, but you have a mild case."
C. "The condition is self-limiting, and most likely complete recovery will occur."
D. "With suppressive drug therapy, you can minimize the symptoms."

Answers

7–1 Answer C

A carotid bruit heard on auscultation indicates a narrowing of the carotid artery as a result of atherosclerosis of the vessel. Bruits and heart murmurs have similar characteristics and are both caused by turbulent blood flow; however, they arise from different causes. In this case, the turbulent flow is heard as a bruit because the vessel is narrowed as a result of atherosclerotic changes. Auscultation alone cannot diagnose an evolving embolus. If a complete occlusion of the carotid artery were present, no sound would be heard.

7–2 Answer A

The typical perpetrator in a domestic violence situation is one who has a history of being a victim of abuse. Domestic violence abusers may or may not have a criminal record, are typically in a long-term relationship, and are from all socioeconomic backgrounds.

7–3 Answer C

Suggestions for making lifestyle changes that might assist a client in promoting helpful sleep include advising the client to wind down before bedtime by taking a warm bath or by reading for 10 minutes, to try some valerian extract (obtainable from a health food store), and not to read or watch television while in bed. Exercising before going to bed is stimulating, but evidence suggests that an afternoon workout improves sleep quantity and quality. In a large study, people fell asleep twice as fast and slept an extra hour once they began going for brisk walks in the afternoon. Bed should be a place for sleep and sex only. In a recent study of valerian extract, it was found to help troubled sleepers drop off faster and stay asleep longer.

7–4 Answer C

The diagnosis of depression in an older adult is especially difficult when a medical illness is present. Antiparkinsonian agents, hormones, and antihypertensive drugs all have depression as a possible side effect. Cholesterol-lowering agents do not cause depression. Other drugs that also have depression as a possible side effect include analgesics, anti-inflammatory drugs, antianxiety agents, anticonvulsants, antihistamines, antimicrobials, antipsychotics, cytotoxic agents, and immunosuppressants.

7–5 Answer A

The prevalence of depression (5–10%) does not change with age, but depression is often overlooked in the older adult. The diagnosis requires a depressed mood for 2 straight weeks and at least 4 of the following 8 signs (which can be remembered using the mnemonic SIG E CAPS [like prescribing energy caps]): S for sleep disturbance, I for lack of interest, G for feelings of guilt, E for decreased energy, C for decreased concentration, A for decreased appetite, P for psychomotor agitation or retardation, and S for suicidal ideation.

Dementia and delirium often coexist with depression. Delirium is a confusional state characterized by inattention, rapid onset, and fluctuating course that may persist for months if untreated. The person with delirium has memory impairment, such as inability to learn new material or to remember past events. With dementia, there is a cognitive deterioration with little or no disturbance of consciousness or perception; attention span and short-term memory are impaired, along with judgment, insight, spatial perception, abstract reasoning, and thought process and content.

7–6 Answer C

The older adult with delirium would present with agitated and restless behavior. The older adult with depression would be fatigued, apathetic, and occasionally agitated, whereas the person with dementia would be agitated and apathetic and exhibit wandering behavior. Slow and purposeless behavior may indicate either depression or dementia.

7–7 Answer C

The key phrase is the time of onset of the symptoms. Dave's wife stated that her husband's complaints occurred within the past few days, which is characteristic of delirium. In a depressive state, the onset may be weeks to months, whereas with dementia, the onset is usually insidious and gradual.

7–8 Answer D

Grandiose delusions refer to exaggerated beliefs of one's importance or identity, which is the opposite of depression. Criteria for a major depressive episode include weight loss or gain, insomnia or hypersomnia, and diminished ability to think or concentrate. Others may include feelings of worthlessness, excessive or inappropriate feelings of guilt, indecisiveness, recurrent thoughts of death, and suicidal ideation.

7–9 Answer C

Although Bob is experiencing anxiety with his unpleasant dreams, they are a component of post-traumatic stress disorder (PTSD). One of the specific diagnostic criteria of PTSD is reexperiencing the traumatic event in recurrent, intrusive, and distressing images, thoughts, or perceptions. Depersonalization can be seen in depression and schizophrenia, but not PTSD. With schizophrenia, there may or may not be a history of a major disruption in the person's life, but eventually gross psychotic deterioration is evident.

7–10 Answer C

Middle-aged men get cluster headaches more frequently than women. Ed's presentation (a chronic, episodic headache that can wake the client up at night; lasts 15 minutes to 3 hours; and occurs daily over a period of 4–8 weeks) is a classic instance of a cluster headache. A tension headache may also be chronic and episodic, but it usually lasts from 30 minutes to 7 days. A migraine headache may last from 4–72 hours. Organic disease, such as a brain tumor, would be ruled out once the practitioner looked for signs or symptoms of organic disease, such as abnormal vital signs, altered consciousness, unequal pupils, weakness, and reflex asymmetry. The headache pain in a person with a brain tumor is constant because of increased intracranial pressure.

7–11 Answer A

Although systemic steroids have been shown to possibly prevent the development of postherpetic neuralgia if given early in the course of herpes zoster, once postherpetic neuralgia is present, tricyclic antidepressants such as amitriptyline (Elavil) have been shown to be effective in relieving the pain. Beta blockers and nonsteroidal anti-inflammatory drugs offer minimal relief.

7–12 Answer C

A phobia is a persistent, excessive, or unreasonable fear of a specific object or situation such as elevators, airplanes, dogs, injections, etc. A panic disorder presents as a discrete episode of intense anxiety that begins abruptly and reaches a peak in about 10 minutes. Agoraphobia occurs in crowds, or being in a place from which the individual cannot escape. Obsessive-compulsive disorder is an occurrence of recurrent thoughts, images, or impulses that are intrusive and inappropriate and that cause anxiety—the "obsessions"—along with repetitive behaviors that try to allay the anxiety—the "compulsions."

7–13 Answer B

Parkinson's disease is a slowly progressing neurological movement disorder affecting nearly 1% of the population over age 65. It affects more men than women, in a ratio of 3:2. The average age of onset is 57 years. The treatment is primarily pharmacological; however, surgical procedures (pallidotomy, thalamotomy, and tissue implants) may be used for clients who have failed to respond satisfactorily to drug therapy.

7–14 Answer C

Although rigidity, bradykinesia, and flexed posture are associated with Parkinson's disease, rest tremor is usually the first symptom seen. Rest tremor disappears with action, but recurs when the limbs maintain a posture.

7–15 Answer B

The goal of therapy for the client with Parkinson's disease is to keep the client functioning independently as long as possible. There is no drug or surgical approach that will prevent the progression of the disease. Treatment is aimed at controlling symptoms. Depression occurs in more than 50% of clients with Parkinson's disease, and it is undetermined whether it is a reaction to the illness or a part of the illness itself.

7–16 Answer C

Decreased facial strength indicates a lesion of cranial nerve (CN) VII. A CN III lesion would cause diplopia; a CN V lesion would cause decreased facial sensation; and a CN VIII lesion would cause dizziness and deafness.

7–17 Answer A

Although the client with a cerebellar problem may have difficulty driving a car with a standard shift, walking up stairs, and eating, inserting a key into the narrow slot of a lock requires the most finely coordinated movement and therefore would be the most difficult.

7–18 Answer A

The total possible score on the MMSE is 30. The median score for persons age 18–59 is 29. For persons aged 80 and above, the median score is 25. A score of 20–25 indicates early Alzheimer's disease; a score of 10–19 indicates middle-stage Alzheimer's disease. Someone with late-stage Alzheimer's disease may score below 10.

7–19 Answer D

Munchausen syndrome, named after a fictional German baron and storyteller, is a psychiatric condition, occurring more frequently in women, in which the history often includes multiple invasive procedures with negative findings. When the client is someone other than the person requesting or causing the problem, it is called Munchausen syndrome by proxy. Malingering is a conscious intent to deceive. There is no masochist syndrome.

7–20 Answer C

Naloxone (Narcan) is the antidote for an overdose of narcotics. It is given at a dose of 0.4–2.0 mg IV and may be repeated every 2–3 minutes. For an acetaminophen overdose, a loading dose of acetylcysteine, 140 mg/kg followed by 70 mg/kg every 4 hours for 72 hours, is given. Flumazenil (Romazicon) is the antidote for an overdose of benzodiazepines. Activated charcoal is the antidote for phenothiazine overdose.

7–21 Answer C

Bell's palsy, a demyelinating viral inflammatory disease, affects cranial nerve VII (the facial nerve) and results in a unilateral loss of facial expression with difficulty in chewing and diminished taste.

7–22 Answer B

The diagnosis of Guillain-Barré syndrome is confirmed by a rapidly progressive weakness, usually in an ascending pattern from the legs up to the trunk, then to the arms and face. There is no significant sensory loss and the reflexes are usually hyporeflexive or absent.

Guillain-Barré syndrome is a form of peripheral neuropathy. Peripheral neuropathy, which usually involves the distal extremities, does not have the ascending pattern just described. Peripheral neuropathy is also caused by diabetes, alcohol abuse, nutritional deficiencies, trauma, and syphilis.

Myasthenia gravis is an autoimmune neuromuscular junction disease in which the client produces antibodies that destroy the acetylcholine receptors on muscle.

Radiculopathies are usually caused by mechanical compression and cause neck and low back pain.

7–23 Answer D

Alcoholism is the most common cause of cerebellar disease. Hypothyroidism, use of drugs such as 5-fluorouracil and phenytoin, cerebellar neoplasms, hemorrhages, and infarcts also cause cerebellar disease, but alcoholism is the most frequent offender.

7–24 Answer A

Thrombotic strokes comprise 40% of all strokes, followed by embolic strokes (30%), lacunar strokes (20%), and hemorrhagic strokes (10%). Thrombotic and lacunar strokes usually have a gradual onset, whereas embolic and hemorrhagic strokes usually have a sudden onset.

7–25 Answer A

The leading cause of death after a stroke is pneumonia as a complication. The second and third most common causes of death, respectively, are pulmonary embolus resulting from immobilization and ischemic heart disease (because atherosclerosis affects the coronary arteries as well as the cerebral vasculature). Septicemia does not usually occur after a stroke.

7–26 Answer A

Generalized absence seizures (petit mal seizures) almost always occur in children. With generalized absence seizures, there is usually no aura or postictal state. The seizure usually lasts just a few seconds and consists of staring, accompanied by an altered mental state.

7–27 Answer D

When you ask a client to walk a straight line placing heel to toe, you are assessing the proprioceptive aspect of the nervous system, which controls posture, balance, and coordination. Assessing dermatomes and the major peripheral nerves tests sensory function. The cerebellum is one of the neural structures involved in proprioception and can be assessed by coordination functions. Cranial nerves are assessed in many ways, but not by walking.

7–28 Answer A

When you place a key in a client's hand while the client's eyes are closed and ask him or her to identify it, you are assessing stereognosis. Stereognosis is the ability to recognize objects by touching and manipulating them. Graphesthesia is the ability to identify letters or numbers written on each palm with a blunt point. Two-point discrimination is the ability to sense whether one or two areas of the skin are being touched at the same time. Position sense (kinesthetic sensation) is the ability to recognize what position parts of the body are in when the eyes are closed, and is tested by actions such as moving a digit.

7–29 Answer A

A grade of 3+ for deep tendon reflexes indicates that the reflexes are brisker than normal, but is not necessarily indicative of disease. A grade of 4+ is brisk and hyperactive, with clonus of the tendon, and is associated with disease. A grade of 2+ is normal. A grade of 1+ is low normal, indicating a slightly diminished response. A grade of zero indicates that there is no reflex response.

7–30 Answer C

Syncope is a temporary loss of consciousness that is associated with an increased rate of respiration, tachycardia, pallor, perspiration, and coolness of the skin. Lethargy is drowsiness from which the client may be aroused; the client responds appropriately, then may immediately fall asleep again. Delirium is confusion, with disordered perception and a decreased attention span. Delirium may also involve motor and sensory excitement, inappropriate reactions to stimuli, and marked anxiety. A fugue state is a dysfunction of consciousness in which the individual carries on purposeful activity that he or she does not remember afterward.

7–31 Answer A

The facial nerve (cranial nerve [CN] VII) is tested by applying a small amount of sugar or salt to the anterior two-thirds of the tongue. Sensory function of the trigeminal nerve (CN V) is tested by tactile and pain sensation in all three divisions on the face. The motor function is tested by feeling the two masseter muscles as the client bites down. The abducens nerve (CN VI) is tested by extraocular eye movements. The motor portion of the glossopharyngeal nerve (CN IX) is tested by touching the pharynx with a cotton applicator, and the sensory portion is tested by taste on the posterior third of the tongue.

7–32 Answer B

Cranial nerve (CN) XI is the accessory nerve. It is tested by having the client shrug his or her shoulders while you resist the movement. Having the client say "ah" tests CN X, the vagus nerve. Having the client stick out his or her tongue and move it from side to side tests CN XII, the hypoglossal nerve. Touching the pharynx with a cotton applicator tests CN IX, the glossopharyngeal nerve.

7–33 Answer D

Alternately touching the nose with the index finger of each hand and repeating the motion faster and faster with the eyes closed tests cerebellar function, which integrates muscle contractions to maintain posture. Cranial nerve (CN) X is assessed by eliciting the gag reflex and observing for uvula movement, CN XI by checking for the strength of the trapezius muscles, and CN XII by assessing tongue movement.

7–34 Answer D

Remote memory is verbalized after hours, days, or years and may be assessed by asking a client his or her mother's maiden name. Asking questions about things that happened today, such as how long the client has been at your office, what time the client arrived, and what he or she ate for breakfast, tests recent memory.

7–35 Answer A

Asking the client the meaning of a familiar proverb assesses abstraction ability. It must be kept in mind that many proverbs are culturally derived, and the client may not have heard them before. Asking the client to subtract numbers tests computational ability. Asking clients what they think is the best treatment for their problem elicits information about their mental representation or beliefs about the illness. Asking clients what they would do if a fire broke out in a restaurant assesses their judgment.

7–36 Answer C

The Glasgow coma scale is an assessment tool that rates the level of consciousness by assigning a numerical score to the behavioral components of eye opening, verbal response, and motor response. The Mini-Mental State Examination (MMSE) tests orientation, registration, attention and calculation, recall, and language. Brudzinski's sign tests nuchal rigidity, which indicates meningeal irritation. The CAGE questionnaire is a screening tool for alcoholism.

7–37 Answer B

Anosmia is the inability to smell. Hyposmia is a diminished sense of smell. Ageusia is the loss of the sensation of taste or the ability to discriminate sweet, sour, salty, and bitter tastes. Agnosia is the inability to discriminate sensory stimuli.

7–38 Answer B

Although all the questions are important, suicidal ideation is an emergency situation, and if it is present, the client needs immediate admission, preferably to a psychiatric hospital. The next most appropriate question would be to ask him what he thinks is causing the problem, but certainly assessing suicide risk takes priority.

7–39 Answer A

Obsessive-compulsive disorder symptoms usually occur before age 15. Young people in their early teens with obsessive-compulsive disorder are inflexible, lack spontaneity, are ambivalent, and are in a constant state of conflict while harboring hostile feelings. The condition is manifested in this age group when parents of these individuals expect their children to live up to their expectations and condemn them if they fail to achieve the imposed standards of conduct.

7–40 Answer C

The medication of choice for obsessive-compulsive disorders is clomipramine (Anafranil), a tricyclic antidepressant. It seems to have a much better effect than alprazolam (Xanax), an antianxiety agent; carbamazepine (Tegretol), an anticonvulsant; or buspirone (Buspar), a nonbenzodiazepine anxiolytic.

7–41 Answer D

Hallucinations are not extrapyramidal symptoms. Extrapyramidal side effects of antipsychotic medications include akathisia (continuous restlessness and fidgeting); dystonia (involuntary muscular movements or spasms of the face, arms, legs, and neck); and parkinsonism (tremors, shuffling gait, drooling, and rigidity, all characteristic of Parkinson's disease).

7–42 Answer C

Methylphenidate (Ritalin) is a central nervous system stimulant commonly used for children with attention deficit-hyperactivity disorder (ADHD). Drugs used to counteract extrapyramidal side effects include anticholinergic agents, such as benztropine (Cogentin) and trihexyphenidyl (Artane), and dopaminergic agonists such as amantadine (Symmetrel).

7–43 Answer C

Altered mental status is the most sensitive indicator of increased intracranial pressure and is the first symptom to change as the pressure rises. As the pressure continues to rise, brainstem herniation occurs, along with dilatation of the pupil, hyperventilation, and focal neurological signs such as hemiparesis.

7–44 Answer A

Temporal arteritis, also called giant cell arteritis, presents as a systemic illness with generalized symptoms such as fever, myalgia, arthralgia, anemia, and elevated liver function tests. The headache is a new, mild to moderate one with diffuse pain, not necessarily confined to the temples or frontal region of the head. The erythrocyte sedimentation rate, which can be used as a screening tool, is usually very elevated (greater than 100 mm/min). A temporal artery biopsy shows granulomatous arteritis. A client with meningitis would show signs of irritation of the brain and meninges, such as a stiff neck. The client with subarachnoid and intracerebral hemorrhage would have an altered mental status.

7–45 Answer D

An electroencephalogram (EEG) is not useful in the routine evaluation of George's headache. His headache is most likely a tension headache because it is a weekly occurrence. A CT scan or MRI study is only recommended if the headache pattern is atypical, has changed in pattern, or is accompanied by other symptoms. The nurse practitioner should discuss with George strategies to avoid possible triggers, how to abort an attack, how to obtain relief from pain, and how to decrease the frequency and severity of attacks. The initial focus should be on the use of NSAIDs, cool compresses, and stress reduction techniques.

7–46 Answer D

Hypertension in the majority of cases in older adults with strokes is the body's attempt to maintain perfusion. More than two-thirds of these clients become normotensive without any intervention within several days after the stroke. If they had been treated, they would have become hypotensive. If the systolic blood pressure (BP) is greater than 220 mm Hg in a client with an ischemic stroke, treatment should be considered.

7–47 Answer C

When a diagnosis of encopresis is made, a physical exam should rule out a neurological disorder affecting the lumbosacral spinal cord. Encopresis, repeated involuntary defecation into the clothing, is more common in boys, usually over 4 years of age. Almost half of the children with this condition have abnormal or prolonged external anal sphincter contraction while straining to defecate.

7–48 Answer A

Ticlopidine (Ticlid), an antiplatelet agent, has been shown to be effective in preventing recurrent strokes in clients with transient ischemic attacks (TIAs) or mild strokes. It is a little more effective than aspirin in preventing recurrent strokes in clients with TIAs and those with moderate or large strokes. The benefit of aspirin in women has not been clearly proven. Aspirin also has more side effects than ticlopidine. The desired effect is decreased platelet aggregation rather than anticoagulation, which warfarin would accomplish. Nitroglycerin has no effect on platelets.

7–49 Answer B

A classic migraine (20% of all migraines) is preceded by either a visual aura, a sensory aura, unilateral weakness, or a speech disturbance. Tension headaches are not accompanied by nausea, vomiting, photophobia, or phonophobia. Cluster headaches occur more often in middle-aged men; cause severe unilateral orbital, supraorbital, or temporal pain; and occur in clusters on a seasonal basis, with 3- to 18-month periods of no headaches.

7–50 Answer C

Naproxen sodium (Anaprox DS) is a nonsteroidal anti-inflammatory drug (NSAID) that can cause gastrointestinal (GI) distress and must be taken with food. Ergot preparations such as Cafergot may cause nausea and vomiting, but not the GI distress caused by an NSAID. Sumatriptan may cause fatigue and drowsiness, and nadolol may cause hypotension and bradycardia, but neither causes GI distress.

7–51 Answer C

Of clients with generalized myasthenia gravis, 80–90% have antibodies to acetylcholine receptors. Electromyography nerve conduction tests are a way to categorize peripheral neuropathies as being demyelinating or axonal. A magnetic resonance imaging scan of the brain and brainstem is useful in helping to diagnose amyotrophic lateral sclerosis. A lumbar puncture is crucial in diagnosing suspected bacterial meningitis.

7–52 Answer C

Interferon B (Betaseron) was approved in 1993 for the treatment of multiple sclerosis because it decreases the frequency of exacerbations in clients with the relapsing-remitting type of multiple sclerosis. High-dose steroids (for acute exacerbations) and baclofen (Lioresal) or diazepam (Valium) (for excessive spasticity and spasms) were used before 1993. Benzodiazepines are ordered in a small dosage for anxiety.

7–53 Answer A

An astrocytoma is the most common primary intra-axial (within the substance of the brain) brain tumor. Pituitary adenoma, meningioma, and acoustic neuroma are the three most common extra-axial brain tumors arising from tissues surrounding the brain, such as the meninges or cranial nerves.

7–54 Answer B

Deficiency of vitamin B_{12} usually presents with an insidious onset of paresthesias of the hands and feet that are usually painful. A thiamine deficiency, commonly seen with chronic severe alcoholism or malabsorption, results in Wernicke-Korsakoff syndrome, which manifests as confusion, involuntary eye movements, and gait instability or ataxia. A folic acid deficiency results in neural tube defects in the fetus. A vitamin K deficiency results in coagulation disorders.

7–55 Answer B

A panic attack is characterized by its episodic nature. It is manifested by the sudden onset of intense apprehension, fear, or terror, and the abrupt development of some of the following symptoms: dyspnea, palpitations, chest pain or discomfort, choking or smothering sensations, dizziness, a feeling of being detached, diaphoresis, trembling, and nausea. All of these peak within 10 minutes. Anxiety is manifested for longer periods of time. Although depression may involve some psychomotor agitation—either irritability or anxiety—usually there is decreased energy, lack of motivation, fatigue in the morning, and depressed affect. Agoraphobia is fear of leaving the house because of the association of panic attacks with associated environmental cues.

7–56 Answer D

A phobia is the persistent and irrational fear of a specific object, activity, or situation that results in the compelling desire to avoid the dreaded object, activity, or situation. A depressed person has feelings of hopelessness and helplessness and has no energy to "fight off" the cause of the fear. An obsession is a recurrent and persistent thought or desire, whereas a compulsion is an uncontrollable urge to perform some repetitive and stereotyped action. Agoraphobia is fear of leaving the house or of open spaces.

7–57 Answer D

Clients with post-traumatic stress disorder (PTSD) have experienced some severe catastrophic event (in this case, rape) and re-experience the event by having recurrent, often intrusive images of the trauma and recurrent dreams or nightmares of the event. Clients frequently have combinations of symptoms of PTSD, panic disorder, and major depression, all relating to the initial traumatic stress event.

7–58 Answer C

A client's intent or commitment to the act of suicide by means of a plan suggests a high risk of actually committing the act. A client is at high risk if he or she has a definite plan, considers using more than one method at a time, and has made preparations for death. Also at high risk is the client who is impulsive, psychotic, or frequently intoxicated.

7–59 Answer C

In the depressed client, antidepressants are most effective in alleviating sleep and appetite disturbances. Psychotherapy is most effective in dealing with suicidal feelings and interpersonal problems.

7–60 Answer B

The two most common causes of dementia in older adults are dementia of the Alzheimer type (Alzheimer's disease) and vascular disorders such as hypertension, atherosclerosis, vasculitis, embolic disease, and cardiac disease. Polypharmacy, nutritional disorders, metabolic disorders, space-occupying lesions, and infections affecting the brain are all additional causes of dementia that can be removed or reversed.

7–61 Answer D

The most sensitive diagnostic test for identifying an alcoholic client is the g-glutamyltransferase (GGT) test. GGT is an enzyme produced in the liver after consumption of five or more drinks daily. A GGT of more than 40 units indicates alcoholism. The assay is 70% sensitive and has a similar specificity. The aspartate transaminase, mean corpuscular volume, and alkaline phosphatase levels are all increased in clients who are alcoholics, but the level of sensitivity and specificity is not as impressive as the GTT.

7–62 Answer A

If you suspect that your client abuses alcohol, the most appropriate action would be to confront the client. The first confrontation may be met with one of many responses, but it "keeps the door open" for further conversations. The overall goal of all types of confrontation is to help the client understand the need for abstinence, then discuss interventions to assist with this goal. When the client denies alcoholism, one intervention is to have family and friends confront the client at the same time with reflections of how the client's alcohol problem has affected them personally.

7–63 Answer A

In a study on behavioral change related to cigarette smoking, the first stage is the precontemplation phase, during which the client should not be confronted with actually quitting, but be asked the safe question, "What would it take for you to consider quitting?" In the next stage, the contemplation stage, it would be appropriate to ask, "What would it take for you to quit now?" In the preparation stage, one might ask, "What technique do you think will work best for you?" In the action phase, the healthcare provider might ask, "What do you think will be your biggest challenge to quitting?" In the maintenance stage, when the client has stopped smoking for more than 6 months, it is appropriate to ask, "What have you learned about people, places, events, and emotions that make you want to smoke?"

7–64 Answer A

The Agency for Health Care Policy and Research recommends in their smoking cessation clinical practice guideline that providers ask and record the tobacco-use status of every client at every visit.

7–65 Answer C

Bupropion (Zyban), an aminoketone, has had some success as a smoking cessation aid, either by itself or in conjunction with nicotine patches or gum. Bupropion was first identified in a Virginia hospital under the trade name Wellbutrin. When used as an antidepressant, it also curbed clients' smoking desire. This led to further studies of the drug as a smoking cessation intervention. The trade name was then changed from Wellbutrin to Zyban. Oxazepam (Serax), clorazepate dipotassium (Tranxene), and alprazolam (Xanax) are all benzodiazepines that are helpful with anxiety.

7–66 Answer D

Marijuana tests positive in the urine for up to 30 days after a person stops smoking the drug.

7–67 Answer A

A hypoactive or weaker than normal reflex is scored as 1+. It is present with lower motor neuron involvement, as in a slipped lumbar disk or spinal cord injuries. Hyperactive reflexes, scored as 3+ or 4+, are present with lesions of upper motor neurons, such as a cerebrovascular accident. A normal reflex is scored as 2+.

7–68 Answer A

The position with the client supine, flexing the head to the chest, is referred to as Brudzinski's sign. Pain, resistance, and flexion of the hips and knees occurs with meningeal irritation. Kernig's sign, which also tests for meningeal irritation when there is excessive pain or resistance, is assessed when the client lies supine, the knees and hips are flexed, and then the knee is straightened. Decorticate posturing occurs with lesions of the corticospinal tracts. Decerebrate posturing occurs with lesions of the midbrain, pons, or diencephalon.

7–69 Answer C

When you move a client's head to the left and the eyes move to the right in relation to the head, this is referred to as doll's eyes. This is the normal response to passive head movement and is an indicator of brainstem function. Doll's eyes are absent when the eyes fail to turn together and eventually remain fixed in the midposition as the head is turned to the side.

7–70 Answer B

A subdural hematoma is the most common of the intracranial hematomas, occurring in 10–15% of all head injuries. Clients present with headache, drowsiness, agitation, slowed thinking, and confusion. Epidural hematomas occur in 2–3% of all head injuries. The client usually has a momentary loss of consciousness followed by a lucid period lasting from a few hours to 1–2 days. There is then a rapid deterioration in the level of consciousness. An intracerebral hematoma occurs in 2–3% of all head injuries. The client presents with a headache, consciousness deteriorating to deep coma, and hemiplegia on the contralateral side.

7–71 Answer C

A spinal cord injury at the level of C6 allows clients to self-transfer to a wheelchair. Clients can use their shoulders and extend their wrists but have no finger control. An injury at the level of C4 would involve some sensation in the head and neck and some control of the neck and diaphragm. Mobility is restricted. An injury at the level of C5 would allow clients to control their head, neck, and shoulders and flex their elbows, but they would not be able to self-transfer from the wheelchair to the bed. An injury at C7–C8 would allow clients to extend their elbows, flex their wrists, and have some use of their fingers. They would be able to use a manual wheelchair.

7–72 Answer A

The diagnosis of multiple sclerosis (MS) is often difficult given the large variety of symptoms, but is a strong possibility in this case. Generally, clients age 20–40 who have had two separate lesions in the central nervous system at two separate times have a strong likelihood of having MS. The most common symptoms of MS include focal weakness, optic neuritis, focal numbness, cerebellar ataxia, diplopia, nystagmus, and bowel and bladder changes.

7–73 Answer B

Clients with Parkinson's disease may exhibit "cogwheel rigidity," a condition where there is an increased resistance in muscle tone when the nurse practitioner moves the client's neck, trunk, or limbs. The muscle is stiff and difficult to move. There is a ratchetlike, rhythmic contraction on passive stretching, particularly in the hands.

7–74 Answer B

Fetal alcohol syndrome is most often responsible for developmental delays in children. In descending order, the others are cerebral palsy, Down syndrome, and meningomyelocele.

7–75 Answer C

Bromocriptine and pergolide mimic dopamine. The other mechanisms of antiparkinsonian treatments are as follows: anticholinergics restore acetylcholine-dopamine balance; levodopa restores striatal dopamine; and tolcapone and entacapone reduce systemic degradation of oral dopamine.

7–76 Answer B

A ruptured intervertebral disk at the L5–S1 level affects the first sacral nerve root. The client would have pain in the midgluteal region as well as the posterior thigh and calf to heel area; paresthesias in the posterior calf and lateral heel, foot, and toes; and difficulty walking on the toes. When the L4–5 level (fifth lumbar nerve root) is affected, it manifests as pain in the hip, lower back, posterolateral thigh, anterior leg, dorsal surface of the foot, and great toe. In addition, there would be muscle spasms, paresthesia over the lateral leg and web of the great toe, and decreased or absent ankle reflexes. When the C5–6 level is affected (sixth cervical nerve root), there is pain in the neck, shoulder, anterior upper arm, and radial area of the forearm and thumb; paresthesias of the forearm, thumb, forefinger, and lateral arm; a decreased biceps and supinator reflex; and a triceps reflex that is normal to hyperactive.

7–77 Answer C

A foraminotomy is an enlargement of the opening between the disk and the facet joint to remove bony overgrowth compressing the nerve. A laminectomy is the removal of a part of the vertebral lamina. It relieves pressure on the nerves. A diskectomy is the removal of the nucleus pulposus of an intervertebral disk. Chemonucleolysis is the injection of the enzyme chymopapain into the nucleus pulposus. It hydrolyzes the nucleus pulposus, thus decreasing the size of the protruding herniation.

7–78 Answer B

Sundowning is a common behavioral change in clients with Alzheimer's disease. It is characterized by increased agitation, time disorientation, and wandering behaviors during the afternoon and evening hours. It is frequently worse on overcast days.

7–79 Answer B

It is expected that Marian might be depressed because of her multiple sclerosis (MS). Focusing more on what she has "going for her" rather than the type of MS she has should be the first response. At least partial recovery from acute exacerbations can reasonably be expected, although further relapses can occur. Some disability is likely to result eventually, but usually half of all clients live well without significant disability, even 10 years after the onset of symptoms.

There are many different clinical courses of MS. The chronic-relapsing type is only one type; however, it occurs in the highest percentage (40%) of all cases. In the chronic-relapsing clinical type, remissions are fewer and symptoms more disabling and cumulative between exacerbations compared to the exacerbating-remitting form. More symptoms are evident with each exacerbation. The other types of clinical courses, in descending frequency, are exacerbating-remitting (25%), in which attacks are more frequent and begin earlier, remissions are marked by less clearing of manifestations compared to the benign course, and the remissions last longer with stable manifestations between; benign (20%), in which there are minimum deficits from few mild exacerbations to total or nearly total return to the previous functioning; and chronic-progressive (15%) in which the onset is insidious, there are no remissions, and the disabilities become steadily more severe. It is slower in its progression than the chronic-relapsing type.

7–80 Answer B

Plasmapheresis, or plasma exchange, has successfully induced remission in some clients with multiple sclerosis when used with adrenocorticotropic hormone therapy or other pharmacological therapy. Plasmapheresis is a procedure that removes the plasma component from whole blood, with the goal being to remove inflammatory agents, such as T lymphocytes, through exchanging plasma while suppressing the immune response and inflammation.

7–81 Answer C

A thymectomy is performed in approximately 75% of clients with myasthenia gravis because of dysplasia of the thymus gland. It is usually recommended within 2 years after diagnosis. The thymus gland is usually inactive after puberty, but in about 75% of clients with myasthenia gravis, the gland continues to produce antibodies because of hyperplasia of the gland or tumors. The thymus is a source of autoantigen that triggers an autoimmune response in clients with myasthenia gravis.

7–82 Answer C

Guillain-Barré syndrome (GBS) is an acute demyelinating disorder. It is a peripheral nervous system disorder that usually follows a viral respiratory or gastrointestinal infection. Cytomegalovirus, herpes zoster, and sometimes general anesthesia have been associated with the development of GBS. Trigeminal neuralgia is a chronic disease of the trigeminal cranial nerve.

7–83 Answer C

To help differentiate between depression and dementia, keep in mind that the person with dementia tries to hide problems concerning memory, whereas the person with depression complains about memory and discusses the fact that there is a problem with memory. Also, with depression there is usually a time-specific onset, and affected clients tend to be apathetic and withdrawn and have a poor self-image.

7–84 Answer A

Clients with senile dementia of the Alzheimer's type (SDAT) commonly die of pneumonia (the most common cause of death of clients with Alzheimer's disease). Clients with late-stage Alzheimer's disease have problems related to immobility and usually develop pressure sores. They also have a poor nutritional status and may develop malnutrition. Depressed clients are at more risk for suicide than demented clients.

7–85 Answer B

With the quadriplegic client, the most effective program to stimulate the rectum to evacuate is to insert a rectal suppository, then eventually perform digital stimulation. The rectum will expel a rectal suppository along with the contents of the sigmoid colon. The bowel can be trained by using this stimulus, and eventually all that will be needed will be a digital stimulus. Occasionally, digital evacuation may be necessary. Increasing fluids and roughage in the diet are also part of a bowel program, along with occasional stool softeners or laxatives and, rarely, an enema.

7–86 Answer A

A low cerebrospinal fluid (CSF) glucose level may indicate a specific central nervous system infection such as meningitis. The normal CSF glucose level is 45–80 mg/dL, which is about 20 mg/dL less than the serum glucose level. An elevated CSF pressure may be the result of several problems, not specifically a CNS infection. A few red blood cells in the CSF may be a result of the procedure of the lumbar puncture. Elevated white blood cell levels may be the result of any number of infections, not specifically in the CNS.

7–87 Answer B

A rhizotomy, the surgical severing of a nerve root, performed on the trigeminal nerve, may be performed for the client with tic douloureux (trigeminal neuralgia) if pharmacological treatment is not successful. There is no evidence that surgical decompression of the facial nerve is helpful in Bell's palsy. Surgical implantation of adrenal medullary or specific fetal tissue into the caudate nucleus has been tried in Parkinson's disease with mixed results. A thymectomy is performed in 75% of the clients with myasthenia gravis.

7–88 Answer A

Mental defense mechanisms are the first line of protection or defense against an increase in anxiety. Serotonin is the central mood regulator neurotransmitter. A panic attack is the highest anxiety level. Immature, ineffective defenses such as denial reduce anxiety but undermine effective coping.

7–89 Answer A

A client with Ménière's disease presents with episodic attacks of severe vertigo, usually with associated ear fullness or hearing loss. The duration of the attacks is usually several hours, and the client is well before and after the attack unless hearing loss progresses and persists. The diagnosis is based on a typical history with recurrences. Treatment involves a low-sodium diet, diuretics, and possibly surgery. Vestibular neuronitis has an acute onset with severe vertigo, and sometimes follows a viral respiratory infection. Benign paroxysmal positional vertigo is paroxysmal, brief, and purely positional vertigo. Otosclerosis involves progressive hearing loss, sometimes with intermittent vertigo.

7–90 Answer B

A compulsive eater engages in uncontrolled eating, like the client with bulimia, but does not purge (induce vomiting). Clients with anorexia have an absence of or irregular menstruation. Clients with bulimia have tooth and gum erosion from frequent exposure to gastric enzymes through vomiting. Clients with anorexia and bulimia have compulsive exercising habits; compulsive eaters do not. It is important to distinguish among the types of eating disorders because their treatment differs.

7–91 Answer C

Clients with eating disorders tend to have low self-esteem. Other factors that appear to increase the risk for an eating disorder include female gender, young age, perfectionist personality, family history of eating disorders, attempts to diet, depression, and living in cultures in which thinness is a standard of beauty.

7–92 Answer D

If you suspect anorexia, the best initial approach is to confront Julie with the fact that you suspect an eating disorder. Clients are usually aware that a problem exists but need the extra "push" that confrontation provides. Once they accept the diagnosis, proven treatments include medical monitoring; nutritional counseling; psychotherapy, including behavioral therapy, family counseling, and stress-reduction techniques; medications; and support group participation.

7–93 Answer B

When a client states, "It's the worst headache I've ever had," it is noteworthy. Other findings suggestive of serious underlying causes of headaches include advanced age, onset with exertion, decreased alertness or cognition, radiation of the pain to between the shoulder blades (suggesting spinal arachnoid irritation), nuchal rigidity, any historical or physical abnormality suggesting infection, and worsening under observation.

7–94 Answer B

The Hallpike maneuver is performed to elicit vertigo. It evaluates the effect of head position on the elicitation of vertigo. The client sits with the head to one side with eyes open. The examiner grasps the head and quickly assists the client to a supine position with the head hanging below the level of the table. After 30 seconds, the client is quickly assisted back to the sitting position, the head is rotated to the other side, and the maneuver repeated. Vertigo will be apparent in clients with a peripheral, but not central, cause of vertigo.

7–95 Answer B

Elizabeth Kübler-Ross's stages of anticipatory grieving are shock, denial, anger, bargaining, depression, and acceptance. Each person goes through each stage at his or her own rate, but the stages vary little from person to person.

7–96 Answer A

The CAGE instrument is a widely used questionnaire that has a high degree of accuracy for identifying clients who abuse alcohol. CAGE is an acronym for four questions: the C stands for, "Have you ever felt you should *cut* down on drinking?"; the A for, "Have people *annoyed* you by criticizing your drinking"; the G for "Have you felt bad or *guilty* about your drinking"; and the E for "Have you had a drink first thing in the morning (an "*eye opener*") to steady your nerves or to get rid of a hangover?" There are no such measurements as the HEAT instrument or the DRINK tool. The MMSE is the Mini-Mental State Examination, which can help determine the degree of confusion and therefore help to isolate possible causes.

7–97 Answer B

Any medication that is taken more than three times a week for migraines has the potential for creating daily or "rebound" headaches. The worst offender seems to be ergotamine tartrate.

7–98 Answer A

Beta blockers and calcium channel blockers may be used in the treatment of migraine headaches. Beta blockers, by blocking beta receptors, prevent arterial dilatation. Propranolol (Inderal) is the most frequently prescribed of the beta blockers. Calcium channel blockers are also used to treat migraine headaches by inhibiting arterial vasospasm and blocking the release of serotonin platelets. They also affect cerebral blood flow, neurotransmission, and neuroreceptor blockade to assist in preventing migraines. Verapamil (Calan) is probably the best known of the calcium channel blockers used for this purpose.

7–99 Answer A

Hot showers may exacerbate the symptoms of multiple sclerosis. For the same reason, fevers should be controlled. Teaching points would include avoiding hot showers, controlling fevers, encouraging exercise and plenty of rest, and seeking psychological and emotional support.

7–100 Answer C

The FAQ (Functional Activities Questionnaire) is a measure of functional activities. There are 10 complex, higher-order activities that are appropriate for the initial assessment of Alzheimer's disease. The MMSE (Mini-Mental State Exam) is a test of cognition. The CAGE questionnaire is a screening tool for alcoholism. The Holmes and Rahe Social Readjustment Scale measures major life changes for identifying the impact of stress on an individual.

7–101 Answer D

Sixty percent of clients suffer major depression during their first year after a stroke. Other depressive symptoms as well as major depression may also occur, although usually less often, with thyroid disorders, Parkinson's disease, heart disease, and dementia.

7–102 Answer D

Direct confrontation should be used when suspecting depression and the possibility of suicide. Fatigue, loss of weight, and insomnia, in combination with the client's history of the death of his spouse should point in the direction of depression with a suicidal potential. Suicidal ideation and plans should be asked as well as the availability of companionship and support. Older white men have the highest incidence of suicide among the entire adult population.

7–103 Answer A

The gait of sensory ataxia includes brusqueness of movements of the leg and stamping of the feet. A Parkinsonian gait involves the trunk bent forward, arms slightly flexed, with an unsteady gait, particularly with turning. The legs are stiff and bent at the knees and hips. The client shuffles forward with an accelerating gait known as festination. An antalgic gait occurs with osteoarthritis of the hip, which causes functional shortening of the leg and produces a characteristic limp. A cerebellar gait is unsteady, with a wide-based stride and an irregular swinging of the trunk. It is more prominent when rising from a chair or turning suddenly.

7–104 Answer A

A client's signs and symptoms may lead the practitioner to suspect which part of the brain has been occluded. The basilar artery branches supply the occipital and temporal lobes, the dorsal surface of the thalamus, the upper part of the cerebellum, and the midbrain. This would result in the client exhibiting limb paralysis, nystagmus, vertigo, nausea, slurred speech, and cerebellar ataxia. The internal carotid artery supplies the anterior cerebral surfaces and an occlusion here would result in unilateral sensory and motor disturbances, visual disturbances, and aphasia with a left-sided lesion. An occlusion of the posterior cerebral surfaces would result in an ipsilateral visual field deficit, contralateral hemiplegia, bilateral motor, sensory, and visual complaints, vertigo, diplopia, and dysphagia. Occlusion of parts of the medulla would result in contralateral impairment of pain and temperature sensation, dysphagia, and vertigo

7–105 Answer C

Viral encephalitis is the most common type of encephalitis with a progressive altered level of consciousness, seizures, motor weakness, and headache. Herpes simplex virus and microbial encephalitis are other major types of encephalitis. Pneumococcal is a type of meningitis.

7–106 Answer C

The peripheral facial palsy of Bell's palsy is self-limiting, and complete recovery usually occurs in several weeks or months in the majority of cases. To cope with self-esteem, clients may be encouraged to change their hairstyle, and men may also be encouraged to grow a beard or mustache. There is no suppressive drug therapy. A course of acyclovir may be ordered. Taking prednisone for 10 days has been found to shorten the recovery period and help with symptoms. Long-term therapy is not warranted because the condition is self-limiting.

Bibliography

Bruckenthal, P: A guide to the diagnosis and management of migraine headaches for the nurse practitioner. Am J Nurs Pract 1:3, 1997.

Clark, CC: Posttraumatic stress disorder: How to support healing. Am J Nurs 97:8, 27, 1997.

Dunphy, L, and Winland-Brown, JE: Primary Care: The Art and Science of Advanced Practice Nursing. FA Davis, Philadelphia, 2001.

Epstein, D: Battling eating disorders: A lifelong struggle you can win. The Female Patient: Total Health Care for Women 8:6, 1997.

Fortinash, KM, and Holoday-Worret, PA: Psychiatric Mental Health Nursing. Mosby, St Louis, 2000.

Frozena, C: Multiple sclerosis. Am J Nurs 97:11, 1997.

Ham, RJ, et al.: Primary Care Geriatrics, ed 4. Mosby, St Louis, 2002.

Houde, SC, and Kampee-Leacher, R: Chronic fatigue syndrome: An update for clinicians in primary care. Nurse Pract 22:7, 1997.

McCrone, S: Issues in the measurement of depression in older adults with medical illnesses. Am J Nurs Pract 1:2, 1997.

Mestel, R: Insomnia. Hippocrates 11:9, 1997.

Shea, CA, et al.: Breaking through the barriers to domestic violence intervention. Am J Nurs 97:6, 1997.

Smith, RB: Headache management made painless. Hosp Pract 32:9, 1997.

Tapper, VJ: Pathophysiology, assessment, and treatment of Parkinson's disease. Nurse Pract 22:7, 1997.

Volmink, J, et al.: Treatments for postherpetic neuralgia: A systematic review of randomized controlled trials. Fam Pract 13:84, 1996.

HOW WELL DID YOU DO?
85% AND ABOVE CONGRATULATIONS! THIS SCORE SHOWS APPLICATION OF TEST-TAKING PRINCIPLES AND ADEQUATE CONTENT KNOWLEDGE.
75–85% KEEP WORKING! REVIEW TEST-TAKING PRINCIPLES AND TRY AGAIN.
65–75% HANG IN THERE! SPEND SOME TIME REVIEWING CONCEPTS AND TEST-TAKING PRINCIPLES AND THEN TRY THE TEST AGAIN.

Integumentary Problems

8

JILL E. WINLAND-BROWN

8–1 *The ABCDs of melanoma identification include all the following* ***except:***

A. A (asymmetry): one half does not match the other half.
B. B (birthmark): recently changed in appearance.
C. C (color): pigmentation is not uniform; there may be shades of tan, brown, and black as well as red, white, and blue.
D. D (diameter): greater than 6 mm.

8–2 *The connection between the surface of the skin and an underlying structure is called a(n):*

A. ulcer.
B. sinus.
C. erosion.
D. abscess.

8–3 *A Wood's light is especially useful in diagnosing:*

A. tinea versicolor.
B. herpes zoster.
C. a decubitus ulcer.
D. a melanoma.

8–4 *A darkfield microscopic examination is used to diagnose:*

A. scabies.
B. leprosy.
C. syphilis.
D. *Candida* infections.

8–5 *Jane is the 26-year-old Asian mother of Alysia, age 2 months. She is concerned about the large blue spot covering her infant's entire right lower leg. Jane tells you that Alysia was born with the spot. You tell her that:*

A. when the infant reaches her adult height, the macule can be surgically removed.
B. she should take the infant immediately to a plastic surgeon because this is a rare cancerous lesion.
C. this is a mongolian spot. It is common in Asians and blacks and no treatment is necessary because it will fade with age.
D. she should always keep the spot covered because sunlight will aggravate it.

8–6 *All of the following statements about malignant melanomas are true* ***except:***

A. they usually occur in middle-aged adults of both sexes.
B. the client usually has a family history of melanoma.
C. they are common in blacks.
D. the prognosis is directly related to the thickness of the lesions.

8–7 *Stephen, age 18, presents with a pruritic rash on his upper trunk and shoulders. You observe flat to slightly elevated brown papules and plaques that scale when they are rubbed. You also note areas of hypopigmentation. Your initial diagnosis is:*

A. lentigo syndrome.
B. tinea versicolor.
C. localized brown macules.
D. ochronosis.

8–8 *A client with a platelet abnormality may present with:*

A. red to blue macular plaques.
B. multiple frecklelike macular lesions in sun-exposed areas.
C. numerous small, brown, nonscaly macules that become more prominent with sun exposure.
D. red, flat, nonblanchable petechiae.

8–9 *Which disease usually starts on the cheeks and spreads to the arms and trunk?*

A. Erythema infectiosum (fifth disease)
B. Rocky Mountain spotted fever
C. Rubeola
D. Rubella

8–10 *Debbie, age 29, has a high fever and red, warm, sharply marginated plaques on the right side of her face that are indurated and painful. You diagnose erysipelas. What treatment do you begin?*

A. Systemic steroids
B. Topical steroids
C. Systemic antibiotics
D. Nonsteroidal anti-inflammatory drugs

8–11 *Lance, age 50, is complaining of an itchy rash that occurred about $^1/_2$ hour after putting on his leather jacket. He recalls a slightly similar rash last year when he wore his jacket. The annular lesions are on his neck and both arms. They are erythematous, sharply circumscribed, and both flat and elevated. His voice seems a little raspy, although he states that his breathing is normal. What is your first action?*

A. Order a short course of systemic corticosteroids.
B. Determine the need for 0.5 mL 1:1000 epinephrine subcutaneously.
C. Start daily antihistamines.
D. Tell Lance to get rid of his leather jacket.

8–12 *Margaret, age 32, comes into the clinic. She has painful joints and a distinctive rash in a butterfly distribution on her face. The rash has red papules and plaques with a fine scale. You suspect:*

A. lymphocytoma cutis.
B. relapsing polychondritis.
C. systemic lupus erythematosus.
D. none of the above.

8–13 *Jennifer, age 32, has genital warts (condylomata) and would like to have them treated. All of the following could be applied* ***except:***

A. benzoyl peroxide.
B. podophyllum.
C. trichloroacetic acid.
D. liquid nitrogen.

8–14 *Johnny, age 12, just started taking amoxicillin for otitis media. His mother said that he woke up this morning with a rash on his trunk. What is your first action?*

A. Prescribe systemic antihistamines.
B. Prescribe a short course of systemic steroids.
C. Stop the amoxicillin.
D. Continue the drug; this reaction on the first day is normal.

8–15 *Jim, age 59, presents with recurrent, sharply circumscribed red papules and plaques with a powdery white scale on the extensor aspect of his elbows and knees. You suspect:*

A. actinic keratosis.
B. eczema.
C. psoriasis.
D. seborrheic dermatitis.

8–16 *What is a safe and effective treatment for psoriasis?*

A. Coal tar preparations
B. Topical steroids
C. Topical antibiotics
D. Systemic antihistamines

8–17 *A biopsy of a small, yellow-orange papulonodule on the eyelid will probably show:*

A. fragmented, calcified elastic tissue.
B. mature sebaceous glands.
C. lipid-laden cells.
D. endothelial swelling and an infiltrate rich in plasma cells.

8–18 *Permethrin (Elimite) applied over the body overnight from the neck down is the preferred treatment for:*

A. scabies.
B. eczema.
C. herpes simplex.
D. psoriasis.

8–19 *Elizabeth, age 83, presents with a 3-day history of pain and burning in the left forehead. This morning she noticed a rash with erythematous papules in that site. You suspect:*

A. varicella.
B. herpes zoster.
C. syphilis.
D. rubella.

8–20 *A 70-year-old client with herpes zoster has a vesicle on the tip of the nose. This may indicate:*

A. ophthalmic zoster.
B. herpes simplex.
C. Kaposi's sarcoma.
D. Orf and milker's nodules.

8–21 *Large, flaccid bullae with honey-colored crusts around the mouth and nose are characteristic of:*

A. a burn.
B. Rocky Mountain spotted fever.
C. measles.
D. impetigo.

8–22 *Balanitis is associated with:*

A. diabetes.

B. macular degeneration.
C. *Candida* infection of the penis.
D. measles.

8–23 *Steve, age 29, has a carbuncle on his neck. After an incision and drainage (I&D), an antibiotic is ordered. What is the most common organism involved?*

A. Streptococcus
B. *Moraxella catarrhalis*
C. *Staphylococcus aureus*
D. *Klebsiella*

8–24 *A Gram's stain of which lesion reveals large, square-ended, gram-positive rods that grow easily on blood agar?*

A. Dermatophyte infection
B. Tuberculosis (scrofuloderma)
C. Sarcoidosis
D. Anthrax

8–25 *Sidney, age 72, has just been diagnosed with temporal arteritis. What do you prescribe?*

A. Systemic corticosteroids
B. Topical corticosteroids
C. Antibiotics
D. Antifungal preparations

8–26 *Jamie, age 6, was bitten by a dog. Her mother asks you if the child needs antirabies treatment. You tell her:*

A. "If the dog was a domestic pet that had been vaccinated, the wound should be cleaned and irrigated."
B. "Antirabies treatment must be started immediately."
C. "Rabies can be contracted only through the bites of wild animals."
D. "Wait until you have observed the animal for 2 weeks to determine if it is rabid."

8–27 *Sophie brings in her husband, Nathan, age 72, who is in a wheelchair. On his sacral area he has a deep crater with full-thickness skin loss involving necrosis of subcutaneous tissue that extends down to the underlying fascia. Which pressure ulcer stage is this?*

A. Stage I
B. Stage II
C. Stage III
D. Stage IV

8–28 *The purpose of a transparent dressing such as Tegaderm applied over a pressure ulcer is to:*

A. toughen intact skin and preserve skin integrity.
B. prevent skin breakdown and the entrance of moisture and bacteria, but allow permeability of oxygen and moisture vapor.
C. allow necrotic material to soften.
D. use the proteolytic enzymes in the dressing to serve as a débriding agent.

8–29 *Treatment for a stage I pressure ulcer may include:*

A. an enzymatic preparation.
B. systemic antibiotics.
C. surgical treatment with muscle flaps.
D. A transparent semipermeable membrane dressing.

8–30 *Which structure of the skin is responsible for storing melanin?*

A. Epidermis
B. Dermis
C. Sebaceous glands
D. Eccrine sweat glands

8–31 *When palpating the skin over the clavicle of James, age 84, you notice tenting. This is:*

A. indicative of dehydration.
B. common in thin older adults.
C. a sign of edema.
D. indicative of scleroderma.

8–32 *Thin, spoon-shaped nails are usually seen in:*

A. trauma.
B. a fungal infection.
C. anemia.
D. psoriasis.

8–33 *A secondary skin lesion with a crust may be any of the following* ***except:***

A. eczema.
B. impetigo.
C. psoriasis.
D. herpes.

8–34 *A client with a nutritional deficiency of vitamin C may have:*

A. dry skin and loss of skin color.
B. thickened skin that is dry or rough.
C. flaky skin, sores in the mouth, and cracks at the corners of the mouth.
D. bleeding gums and delayed wound healing.

8–35 *Sandra, age 69, is complaining of dry skin. You advise her to:*

A. bathe every day.
B. use tepid water and a mild cleansing cream.
C. use a dehumidifier.
D. decrease the oral intake of fluids.

8–36 *Ultraviolet light therapy is used to treat psoriasis by:*

A. drying the lesions.

B. killing the bacteria.
C. decreasing the growth rate of epidermal cells.
D. killing the fungi.

8–37 *Mitch, age 18, has tinea pedis. You tell him all the following* ***except:***

A. "Dry between your toes every day."
B. "Wash your socks with bleach."
C. "Use an antifungal powder twice a day."
D. "Wear rubber shoes in the shower to prevent transmission to others."

8–38 *Abe, age 57, has just been given a diagnosis of herpes zoster. He asks you about exposure to others. You tell him that:*

A. once he has been on the medication for a full 24 hours, he is no longer contagious.
B. he should stay away from children and pregnant women who have not had chickenpox.
C. he should wait until the rash is completely gone before going out in crowds.
D. he should be isolated from all persons except his wife.

8–39 *Which form of acne is more common in the middle-aged to older adult and causes changes in skin color, enlarged pores, and thickening of the soft tissues of the nose?*

A. Acne vulgaris.
B. Acne rosacea.
C. Acne conglobata.
D. None of the above; acne does not occur at this age.

8–40 *An excessive amount of collagen that develops during scar formation is called a(n):*

A. keloid.
B. skin tag.
C. angioma.
D. keratosis.

8–41 *Nevi arise from:*

A. plugged follicles.
B. melanocytes.
C. capillary occlusion.
D. epithelium.

8–42 *Which skin lesions are directly related to chronic sun exposure and photodamage?*

A. Skin tags
B. Seborrheic keratoses
C. Actinic keratoses
D. Angiomas

8–43 *Samantha, age 52, has an acrochordon on her neck. She refers to this as a:*

A. nevus.
B. skin tag.
C. lipoma.
D. wart.

8–44 *A basal cell carcinoma is:*

A. an epithelial tumor that originates from either the basal layer of the epidermis or cells in the surrounding dermal structures.
B. a malignant tumor of the squamous epithelium of the skin or mucous membranes.
C. an overgrowth and thickening of the cornified epithelium.
D. lined with epithelium and contains fluid or a semisolid material.

8–45 *A noninvasive method of treating skin cancer (other than melanoma) that uses liquid nitrogen is:*

A. Mohs' micrographic surgery
B. curettage and electrodesiccation.
C. radiation therapy.
D. cryosurgery.

8–46 *Zinc oxide, magnesium silicate, ferric chloride, and kaolin are examples of:*

A. chemical sunscreens.
B. physical sunscreens.
C. agents used in tanning booths.
D. emollients.

8–47 *Amy, age 36, is planning to go skiing with her fiancé. He has warned her about frostbite and she is wondering what to do if frostbite should occur. You tell her she should do all the following* ***except:***

A. remove wet footwear if her feet are frostbitten.
B. rub the area with snow.
C. apply firm pressure with a warm hand to the area.
D. place the hands in the axillae if the hands are frostbitten.

8–48 *Susan states that her fiancé has been frostbitten on the nose while skiing and is fearful that it will happen again. You tell her:*

A. "Don't worry, as long as he gets medical help in the first few hours after being frostbitten again, he'll recover."
B. "Once frostbitten, he should not go out skiing again."
C. "If it should happen again, massage the nose with a dry hand."
D. "Infarction and necrosis of the affected tissue can happen with repeated frostbite."

8–49 *The total loss of hair on all parts of the body is referred to as:*

A. female pattern alopecia.
B. alopecia areata.
C. alopecia totalis.
D. alopecia universalis.

8–50 *All of the following medications may cause alopecia* ***except:***

A. warfarin (Coumadin).
B. minoxidil (Rogaine).
C. levonorgestrel (Norplant).
D. acetylsalicylic acid (aspirin).

8–51 *The morphology of which lesion begins as an inflammatory papule that develops within several days into a painless, hemorrhagic, and necrotic abscess, eventually with a dense, black, necrotic eschar forming over the initial lesion?*

A. Furuncle-carbuncle
B. Hidradenitis suppurativa
C. Anthrax
D. Cellulitis

8–52 *What is the initial emergency measure to limit burn severity?*

A. Stabilize the client's condition.
B. Identify the type of burn.
C. Prevent heat loss.
D. Eliminate the heat source.

8–53 *In a burn trauma, which blood measurement rises as a secondary result of hemoconcentration when fluid shifts from the intravascular compartment?*

A. Hemoglobin
B. Sodium
C. Hematocrit
D. Blood urea nitrogen (BUN)

8–54 *In burn trauma, silver sulfadiazine (Silvadene), a sulfonamide, is the most commonly used topical agent. What is its mechanism of action?*

A. A synthetic antibiotic that appears to interfere with the metabolism of bacterial cells
B. A bacteriostatic agent that inhibits a wide variety of gram-positive and gram-negative organisms by altering the microbial cell wall and membrane
C. A bactericidal agent that acts on the cell membrane and cell wall of susceptible bacteria and binds to cellular DNA
D. A protective covering that prevents light, air, and invading organisms from penetrating its surface

8–55 *Tanisha, a 24-year-old African-American mother of four young children, presents in the clinic today with varicella. She states that three of her children also have it and that her eruption started less than 24 hours ago. Which action may shorten the course of the disease in Tanisha?*

A. Calamine lotion
B. Cool baths
C. Acyclovir (Zovirax)
D. Corticosteroids

8–56 *Your 24-year-old client, whose varicella rash just erupted yesterday, asks you when she can go back to work. You tell her:*

A. "Once all the vesicles are crusted over."
B. "When the rash is entirely gone."
C. "Once you have been on medication for at least 48 hours."
D. "Now, as long as you stay away from children and pregnant women."

8–57 *Jack, age 59, has a nevus on his shoulder that has recently changed from brown to bluish black. You advise him to:*

A. have an excisional biopsy.
B. monitor the nevus for a change at the end of one month.
C. Apply benzoyl peroxide solution.
D. apply hydrocortisone 1% cream.

8–58 *John, age 58, is a farmer. He presents with a painful finger ulcer and a palpable olecranal lymph node. Suspecting an orf skin ulcer, you ask him if he works with:*

A. sheep and goats.
B. horses.
C. metals.
D. tile.

8–59 *All of the following are treatments for psoriasis* ***except:***

A. topical antifungals.
B. systemic medications.
C. phototherapy.
D. topical corticosteroids.

8–60 *The most common rosacea trigger is:*

A. alcohol.
B. cold weather.
C. skin care products.
D. sun exposure.

8–61 *The most effective treatment for urticaria is:*

A. an oral antihistamine.
B. dietary management.
C. avoidance of the offending agent.
D. a glucocorticosteroid.

8–62 *A linear arrangement along a nerve distribution is a description of which type of skin lesion?*

A. Annular
B. Zosteriform
C. Keratotic
D. Linear

8–63 *Pastia lines are present in:*

A. toxic shock syndrome.
B. Rocky Mountain spotted fever.

C. scarlet fever.
D. meningococcemia.

8–64 *The viral exanthem of Koplik's spots is present in:*

A. rubeola.
B. rubella.
C. fifth disease.
D. varicella.

8–65 *A darkfield examination is used to cutaneously diagnose:*

A. syphilis.
B. viral blisters.
C. scabies.
D. candidiasis.

8–66 *Which of the following secondary skin lesions usually results from chronic scratching or rubbing?*

A. Crusts
B. Scales
C. Lichenification
D. Atrophy

8–67 *Which skin lesion is morphologically classified as pustular?*

A. A wart
B. Impetigo
C. Herpes simplex
D. Acne rosacea

8–68 *The "herald patch" is present in almost all cases of:*

A. pityriasis rosea.
B. psoriasis.
C. impetigo.
D. rubella.

8–69 *The five Ps—purple, polygonal, planar, pruritic papules—are present in:*

A. ichthyosis.
B. lichen planus.
C. atopic dermatitis.
D. seborrheic dermatitis.

8–70 *Adverse effects from prolonged or high-potency topical corticosteroid use to an open lesion may include:*

A. epidermal proliferation.
B. striae.
C. vitiligo.
D. easy bruisability.

8–71 *Buddy, age 12, presents with annular lesions with a scaly border and central clearing on his trunk. What do you suspect?*

A. Psoriasis
B. Erythema multiforme
C. Tinea corporis
D. Syphilis

8–72 *Harry uses a high-potency corticosteroid cream for his dermatoses. You tell him the following:*

A. "You must use this for an extended period of time for it to be effective."
B. "It will work better if you occlude the lesion."
C. "It may exacerbate your concurrent condition of tinea corporis."
D. "Be sure to use it daily."

8–73 *Janine, age 29, has numerous transient lesions that come and go and is diagnosed with urticaria. You order the following:*

A. aspirin
B. nonsteroidal anti-inflammatory drugs
C. opioids
D. antihistamines

8–74 *What is the name of the acquired disorder characterized by complete loss of pigment of the involved skin?*

A. Tinea versicolor
B. Vitiligo
C. Tuberous sclerosis
D. Pityriasis alba

8–75 *Which is the drug of choice for tinea capitis?*

A. A topical corticosteroid
B. Oral griseofulvin (Grisactin)
C. A topical antifungal
D. An antibiotic

8–76 *Which of the following therapeutic modalities is not useful for the management of acute atopic dermatitis?*

A. Emollients
B. Compresses
C. Ultraviolet light
D. Tars

8–77 *A mother complains that her newborn infant lying on his or her side may appear red on the dependent side of the body while appearing pale on the upper side. When she picks up the baby, this coloring disappears. You explain to her about:*

A. a temporary hemangioma
B. Hyperbilirubinemia
C. Harlequin sign
D. Mongolian spots

8–78 *Suzanne has a 7-year-old daughter who has had two recent infestations of lice. She asks you what she can do to prevent this. You respond:*

A. "After two days of no head lice, her bedding is lice-free."
B. "Boys are more susceptible, so watch out for her brother also."
C. "After several infestations, she is now immune and is no longer susceptible."
D. "Don't let her share hats, combs, or brushes with anyone."

8–79 *Which treatment would you order for anogenital pruritus?*

A. Suppositories for pain
B. Antifungal cream for itching
C. A high-fiber diet for constipation
D. Zinc oxide ointment

8–80 *Persons with which skin phototype (SPT) sunburn easily after 30 minutes in the sun but never tan?*

A. SPT I
B. SPT II
C. SPT III
D. SPT IV

8–81 *The "gold standard" used to confirm the suspicion of a true food allergy (IgE reaction) in a young child is the:*

A. immediate-reacting IgE skin test.
B. food challenge.
C. double-blind, placebo-controlled food challenge.
D. diagnostic food diet diary and home challenge.

8–82 *Janice states that her son is allergic to eggs and she heard that he should not receive the flu vaccine. How do you respond?*

A. "Although measles, mumps, rubella, and influenza vaccines contain a minute amount of egg, most egg-allergic individuals can tolerate these vaccines without any problems."
B. "Most of the allergic reactions are caused by the actual vaccinations, therefore a skin test should be done first."
C. "You're right. We should not give this vaccination to your son."
D. "He should not have a skin test done if he has this allergy because a serious cellulitis may occur at the testing site."

8–83 *Dry, itchy skin in older adults results from:*

A. the reduction of sweat and oil glands.
B. loss of subcutaneous tissue.
C. dermal thinning.
D. decreased elasticity.

8–84 *Marie asks what she can do for Sarah, her 90-year-old mother, who has extremely dry skin. You respond:*

A. "After bathing every day, use a generous supply of moisturizers."
B. "Use a special moisturizing soap every day."
C. "Your mother does not need a bath every day."
D. "Increase your mother's intake of fluids."

8–85 *Clubbing is defined as:*

A. elongation of the toes.
B. broadening of each thumb.
C. a birth deformity of the feet.
D. a thickening and broadening of the ends of the fingers.

8–86 *The epitrochlear lymph node is located:*

A. in front of the ear.
B. halfway between the angle and the tip of the mandible.
C. in the posterior triangle along the edge of the trapezius muscle.
D. in the inner condyle of the humerus.

8–87 *Gouty pain in the great toe is:*

A. toe gout.
B. hyperuricemia of the toe.
C. podagra.
D. tophus.

8–88 *Jerry, age 52, has gout. You suggest:*

A. using salicylates for an acute attack.
B. limiting consumption of purine-rich foods.
C. testing his uric acid level every 6 months.
D. decreasing fluid intake.

8–89 *An eczematous skin reaction may result from:*

A. penicillin.
B. allopurinol (Zyloprim).
C. an oral contraceptive.
D. phenytoin (Dilantin).

8–90 *Mary just came from visiting her husband, Sam, age 82, who recently had an ileostomy resulting in a stoma. She did not think that Sam's stoma looked "right." You tell her that the color of the stoma should be:*

A. pale pink.
B. beefy red.
C. dark red or purple.
D. flesh-colored.

8–91 *Your client had a colostomy several weeks ago and is having difficulty finding a permanent appliance that fits. How long do you tell him to wait for the stoma to shrink before buying a permanent appliance?*

A. 2–4 weeks
B. 4–6 weeks

C. 6–8 weeks
D. Just over 2 months

8–92 *Silas, age 82, comes to your office with a fairly new colostomy. Around the stoma he has a papular rash with satellite lesions. What does this indicate?*

A. A fungal infection, usually *Candida albicans*
B. An allergic reaction to the appliance
C. A normal reaction to fecal drainage
D. A fluid volume deficit

8–93 *Which type of hemangioma in a newborn occurs on the nape of the neck and is usually not noticeable when it becomes covered by hair?*

A. Nevus flammeus (port-wine stain)
B. Stork's beak mark
C. Strawberry hemangioma
D. Cavernous hemangioma

8–94 *Which of the following is not one of the predisposing conditions for furunculosis?*

A. Diabetes mellitus
B. Hypertension
C. Human immunodeficiency virus (HIV)
D. Injectable drug use

8–95 *The treatment for thrush is:*

A. nystatin oral suspension for 2 weeks, 2–3 mL in each side of the mouth, held as long as possible.
B. clotrimazole oral troches (10 mg) 2 times per day for 7 days.
C. fluconazole (100 mg) twice daily for 1 week.
D. antiseptic mouth rinses after each meal.

8–96 *Justin, an obese 42-year-old, cut his right leg 3 days ago while climbing a ladder. Today his right lower leg is warm, reddened, and painful without a sharply demarcated border. You suspect:*

A. diabetic neuropathy.
B. cellulitis.
C. peripheral vascular disease.
D. a beginning stasis ulcer.

8–97 *Psoriasis may occur after months of using:*

A. vitamins.
B. hormone replacement therapy.
C. nonsteroidal anti-inflammatory drugs.
D. antihistamine nasal sprays.

8–98 *The drug of choice for acute anaphylaxis is:*

A. diphenhydramine (Benadryl) 25–100 mg PO qid for adults.
B. epinephrine 1:1000 subcutaneously (0.3–0.5 ml) for adults.
C. prednisone (2 mg/kg q 24 hours) PO in one initial daily dose, tapered off over 1 to 2 weeks.
D. amlodipine besylate (Norvasc) 5 mg qid for 4 weeks.

8–99 *What is the most important thing a woman can do to have youthful, attractive skin?*

A. Keep well hydrated.
B. Use sunscreen with an SPF of at least 45.
C. Avoid smoking.
D. Use mild defatted or glycerin soaps.

8–100 *The majority of malignant melanomas are:*

A. superficially spreading.
B. lentigo maligna.
C. acral-lentiginous.
D. nodular.

8-101 *Susie asks you about the "blackheads" on her face. You tell her these are referred to as:*

A. open comedones.
B. closed comedones.
C. papules.
D. pustules.

8–102 *Which of the following warts (HPV) looks like a cauliflower and is usually found in the anogenital region?*

A. Plantar warts
B. Filiform and digitate warts
C. Condyloma acuminata
D. Verruca plana

8–103 *Susan, a new mother, states that when she pushes her index finger on one of her baby's skull bones, it presses in and then returns to normal when she removes her finger. She is concerned about this. You tell her that it's common and is called:*

A. craniotabes
B. molding
C. caput succedaneum
D. cephalhematoma

8–104 *Candidiasis may occur in many parts of the body. James, age 29, has it in the glans of his penis. What is your diagnosis?*

A. Balanitis
B. Thrush
C. Candidal paronychia
D. Subungual candida

8–105 *Shelby has a blister filled with clear fluid on her arm. It is the result of contact with a hot iron. How do you document this?*

A. Bulla
B. Wheal

C. Cyst
D. Pustule

8–106 *You are teaching Harvey about the warts on his hands. What is included in your teaching?*

A. Treatment is usually effective and most warts will not recur afterwards.
B. Because warts have roots, it is difficult to remove them surgically.
C. Warts are caused by the human papillomavirus.
D. Shaving the wart may prevent its recurrence.

Answers

8–1 Answer B

Although one of the warning signs of cancer is a lesion that does not heal or one that changes in appearance, the B in the ABCDs of melanoma identification stands for border irregularity. The edges of a melanoma are ragged, notched, or blurred. The A is for asymmetry: one half does not match the other half. The C is for color: pigmentation is not uniform; there may be shades of tan, brown, and black as well as red, white, and blue.The D is for diameter: greater than 6 mm.

8–2 Answer B

The connection between the surface of the skin and an underlying structure is called a sinus. An ulcer is a depressed lesion in which the epidermis and part of the dermis have been lost. An erosion is a moist, red, shiny, circumscribed lesion that lacks the upper layer of the skin. An abscess is a circumscribed collection of pus that involves the deeper layers of the skin.

8–3 Answer A

A Wood's light is especially useful in diagnosing tinea versicolor or other fungal infections. A Wood's light produces a "black light" through long-wave ultraviolet rays. It accentuates minor losses of melanin, which makes it useful in diagnosing tinea versicolor or vitiligo, in which there is hypopigmentation.

8–4 Answer C

A darkfield microscopic examination is used to diagnose syphilis. A darkfield examination, with its special condenser, causes an oblique beam of light to refract off objects too small to be seen by conventional microscopes, such as the narrow organism causing syphilis, *Treponema pallidum*. Application of a special tetracycline solution followed by shining a Wood's light on the skin may accentuate the burrow of scabietic mites, thus helping to diagnose scabies. A direct acid-fast stain is used to diagnose leprosy. A potassium hydroxide (KOH) stain helps diagnose *Candida* infections.

8–5 Answer C

Mongolian spots (congenital dermal melanocytosis) are poorly defined, blue to blue-black flat lesions that usually occur on the trunk and buttocks but may occur anywhere. They are present at birth and are asymptomatic. No treatment is necessary because the spots fade with age.

8–6 Answer C

Malignant melanomas usually occur in middle-aged adults of both sexes. The client usually has a family history of melanoma, and the prognosis is directly related to the thickness of the lesions. Melanomas occur rarely in blacks; when they do, the lesions usually develop on the palms and soles and under the nails.

8–7 Answer B

If a client presents with a pruritic rash on his upper trunk and shoulders and you observe areas of hypopigmentation and flat to slightly elevated brown papules and plaques that scale when they are rubbed, suspect tinea versicolor. Lentigines are macular tan to black lesions, ranging from 1 mm to 1 cm in size. They do not increase in color with exposure to the sun. One or more lentigines are seen in normal individuals. Multiple ones need to be further assessed. Localized brown macules are freckles. Ochronosis is a condition with poorly circumscribed, blue-black macules.

8–8 Answer D

A client with a platelet abnormality may present with red, flat, nonblanchable petechiae. Red to blue macular plaques describe ecchymoses; multiple frecklelike macular lesions in sun-exposed areas indicate xeroderma pigmentosum; and numerous small, brown, nonscaly macules that become more prominent with sun exposure are freckles.

8–9 Answer A

Erythema infectiosum (fifth disease) usually starts on the cheeks and spreads to the arms and trunk. Rocky Mountain spotted fever is associated with a history of tick bites and starts as a maculopapular rash with erythematous borders appearing first on the wrists, ankles, palms, soles, and forearms. Rubeola (measles) starts as a brownish-pink maculopapular rash around the ears, face, and neck and then progresses over the trunk and limbs. Rubella (German measles) starts as a fine, pinkish, macular rash that becomes confluent and pinpoint after 24 hours.

8–10 Answer C

Erysipelas is caused by *Streptococcus hemolyticus* and must be treated with appropriate antibiotics. A 7-day course of therapy is recommended: penicillin VK 250 mg, dicloxacillin 250 mg, or a first-generation cephalosporin 250 mg PO qid. In penicillin-allergic clients, either erythromycin 250 mg qid for 7–14 days or clarithromycin 250 mg bid for 7–14 days is a good choice.

8–11 Answer B

Lance has hives. Although all the actions are appropriate, the first step is to determine the need for 0.5 mL 1:1000 epinephrine subcutaneously (SQ). With Lance's neck involvement, it is most important to determine if respiratory distress is imminent, in which case the epinephrine must be administered.

8–12 Answer C

If a client comes into the clinic complaining of painful joints and has a distinctive rash in a butterfly distribution on the face that has red papules and plaques with a fine scale, suspect systemic lupus erythematosus. Acute lupus erythematosus occurs most often in young adult women and has a classic presentation of a rash in a butterfly distribution. The lesions are red papules and plaques with a fine scale. In the acute phase, the client is febrile and ill. The presence of these skin lesions in a client with neurological disease, arthritis, renal disease, or neuropsychiatric disturbances also supports the diagnosis. Lymphocytoma cutis is also most common on the face and neck. It occurs in both sexes and has smooth, red to yellow-brown papules up to 5 cm in diameter. Relapsing polychondritis occurs in adults with a history of arthritis. It appears as a macular erythema, tenderness, and swelling over the cartilaginous portions of the ear.

8–13 Answer A

If a client has genital warts (condylomata), they may be treated using podophyllin (contraindicated in pregnant clients), trichloroacetic acid, or liquid nitrogen. Benzoyl peroxide is used for acne.

8–14 Answer C

If you suspect a drug reaction to amoxicillin, stop the amoxicillin. Symptomatic relief may be obtained by systemic antihistamines and steroids. Systemic steroids may be necessary with severely symptomatic clients, although topical steroids may help clients with the pruritus.

8–15 Answer C

If a client presents with recurrent, sharply circumscribed red papules and plaques with a powdery white scale on the extensor aspect of his elbows and knees, suspect psoriasis. This is a classic presentation of psoriasis. Besides the extensor aspect of the elbows and knees, it occurs frequently in the presacral area and scalp, although lesions may occur anywhere. Actinic keratosis is distributed on sun-exposed areas such as the face, head, neck, and dorsum of the hand, and appears as poorly circumscribed, pink to red, slightly scaly lesions. Eczema presents as a group of pinpoint pruritic vesicles and papules on a coin-shaped erythematous base that usually worsens in winter. Seborrheic dermatitis has a symmetric appearance of raised, scaly, red, greasy papules and plaques that may be sharply or poorly circumscribed.

8–16 Answer A

A safe and effective treatment for psoriasis is the use of coal tar preparations. The concentration is increased every few days from 0.5% to a maximum of 10%. A contact period of several hours is required and the odor is unpleasant. Topical steroids are used in the treatment of atopic dermatitis; topical antibiotics are indicated for acne rosacea; and systemic antihistamines are indicated for pityriasis rosea.

8–17 Answer C

A biopsy of a small, yellow-orange papulonodule on the eyelid will probably show lipid-laden cells. This is a description of a noneruptive xanthoma of the eyelid (xanthelasma). Fragmented, calcified elastic tissue is diagnostic of pseudoxanthoma elasticum. A biopsy of sebaceous hyperplasia will show large, mature sebaceous glands. A biopsy revealing endothelial swelling and perivascular round-cell infiltrate that is rich in plasma cells is diagnostic of syphilis.

8–18 Answer A

Permethrin (Elimite) applied over the body overnight from the neck down is the preferred treatment for scabies. Lindane (Kwell) is also often effective. Topical corticosteroids or systemic antihistamines are indicated for eczema. Acyclovir (Zovirax) is the treatment for herpes simplex, and coal tar preparations are used to treat psoriasis.

8–19 Answer B

The rash of herpes zoster is characteristic in that it appears on only one side of the body. Herpes zoster begins in a dermatomal distribution, most commonly in the thoracic, cervical, and lumbosacral areas, although it also occurs on the face. Although it is caused by the reactivation of latent varicella virus in the distribution of the affected nerve, varicella (chickenpox) presents with a scattered rash on both sides of the body. A client with syphilis would present with sharply circumscribed, ham-colored papules with a slight scale and lesions over the entire body, especially on the palms and soles. Rubella (German measles) occurs in childhood. It begins on the face and rapidly (in hours) spreads down to the trunk.

8–20 Answer A

Ophthalmic zoster (herpes zoster ophthalmica) involves the ciliary body and may appear clinically as vesicles on the tip of the nose. The client with a herpetic lesion on the nose indicating ophthalmic zoster needs to be referred to an ophthalmologist to preserve the eyesight. Herpes simplex primarily occurs on the perioral, labial, and genital areas of the body. Kaposi's sarcoma in the older adult usually occurs in the lower extremities. Orf and milker's nodules almost always appear on the hands.

8–21 Answer D

Large, flaccid bullae with honey-colored crusts around the mouth and nose are characteristic of impetigo. These weeping erosions can appear anywhere, but usually appear on the face and nose and around the mouth. Hemorrhagic blisters may be present with a burn. Rocky Mountain spotted fever presents with petechiae beginning at the wrist and ankles and going to the palms and soles, then centrally to the face. Measles begins with red macules on the back of the neck, then spreads over the face and upper trunk. The lesions then become papular and may be confluent over the face.

8–22 Answer C

Balanitis is associated with *Candida* infection of the penis. Candidiasis (moniliasis) may affect the mouth (thrush), penis (balanitis), or vagina (vaginitis).

8–23 Answer C

Treatment for a furuncle (boil) or carbuncle (cluster of boils) may involve systemic antibiotics. The most common offending organism is *Staphylococcus aureus*. Streptococcus, *klebsiella*, and *Moraxella catarrhalis*, as well as *Staphylococcus aureus*, are all causative organisms of pneumonia.

8–24 Answer D

Anthrax is diagnosed with a Gram's stain of the lesion, which reveals large, square-ended gram-positive rods that grow easily on blood agar. A dermatophyte infection is diagnosed with a potassium hydroxide preparation which reveals hyphae and spores. In addition, fungal cultures demonstrate different fungi. Tuberculosis (scrofuloderma) is diagnosed with a histologic examination that reveals caseation necrosis and acid-fast bacilli. Sarcoidosis is diagnosed with a biopsy revealing noncaseating granulomas.

8–25 Answer A

Treatment for temporal arteritis involves systemic corticosteroids and immunosuppressives. The erythrocyte sedimentation rate is frequently elevated and a biopsy reveals granulomas and giant cells. Antibiotics and antifungal preparations are not indicated.

8–26 Answer A

Dogs are responsible for 80–90% of animal bites to humans. Annually, 10–20 deaths occur from dog bites. Most of these deaths result from the exsanguination associated with head and neck bites in children under age 4. The wound should be washed thoroughly with soap and water, then treated like any other wound. Because rabies may be contracted from domestic dogs and cats that have not been vaccinated, the animal should be confined for observation. A rabid animal has an initial anxiety stage followed by a furious stage. Preventive treatment of suspected rabies is based on immunization by a series of vaccine and immune serum injections. Domestic pets that do not appear rabid are assumed to have been vaccinated against rabies; this needs to be confirmed by the owner. Biting animals with an unknown vaccination record that appear healthy should be kept under observation for 7–10 days. Sick or dead animals should be examined for rabies. Because rabies is almost always fatal, when in doubt, treat. The type of immunization determines the timing of the treatment. If immune globulin is given, half of it is infiltrated around the wound and the remainder is administered intramuscularly. Inactivated human diploid cell rabies vaccine (HDCV) is given as a series of five injections beginning immediately and ending on day 28.

8–27 Answer C

A stage III pressure ulcer is one that has a deep crater with full-thickness skin loss and that involves necrosis of subcutaneous tissue extending down to the underlying fascia. Stage I is nonblanchable erythema of intact skin. Stage II is partial-thickness skin loss involving the epidermis or dermis. It may appear as an abrasion, blister, or shallow ulcer. Stage IV involves full-thickness skin loss with extensive destruction, tissue necrosis, or damage to muscle, bone, or supporting structures.

8–28 Answer B

A transparent dressing is applied over a pressure ulcer to prevent skin breakdown and the entrance of moisture and bacteria, but allow permeability of oxygen and moisture vapor. A liquid preparation such as benzoin is used to toughen intact skin and preserve skin integrity. Wet-to-dry gauze dressings allow necrotic material to soften. They adhere to the gauze, so the wound is débrided. A proteolytic enzyme such as Elase may serve as a débriding agent in inflamed and infected lesions.

8–29 Answer D

Treatment for a stage I pressure ulcer may include a hydrocolloid or transparent semipermeable membrane. An enzymatic preparation is used for a stage IV ulcer, surgery may possibly be necessary. The use of antibiotics is recommended only for patients with clinical signs of sepsis. Antibiotics are not indicated when signs of infection are localized.

8–30 Answer A

Besides storing melanin, which protects tissues from

the harmful effects of ultraviolet radiation in sunlight, the epidermis protects tissues from physical, chemical, and biological damage, prevents water loss, converts cholesterol molecules to vitamin D when exposed to sunlight, and contains phagocytes, which prevent bacteria from penetrating the skin. The dermis is the second layer of the skin. Its fibrous connective tissue gives the skin its strength and elasticity. The sebaceous glands are sebum-producing glands that assist in retarding evaporation and water loss from the epidermal cells. The eccrine sweat glands open directly onto the skin's surface and are widely distributed throughout the body in the subcutaneous tissue.

8–31 Answer B

Tenting, which occurs when pinched skin over the clavicle remains pinched for a few moments before resuming its normal position, is common in thin older adults. Skin turgor is decreased with dehydration and increased with edema and scleroderma.

8–32 Answer C

Thin, spoon-shaped nails are usually seen in anemia. Causes of thick nails include trauma, fungal infections, psoriasis, and decreased peripheral vascular blood supply.

8–33 Answer C

Crusts are dried blood, serum, or pus left on the skin surface when vesicles or pustules burst. They can be red-brown, orange, or yellow. Examples include eczema, impetigo, herpes, or scabs following abrasions. Psoriasis results in scales or shedding flakes of greasy, keratinized skin tissue. The color may be white, gray, or silver and the texture may vary from fine to thick.

8–34 Answer D

A vitamin C deficiency results in bleeding gums and delayed wound healing. A protein deficiency results in dry skin and loss of skin color. A vitamin A deficiency results in thickened skin that is dry or rough. A vitamin B_6 deficiency results in flaky skin, sores in the mouth, and cracks at the corners of the mouth.

8–35 Answer B

If a client is complaining of dry skin, the client should use tepid water and a mild cleansing cream or soap, use a humidifier to humidify the air, and increase the oral intake of fluids to assist in replacing some of the fluids lost from the skin. Advise the client that it is not necessary to take a bath every day because soaps and hot water are drying.

8–36 Answer C

Ultraviolet light therapy is used to treat psoriasis to decrease the growth rate of epidermal cells. This assists in decreasing the hyperkeratosis. Treatments are given daily and last only for seconds.

8–37 Answer D

If a client has tinea pedis, tell the client to dry between the toes every day, wash socks with bleach, and use an antifungal powder twice per day. Rubber- or plastic-soled shoes can harbor the fungus and therefore should not be worn. The shower should be washed with bleach to kill the fungi.

8–38 Answer B

If a client has just been given a diagnosis of herpes zoster, advise the client to stay away from children and pregnant women who have not had chickenpox until crusts have formed over the blistered areas. Herpes zoster is contagious to people who have not had chickenpox.

8–39 Answer B

Acne rosacea is a chronic type of facial acne that occurs in middle-aged to older adults. Over time, the skin changes in color to dark red, pores become enlarged, and the soft tissue of the nose may exhibit rhinophyma, an irregular bullous thickening. Acne vulgaris is the form of acne common in adolescents and young to middle-aged adults. Acne conglobata begins in middle adulthood and causes serious skin lesions such as comedones, papules, pustules, nodules, cysts, and scars primarily on the back, buttocks, and chest.

8–40 Answer A

A keloid is an elevated, irregularly shaped, and progressively enlarging scar that arises from excessive amounts of collagen during scar formation. A skin tag is a soft papule on a pedicle. An angioma is a benign vascular tumor. A keratosis is any skin condition in which there is a benign overgrowth and thickening of the cornified epithelium.

8–41 Answer B

Nevi, commonly called moles, are flat or raised macules or papules that arise from melanocytes during early childhood. A nevus flammeus (port-wine stain) is an angioma, a congenital vascular lesion that involves the capillaries.

8–42 Answer C

Actinic keratoses, also called senile or solar keratoses, are epidermal skin lesions that are directly related to chronic sun exposure and photodamage. Skin tags occur in middle-aged adults of both genders and may be associated with acromegaly or acanthosis nigricans. Seborrheic keratoses are lesions most often seen in older adults and do not appear to be related to damage from sun exposure. Angiomas are common small red to purple papules unrelated to sun exposure.

8–43 Answer B

Skin tags (acrochordons) are benign overgrowths of skin, commonly seen after middle age and usually found on the neck, axilla, groin, upper trunk, and eyelid. A nevus is a mole, and a lipoma is a benign subcutaneous tumor that consists of adipose tissue.

8–44 Answer A

A basal cell carcinoma is an epithelial tumor that originates from either the basal layer of the epidermis or cells in the surrounding dermal structures. A squamous cell carcinoma is malignant and originates in the squamous epithelium. An overgrowth and thickening of the cornified epithelium is a keratosis. A cyst is a benign closed sac in or under the skin surface that is lined with epithelium and contains fluid or a semisolid material.

8–45 Answer D

Cryosurgery is a noninvasive method of treating skin cancer other than melanoma in which liquid nitrogen is used to freeze and destroy the tumor tissue. Mohs' micrographic surgery involves shaving thin layers of the tumor tissue horizontally, then taking a frozen section to determine tumor margins. Curettage and electrodesiccation are used to treat basal cell cancers less than 2 cm in diameter and primary squamous cell cancers that are less than 1 cm in diameter. Radiation therapy is used for lesions that are inoperable because of their location.

8–46 Answer B

Zinc oxide, magnesium silicate, ferric chloride, and kaolin are examples of physical sunscreens that reflect and scatter ultraviolet light. Chemical sunscreens such as PABA, benzophenones, and salicylates absorb ultraviolet light and act as a radiation filter. Tanning booths should be avoided because ultraviolet (UVA) radiation emitted by tanning booths damages the deep skin layers.

8–47 Answer B

Rubbing or massaging the frostbitten areas, especially with snow, may cause permanent tissue damage. Advise the client to remove wet footwear if the feet are frostbitten; apply firm pressure with a warm hand to the area; and place the hands in the axillae if the hands are frostbitten.

8–48 Answer D

Permanent tissue damage can occur with a second episode of frostbite on the same skin surface. Susan's fiancé should be extremely careful and wear a warm knit mask covering the entire face with only small holes for his orifices if he insists on skiing. With continued exposure, vasoconstriction and increased viscosity of the blood can cause infarction and necrosis of the nose. Massaging a frostbitten nose may cause tissue damage.

8–49 Answer D

Alopecia universalis is the loss of hair on all parts of the body. Female-pattern alopecia is progressive thinning and loss of hair over the central part of the scalp. Alopecia areata appears as round or oval bald patches on the scalp and other hairy parts of the body. Alopecia totalis is the loss of all hair on the scalp.

8–50 Answer B

Minoxidil (Rogaine) is a vasodilator and may stimulate vertex hair growth. Anticoagulants, oral contraceptives, and salicylates may cause alopecia. Other drugs that may also cause alopecia include antithy roid drugs, allopurinol, propranolol, amphetamines, and levodopa.

8–51 Answer C

Although cellulitis, furuncle-carbuncles, and hidradenitis suppurativa are all distinctive abscesses, only anthrax has this morphology, which results in a dense, black, necrotic eschar gradually forming over the initial lesion. A furuncle-carbuncle is a pustular lesion surrounding one or several hair follicles, and a hidradenitis suppurativa lesion results in scarring and fibrotic bands.

8–52 Answer D

The first intervention is to eliminate the heat source, then stabilize the client's condition, identify the type of burn, prevent heat loss, reduce wound contamination, and then prepare for emergency transportation.

8–53 Answer C

In burn trauma, the hematocrit rises as fluid, not blood, shifts from the intravascular compartment. The hemoglobin level decreases secondary to hemolysis; the sodium level decreases secondary to massive fluid shifts into the interstitium; and the blood urea nitrogen level increases secondary to dehydration.

8–54 Answer C

Silver sulfadiazine (Silvadene), the most commonly used topical agent for burn trauma, is a bactericidal agent that acts on the cell membrane and cell wall of susceptible bacteria and binds to cellular DNA. It is effective against a wide variety of both gram-negative and gram-positive organisms. Mafenide acetate (Sulfamylon) is a synthetic antibiotic that interferes with the metabolism of bacterial cells. Approximately 3–5% of clients develop a hypersensitivity to mafenide. Silver nitrate is a bacteriostatic agent that alters the microbial cell wall and membrane. It has limited penetrating ability and is ineffective if used more than 72 hours after a burn injury.

8–55 Answer C

Although the treatment of varicella (chickenpox) in children consists of cool baths with Aveeno for pruritus and calamine lotion to dry the lesions, acyclovir (Zovirax) is not recommended. In adolescents and young adults, however, if started within the first

24–48 hours after the rash first appears, acyclovir may shorten the course of the disease.

8–56 Answer A

A client who has a varicella rash can return to work once all the vesicles are crusted. Varicella is contagious from 48 hours before the onset of the vesicular rash, during the rash formation (usually 4–5 days), and during the several days while the vesicles dry up. The characteristic rash appears 2–3 weeks after exposure. Treatment is effective only if started within the first few days, and then only to shorten the course of the disease. Clients should avoid contact with pregnant women and children who have not been exposed to varicella.

8–57 Answer A

The ABCDs (asymmetry, border irregularity, color changes, diameter) of melanomas should be taught to all clients. A change in the color variation may indicate a melanoma, and an excisional biopsy should be done. Monitoring for a month may enable a melanoma to extend extensively, resulting in death. Benzoyl peroxide and hydrocortisone may be used with folliculitis.

8–58 Answer A

An orf skin ulcer results from a *Parapoxvirus* infection, which causes a common skin disease of sheep and goats. It is occasionally transmitted to humans.

8–59 Answer A

Antifungal agents are ineffective against psoriasis. The most common form of treatment is corticosteroids applied topically. Systemic treatments are used in more severe cases, and phototherapy, from either natural or artificial light, may also be helpful.

8–60 Answer D

Patients with rosacea usually have a long history of flushing in response to sun exposure. Alcohol, cold weather, and skin-care products may also be triggers, but not nearly as often. Other triggers may include emotional stress, spicy foods, exercise, wind, hot baths, and hot drinks.

8–61 Answer C

The most effective treatment for urticaria (hives) is avoidance of the offending agent. Usually the offending antigen is identifiable and exposure is self-limited. Treatment with oral antihistamines is usually effective for symptomatic relief of itching, swelling, and nasal symptoms. Dietary management may sometimes be helpful if the cause of the problem is a known offending agent, such as shellfish, nuts, fish, eggs, chocolate, or cheese. Glucocorticoids have a minimal role in treating urticaria. A brief trial may be indicated for temporary relief in a difficult case.

8–62 Answer B

A zosteriform lesion is a linear arrangement along a nerve distribution and typifies herpes zoster. An annular lesion is ring shaped. Linear simply implies that the lesion appears in lines. A keratotic lesion has horny thickenings.

8–63 Answer C

Pastia lines are present in scarlet fever. All of the diseases listed are caused by bacteria. In scarlet fever, there is diffuse erythema with a sandpaper texture and gooseflesh appearance, and accentuation of erythema in the flexural creases referred to as Pastia lines. In toxic shock syndrome, there is a diffuse sunburnlike erythroderma. In Rocky Mountain spotted fever, there is an early maculopapular rash, then petechial or, rarely, purpuric lesions present on the extremities. In meningococcemia, there are erythematous, nonconfluent, discrete papules early in the disease.

8–64 Answer A

The viral exanthem of Koplik's spots is present in rubeola (measles). Koplik's spots are observed on the buccal mucosa before the rash appears in rubeola. There are variable erythematous macules on the soft palate in rubella (German measles). There is no exanthem in fifth disease (erythema infectiosum). In varicella (chickenpox), there may be sparse lesions on the mucosal surfaces, especially the hard palate.

8–65 Answer A

A darkfield examination is used to cutaneously diagnose syphilis. Viral blisters can be diagnosed cutaneously by the Tzanck smear; a scraping can be done to look for scabies; and a potassium hydroxide preparation and culture are used to diagnose candidiasis.

8–66 Answer C

Lichenification is a thickening of the skin that usually results from chronic scratching or rubbing. Crusts represent dried serum, blood, pus, or exudate. Scales are yellow, white, or brownish flakes on the surface of the skin that represent desquamation of stratum corneum. Atrophy represents loss of substance of the skin.

8–67 Answer D

Acne rosacea, acne vulgaris, folliculitis, candidiasis, and miliaria are classified as pustular lesions. Papular lesions include warts, corns, Kaposi's sarcoma, basal cell carcinoma, and scabies. Vesicular lesions include herpes simplex, varicella, and herpes zoster. Erosive lesions include impetigo, lichen planus, and erythema multiforme.

8–68 Answer A

The "herald patch" is present in almost all cases of pityriasis rosea. Pityriasis rosea is a common, acute, viral, self-limited eruption that usually begins with a solitary oval, pink, scaly plaque, approximately 3–5 cm in diameter, on the trunk or proximal extremities. It is referred to as the herald patch because it has an elevated red border and a central clearing.

8–69 Answer B

The five Ps—purple, polygonal, planar, pruritic papules—are present in lichen planus. Lichen planus occurs in clients of all ages but is more common in adults. It has a primary skin lesion with the five Ps that looks like a shiny, violaceous flat-topped papule that is very pruritic. Ichthyosis vulgaris lesions are fine, small, flaky white scales with minimal underlying erythema that can be found anywhere, but are more prominent on the extensor aspects of the extremities. Atopic dermatitis (eczema) presents differently at different ages and in persons of different races, but usually starts as red, weepy, shiny patches. Seborrheic dermatitis presents as dry scales with underlying erythema.

8–70 Answer D

Adverse effects from prolonged or high-potency topical corticosteroid use may include cutaneous atrophy, telangiectases, and easy bruisability, as well as systemic absorption, which may include growth retardation, electrolyte abnormalities, hyperglycemia, hypertension, and increased susceptibility to infection. Vitiligo is caused by loss of melanin. Striae may occur after oral corticosteroids, or occlusive topical corticosteroid therapy.

8–71 Answer C

Psoriasis, erythema multiforme, tinea corporis, and syphilis all have lesions with annular configurations. Tinea corporis (ringworm) has ring-shaped lesions with a scaly border and central clearing or scaly patches with a distinct border on exposed skin surfaces or on the trunk. Psoriasis has annular lesions on the elbows, knees, scalp, and nails. Erythema multiforme has annular lesions that are mostly acral in distribution and are often associated with a recent herpes simplex infection. Secondary syphilis lesions are usually on the palmar, plantar, and mucous membrane surfaces.

8–72 Answer C

If a client uses a high-potency corticosteroid cream for a dermatosis, tell the client that it may exacerbate concurrent conditions such as tinea corporis and acne. Topical corticosteroids should not be used indiscriminately on all cutaneous eruptions. They should not be used for an extended period of time, and the lesion should not be occluded. Intermittent therapy with high-potency agents, such as every other day, or 3–4 consecutive days per week, may be more effective and cause fewer adverse effects than continuous regimens. This is also true of lower-potency corticosteroids.

8–73 Answer D

Transient urticaria requires antihistamines on a regular basis. Aspirin, nonsteroidal anti-inflammatory drugs, and opioids are to be avoided.

8–74 Answer B

Vitiligo, which usually appears in childhood, is an acquired disorder characterized by complete loss of pigment of the involved skin. Although tinea versicolor does have areas of hypopigmentation, they are scattered and do not have complete loss of pigment. In tuberous sclerosis, ash-leaf spots, which are hypopigmented macules, about 2–3 cm in size, are present at birth. Pityriasis alba is also an acquired disorder of hypopigmentation characterized by poorly demarcated, slightly scaly, oval hypopigmented macules that vary from 1.5–2 cm in size.

8–75 Answer B

The drug of choice for tinea capitis is oral griseofulvin (Grisactin), taken for 6–8 weeks. It should be administered with fat-containing foods because fat is required for optimal absorption. Although topical antifungal agents are effective, they take an extremely long time to work. Topical corticosteroids and antibiotics are not effective for fungal lesions.

8–76 Answer D

Therapeutic modalities useful for the management of acute atopic dermatitis include emollients, compresses, and ultraviolet light. Although tars are useful for chronic, dry, lichenified lesions, they are not helpful for acute dermatitis. Emollients are best applied and most helpful if used immediately after bathing or showering. Compresses are indicated for acute weeping lesions to help cool and dry the skin, which reduces inflammation. Ultraviolet light is useful for severe, uncontrollable atopic dermatitis.

8–77 Answer C

The harlequin sign is a transient phenomenon in a newborn who has been lying on his or her side. The dependent side is red while the upper side is pale, as if a line has been drawn down the middle of the body. This disappears when the infant's position is changed. Hyperbilirubinemia results in jaundice. Hemangiomas and mongolian spots are birthmarks.

8–78 Answer D

Head lice may be transmitted by sharing hats, combs, or brushes, so these practices should be discouraged. The louse can survive for more than 2 days off the scalp, so it can still survive in the bed linen. Girls are more susceptible than boys, and lice occur more often in whites. Immunity against head lice is never acquired.

8–79 Answer C

Treating constipation, preferably with a high-fiber diet, may help anogenital pruritus. Most cases of anogenital pruritus have no obvious cause and chiefly cause nocturnal itching without pain. Although the condition is benign, it may be persistent and recurrent. Hydrocortisone-pramoxine (Pramosone) 1% or 2.5% cream, lotion, or ointment helps with pruritus. Suppositories are not necessary. Anogenital hygiene needs to be stressed. Potent fluorinated topical corticosteroids and antifungals may lead to atrophy and striae after several days and should be avoided.

8–80 Answer A

Skin phototyping (SPT) is a risk classification system designed to estimate one's risk for sun damage. SPT ranges from I to VI. A person with SPT I sunburns easily but never tans. Persons with black skin are termed SPT VI. Persons in the middle types tan easily with minimal sunburn.

8–81 Answer C

The "gold standard" used to confirm the suspicion of a true food allergy (IgE reaction) in a young child is the double-blind, placebo-controlled food challenge. It is necessary in research studies and in all unclear clinical situations to confirm the suspicion of a true allergy. An immediate-reacting IgE skin test is a good screening test that can virtually rule out the allergy. A positive result indicates likelihood of an allergy. A food challenge is the only method to confirm the suspicion of a food reaction regardless of the mechanism (allergy or otherwise). A diagnostic food diet diary and home challenge are possibly helpful when the reactions are not life threatening.

8–82 Answer A

If a client is allergic to eggs and does not think that he or she should receive the flu vaccine, advise the client that, although measles, mumps, rubella, and influenza vaccines contain a minute amount of egg, most individuals who are allergic to eggs can tolerate these vaccines without any problems; that some of the allergic reactions are caused by the gelatins in the vaccinations and not the actual vaccinations; and that if the client can eat a whole egg with no reaction, he or she should have no problem with the vaccination. If the history of the allergy is questionable, it is safest to perform a skin test using the vaccine in dilute amounts and then administer the vaccine under strict observation, allowing a 2-hour wait to observe for any reaction.

8–83 Answer A

Dry, itchy skin in older adults results from the reduction of sweat and oil glands. Loss of subcutaneous tissue, dermal thinning, and decreased elasticity are the normal changes, and they may cause wrinkles and sagging of the skin.

8–84 Answer C

Although increasing fluids and a moisturizing cream will help the general problem, Sarah does not need a bath every day, because that will exacerbate the dryness of her skin. Plain water should be used rather than special soap.

8–85 Answer D

Clubbing is defined as a thickening and broadening of the ends of the fingers. Clubbing is a bulbous appearance and swelling of the terminal phalanges, increasing the normal 160-degree angle between the nailbed and the digit to 180 degrees. In adults, it is usually caused by pulmonary disease and the resultant hypoxia.

8–86 Answer D

The epitrochlear lymph node is located in the inner condyle of the humerus. The preauricular lymph node is located in front of the ear; the submaxillary (submandibular) lymph node is halfway between the angle and the tip of the mandible; and the posterior cervical lymph node is in the posterior triangle along the edge of the trapezius muscle.

8–87 Answer C

Podagra is gouty pain in the great toe. Hyperuricemia results in deposits of urate crystals called tophi.

8–88 Answer B

For the client with gout, the consumption of purine-rich foods, such as organ meats, should be limited to prevent uric acid buildup. Alcohol should also be limited and fluids increased to 2 liters per day. Salicylates should be avoided because they block renal excretion of uric acid. An annual testing of the serum uric acid level is sufficient.

8–89 Answer A

Penicillin, neomycin, phenothiazines, and local anesthetics may cause an eczematous type of skin reaction. Exfoliative dermatitis may be caused by allopurinol (Zyloprim) and sulfonamides. Oral contraceptives may cause erythema nodosum. Drug-related systemic lupus erythematosus may result from the use of procainamide (Pronestyl) or phenytoin (Dilantin).

8–90 Answer B

A normal stoma is moist and beefy red. A pale pink color may indicate a low hemoglobin level. A dark-red or purple stoma may indicate early ischemia. A black stoma is the result of necrosis. Stomas are never flesh colored.

8–91 Answer C

Stomas shrink within 6–8 weeks after surgery. At that time it is safe to buy a permanent appliance. Before that, the stoma needs to be measured weekly to find a well-fitting appliance.

8–92 Answer A

A papular rash with satellite lesions around a stoma indicates a fungal infection. It may be a consequence of persistent skin moisture or an adverse effect of antibiotic therapy. If Silas were having an allergic reaction to the appliance, he would have an erythematous vesicular rash limited to the site of the faceplate of the appliance. If the appliance fits properly, fecal drainage should not come in contact with the skin. Fluid and electrolyte imbalances may occur, but the signs and symptoms would be systemic in nature.

8–93 Answer B

A stork's beak mark usually occurs on the nape of the neck and blanches on pressure. Although it does not fade, when it is covered by hair it is usually not noticeable. A nevus flammeus (port-wine stain) is deep red to purple, does not blanch on pressure, and does not fade with age. A strawberry hemangioma is the result of dilated capillaries in the entire dermal and subdermal layers of the skin. Although it continues to enlarge after birth, it usually disappears by 10 years of age. A cavernous hemangioma is the result of a communicating network of venules in the subcutaneous tissue and does not fade with age.

8–94 Answer B

Hypertension is not one of the predisposing conditions for furunculosis or carbuncles. Predisposing conditions include diabetes mellitus, human immunodeficiency virus disease, and injection drug use. Furunculosis (boils) and carbuncles are very painful inflammatory swellings of a hair follicle that result in an abscess, caused by coagulase-positive *Staphylococcus aureus*.

8–95 Answer A

One treatment for thrush includes nystatin oral suspension for 2 weeks, 2–3 mL in each side of the mouth, held as long as possible. When clotrimazole oral troches (10 mg) are used, they should be used 5 times per day for 14 days (not 2 times per day for 7 days). Fluconazole 100 mg may be given as a single dose (not twice per day for 1 week). Antiseptic mouthwashes are not effective for thrush.

8–96 Answer B

Cellulitis is a spreading infection of the epidermis and subcutaneous tissue that usually begins after a break in the skin. The skin is warm, red, and painful. Although Justin may have diabetic neuropathy, peripheral vascular disease, or a stasis ulcer, the information is not complete enough. The information and assessment data given fully support a diagnosis of cellulitis.

8–97 Answer C

Psoriasis may occur after extended therapy with many medications, including beta blockers, lithium, nonsteroidal anti-inflammatory drugs, gold, antimalarials, angiotensin-converting enzyme inhibitors, and heavy alcohol intake.

8–98 Answer B

The drug of choice for acute anaphylaxis is epinephrine 1:1000 subcutaneously (0.3–0.5 mL) for adults. Diphenhydramine IV (Benadryl) is a second-line emergency drug; the oral form would work well as an antihistamine. Prednisone is beneficial in severe or refractory urticaria. Calcium channel blockers, such as amlodipine besylate (Norvasc), may be of value in clients with chronic urticaria unresponsive to antihistamines when used for at least 4 weeks.

8–99 Answer C

The most important thing a woman can do to have youthful, attractive skin is not smoke. Smokers develop more wrinkles and have elastosis, decreased tissue perfusion and oxygenation, and an adverse exposure to free radicals on elastic tissue. Other important things to promote the health of the skin are use of a sunscreen with a sun protective factor of at least 15 and keeping the skin well hydrated. Although keeping the skin well hydrated promotes skin health, it does not prevent wrinkles. Using mild defatted glycerin soaps maintains texture and hydration but does not help prevent wrinkles.

8–100 Answer A

The majority (70%) of malignant melanomas are superficially spreading. These have a good prognosis because they tend to spread superficially before invading the tissues. The next most common type (10%) presents as a black nodule; 5% of melanomas present as lentigo maligna, which arise from precursor lesions, and another 5% are acral-lentiginous. These arise on the hands or feet and are the most common type seen in Asians and African-Americans.

8–101 Answer A

Open comedones are known as blackheads. A person with acne vulgaris may have open comedones, closed comedones (whiteheads), papules, pustules, cysts, and even scars.

8–102 Answer C

Condyloma acuminata is a cauliflower-like wart usually found in anogenital regions and is usually sexually transmitted. Plantar warts appear at maximum points of pressue such as the heads of metatarsal bones or heels; filiform or digitate warts are fingerlike, flesh-colored projections emanating from a narrow or broad base, usually in the facial region; and verruca plana are flat warts that are pink, light brown or yellow with slightly elevated papules that may undergo spontaneous remission.

8–103 Answer A

Craniotabes is localized softening of the cranial bones that are so soft that they may be indented by the pressure of a finger. When the pressure is removed, the bone returns to its normal position. This condition corrects itself in a matter of months without treatment. Molding is when the vertex of the head is molded to fit the cervix contours during delivery. The head usually returns to its normal shape within a few days. Caput succedaneum is edema of the scalp that is usually absorbed and disappears by the third day of life without treatment. A cephalhematoma is a collection of blood on the skull bone caused by rupture of a periosteum capillary due to the pressure of birth and usually occurs 24 hours after birth and may take weeks to be absorbed.

8–104 Answer A

Candidiasis of the glans of the penis is balanitis. Thrush is oral candidiasis; candidal paronychia involves the tissue surrounding the nail; and subungual candida is candidiasis under the nail.

8–105 Answer A

A bulla is a primary skin lesion filled with fluid, also called a vesicle, which is larger than 1 cm in diameter. A wheal is also a primary skin lesion larger than 1 cm in diameter that is transient, elevated, and hive-like, with local edema and inflammation. A cyst is filled with fluid and may occur in a variety of sizes. A pustule is a superficial elevated lesion filled with purulent fluid.

8–106 Answer C

Warts are caused by the human papillomavirus. One in four people is infected with this virus and, despite treatment, most warts recur. Broken or abraded skin can spread the transport of the virus as well as vigorous rubbing, shaving, nail biting, and sexual intercourse. Warts do not have roots, contrary to popular opinion. The underside of a wart is smooth and round.

Bibliography

Anderson, JA: Milk, eggs and peanuts: Food allergies in children. Am Fam Physician 56:5, 1997.

Bradley, M, and Pupiales, M: Essential elements of ostomy care. Am J Nurs 97:7, 1997.

Bynum, DT: Gout. Am J Nurs 97:7, 1997.

Clinical Evidence Concise, issue 7. BMJ Publishing Group, London, 2002.

Fleming, DT, et al.: Herpes simplex virus type 2 in the United States, 1976 to 1994. N Engl J Med 337:16, 1997.

Goldsmith, LA, et al: Adult and Pediatric Dermatology: A Color Guide to Diagnosis and Treatment. FA Davis, Philadelphia, 1997.

Hayes, KVD: Skin wellness and illness. In Condon, MC (ed): Woman's Health. Prentice Hall

Leik, M: Skin problems. In Dunphy, L, and Winland-Brown, J (eds): Primary Care: The Art and Science of Advanced Practice Nursing. FA Davis, Philadelphia, 2001.

McEldowney, S: Malignant melanoma: Familial, genetic, and psychosocial risk factors. Clinician Rev 7:7, 1997.

Ringel, M: Facing acne or rosacea as an adult. The Female Patient: Total Health Care for Women (suppl) 1997.

Roingeard, P, and Machet, L: Orf skin ulcer. N Engl J Med 337:16, 1997.

Taylor, RB: Manual of Family Practice. Little, Brown, Boston, 1997.

Tierney, LM, et al: Current Medical Diagnosis and Treatment. Appleton & Lange, Stamford, CT, 1998.

Youngkin, EQ et al: Pharmacotherapeutics: A Primary Care Clinical Guide. Appleton & Lange, Stamford, CT, 1999.

HOW WELL DID YOU DO?

85% AND ABOVE CONGRATULATIONS! THIS SCORE SHOWS APPLICATION OF TEST-TAKING PRINCIPLES AND ADEQUATE CONTENT KNOWLEDGE.

75–85% KEEP WORKING! REVIEW TEST-TAKING PRINCIPLES AND TRY AGAIN.

65–75% HANG IN THERE! SPEND SOME TIME REVIEWING CONCEPTS AND TEST-TAKING PRINCIPLES AND THEN TRY THE TEST AGAIN.

9 Head and Neck Problems

JILL E. WINLAND-BROWN

9–1 *At birth, a neonate's head size comprises what fraction of the neonate's total body length?*

A. 1/4
B. 1/3
C. 1/8
D. 3/8

9–2 *Tara was born with a cleft lip and palate. When should treatment begin for this condition?*

A. Immediately after birth
B. At age 3 months
C. At age 6 months
D. When Tara is ready to drink from a cup

9–3 *The trachea deviates toward the unaffected side in all of the following conditions* ***except:***

A. aortic aneurysm.
B. unilateral thyroid lobe enlargement.
C. large atelectasis.
D. pneumothorax.

9–4 *A child's head circumference is measured at each well-child visit until age:*

A. 12 months.
B. 18 months.
C. 2 years.
D. 5 years.

9–5 *Jim, age 49, comes to the office with a rapid-onset complete paralysis of one-half of his face. He is unable to raise his eyebrow, close his eye, whistle, or show his teeth. You suspect a lower motor neuron lesion resulting in cranial nerve VII paralysis. What is your working diagnosis?*

A. Cerebrovascular accident
B. Trigeminal neuralgia
C. Bell's palsy
D. Tic douloureux

9–6 *A child's central visual acuity is 20/30 by age:*

A. 18 months.
B. 2 years.
C. 3 years.
D. 4 years.

9–7 *When Judith, age 15, asks you to explain the 20/50 vision in her right eye, you respond:*

A. "You can see at 20 feet with your left eye what the normal person can see at 50 feet."
B. "You can see at 20 feet with your right eye what the normal person can see at 50 feet."
C. "You can see at 50 feet with your right eye what the normal person can see at 20 feet."
D. "You can see at 50 feet with the left eye what the normal person can see at 20 feet."

9–8 *Which assessment test is a gross measurement of peripheral vision?*

A. The cover test
B. The corneal light reflex test
C. The confrontation test
D. The Snellen eye-chart test

9–9 *The normal ratio of the artery-to-vein width in the retina as viewed through the ophthalmoscope is:*

A. 2:3.
B. 3:2.

C. 1:3.
D. 3:1.

9–10 *You observe a mother showing her infant a toy. You note that the infant can fixate on, briefly follow, and then reach for the toy. You suspect that the infant is*

A. 2 months old.
B. 4 months old.
C. 6 months old.
D. 8 months old.

9–11 *June, age 50, presents with soft, raised yellow plaques on her eyelids at the inner canthus. She is concerned that they may be cancerous skin lesions. You tell her that they are probably:*

A. xanthelasmas.
B. pingueculae.
C. the result of arcus senilis.
D. actinic keratoses.

9–12 *Which cranial nerve (CN) is affected in sensorineural or perceptive hearing loss?*

A. CN II
B. CN IV
C. CN VIII
D. CN XI

9–13 *Regular ocular pressure testing is indicated for older adults taking:*

A. high-dose inhaled glucocorticoids.
B. nonsteroidal anti-inflammatory drugs.
C. angiotensin-converting enzyme inhibitors.
D. insulin.

9–14 *What condition occurs in almost all persons beginning around age 42–46?*

A. Arcus senilis
B. Presbyopia
C. Cataracts
D. Glaucoma

9–15 *In older adults, the most common cause of decreased visual functioning is:*

A. cataract formation.
B. glaucoma.
C. macular degeneration.
D. arcus senilis.

9–16 *How should Tommy, age $2^1/_2$, have his vision screened?*

A. Using a Snellen letter chart
B. Using the Allen test
C. Using a Snellen E chart
D. Using a Rosenbaum chart

9–17 *Leah, 4 months old, has both eyes turning inward. What is this called?*

A. Pseudostrabismus
B. Strabismus
C. Esotropia
D. Exotropia

9–18 *Maury, age 52, has throbbing pain in the left eye, an irregular pupil shape, marked photophobia, and redness around the iris. What is your initial diagnosis?*

A. Conjunctivitis
B. Iritis
C. Subconjunctival hemorrhage
D. Acute glaucoma

9–19 *Purulent matter in the anterior chamber of the eye is called:*

A. hyphema.
B. hypopyon.
C. anisocoria.
D. pterygium.

9–20 *A common cause of conductive hearing loss in adults age 20–40 is:*

A. trauma.
B. otitis media.
C. presbycusis.
D. otosclerosis.

9–21 *If a client presents with a red eye and there is no discharge, you should suspect:*

A. bacterial conjunctivitis
B. viral conjunctivitis
C. allergic conjunctivitis
D. iritis

9–22 *Acute otitis media is diagnosed when there is:*

A. fluid in the middle ear without signs or symptoms of an ear infection.
B. a diagnosis of three or more episodes of otitis media within 1 year.
C. fluid in the middle ear accompanied by signs or symptoms of an ear infection.
D. fluid within the middle ear for at least 3 months.

9–23 *Judy, age 67, complains of a sudden onset of impaired vision, severe eye pain, vomiting, and a headache. You diagnose the following condition and refer for urgent treatment:*

A. Cataracts
B. Macular degeneration
C. Presbyopia
D. Acute glaucoma

9–24 *Clonazepam (Klonopin) is occasionally ordered for temporal mandibular joint disease. The following statement applies to this medicine:*

A. It is ordered for inflammatory pain.
B. It is ordered for neuropathic pain.

C. It is ordered for a short course of therapy for 1–2 weeks only.
D. It is ordered for muscle relaxation.

9–25 *The antibiotic of choice for beta-lactamase coverage of otitis media is:*

A. amoxicillin (Amoxil).
B. amoxicillin and potassium clavulanate (Augmentin).
C. azithromycin (Zithromax).
D. prednisone (Deltasone).

9–26 *Sam, age 4, is brought into the clinic by his father. His tympanic membrane is perforated from otitis media. His father asks about repair of the eardrum. How do you respond?*

A. "The eardrum, in most cases, heals within several weeks."
B. "We need to schedule Sam for a surgical repair."
C. "He must absolutely stay out of the water for 3–6 months."
D. "If the eardrum is not healed in several months, we will then surgically repair it."

9–27 *What significant finding(s) in a child with otitis media with effusion would prompt more aggressive treatment?*

A. A change in the child's hearing threshold to less than or equal to 20 dB.
B. The child becomes a fussy eater.
C. The child's speech and language skills seem slightly delayed.
D. Persistent rhinitis is present.

9–28 *The immediate goal of myringotomy and tube placement in a child with recurrent episodes of otitis media is to:*

A. prevent future infections.
B. have an open access to the middle ear for irrigation and instillation of antibiotics.
C. allow removal of suppurative or mucoid material.
D. relieve pain.

9–29 *Marcia, age 4, is brought into the office by her mother. She has a sore throat, difficulty swallowing, copious oral secretions, respiratory difficulty, stridor, and a temperature of 102°F, but no pharyngeal erythema or cough. What do you suspect?*

A. Epiglottitis
B. Group A beta-hemolytic streptococcal infection pharyngitis
C. Tonsillitis
D. Diphtheria

9–30 *John, age 19, has just been given a diagnosis of mononucleosis (Epstein-Barr virus). In teaching John about his condition, you include all the following directions* ***except:***

A. "Complete the antibiotic course regardless of symptom response."
B. "Avoid contact sports and heavy lifting."
C. "Convalescence may take several weeks."
D. "Avoid stress."

9–31 *When assessing Lenore, age 59, who has a sore throat, you note that she has a positive history of diabetes and rheumatic fever. These facts increase the likelihood that which of the following agents caused her sore throat?*

A. *Neisseria gonorrhoeae*
B. Epstein-Barr virus
C. *Haemophilus influenzae*
D. Group A beta-hemolytic streptococcus

9–32 *The first-line antibiotic therapy for an adult with no known allergies and suspected group A beta-hemolytic streptococcal pharyngitis is:*

A. penicillin.
B. erythromycin (E-Mycin).
C. azithromycin (Zithromax).
D. cephalexin (Keflex).

9–33 *Tee, age 64, presents with a sore throat. Your assessment reveals tonsillar exudate, anterior cervical adenopathy, presence of a fever, and absence of a cough. There is a high probability of which causative agent?*

A. *Haemophilus influenzae*
B. Group A beta-hemolytic streptococcus
C. Epstein-Barr virus
D. Rhinovirus

9–34 *Which of the following symptom(s) is (are) most indicative of mononucleosis (Epstein-Barr virus)?*

A. Rapid onset of anterior cervical adenopathy, fatigue, malaise, and headache
B. Gradual onset of fatigue, posterior cervical adenopathy, and palatine petechiae
C. Gradual and seasonal onset of pharyngeal erythema
D. Rapid onset of cough, congestion, and headache

9–35 *Which method can be safely used to remove cerumen in a 12-month-old child's ear?*

A. A size 2 ear curette.
B. Irrigation using hot water from a 3 cc syringe.
C. A commercial jet tooth cleanser.
D. Cerumen should not be removed from a child this young.

9–36 *Mark, age 18, has a persistent sore throat, fever, and malaise not relieved with penicillin therapy. What would you order next?*

A. A throat culture
B. A monospot test
C. A rapid antigen test
D. A Thayer-Martin plate test

9–37 *A sexual history of oral-genital contact in a client presenting with pharyngitis is significant when which of the following organisms is suspected?*

A. *Escherichia coli*
B. *Haemophilus influenzae*
C. *Neisseria gonorrheae*
D. *Streptococcus pneumoniae*

9–38 *When a practitioner places a vibrating tuning fork in the midline of a client's skull and asks if the tone sounds the same in both ears or is better in one, the examiner is performing:*

A. the Rinne test.
B. the Weber test.
C. the caloric test.
D. a hearing acuity test.

9–39 *Sharon, age 29, is pregnant for the first time. She complains of nasal stuffiness and occasional epistaxis. What do you do?*

A. Order extensive lab tests, such as a complete blood count with differential, hemoglobin, and hematocrit.
B. Prescribe an antihistamine.
C. Nothing, except for client teaching.
D. Refer the client to an ear, nose, and throat specialist.

9–40 *You note a completely split uvula in Noi, a 42-year-old Asian. What is your next course of action?*

A. Do nothing.
B. Refer Noi to a specialist.
C. Perform a throat culture.
D. Order a complete blood count.

9–41 *Monique brings her 4-week-old infant into the office because she noticed small, yellow-white, glistening bumps on her infant's gums. She says they look like teeth, but she is worried that they may be cancer. You diagnose these bumps as:*

A. Bednar's aphthae.
B. Epstein's pearls.
C. buccal tumors.
D. exostosis.

9–42 *Mattie says she has heard that it is not good to let a baby go to bed with a bottle. She says that she has always done this with her other children and wonders why it is not recommended. How do you respond?*

A. "A bottle in the baby's mouth forces the baby to breathe through the nose. If the nose is clogged, the baby will not get enough oxygen."
B. "A nipple, when placed in the mouth for long periods of time, can cause tooth displacement. This will also affect the adult teeth not grown in yet, and will necessitate braces in the teen years."
C. "Mouth bacteria act on the carbohydrates in the bottle contents to form acids, which will break down the tooth enamel and destroy its protein."
D. "This encourages the baby to continually want to drink at night, and when the child is older, it will become a habit, and the child will end up wearing diapers into the preschool years."

9–43 *When the Weber test is performed with a tuning fork to assess hearing and there is no lateralization, this indicates:*

A. conductive deafness.
B. perceptive deafness.
C. a normal finding.
D. nerve damage.

9–44 *A smooth tongue may indicate:*

A. a normal finding.
B. alcohol abuse.
C. a vitamin deficiency.
D. nicotine addiction.

9–45 *Signs and symptoms of acute angle-closure glaucoma include:*

A. painless redness of the eyes.
B. loss of peripheral vision.
C. translucent corneas.
D. halos around lights.

9–46 *Greg, age 72, is brought to the office by his son, who states that his father has been unable to see clearly since last night. Greg reports that his vision is "like looking through a veil." He also sees floaters and flashing lights, but is not having any pain. What do you suspect?*

A. Cataracts
B. Glaucoma
C. Retinal detachment
D. Iritis

9–47 *The most common offending allergens causing allergic rhinitis are:*

A. pollens of grasses, trees, and weeds.
B. fungi.
C. animal allergens.
D. dust mites.

9–48 *Shelley, age 47, is complaining of a red eye. You are trying to decide between a diagnosis of conjunctivitis and iritis. The one distinguishing characteristic between the two is:*

A. eye discomfort.
B. slow progression.
C. photophobia.
D. no change in or slightly blurred vision.

9–49 *Clients with allergic conjunctivitis have which type of discharge?*

A. Purulent
B. Serous or clear
C. Stringy and white
D. Profuse, mucoid, or mucopurulent

9–50 *Which is the most common localized infection of one of the glands of the eyelids?*

A. Hordeolum
B. Chalazion
C. Bacterial conjunctivitis
D. Herpes simplex

9–51 *Amy, age 26, has been wearing her contact lenses longer than usual. This morning, she woke up with severe eye pain and tearing. You observe an edematous cornea with some epithelial defects. Your next action is to:*

A. refer her to an ophthalmologist.
B. reassure her and schedule an appointment for the next day.
C. send her to the emergency room.
D. reassure her that this is common and there should not be any problems.

9–52 *The most common cause of a white pupil (leukokoria) in a newborn is:*

A. a cataract.
B. retinoblastoma.
C. persistent hyperplastic primary vitreous.
D. retinal detachment.

9–53 *Natasha, age 4, has amblyopia. How do you respond when her mother asks about treatment?*

A. "We'll wait until she's 7 years old before starting treatment."
B. "Treatment needs to be started now. We'll cover her 'bad' eye."
C. "Treatment needs to be started now. We'll cover her 'good' eye."
D. "No treatment is necessary. She'll outgrow this."

9–54 *How do you respond when Lynne, age 29, asks why she gets sores on her lips every time she sits out in the sun for an extended period of time?*

A. "You are allergic to the sun and must wear sunblock on your lips."
B. "Your lips are dry to begin with and you must keep them moist at all times."
C. "You have herpes simplex that recurs with sunlight exposure."
D. "You're probably allergic to your lip balm."

9–55 *Mavis has persistent pruritus of the external auditory canal. External otitis and dermatological conditions such as seborrheic dermatitis and psoriasis have been ruled out. What can you advise her to do?*

A. Use a cotton-tipped applicator daily to remove all moisture and potential bacteria.
B. Wash daily with soap and water.
C. Apply mineral oil to counteract dryness.
D. Avoid topical corticosteroids.

9–56 *How do you test for near vision?*

A. By using the Snellen eye chart
B. By using the Rosenbaum chart
C. By asking the client to read from a magazine or newspaper
D. By testing the cardinal fields

9–57 *When assessing the corneal light reflex, an abnormal finding indicates:*

A. possible use of eye medications.
B. a neurological problem.
C. improper alignment of the eyes.
D. strabismus.

9–58 *When assessing the internal structure of the eye, absence of a red reflex may indicate:*

A. a cataract or a hemorrhage into the vitreous humor.
B. acute iritis.
C. nothing; this is a normal finding in older adults.
D. diabetes or long-standing hypertension.

9–59 *Mavis is 70 years old and wonders if she can donate her corneas when she dies. How do you respond?*

A. "As long as you don't have any chronic illness, your corneas may be harvested."
B. "They will use corneas only from persons under age 65."
C. "What makes you feel like you are dying?"
D. "Don't think about such terrible things now."

9–60 *Justin, age 69, is going home 1 hour after having a lens implant after cataract removal in his left eye. In teaching him, you include all of the following points* ***except:***

A. "Keep the eye shield on until you see the doctor tomorrow."
B. "Sleep on the operative side."
C. "Take acetaminophen for discomfort."
D. "Avoid reading, lifting, or strenuous activity."

9–61 *Barbara, age 72, states that she was told she had atrophic macular degeneration and asks you if there is any treatment. How do you respond?*

A. "No, but 5 years from the time of the first symptoms, the process usually stops."
B. "Yes, there is a surgical procedure that will cure this."
C. "If we start medications now, they may prevent any further damage."
D. "Unfortunately, there is no effective treatment."

9–62 *Nathan, age 19, is a college swimmer. He frequently gets swimmer's ear and asks if there is* *anything he can do to help prevent it other than wearing earplugs, which don't really work for him. What do you suggest?*

A. Use a cotton-tipped applicator to dry the ears after swimming.
B. Use eardrops made of a solution of equal parts of alcohol and vinegar in each ear after swimming.
C. Use a hair dryer on the highest setting to dry the ears.
D. Tell Nathan that he must change his sport.

9–63 *Harry, age 69, has had Ménière's disease for several years. He has some hearing loss, but now has persistent vertigo. What treatment might be instituted to relieve the vertigo?*

A. A labyrinthectomy
B. Pharmacological therapy
C. A vestibular neurectomy
D. Wear an earplug in the ear with the most hearing loss

9–64 *Marvin has sudden eye redness that occurred after a strenuous coughing episode. You diagnose a subconjunctival hemorrhage. Your next step is to:*

A. refer him to an ophthalmologist.
B. order antibiotics.
C. do nothing other than provide reassurance.
D. consult with your collaborating physician.

9–65 *The leading cause of blindness in persons ages 20–60 in the United States is:*

A. macular degeneration.
B. glaucoma.
C. diabetic retinopathy.
D. trauma.

9–66 *Samantha, age 12, appears with ear pain. When you begin to assess her ear, you tug on her normal-appearing auricle, eliciting severe pain. This leads you to suspect:*

A. otitis media.
B. otitis media with effusion.
C. otitis externa.
D. primary otalgia.

9–67 *David, age 32, states that he thinks he has an ear infection because he just flew back from a business trip and feels unusual pressure in his ear. You diagnose barotrauma. What is your next action?*

A. Prescribe nasal steroids and oral decongestants.
B. Prescribe antibiotic eardrops.
C. Prescribe systemic antibiotics.
D. Refer David to an ear, nose, and throat specialist.

9–68 *Jill states that her 5-year-old daughter continually grinds her teeth at night. You document this as:*

A. temporal mandibular joint malocclusion.
B. bruxism.
C. a psychosis.
D. an oropharyngeal lesion.

9–69 *The most common cause of sensorineural hearing loss is:*

A. trauma.
B. tympanic membrane sclerosis and scarring.
C. otosclerosis.
D. presbycusis.

9–70 *In a young child, unilateral purulent rhinitis is most often caused by:*

A. a foreign body.
B. a viral infection.
C. a bacterial infection.
D. an allergic reaction.

9–71 *Claude, age 78, is being treated with timolol maleate (Timoptic) drops for his chronic open-angle glaucoma. While performing a new client history and physical, you note that he is taking other medications. Which medication would you be most concerned about?*

A. Aspirin therapy as prophylaxis for heart attack
B. Ranitidine (Zantac) for gastroesophageal reflux disease
C. Alprazolam (Xanax), an anxiolytic for anxiety
D. Atenolol (Tenormin), a beta blocker for high blood pressure

9–72 *Manny, age 16, was hit in the eye with a baseball. He developed pain in the eye, decreased visual acuity, and injection of the globe. You confirm the diagnosis of hyphema by finding blood in the anterior chamber. What treatment would you recommend while Manny is waiting to see the ophthalmologist?*

A. Application of bilateral eye patches.
B. Have Manny lie flat.
C. Refer him to an ophthalmologist within a week.
D. Make sure Manny is able to be awakened every 30 minutes.

9–73 *Jill presents with symptoms of hay fever and you assess the nasal mucosa of her turbinates to be pale. What diagnosis do you suspect?*

A. Allergic rhinitis
B. Viral rhinitis
C. Nasal polyps
D. Nasal vestibulitis from folliculitis

9–74 *Joy, age 36, has a sudden onset of shivering, sweating, headache, aching in the orbits, and general malaise and misery. Her temperature is 102°F. You diagnose influenza (flu). What is your next course of action?*

A. Order amoxicillin (Amoxil) 500 mg every 12 hours for 7 days.
B. Prescribe rest, fluids, acetaminophen (Tylenol), and possibly a decongestant and an antitussive.
C. Order a complete blood count.
D. Consult with your collaborating physician.

9–75 *Mandy was given a diagnosis of flu 3 days ago and wants to start on the "new flu medicine" right away. What do you tell her?*

A. "The medication is effective only if started within the first 48 hours after symptoms begin."
B. "If you treat a cold, it goes away in 7 days; if you don't treat it, it goes away in 1 week."
C. "The medicine has not proven its effectiveness."
D. "Good idea; I'll start you on amantadine."

9–76 *Matthew, age 52, has allergic rhinitis and would like some medicine to relieve his symptoms. He is taking cimetidine (Tagamet) for gastroesophageal reflux disease. Which medication would you* **not** *order?*

A. A first-generation antihistamine
B. A second-generation antihistamine
C. A decongestant
D. A topical nasal corticosteroid

9–77 *Sara, age 29, states that she has painless, white, slightly raised patches in her mouth. They are probably caused by:*

A. herpes simplex.
B. aphthous ulcers.
C. candidiasis.
D. oral cancer.

9–78 *Mycostatin (Nystatin) is ordered for Michael, who has an oral fungal infection. What instructions do you give Michael for taking the medication?*

A. "Don't swallow the medication because it's irritating to the gastric mucosa."
B. "Take the medication with meals so that it's absorbed better."
C. "Swish and swallow the medication."
D. "Apply the medication only to the lesions."

9–79 *Risk factors for oral cancers include:*

A. a family history, poor dental habits, and use of alcohol.
B. obesity, sedentary lifestyle, and chewing tobacco.
C. a history of diabetes, smoking, and a high fat intake.
D. smoking, use of alcohol, and chewing tobacco.

9–80 *Your neighbor calls you because her son, age 9, fell on the sidewalk while playing outside and a tooth fell out. She wants to know what she should put the tooth in to transport it to the dentist. You tell her that the best solution to put it in is:*

A. salt water.
B. saliva.
C. milk.
D. water.

9–81 *Because of Martha's history and the fact that she complains of pain behind her eye and high on her nose, you have made a diagnosis of acute sinusitis. Which sinuses are affected?*

A. Maxillary
B. Ethmoid
C. Frontal
D. Sphenoid

9–82 *You diagnose acute epiglottitis in Sally, age 5, and immediately send her to the local emergency room. All of the following symptoms would indicate that an airway obstruction is imminent* **except:**

A. stridor.
B. restlessness.
C. elevated temperature.
D. nasal flaring.

9–83 *Darren, age 26, has AIDS and presents with a painful tongue covered with what looks like creamy-white curd-like patches overlying erythematous mucosa. You are able to scrape off these "curds" with a tongue depressor, which assists you in making which of the following diagnoses?*

A. Leukoplakia
B. Lichen planus
C. Oral candidiasis
D. Oral cancer

9–84 *What is the easiest way to differentiate between otitis externa and otitis media?*

A. With otitis media, tender swelling is usually visible.
B. With otitis media, there is usually bilateral pain in the ears.
C. With otitis media, there is usually tenderness on palpation over the mastoid process.
D. With otitis externa, movement or pressure on the pinna is extremely painful.

9–85 *Which of the following refractive errors in vision is a result of the natural loss of accommodative capacity with age?*

A. Presbyopia
B. Hyperopia
C. Myopia
D. Astigmatism

9–86 *The most frequent cause of laryngeal obstruction in an adult is:*

A. a piece of meat.
B. a tumor.

C. mucosal swelling from an allergic reaction.
D. inhalation of a carcinogen.

9–87 *Marnie, who has asthma, has been told that she has nasal polyps. What do you tell her about them?*

A. Nasal polyps are usually precancerous.
B. Nasal polyps are benign growths.
C. The majority of nasal polyps are neoplastic.
D. They are probably inflamed turbinates, not polyps, because polyps are infrequent in clients with asthma.

9–88 *Mary, age 82, presents with several eye problems. She states that her eyes are always dry and look "sunken in." What do you suspect?*

A. Hypothyroidism
B. Normal age-related changes
C. Cushing's syndrome
D. A detached retina

9–89 *Marian, age 79, is at a higher risk than a middle-aged client for developing an eye infection because of which age-related change?*

A. Increased eyestrain
B. Loss of subcutaneous tissue
C. Change in pupil size
D. A decrease in tear production

9–90 *Marty has a hordeolum in his right eye. You suspect that the offending organism is:*

A. Herpes simplex virus.
B. *Staphylococcus*.
C. *Candida albicans*.
D. *Escherichia coli*.

9–91 *Henry is having difficulty getting rid of a corneal infection. He asks you why. How do you respond?*

A. "We can't determine the causative agent."
B. "Antibiotics have difficulty getting to that area."
C. "Because the infection was painless, it was not treated early enough."
D. "Because the cornea doesn't have a blood supply, an infection can't be fought off as usual."

9–92 *Sylvia has glaucoma and has started taking a medication that acts as a diuretic to reduce the intraocular pressure. Which medication is she taking?*

A. A carbonic anhydrase inhibitor
B. A beta-adrenergic receptor blocker
C. A miotic
D. A mydriatic

9–93 *Cydney, age 7, is complaining that she feels as though something is stuck in her ear. What action is contraindicated?*

A. Inspecting the ear canal with an otoscope
B. Using a small suction device to try to remove the object
C. Flushing the ear with water
D. Instilling several drops of mineral oil in the ear

9–94 *Ty, age 68, has a hearing problem. He tells you that he is ready for a drastic solution to the problem because he likes to play bingo but cannot hear the calls. What can you do for him?*

A. Refer him to a hearing aid specialist.
B. Refer him for further testing.
C. Perform a gross hearing test in the office, then repeat it in 6 months to determine if there is any further loss.
D. Nothing. Tell him that a gradual hearing loss is to be expected with aging.

9–95 *How would you describe the cervical lymphadenopathy associated with asymptomatic human immunodeficiency virus infection?*

A. Movable, discrete, soft, and nontender lymph nodes
B. Enlarged, warm, tender, firm, but freely movable lymph nodes
C. Hard, unilateral, nontender, and fixed lymph nodes
D. Firm but not hard, nontender, and mobile lymph nodes

9–96 *Microtia refers to the size of the:*

A. ears.
B. skull.
C. pupils.
D. eyes.

9–97 *With a chronic allergy, a client's nasal mucosa appear:*

A. swollen and red.
B. swollen, boggy, pale, and gray.
C. hard, pale, and inflamed.
D. bright pink and inflamed.

9–98 *Which manifestation is noted with carbon monoxide poisoning?*

A. Circumoral pallor of the lips
B. Cherry-red lips
C. Cyanosis of the lips
D. Pale pink lips

9–99 *Which manifestation of the buccal mucosa is present in a client with mumps?*

A. Pink, smooth, moist appearance with some patchy hyperpigmentation
B. Dappled brown patches
C. The orifice of Stensen's duct appearing red
D. Koplik's spots

9–100 *How would you grade tonsils that touch the uvula?*

A. Grade 1+
B. Grade 2+
C. Grade 3+
D. Grade 4+

9–101 *Sara, age 92, presents with dry eyes, redness, and a scratchy feeling. You note that this is one of the most common disorders, particularly in older women, and diagnose this as:*

A. viral conjunctivitis.
B. keratoconjunctivitis sicca.
C. allergic eye disease.
D. corneal ulcer.

9–102 *Mattie, age 64, presents with blurred vision in one eye and states that it felt like "a curtain came down over my eye." She doesn't have any pain or redness. What do you suspect?*

A. Retinal detachment
B. Acute angle-closure glaucoma
C. Open-angle glaucoma
D. Cataract

9–103 *Martin, age 24, presents with an erythematous ear canal, pain, and a recent history of swimming. What do you suspect?*

A. Acute otitis media
B. Chronic otitis media
C. External otitis
D. Temporomandibular joint syndrome

9–104 *Which pharmacological therapy has proved the most beneficial for long-term symptom relief of tinnitus?*

A. Aspirin
B. Lidocaine
C. Nortriptyline at bedtime
D. Corticosporin otic gtts prn

9–105 *Sally, age 19, presents with pain and pressure over her cheeks and discolored nasal discharge. You cannot transilluminate the sinuses. You suspect which common sinus to be affected?*

A. Maxillary sinus
B. Ethmoid sinus
C. Temporal sinus
D. Frontal sinus

9–106 *While doing a face, head, and neck exam, you note that the palpebral fissures are abnormally narrow. What are you examining?*

A. Nasolabial folds
B. The openings between the margins of the upper and lower eyelids
C. The thyroid gland in relation to the trachea
D. The distance between the trigeminal nerve branches

Answers

9–1 Answer A

At birth, a neonate's head size is 25% of the neonate's total body length, and the head size is greater than the chest circumference. When a child is age 6, the head is 90% of its final size. By adulthood, the head size is 12.5% of the adult's overall height.

9–2 Answer A

Treatment for cleft lip and palate needs to be instituted immediately after birth by constructing a palatal obturator to help the infant feed. Cleft lip and palate rehabilitation is an extensive program involving multiple procedures. A cleft lip may be unilateral or bilateral and complete or incomplete. It may also occur with a cleft in the entire palate or just the anterior or posterior palate.

9–3 Answer C

The trachea deviates toward the affected side with a large atelectasis or fibrosis. It deviates toward the unaffected side with an aortic aneurysm, unilateral thyroid lobe enlargement, and pneumothorax.

9–4 Answer C

A child's head circumference is measured, using a measuring tape, at each well-child visit until age 2 years. At birth, head circumference measures about 32–38 cm and is 2 cm larger than the chest circumference. At age 2, both the head and chest measurements are equal. During childhood, the chest circumference exceeds the head circumference by 5–7 cm.

9–5 Answer C

Bell's palsy should be suspected if a client presents with a rapid-onset, complete paralysis of one-half of the face and the inability to raise the eyebrow, close the eye, whistle, or show the teeth. Bell's palsy is a lower-motor-neuron lesion resulting in cranial nerve VII paralysis. It is often a self-limiting condition lasting a few days or weeks. Occasionally, facial paralysis may result from a tumor or physical trauma compromising the facial nerve. A cerebrovascular accident (CVA) would affect more than just the face. Trigeminal neuralgia, also called tic douloureux, is a painful disorder of the trigeminal nerve. It causes severe pain in the face and forehead on the affected side and is triggered by stimuli such as cold drafts, chewing, and drinking cold liquids.

9–6 Answer C

A child's central visual acuity is 20/30 by age 3 years. At birth, an infant can see about 12 inches away, an approximate 20/300 central visual acuity. It improves to 20/40 by age 2, 20/30 by age 3, and 20/20 by age 4.

9–7 Answer B

An explanation of 20/50 vision in a client's right eye would be: "You can see at 20 feet with your right eye what the normal person can see at 50 feet." Normal visual acuity is 20/20 on a Snellen eye chart. The larger the denominator, the poorer the vision. If vision is greater than 20/30, refer the client to an ophthalmologist or optometrist.

9–8 Answer C

The confrontation test is a gross measure of peripheral vision. It compares the client's peripheral vision with the practitioner's, assuming that the practitioner has normal peripheral vision. The cover test detects small degrees of deviated alignment by interrupting the fusion reflex that normally keeps both eyes parallel. The corneal light reflex test assesses the parallel alignment of the eye axes. The Snellen eye chart test assesses visual acuity.

9–9 Answer A

The normal ratio comparing the artery-to-vein ratio in the retinal vessels is 2:3 or 4:5, with the arterioles being a brighter red than the veins when viewed through the ophthalmoscope. The arterioles have a narrow light reflex from the center line of the vessel. Veins do not normally show a light reflex. Both arterioles and veins show a gradual and regularly diminishing diameter as you look at them from the disc to the periphery. When hypertension is present, the arterioles may be only about one-half the size of the corresponding vein, and they may appear opaque and lighter. With long-standing hypertension, nicking is present. This occurs when the underlying veins are concealed to some degree by the abnormally opaque arteriole wall at the vessel crossings.

9–10 Answer B

By age 3–4 months, an infant can fixate on, briefly follow, and then reach for a toy when the toy is placed in the infant's line of vision. At age 2–4 weeks, an infant can fixate on an object. By age 1 month, an infant can fixate on and follow a light or a bright toy. By age 6–10 months, an infant can fixate on and follow a toy in all directions.

9–11 Answer A

Xanthelasmas are soft, raised yellow plaques on the eyelids at the inner eye canthus. They appear most frequently in women, beginning in the 50s. Xanthelasmas occur with both high and normal lipid levels and have no pathologic significance. Pingueculae are yellowish, elevated nodules appearing on the sclera. They are caused by a thickening of the bulbar conjunctiva from prolonged exposure to the sun, wind, and dust. Arcus senilis appears as gray-white arcs or circles around the limbus as a result of deposits of lipid material that make the cornea look cloudy. Actinic keratoses are wartlike growths on the skin that occur in middle-aged or older adults and are caused by excessive exposure to the sun.

9–12 Answer C

Cranial nerve (CN) VIII, the vestibulocochlear nerve, is affected by sensorineural or perceptive hearing loss. Both the cochlear and vestibular branches have sensory pathways. CN II, the optic nerve, has sensory pathways. CN IV, the trochlear nerve, has both sensory and motor pathways. CN XI, the accessory nerve, has motor pathways.

9–13 Answer A

Although regular ocular pressure testing is indicated for all older adults on a routine basis, it is especially important for clients taking an extended regimen of high-dose inhaled glucocorticoids because prolonged continuous use increases the risk of ocular hypertension or open-angle glaucoma. Nonsteroidal anti-inflammatory drugs and angiotensin-converting enzyme inhibitors do not require ocular pressure monitoring. Older adults taking insulin need to have regular eye examinations because they are diabetic and have a risk of diabetic retinopathy, not because they are taking insulin.

9–14 Answer B

Presbyopia occurs in almost all persons beginning about the mid-40s. The lens loses elasticity and becomes hard and glasslike, decreasing the lens's ability to change shape to accommodate for near vision. Arcus senilis, a gray-white arc or circle around the limbus from deposition of lipid material, does not affect vision. Cataracts and glaucoma may occur around age 50 or above.

9–15 Answer A

In older adults, the most common cause of decreased visual functioning is cataract formation (lens opacity), which should be expected by age 70. Glaucoma (increased ocular pressure) is the second most common cause of decreased visual functioning. It increases from age 46–60, then levels off. Macular degeneration (loss of central vision), which affects 30% of persons over age 65, affects a person's ability to read fine print and do handiwork. Arcus senilis does not affect vision.

9–16 Answer B

Children aged $2^1/_2$–3 years should have their vision screened using the Allen test, which uses picture cards. The Snellen E chart is used for preschoolers age 3–6, whereas the Snellen letter chart is used for school-age and older clients. The Rosenbaum chart is used for a gross assessment of near vision by having the client hold reading material approximately 12–14 inches away.

9–17 Answer C

Esotropia is the inward turning of the eyes. Exotropia is the outward turning of the eyes. Strabismus, also called tropia, is the constant malalignment of the eye axes. It is likely to cause amblyopia. Pseudostrabismus has the appearance of strabismus because of the presence of epicanthic folds, but is normal in young children.

9–18 Answer B

If a client has throbbing pain in the eye, an irregular pupil shape, marked photophobia, and redness (a deep, dull, red halo) around the iris and/or cornea, suspect iritis. An immediate referral is warranted. The client may also have blurred vision. The client with conjunctivitis has redness more prominently at the periphery of the eye, along with tearing and itching. The client may also complain of a scratchy, burning, or gritty sensation, but not pain, although photophobia may be present. The client with subconjunctival hemorrhage presents with a sudden onset of a painless, bright-red appearance on the bulbar conjunctiva that usually results from pressure exerted during coughing, sneezing, or Valsalva's maneuver. Other conditions that may result in a subconjunctival hemorrhage include uncontrolled hypertension and the use of anticoagulant medication. The client with acute glaucoma presents with circumcorneal redness, with the redness radiating around the iris, and a dilated pupil.

9–19 Answer B

Hypopyon is purulent matter in an inflamed anterior chamber. A hyphema is blood in the anterior chamber, the result of trauma or spontaneous hemorrhage. Anisocoria, common in 5% of the population, refers to unequal pupil size. In 95% of these persons, it indicates central nervous system disease. A pterygium is a painless, unilateral or bilateral, triangle-shaped encroachment onto the conjunctiva that appears on the nasal side and is caused by excessive ultraviolet light exposure.

9–20 Answer D

A common cause of conductive hearing loss in adults ages 20–40 is otosclerosis, a gradual hardening of the tympanic membrane that causes the footplate of the stapes to become fixed in the oval window. Presbycusis, a progressive, bilaterally symmetrical perceptive hearing loss arising from structural changes in the hearing organs, usually occurs after age 50. Trauma may result in a conductive hearing loss, but this is certainly not common.

9–21 Answer D

With bacterial conjunctivitis there is purulent, thick discharge; with allergic conjunctivitis, a stringy mucoid discharge; and with viral conjunctivitis, there is usually a watery discharge. In a client with iritis, there is rarely a discharge.

9–22 Answer C

Acute otitis media is diagnosed when there is fluid in the middle ear accompanied by signs or symptoms of an ear infection. During the acute stage, acute otitis media is very painful. Inappropriate or ineffective treatment can lead to otitis media with effusion, which is often painless. An acute infection implies a current, not chronic, problem.

9–23 Answer D

A client with acute glaucoma requires urgent treatment and usually presents with sudden onset of impaired vision, severe eye pain, vomiting, and headache. You may assess injected conjunctiva, steamy corneas, a fixed, partially dilated pupil and a narrow chamber angle. A client with cataracts may present with decreased vision, and you would see an opacity, a cloudy lens, and a decreased view of the fundus. With macular degeneration there is decreased central vision, and with presbyopia, there may be blurred vision, but with a gradual onset. Only acute-angle glaucoma requires urgent treatment.

9–24 Answer C

Benzodiazepines like Clonazepam (Klonopin) may be ordered for temporal mandibular joint disorders for a short course of therapy only (1–2 weeks). They may be helpful for acute pain secondary to masticatory muscle spasm or temporomandibular joint pain. Monopioid analgesics may be ordered for inflammatory pain; anticonvulsants may be ordered for neuropathic pain; and skeletal muscle relaxants may be ordered for muscle relaxation.

9–25 Answer B

The antibiotic of choice for beta-lactamase coverage of otitis media is amoxicillin and potassium clavulanate (Augmentin). It is the first-line treatment for otitis media because it is effective against a wide range of bacteria including beta lactamase. Amoxicillin (Amoxil) is not effective against beta lactamase. Azithromycin (Zithromax) for otitis media is usually reserved for more resistant strains of the common bacterial pathogens. Prednisone (Deltasone) is reserved for otitis media with effusion.

9–26 Answer A

Most perforated tympanic membranes seen with acute otitis media heal within several weeks. If it has not healed within 3–6 months, a surgical repair can be done, but not until age 7–9 years. Sam can swim on the surface with the use of an ear mold, but must not dive, jump, or swim under water.

9–27 Answer A

If a child with otitis media with effusion has a change in the hearing threshold to less than or equal to 20 dB and has notable speech and language delays, more aggressive treatment is indicated. When the child's hearing examination reveals a change in the hearing threshold, it is extremely important that the provider evaluate the child's achievement of developmental milestones in speech and language. Any abnormal findings warrant referral.

9–28 Answer C

The immediate goal of myringotomy and tube placement in a child with recurrent episodes of otitis media is to allow removal of suppurative and mucoid material, thus releasing the pressure. This also prolongs the period of ventilation, allowing the middle ear mucosa to return to normal. Ventilation of the middle ear must be done to restore hearing and prevent aberrations in growth and development associated with hearing loss.

9–29 Answer A

A symptom cluster of severe throat pain with difficulty swallowing, copious oral secretions, respiratory difficulty and stridor, and fever, but without pharyngeal erythema or cough is indicative of epiglottitis. Streptococcal pharyngitis presents with cervical adenitis, petechiae, a beefy-red uvula, and a tonsillar exudate. A mild case of tonsillitis may appear to be only a slight sore throat. A more severe case would involve inflamed, swollen tonsils, a very sore throat, and a high fever. Diphtheria starts with a sore throat, fever, headache, and nausea, then progresses to patches of grayish or dirty-yellowish membranes in the throat that eventually grow into one membrane.

9–30 Answer A

When teaching clients about mononucleosis (Epstein-Barr virus [EBV]), tell them to avoid contact sports, heavy lifting, and stress, and that convalescence may take several weeks. Antibiotic therapy is not indicated for EBV. Bedrest is necessary only in severe cases.

9–31 Answer D

If a client has a sore throat and a history of diabetes or rheumatic fever, it is very likely that the infection is a result of group A beta-hemolytic streptococcus).

9–32 Answer A

The first-line antibiotic therapy for an adult with no known allergies and suspected group A beta-hemolytic streptococcus pharyngitis is penicillin.

9–33 Answer B

When the following four symptoms present as a cluster, there is a high probability (43%) that the infection is caused by group A beta-hemolytic streptococcus: throat pain with tonsillar exudate, anterior cervical adenopathy, presence of fever, and absence of cough.

9–34 Answer B

Symptoms most indicative of mononucleosis (Epstein-Barr virus) are gradual onset of fatigue, posterior cervical adenopathy, palatine petechiae, and hepatosplenomegaly.

9–35 Answer C

Irrigation with a soft bulb syringe or a commercial jet tooth cleanser may be used to remove cerumen. Irrigation using lukewarm water should be done when the cerumen is dry and hard but not if the tympanic membrane might be perforated. Cerumen can be safely removed from an infant's ear by the practitioner for adequate visualization of the tympanic membrane by using an ear curette through an operating otoscope, or if an operating otoscope is not available, by using a size 00 ear curette through a size 3-mm speculum.

9–36 Answer B

If a client has a persistent sore throat, fever, and malaise not relieved with penicillin therapy, a monospot test should be performed to rule out mononucleosis (Epstein-Barr virus). A throat culture and rapid antigen test are performed to help diagnose group A beta-hemolytic streptococci infection. A Thayer-Martin plate test is performed to diagnose a gonococcal infection.

9–37 Answer C

A sexual history of oral-genital contact in a client presenting with pharyngitis is significant when infection with *Neisseria gonorrhoeae* is suspected. *N. gonorrhoeae* pharyngitis is a common sexually transmitted disease. *Escherichia coli, Haemophilus influenzae,* and *Streptococcus pneumoniae* all cause acute bacterial meningitis.

9–38 Answer B

When a practitioner places a vibrating tuning fork in the midline of a client's skull and asks if the tone sounds the same in both ears or is better in one, the examiner is performing the Weber test. The Weber test is valuable when a client states that hearing is better in one ear than the other. The Rinne test compares air conduction and bone conduction sound. The stem of a vibrating tuning fork is placed on the client's mastoid process and the client is asked to signal when the sound disappears. The fork is then quickly inverted so that the vibrating end is near the ear canal, at which time the client should still hear a sound. Normally, sound is heard twice as long by air conduction as by bone conduction. The caloric test, or oculovestibular test, assesses cranial nerves III, VI, and VIII. Ice water is instilled into the ear; if nerve function is normal, the eyes will deviate to that side. A hearing acuity test assesses the client's ability to hear the spoken word.

9–39 Answer C

Nasal stuffiness and epistaxis may occur during a normal pregnancy because of increased vascularization in the upper respiratory tract. The gums may also be soft and hyperemic and may bleed with normal toothbrushing. No treatment, other than teaching the client what to expect and do, is indicated.

9–40 Answer A

Bifid uvula, a condition in which the uvula is either partially or completely split, occurs in 18% of Native Americans and 10% of Asians and is rare in whites and blacks. There is no need for treatment.

9–41 Answer B

Epstein's pearls are a normal finding in newborns and infants. They appear as small, yellow-white, glistening, pearly papules along the median raphe of the hard palate and on the gums. They look like teeth, but are small retention cysts that disappear after a few weeks. Bednar's aphthae are traumatic areas or ulcers that appear on the posterior hard palate on either side of the midline. They result from abrasions while sucking. A buccal tumor is a tumor on the inside of the cheek. Exostosis (torus palatinus) is found in the midline of the posterior 2/3 of the hard palate and is benign. It is a smooth, symmetrical bony structure.

9–42 Answer C

Baby bottle caries is a destruction of the upper deciduous teeth that occurs in older infants and toddlers who take a bottle of milk, juice, or sweetened liquid to bed. The liquid pools around the upper front teeth and the mouth bacteria act on the carbohydrates, especially sucrose, in the drink, forming metabolic acids that break down the tooth enamel and destroy its protein.

9–43 Answer C

A Weber test assesses hearing by bone conduction. With normal hearing, sound is heard equally well in both ears, meaning there is no lateralization. With conductive deafness, sound lateralizes to the defective ear because it is transmitted through bone rather than air. With perceptive deafness, sound lateralizes to the better ear.

9–44 Answer C

A smooth tongue may result from a vitamin deficiency. Normally, the dorsal surface of the tongue is rough because of papillae. The ventral surface near the floor of the mouth is smooth and shows large veins.

9–45 Answer D

Signs and symptoms of acute angle-closure glaucoma include seeing halos around lights, severe eye pain and redness, nausea and vomiting, headache, blurred vision, conjunctival injection, cloudy cornea, mid-dilated pupil, and an increased intraocular pressure. Acute angle-closure glaucoma is less common than primary open-angle glaucoma, accounting for about 10% of all glaucoma cases in the United States. Emergency treatment is indicated, so a prompt referral is necessary when these signs and symptoms occur.

9–46 Answer C

A client with retinal detachment complains of a sudden change in vision (either blurry vision, flashing lights, or floaters), but has no pain. On ophthalmoscopy, the retina appears pale, opaque, and folds in and undulates freely as the eye moves. Retinal detachment is an emergency and requires immediate surgery, usually scleral buckling, in which an encircling silicon band is used to keep the choroid in contact with the retina to promote attachment. Iritis is characterized by severe pain.

9–47 Answer A

The most common offending allergens causing allergic rhinitis are, in descending order, pollens of grasses, trees, and weeds; fungi; animal allergens; and dust mites. Rhinitis is the most troublesome allergic problem and affects 20% of the population.

9–48 Answer C

When trying to decide between a diagnosis of conjunctivitis and iritis, the one distinguishing characteristic between the two is photophobia. Photophobia occurs with corneal inflammation, iritis, and angle-closure glaucoma. Clients who have conjunctivitis usually do not have photophobia. Clients with iritis and conjunctivitis complain of eye discomfort, although in iritis the pain is moderately severe with intermittent stabbing. Both conditions generally produce a slowly progressive redness. Vision is normal with conjunctivitis and blurred with iritis.

9–49 Answer C

Clients with allergic conjunctivitis have a stringy, white discharge. Clients with bacterial conjunctivitis have a purulent discharge; those with viral conjunctivitis have serous or clear drainage and preauricular lymph node enlargement. A profuse mucoid or mucopurulent discharge is indicative of chlamydial conjunctivitis.

9–50 Answer A

Hordeolum (stye) is the most common localized infection of one of the glands of the eyelids. Treatment includes warm compresses for 15 minutes 4 times a day and topical antibiotics. A chalazion is a chronic swelling of the eyelids not associated with conjunctivitis. Bacterial conjunctivitis does not involve one of the glands of the eyelids. Primary herpes simplex of the eye usually presents as conjunctivitis with a clear, watery discharge; vesicles on the lids; and preauricular lymphadenopathy.

9–51 Answer B

If a client has been wearing his or her contact lenses longer than usual and has severe eye pain and tearing and an edematous cornea with some epithelial defects, he or she should be reassured and scheduled for an appointment the next day. If there is no improvement when the client is seen the following day, referral to an ophthalmologist is indicated. Reassure the client that the condition is usually not serious even though there is severe pain. Occasionally, contact lens-induced corneal abrasions, especially those associated with soft lenses, can progress rapidly to severe corneal infection; therefore, follow-up the next day is necessary. Clients may resume wearing their contact lenses after complete healing of the corneal epithelium has occurred.

9–52 Answer A

The most common cause of a white pupil (leukokoria) in a newborn is a congenital cataract. The incidence may be as high as 1 in every 500–1000 live births, and there is usually a family history. Some infants require no treatment; however, surgery may be performed on others during the first few weeks of life. Retinoblastoma, a common intraocular malignancy, is detected within the first few weeks of life and is the second most common cause of white pupil. Persistent hyperplastic primary vitreous is the third most common cause of white pupil and is a congenital developmental abnormality. Retinal detachment may occur as a result of trauma or disease and only rarely occurs in infancy.

9–53 Answer C

Treatment of amblyopia ("lazy eye") includes occluding the client's "good" (or better-seeing) eye and treating any underlying conditions such as cataracts or refractive errors. Treatment must be started by age 3 or 4 because amblyopia is irreversible after age 7. Amblyopia occurs in 50% of clients who have strabismus or misalignment of the eye muscles. Adults with strabismus frequently have double vision; however, young children learn to suppress or ignore double vision. As a result, young children have reduced central vision in the crossed eye from lack of use.

9–54 Answer C

Herpes simplex is associated with vesicular lesions on the lips and oral mucosa. The virus remains latent and may recur with sunlight exposure, stressful times, fever, trauma, and treatment with immunosuppressive drugs.

9–55 Answer C

Pruritus of the external ear canal is a common problem. In most cases, the pruritus is self-induced from enthusiastic cleaning or excoriation. The protective cerumen covering must be allowed to regenerate and may be helped to do so by application of a small amount of mineral oil, which helps to counteract dryness and reject moisture. The use of soap and water, as well as cotton-tipped swabs, should be avoided. The old adage "you shouldn't put anything smaller than your elbow in your ear" holds true today. If an inflammatory component is present, a topical corticosteroid may be applied. Often, isopropyl alcohol may relieve ear canal pruritus.

9–56 Answer B

Test for near vision by using the Rosenbaum chart. Hold it about 12–14 inches from the client's eyes. A gross estimate of near vision may also be assessed by asking the client to read from a magazine or newspaper held about 12–14 inches away from the eyes. The Snellen eye chart tests vision at a distance of 20 feet. Testing the cardinal fields of gaze does not test for vision, but rather for extraocular eye movements.

9–57 Answer C

When assessing the corneal light reflex, an abnormal finding indicates improper alignment of the eyes. It is noted when the reflections of the light are on different sites on the eyes. Some eye medications may cause unequal dilation, constriction, or inequality of pupil size and may be noted when assessing for direct and consensual pupil response. A neurological problem may be suspected if the pupils are unequal in size. Strabismus is noted during the cover-uncover test.

9–58 Answer A

When assessing the internal structure of the eye, absence of a red reflex may indicate the total opacity of the pupil because of a cataract or a hemorrhage into the vitreous humor. It may also be a result of improper positioning of the ophthalmoscope. Acute iritis is noted by constriction of the pupil accompanied by pain and circumcorneal redness. When inspecting the retina, if areas of hemorrhage, exudate, and white patches are present, they are usually a result of diabetes or long-standing hypertension.

9–59 Answer B

Corneas are harvested from the cadavers of uninfected persons under age 65 who die as the result of an acute trauma or illness. The client's question does not necessarily mean that she is thinking about dying, but it is natural for older adults to think about death, and their thoughts and feelings should be explored.

9–60 Answer B

After cataract surgery, clients should be instructed to avoid sleeping on the operative side to reduce edema and intraocular pressure. In addition, they should keep the eye shield or dressing in place until they see the doctor the following day for evaluation and dressing removal; take acetaminophen for discomfort; and avoid reading, lifting, or strenuous activity, which may also increase the intraocular pressure.

9–61 Answer D

Currently, there is no effective treatment for atrophic macular degeneration. Laser photocoagulation may slow the exudative form of macular degeneration if performed early in the course of the disease. It seals leaking capillaries and stops the exudation. Clients cope with the disease by using large-print books and magazines, magnifying glasses, and high-intensity lighting.

9–62 Answer B

Using eardrops made of a solution of equal parts of alcohol and vinegar in each ear after swimming is effective in drying the ear canal and maintaining an acidic environment and therefore preventing a medium for bacteria, the cause of swimmer's ear, to grow. It was previously mentioned that nothing smaller than your elbow should go in the ear. A hair dryer on the lowest setting several inches from the ear may be used to dry the canal.

9–63 Answer C

For a client who has had Ménière's disease for several years with some hearing loss, but now has persistent vertigo, treatment by vestibular neurectomy might relieve the vertigo. In vestibular neurectomy, the portion of cranial nerve VIII controlling balance and sensations of vertigo is severed. Vertigo is usually relieved in 90% of the cases. A labyrinthectomy is the surgery of last resort for a client with Ménière's disease because the labyrinth is completely removed and cochlear function destroyed. This procedure is used only when hearing loss is nearly complete. Oral diuretics and a low-sodium diet may aid in maintaining a lower labyrinth pressure, which may help slightly. Wearing an earplug will not help, and may aggravate the condition.

9–64 Answer C

There is no treatment for a subconjunctival hemorrhage other than to reassure the client that the blood will be reabsorbed within 2 weeks.

9–65 Answer C

The leading cause of blindness in persons ages 20–60 in the United States is diabetic retinopathy, a progressive microangiopathy with small-vessel damage and occlusion. Macular degeneration is the leading cause of blindness in persons over age 60. Glaucoma may eventually lead to loss of vision, but the symptoms have a slow progression, usually leading the client to eventual surgery to correct the problem. Trauma rarely leads to blindness.

9–66 Answer C

When severe pain is elicited by tugging on a normal-appearing auricle, an acute infection of the external ear canal (otitis externa) is suspected. Otitis media, with or without effusion, cannot be diagnosed without examining the tympanic membrane. Otalgia is simply ear pain.

9–67 Answer A

Barotrauma of the auditory canal causing abnormal middle ear pressure may be relieved by the use of nasal steroids and oral decongestants. With barotrauma, there is no infection, just swelling of the airways, which causes the abnormal pressure sensation; therefore, antibiotics are not indicated. This is certainly within the practitioner's scope of practice, and a referral is not indicated.

9–68 Answer B

Bruxism is grinding the teeth while sleeping and frequently occurs in young children. Bite blocks will prevent this until the child grows out of it.

9–69 Answer D

The most common cause of sensorineural hearing loss is presbycusis, a gradual decrease in cochlear function that occurs in most persons with advancing age. Otosclerosis (stapes fixation) and tympanic membrane sclerosis and scarring both result in a conductive hearing loss. Trauma would also result in a conductive hearing loss.

9–70 Answer A

In a young child, unilateral purulent rhinitis is most often caused by a foreign body. The key word is unilateral. Viral and bacterial infections and allergic reactions usually affect both nares.

9–71 Answer D

If a client is taking timolol maleate (Timoptic) drops for chronic open-angle glaucoma, you should be most concerned if the client is also taking atenolol (Tenormin), a beta blocker, for high blood pressure. Because timolol maleate drops are beta-adrenergic blockers, additional beta blockers can cause worsening of congestive heart failure or reactive airway disease, as well as acute delirium. Aspirin therapy as prophylaxis for heart attack, ranitidine (Zantac) for gastroesophageal reflux disease, and alprazolam (Xanax), an anxiolytic for anxiety, do not interact adversely with eye drops for glaucoma.

9–72 Answer A

The treatment for hyphema is strict bed rest, with the head elevated at least 20 degrees. The client needs to see an ophthalmologist within 24 hours. In the meantime, the application of bilateral eye patches to minimize eye movement, the instillation of atropine 1%, 2 drops b.i.d. to reduce ciliary spasm, and the administration of appropriate aspirin-free pain medications are indicated.

9–73 Answer A

The symptoms of hay fever, also called allergic rhinitis, are similar to those of viral rhinitis, but usually persist and are seasonal in nature. When assessing the nasal mucosa, you will observe that the turbinates are usually pale or violaceous because of venous engorgement with allergic rhinitis. With viral rhinitis, the mucosa is usually erythematous, and with nasal polyps, there are usually yellowish boggy masses of hypertrophic mucosa. Nasal vestibulitis usually results from folliculitis of the hairs that line the nares.

9–74 Answer B

Management of influenza (flu) is generally symptomatic and includes rest, fluids, acetaminophen (Tylenol), and possibly a decongestant and an antitussive. The client should be advised to call in 4 days if symptoms have not resolved.

9–75 Answer D

For the client with flu, amantadine (Symmetrel) or rimantadine (Flumadine) may be given. The dosage for adults is 100 mg twice a day, except for older adults with poor renal function; then the dosage is 100 mg once daily. The dosage in children up to age 10 is 5 mg/kg per day as a single dose. If the virus causing flu is type A influenza, the client may benefit from either one of these drugs. They are most effective if started early in the course of the disease, although reduction of symptoms and shortening the course of illness are still possible even if started 3–5 days after symptoms begin.

9–76 Answer B

Caution needs to be used when ordering a second-generation antihistamine for a client taking drugs such as cimetidine (Tagamet), erythromycin (E-Mycin), clarithromycin (Biaxin), and ketoconazole (Nizoral) that can block cytochrome P450 metabolism or if the client has serious hepatic impairment. There is also a rare causal link between terfenadine (Seldane) and astemizole (Hismanal) and torsade de pointes when given with some of these medications.

9–77 Answer C

Painless, white, slightly raised patches in a client's mouth are probably caused by candidiasis (thrush). Aphthous ulcers (canker sores) are extremely painful. Herpes simplex (a viral infection), canker sores, and cancerous lesions are usually discrete and not spread over a large area.

9–78 Answer C

When ordering mycostatin (Nystatin) for an oral fungal infection, tell the client to swish the medication in the mouth to coat all the lesions, then swallow it.

9–79 Answer D

Risk factors for oral cancers include smoking, use of alcohol, and chewing tobacco.

9–80 Answer C

Milk is the best storage and transport solution for avulsed teeth when one is planning on re-implanting them. If milk is not available, other solutions that might be used include saline (salt water), water, and saliva.

9–81 Answer B

With ethmoid sinus problems, the pain is behind the eye and high on the nose. Maxillary sinus pain is over the cheek and into the upper teeth; frontal sinus pain is over the lower forehead; and sphenoid sinus pain is in the occiput, vertex, or middle of the head.

9–82 Answer C

In a client with acute epiglottitis, the following symptoms would indicate that an airway obstruction is imminent: stridor, restlessness, nasal flaring, and use of accessory muscles for breathing. An elevated temperature would not indicate an imminent airway obstruction.

9–83 Answer C

Oral candidiasis (thrush) is distinctive because of the ability to rub off the white areas on the tongue with a tongue depressor. Leukoplakia cannot be removed by rubbing the mucosal surface. It appears as little white lesions on the tongue. Oral lichen planus is a chronic inflammatory autoimmune disease. It also has white lesions that do not rub off. Oral cancer must be ruled out in any lesion because early detection is the key to successful management and a good prognosis. Thrush may be seen in denture wearers; debilitated clients; and those who are immunocompromised, on corticosteroids, or on broad-spectrum antibiotics.

9–84 Answer D

The easiest way to differentiate between otitis externa and otitis media is that with otitis externa, movement or pressure on the pinna is extremely painful. With otitis externa, there may also be tender swelling of the outer ear canal. Bilateral pain in the ears is more suggestive of otitis externa. Clients with acute mastoiditis present with severe pain in, and especially behind, the ear.

9–85 Answer A

Presbyopia is the natural loss of accommodative capacity with age. About the mid-40s, persons note the inability to focus on objects at a normal reading distance. With hyperopia, objects at a distance are not seen clearly unless accommodation is used, and near objects may not be seen. This is corrected with plus or convex lenses. With myopia, the person is able to focus on very near objects without glasses. Far vision is difficult without the aid of corrective or minus, concave lenses. With astigmatism, the refractive errors are different in the horizontal and vertical axes.

9–86 Answer A

The most frequent cause of laryngeal obstruction in an adult is a piece of meat that lodges in the airway. With a tumor, there would be a gradual growth, and treatment would probably be sought before there is a complete obstruction. Mucosal swelling from an allergic reaction may result in an obstruction, but this does not occur as frequently as a laryngeal obstruction from a piece of meat. Inhalation of a carcinogen would result only in an irritation of the mucosa, if anything.

9–87 Answer B

Nasal polyps are benign growths that occur frequently in clients with sinus problems, asthma, and allergic rhinitis. Polyps are neither neoplastic growths nor precancerous, but do have the potential to affect the flow of air through the nasal passages. Clients who have asthma and have nasal polyps may have an associated allergy to aspirin, a syndrome that is referred to as Samter's triad.

9–88 Answer B

Dryness of the eyes and the appearance of "sunken" eyes are normal age-related changes. With hyperthyroidism, the eyes appear to bulge out (exophthalmos), but in hypothyroidism, the eyes do not appear any different. A moon face is apparent with Cushing's syndrome, and this might make the eyes appear to be sunken in, although on close examination, they are not. With a detached retina, the outward appearance is normal, but the client complains of seeing floaters or spots in the visual field and describes the sensation as like a curtain being drawn across the vision.

9–89 Answer D

Older adults are at a higher risk than middle-aged adults for developing an eye infection because of a decrease in tear production, which results in the inability of the tear ducts to wash out infectious organisms.

9–90 Answer B

A hordeolum (stye) is an abscess that may occur on the external or internal margin of the eyelid. It is typically caused by *Staphylococcus* bacteria.

9–91 Answer D

Because the cornea is an avascular organ, immune defenses have difficulty fighting off infections.

9–92 Answer A

Carbonic anhydrase inhibitors, such as acetazolamide (Diamox), act as diuretics to reduce the intraocular pressure in clients with glaucoma. A miotic causes contraction of the pupil and a mydriatic dilates the pupil. Because of the effect of pupil dilation on aqueous outflow in angle-closure glaucoma, medications such as atropine and other anticholinergics that have a mydriatic effect should be avoided. Miotics such as pilocarpine (Pilocar) may be given to cause contraction of the sphincter of the iris and to contract the ciliary muscle, which promotes accommodation for near vision and facilitates aqueous humor outflow by increasing drainage through the trabecular meshwork in open-angle glaucoma. But the question is asked about diuretics, which pilocarpine is not. It is a cholinergic agent.

9–93 Answer C

Flushing the ear with water is contraindicated when a client has a probable foreign body or insect in it. The water may cause the object to swell, making removal more difficult. Actions that may be taken include inspecting the ear canal with an otoscope, using a small suction device to try to remove the object, or instilling several drops of mineral oil in the ear.

9–94 Answer B

Approximately 10% of clients with a hearing loss are helped by medical or surgical treatment. If clients are sent for a hearing aid and not correctly identified as having a hearing loss, the underlying problem may not be resolved.

9–95 Answer D

The cervical lymphadenopathy associated with asymptomatic human immunodeficiency virus infection may be described as cervical lymph nodes that are firm but not hard, nontender, and mobile. In a healthy person, cervical nodes are often palpable, and are movable, discrete, soft, and nontender. In a client with an acute infection, the cervical nodes are bilateral, enlarged, warm, tender, and firm, but freely movable. Cancerous nodes are hard, unilateral, nontender, and fixed. In a client with a chronic inflammation, such as tuberculosis, the nodes are clumped.

9–96 Answer A

Microtia refers to the size of the ears, specifically ears smaller than 4 cm vertically.

9–97 Answer B

With a chronic allergy, a client's mucosa appears swollen, boggy, pale, and gray.

9–98 Answer B

Cherry-red lips are a manifestation of carbon monoxide poisoning. They also occur with acidosis from aspirin poisoning or ketoacidosis. In light-skinned clients, circumoral pallor of the lips occurs with shock and anemia and cyanosis of the lips occurs with hypoxemia and chilling. Some lips are normally pale pink.

9–99 Answer C

In a client with mumps, the orifice of Stensen's duct appears red. The buccal mucosa in a normal client appears pink, smooth, and moist, although there may be some patchy hyperpigmentation in dark-skinned clients. Dappled brown patches are present with Addison's disease. Koplik's spots are a prodromal sign of measles.

9–100 Answer C

Tonsils that touch the uvula are graded 3+. A grade of 1+ indicates that the tonsils are visible; a 2+ indicates that the tonsils are halfway between tonsillar pillars and uvula; and 4+ indicates that the tonsils touch each other. Tonsils are enlarged to 2+, 3+, or 4+ with an acute infection.

9–101 Answer B

Keratoconjunctivitis sicca is dry eyes, a common disorder among older women. It is associated with dryness, redness, or a scratchy feeling in the eyes. On rare severe occasions, there is marked discomfort and photophobia. Typically, it is caused by subtle abnormalities of the tear film and a reduced volume of tears. In most cases, tears can be replenished with the aqueous component of tears with over-the-counter artificial tears. Occasionally mucomimetics are indicated when there is mucin deficiency. Viral conjunctivitis is caused by a virus and is associated with pharyngitis, fever, malaise, and preauricular lymph node enlargement. Allergic eye disease is benign and usually occurs in late adolescence or early adulthood. It is usually seasonal, and allergy treatment may be effective. A corneal ulcer is most commonly the result of a bacterial, viral, or fungal infection.

9–102 Answer A

The classic sign of retinal detachment is a client stating that "a curtain came down over my eye." Typically, the person presents with blurred vision in one eye that becomes progressively worse, with no pain or redness. With acute angle-closure glaucoma there is a rapid onset in older adults, with severe pain and profound visual loss. The eye is red, with a steamy cornea and a dilated pupil. With open angle-glaucoma, there is an insidious onset in older adults, a gradual loss of peripheral vision over a period of years, and perception of "halos" around lights. With a cataract, there is blurred vision that is progressive over months or years and no pain or redness.

9–103 Answer C

With external otitis there is pain, an erythematous ear canal, and usually a history of recent swimming. Acute otitis media is also painful, is usually a result of cotton swab use or physical trauma, and usually follows an upper respiratory infection. Chronic otitis media is usually not painful, although during an exacerbation the ear may be painful. Ear pain may also be the result of temporomandibular joint dysfunction. It is usually made worse by chewing or grinding the teeth.

9–104 Answer C

Antidepressants, such as nortriptyline 50 mg at bedtime, have proven to be the most efficacious for chronic tinnitus. High doses of aspirin over a sustained period of time may actually cause tinnitus. Lidocaine given intravenously suppresses tinnitus in some individuals, but is not suitable for long-term suppression. Corticosporine eardrops have proven to have no effect.

9–105 Answer A

The maxillary sinus is the largest of the paranasal sinuses and is the most commonly affected sinus. There is usually pain and pressure over the cheek. Inability to transilluminate the cavity usually indicates a cavity filled with purulent material. Discolored nasal discharge, as well as a poor response to decongestants, may also indicate sinusitis. The ethmoid sinuses are usually nonpalpable and may not be transilluminated. The frontal sinuses are just below the eyebrows. Frontal sinusitis also includes pain and tenderness of the forehead.

9–106 Answer B

The palpebral fissures are the openings between the margins of the upper and lower eyelids. Someone who appears to be squinting is said to have narrow palpebral fissures. The nasolabial folds are the skin creases that extend from the angle of the nose to the corner of the mouth.

Bibliography

Berman, S: Otitis media in children. N Engl J Med 332:23, 1997.

Chaudhry, I, and Wong, S: Recognizing glaucoma: A guide for the primary care physician. Postgrad Med 99:5, 1997.

Dillon, PM: Nursing Health Assessment: A Critical Thinking, Case Studies Approach. FA Davis, Philadelphia, 2003.

Dunphy, LM, and Winland-Brown, JE: Primary Care: The Art and Science of Advanced Practice Nursing. FA Davis, Philadelphia, 2001.

Editorial: Inhaled and nasal steroids and the risk of glaucoma. Emerg Med 29:9, 1997.

Kearney, KM: Retinal detachment. Am J Nurs 97:8, 1997.

Naclerio, R, and Solomon, W: Rhinitis and inhalant allergens. JAMA 278:22, 1997.

Perkins, A: An approach to diagnosing the acute sore throat. Am Fam Physician 55:1, 1997.

Rubin, RH, et al: Medicine: A Primary Care Approach. WB Saunders, Philadelphia, 1996.

Ruppert, S: Differential diagnosis of common causes of pediatric pharyngitis. Nurse Pract 21:4, 1996.

Taylor, RB: Manual of Family Practice. Little, Brown, Boston, 1997.

Tierney, LM, et al. (eds): Current Medical Diagnosis & Treatment. Lange Medical Books–McGraw-Hill, New York, 2002.

HOW WELL DID YOU DO?

85% AND ABOVE CONGRATULATIONS! THIS SCORE SHOWS APPLICATION OF TEST-TAKING PRINCIPLES AND ADEQUATE CONTENT KNOWLEDGE.

75–85% KEEP WORKING! REVIEW TEST-TAKING PRINCIPLES AND TRY AGAIN.

65–75% HANG IN THERE! SPEND SOME TIME REVIEWING CONCEPTS AND TEST-TAKING PRINCIPLES AND THEN TRY THE TEST AGAIN.

Respiratory Problems 10

JILL E. WINLAND-BROWN
and
GRETCHEN HOPE MILLER HEERY

10–1 *Jessica, age 9 months, is brought into the clinic by her mother. She has a low-grade fever, stridor with agitation, some retractions, and a cough, but no drooling. You diagnose viral croup. Your next step would be to:*

A. hospitalize Jessica.
B. start antibiotic therapy.
C. order supportive treatment.
D. begin treatment with inhaled corticosteroids.

10–2 *Mr. Marks, age 54, has chronic obstructive pulmonary disease (COPD). He has recently been experiencing difficulty in breathing. His arterial blood gas screening reveals: pH 7.3; PaO_2 57 Hg; $PaCO_2$ 54 mm Hg; and oxygen saturation 84%. Mr. Marks has:*

A. respiratory acidosis.
B. respiratory alkalosis.
C. metabolic acidosis.
D. metabolic alkalosis.

10–3 *When teaching a mother who has a child with cystic fibrosis, you emphasize that the most important therapeutic approach to promote the child's pulmonary function is to:*

A. continuously administer low-flow oxygen.
B. administer bronchodilators on a regular basis.
C. perform chest physiotherapy with postural drainage, percussion, and vibration.
D. use maintenance antibiotic prophylactic therapy.

10–4 *Risk factors for pulmonary embolism in women include all of the following* ***except:***

A. obesity.
B. alcohol intake.
C. cigarette smoking.
D. hypertension.

10–5 *What is the normal ratio of the anteroposterior chest diameter to the transverse chest diameter?*

A. 1:1
B. 1:2
C. 2:3
D. 2:1

10–6 *To ease their breathing, clients with chronic obstructive pulmonary disease often position themselves in:*

A. an erect sitting position.
B. a tripod position.
C. a supine position.
D. a prone position.

10–7 *Increased tactile fremitus occurs with:*

A. pleural effusion.
B. lobar pneumonia.
C. pneumothorax.
D. emphysema.

10–8 *Hyperresonance on percussion of the chest occurs with:*

A. emphysema.
B. pneumonia.
C. pleural effusion.
D. lung tumor.

10–9 *The inspiratory rate equals the expiratory rate with which breath sound?*

A. Bronchial
B. Bronchovesicular
C. Vesicular
D. Tracheal

10–10 *With which voice sound technique do you normally hear a muffled "eeee" through the stethoscope on auscultating the chest when the client says "eeee"?*

A. Bronchophony
B. Egophony
C. Whispered pectoriloquy
D. Tonometry

10–11 *What is the name of the horizontal groove in the rib cage at the level of the diaphragm, extending from the sternum to the midaxillary line, that occurs normally in some children as well as in children with rickets?*

A. The sternal groove
B. The rickettsial groove
C. The manubrial groove
D. Harrison's groove

10–12 *What would be the 1-minute Apgar score for a newborn in good condition who needs only suctioning of the nose and mouth and otherwise routine care?*

A. 7–10
B. 6–8
C. 3–6
D. 0–2

10–13 *With respiratory retraction, in which age group does it occur more often?*

A. Newborn and infant
B. School-age child
C. Young adult
D. Older adult

10–14 *An infant who has periodic breathing with persistent or prolonged apnea (greater than 20 seconds) may have an increased risk of:*

A. pneumonia.
B. left-sided congestive heart failure.
C. sudden infant death syndrome.
D. anemia.

10–15 *Stridor can be heard on auscultation when a client has:*

A. atelectasis.
B. asthma.
C. diaphragmatic hernia.
D. acute epiglotitis.

10–16 *The nursing diagnosis of "impaired gas exchange" may be demonstrated by:*

A. clubbing of the fingers.
B. nasal flaring.
C. the use of accessory muscles.
D. a cough.

10–17 *Which irregular respiratory pattern has a series of three to four normal respirations followed by a period of apnea and is seen with head trauma, brain abscess, heat stroke, spinal meningitis, and encephalitis?*

A. Cheyne-Stokes respiration
B. Biot's respiration
C. Kussmaul's respiration
D. Hypoventilation

10–18 *What is the definition of the spirometric assessment of residual volume?*

A. The sum of the vital capacity and the residual volume
B. The amount of gas left in the lung after exhaling all that is physically possible
C. The volume that can be maximally exhaled after a passive exhalation
D. The measurement of the maximum flow rate achieved during the forced vital capacity maneuver

10–19 *Which of the following conditions is characterized by intermittent episodes of airway obstruction caused by bronchospasm, excessive bronchial secretion, or edema of bronchial mucosa?*

A. Asthma
B. Atelectasis
C. Acute bronchitis
D. Emphysema

10–20 *In which condition would you assess vesicular breath sounds, moderate vocal resonance, and localized crackles with sibilant wheezes?*

A. Bronchiectasis
B. Acute bronchitis
C. Emphysema
D. Asthma

10–21 *In which condition would the trachea be deviated toward the normal side?*

A. Pleural effusion and thickening
B. Pneumonia
C. Bronchiectasis
D. Pulmonary fibrosis

10–22 *Which sympathomimetic agents are the drugs of choice for asthma?*

A. Alpha agonists
B. Beta$_1$ agonists
C. Beta$_2$ agonists
D. Alpha antagonists

10–23 *Jamie has her asthma well controlled by using only a beta-adrenergic metered-dose inhaler. Lately, however, she has had difficulty breathing during the night and her sleep has been interrupted about three times a week. What do you do?*

A. Prescribe a short course of steroid therapy.
B. Prescribe an inhaled steroid.
C. Prescribe a longer-acting bronchodilator.
D. Prescribe oral theophylline.

10–24 *Community-acquired bacterial pneumonia is most commonly caused by:*

A. *Streptococcus pneumoniae.*
B. *Mycoplasma pneumoniae.*
C. *Haemophilus influenzae.*
D. *Staphylococcus aureus.*

10–25 *The antibiotic of choice for the treatment of* Streptococcus pneumoniae *infection is:*

A. dicloxacillin.
B. erythromycin.
C. penicillin.
D. ampicillin clavulanate.

10–26 *Martin, age 76, has just been given a diagnosis of pneumonia. Which of the following is an indication that he should be hospitalized?*

A. Inability to take oral medications and multilobar involvement on chest x ray.
B. Alert and oriented status, slightly high but stable vital signs, and no one to take care of him at home
C. Sputum with gram-positive organisms
D. A CBC showing leukocytosis

10–27 *Which of the following statements is true regarding pulmonary tuberculosis?*

A. Manifestations are usually confined to the respiratory system.
B. Dyspnea is usually present in the early stages.
C. Crackles and bronchial breath sounds are usually present in all phases of the disease.
D. Night sweats are often noted as a manifestation of fever.

10–28 *Groups at high risk for tuberculosis include:*

A. racial and ethnic minorities
B. foreign-born individuals
C. substance abusers
D. all of the above

10–29 *Which of the following individuals most likely will not have a false-negative reaction to the Mantoux test?*

A. Marvin, age 72
B. Jane, who is on corticosteroid therapy for an acute exacerbation of asthma
C. Jerry, who has lymphoid leukemia
D. Mary, who recently was exposed to someone coughing

10–30 *The diagnosis of tuberculosis does not need to be reported when:*

A. the client's Mantoux test shows an induration of 15 mm.
B. a case of tuberculosis is only suspected.
C. an asymptomatic client has a positive chest x ray for pulmonary tuberculosis.
D. the Mantoux test shows a raised injected or red area without induration.

10–31 *Marisa, who is pregnant, has just been given a diagnosis of tuberculosis. What do you do?*

A. Wait until Marisa delivers, then begin therapy immediately.
B. Begin therapy with isoniazid (Nydrazid), rifampin (Rimactane), and pyrazinamide now.
C. Begin therapy with isoniazid, rifampin, and ethambutol (Myambutol) now.
D. Begin therapy with isoniazid now, wait to see how Marisa tolerates it, then add rifampin, pyrazinamide, or ethambutol.

10–32 *Which statement about chronic obstructive pulmonary disease (COPD) is true?*

A. The prevalence of COPD is directly related to increasing age.
B. The incidence of COPD is about equal in men and in women.
C. Cigar or pipe smoking does not increase the risk of developing COPD.
D. Environmental factors such as smoke do not affect the potential for COPD.

10–33 *Theophylline (Theo-Dur) acts:*

A. as a bronchodilator.
B. to decrease dyspnea.
C. to impede mucociliary clearance.
D. by doing all of the above.

10–34 *The following major bacterial pathogen does not cause an infectious exacerbation in a client with chronic obstructive pulmonary disease:*

A. *Streptococcus pneumoniae.*
B. *Haemophilus influenzae.*
C. *Branhamella catarrhalis.*
D. *Pneumococcus coli.*

10–35 *Which statement is false regarding primary spontaneous pneumothorax?*

A. It usually occurs in healthy individuals without pre-existing lung disease.
B. It occurs more commonly in young, tall, asthenic men.

C. It is an accumulation of air in the normally airless pleural space between the lung and chest wall.
D. It frequently occurs in Marfan's syndrome.

10–36 *Which of the following is not a leading contributor to the incidence of carcinoma of the lung?*

A. Cigarette smoking.
B. Exposure to materials such as asbestos, uranium, and radon.
C. Chronic interstitial lung diseases.
D. Chronic pneumonia.

10–37 *What would the TNM (tumor, node, metastasis) classification be for a lung tumor that had carcinoma in situ, metastasis to the lymph nodes in the peribronchial or the ipsilateral hilar region, and distant metastasis to the spine?*

A. T1SN1M1
B. T2N0M0
C. T3N1M1
D. T0N1M0

10–38 *Tina, age 49, is on multiple drug therapy for tuberculosis. She asks you how long she needs to take the drugs. You respond:*

A. "6 weeks to 2 months."
B. "4–6 months."
C. "6–9 months."
D. "1 year."

10–39 *When should well individuals be screened for tuberculosis?*

A. Every year.
B. Every other year.
C. At age 1 year, then again at entry to preschool or kindergarten, and then at some point during adolescence.
D. Every 4 years.

10–40 *What change(s) in the lungs account for decreased cough effectiveness in older adults?*

A. A decrease in vital capacity
B. An increase in the residual volume
C. Less lung elasticity
D. All of the above

10–41 *Clinical manifestations of cancer of the larynx include all of the following* ***except:***

A. earache.
B. halitosis.
C. hoarseness.
D. frequent swallowing.

10–42 *After a total laryngectomy for laryngeal cancer, the client will have a:*

A. permanent tracheostomy.
B. temporary tracheostomy until the internal surgical incision heals.
C. temporary tracheostomy until an implant can be done.
D. patent normal airway.

10–43 *Michael, age 52, has a dry cough, dyspnea, chills, fever, general malaise, headache, confusion, anorexia, diarrhea, myalgias, and arthralgias. Which diagnosis do you suspect?*

A. Bronchopneumonia.
B. Legionnaires' disease.
C. Primary atypical pneumonia.
D. *Pneumocystis carinii* pneumonia.

10–44 *In trying to differentiate between chronic bronchitis and emphysema, you know that chronic bronchitis:*

A. usually occurs after age 50 and has insidious progressive dyspnea.
B. usually presents with a cough that is mild and scant clear sputum, if any.
C. presents with adventitious sounds, wheezing and rhonchi, and a normal percussion note.
D. results in an increased total lung capacity with a markedly increased residual volume.

10–45 *James, age 12, just moved here from Texas. He presents with a headache, cough, fever, rash on the legs and arms, myalgias, and dysuria. His white blood cell count is 12.9 with 8% bands and 7–10% eosinophils. Electrolyte levels are normal. Blood cultures are negative. Sputum is not available. A Mantoux skin test so far is negative. What do you suspect?*

A. Pulmonary tuberculosis
B. Lymphoma
C. Asthma
D. Coccidioidomycosis

10–46 *In inner-city children, an important cause of asthma-related illness and hospitalizations is:*

A. heredity and genetics.
B. vitamin deficiencies.
C. cockroaches.
D. playing on asphalt playgrounds.

10–47 *Jill, age 49, has daily symptoms of asthma. She uses her inhaled short-acting beta$_2$ agonist daily. Her exacerbations affect her activities, and they occur at least twice weekly and may last for days. She is affected more than once weekly during the night with an exacerbation. Which category of asthma severity is Jill in?*

A. Step 1: mild intermittent
B. Step 2: mild persistent
C. Step 3: moderate persistent
D. Step 4: severe persistent

10–48 *What should be considered in all clients with adult-onset asthma or in clients with asthma that worsens in adulthood?*

A. Occupational asthma
B. A suppressed immune system
C. Another immunologic disease
D. Concurrent chronic obstructive pulmonary disease

10–49 *How does pregnancy affect asthma?*

A. During pregnancy, asthma usually improves.
B. During pregnancy, asthma usually worsens.
C. Symptoms in about one-third of pregnant women with asthma improve, about one-third are unchanged, and about one-third worsen.
D. Symptoms in about one-half of pregnant women improve; those of the other half worsen.

10–50 *Associated pathophysiology in clients with chronic bronchitis include all* ***except:***

A. dysfunctional cilia.
B. increased numbers of neutrophils and macrophages.
C. increased permeability of the pulmonary epithelium.
D. hypoplasia of the mucus glands.

10–51 *The bacterial pathogen(s) common in exacerbations of chronic bronchitis is (are):*

A. influenza.
B. rhinovirus.
C. coronavirus.
D. streptococcus pneumoniae.

10–52 *When should a rescue course of prednisolone be initiated for an attack of asthma?*

A. When the client is in step 1 (intermittent stage)
B. When the client is in step 2 (mild persistent stage)
C. When the client is in step 4 (severe persistent stage)
D. Whenever the client needs it, at any time and at any step

10–53 *You are teaching Shawna, age 14 with asthma, to use a home peak expiratory flow meter daily to measure gross changes in peak expiratory flow. Which "zone" would rate her expiratory compliance as 50-80% of her personal best?*

A. white zone
B. green zone
C. yellow zone
D. red zone

10–54 *Which percentage of individuals for whom it is indicated typically receive the pneumococcus vaccine?*

A. 10%
B. 30%
C. 60%
D. 90%

10–55 *Of the nearly 46 million adults who smoke, 34% try to quit each year, but how many actually succeed?*

A. 2.5%
B. 10%
C. 20%
D. 50%

10–56 *What is the first-line bronchodilator therapy for chronic obstructive pulmonary disease?*

A. An inhaled beta_2 agonist.
B. Inhaled ipratropium (Atrovent).
C. A long-acting bronchodilator such as salmeterol (Serevent).
D. A short course of corticosteroids.

10–57 *For a diagnosis of asthma to be made, the client must do all of the following* ***except:***

A. demonstrate episodic symptoms of airflow obstruction.
B. show evidence that the airflow obstruction is at least partly reversible.
C. have other conditions excluded from the differential diagnosis.
D. after a trial course of Proventil.

10–58 *Sally, age 49, has had asthma for several years, but has never used a peak flow meter. Should you now recommend it?*

A. No, she has been managing fine without it.
B. Yes, she might recognize early signs of deterioration.
C. Present the options and let Sally decide.
D. No, at her age it is not recommended.

10–59 *In counseling your client with asthma, you suggest that she does all of the following to help control her allergy to dust mites* ***except:***

A. cover the mattress and pillows in airtight, dust-proof covers.
B. wash the bedding weekly and dry it on a hot setting for 20 minutes.
C. Avoid sleeping on natural fibers such as wool or down.
D. Open the windows and air out the room daily.

10–60 *Which of the following is not an indication for a bronchoscopy?*

A. To evaluate indeterminate lung lesions
B. To stage cancer preoperatively
C. To determine the extent of injury secondary to burns, inhalation, or other trauma
D. To widen a severe tracheal stenosis

10–61 *Which of the following statements is true regarding the recurrence of a spontaneous pneumothorax?*

A. A primary spontaneous pneumothorax is more likely to recur than a secondary one.
B. A secondary spontaneous pneumothorax is more likely to recur than a primary one.
C. Recurrence rates for both primary and secondary spontaneous pneumothorax are similar.
D. Spontaneous pneumothorax rarely reoccurs.

10–62 *Which of the following underlying lung diseases may cause a secondary spontaneous pneumothorax?*

A. Chronic obstructive pulmonary disease
B. Lung abscess
C. Cystic fibrosis
D. All of the above

10–63 *What is the term describing an auscultation sound at the mediastinum in the presence of a mediastinal "crunch" that coincides with cardiac systole and diastole?*

A. Homans' sign
B. Hamman's sign
C. Manubrium's sign
D. Louis's sign.

10–64 *The causative agent of the community-acquired pneumonia seen most often in the client with an alcohol problem is:*

A. pneumococcus.
B. mycoplasma.
C. legionella.
D. *Haemophilus influenzae.*

10–65 *Increased severity of underlying illness, presence of an indwelling urethral catheter, and use of broad-spectrum antibiotics are risk factors predisposing clients to the development of:*

A. tuberculosis.
B. decreased mobility.
C. pressure ulcers.
D. nosocomial pneumonia.

10–66 Which organism most commonly causes nosocomial pneumonia?

A. *Candida*
B. A methicillin-resistant organism
C. *Pseudomonas aeruginosa*
D. *Staphylococcus aureus*

10–67 *Mark, age 72, has been living in a shelter for 4 months. Today he appears at the clinic complaining of productive cough, weight loss, weakness, anorexia, night sweats, and generalized malaise. These have been bothering him for 8 weeks. What would be one of the first tests you order?*

A. Mantoux test
B. Chest x ray
C. Complete blood work
D. Sputum culture

10–68 *Harvey is taking theophylline for his chronic obstructive pulmonary disease. Which of the following increases the clearance rate and might indicate the need for a higher dosage of theophylline to be ordered?*

A. Cigarette smoking
B. Hepatic insufficiency
C. Allopurinol (Zyloprim)
D. Cimetidine (Tagamet)

10–69 *Which of the following statements about sarcoidosis is true?*

A. It commonly occurs in persons in their 50s.
B. It is more common in whites than in blacks.
C. Many organs may be involved, but the most involved organ is the lung.
D. It occurs more frequently in men than in women.

10–70 *Marci, age 15, has been given a diagnosis of step 1 (mild intermittent) asthma. What long-term control therapy is indicated?*

A. None
B. A single agent with anti-inflammatory activity
C. An inhaled corticosteroid with the addition of long-acting bronchodilator if needed
D. Multiple long-term control medications with oral corticosteroids if needed

10–71 *The most common cause of a persistent cough in children of all ages is:*

A. an allergy.
B. recurrent viral bronchitis.
C. asthma.
D. an upper respiratory infection.

10–72 *Chronic cough in children is frequently caused by all of the following* ***except:***

A. allergic rhinitis.
B. chronic sinusitis.
C. enlarged adenoids.
D. cystic fibrosis.

10–73 *Unexplained nocturnal cough in an older adult should suggest:*

A. allergies.
B. asthma.
C. congestive heart failure.
D. viral syndrome.

10–74 *Dyspnea can be caused by:*

A. increased rigidity of lung tissue.
B. increased airway resistance.
C. enhanced ventilation during exercise.
D. all of the above.

10–75 *Which of the following statements is true when trying to differentiate pulmonary from cardiac causes of dyspnea on exertion?*

A. When the cause is pulmonary, the rate of recovery to normal respiration is slow, and dyspnea abates eventually after cessation of exercise.
B. Clients with dyspnea from cardiac causes remain dyspneic much longer after cessation of exercise.
C. In dyspnea arising from cardiac causes, the heart rate will return to pre-exercise levels within a few minutes after cessation of exercising.
D. Clients with pulmonary dyspnea have minimal dyspnea at rest.

10–76 *Laura, age 36, has an acute onset of dyspnea. Associated symptoms include chest pain, faintness, tachypnea, peripheral cyanosis, low blood pressure, crackles, and some wheezes. Her history reveals that she is taking birth control pills and that she smokes. What do you suspect?*

A. Asthma
B. Bronchitis
C. Pulmonary emboli
D. Pneumothorax

10–77 *What percentage of persons who smoke one pack of cigarettes per day or more have a cough?*

A. 10–25%
B. 40–60%
C. 75%
D. 100%

10–78 *The most common reason for a chronic cough in children is:*

A. asthma.
B. a postinfection.
C. a postnasal drip.
D. an irritant.

10–79 *A pulmonary function test, such as spirometry, is helpful in the diagnosis of:*

A. chronic bronchitis.
B. lung cancer.
C. pneumonia.
D. tuberculosis.

10–80 *The three principal triggers for exacerbations of asthma include all the following* ***except:***

A. allergens.
B. infections.
C. weather changes.
D. psychological factors.

10–81 *Mary, age 69, has chronic obstructive pulmonary disease. Her oxygen saturation is less than 89%. She is to start on oxygen therapy to relieve her symptoms. How often must she be on oxygen therapy to actually improve her oxygen saturation?*

A. On an as-needed basis
B. Continuously
C. 6–12 hours per day
D. 18 hours per day

10–82 *Which is the accepted mass screening test for lung cancer?*

A. An annual physical examination.
B. A chest x ray.
C. Sputum cytology.
D. There is no accepted mass screening test for lung cancer.

10–83 *What is effective in the treatment of pneumonia, atelectasis* **and** *cystic fibrosis?*

A. Deep breathing
B. Oxygen
C. Inhalers
D. Chest physiotherapy

10–84 *Which of the following medical conditions is/are known to increase the risk of tuberculosis substantially?*

A. Human immunodeficiency virus infection
B. Jejunoileal bypass
C. Chronic renal failure
D. All of the above

10–85 *Which of the following statements is true regarding weight and smoking cessation?*

A. Smokers weigh 10–20 lbs less than nonsmokers.
B. When smokers quit, 90% of them gain weight.
C. Men gain more weight than women when they quit.
D. Smokers gain weight after smoking cessation because they replace cigarettes with food.

10–86 *When teaching smokers about using nicotine gum to aid in smoking cessation, tell them to:*

A. chew the gum like regular gum.
B. discard the gum after 30 minutes.
C. drink a cup of coffee before chewing the gum because it assists in the nicotine absorption.
D. chew 6–9 pieces daily to help prevent nicotine withdrawal.

10–87 *Which of the following peripharyngeal upper respiratory tract infections occurs most often in children age 2–5 years?*

A. Peritonsillar abscess
B. Epiglottitis
C. Laryngotracheobronchitis (croup)
D. Bacterial tracheitis

10–88 *Susie, age 10, has a cough that characteristically occurs all day long, but never during sleep. You suspect:*

A. a psychogenic cough (or habit).
B. allergic rhinitis.
C. pertussis.
D. postnasal drip.

10–89 *Which of the following drugs causes a cough by inducing mucus production (bronchorrhea)?*

A. Tobacco and/or marijuana
B. Beta-adrenergic blockers
C. Aspirin and nonsteroidal anti-inflammatory drugs
D. Cholinesterase inhibitors

10–90 *The following figure shows a method of assessing for digital clubbing called:*

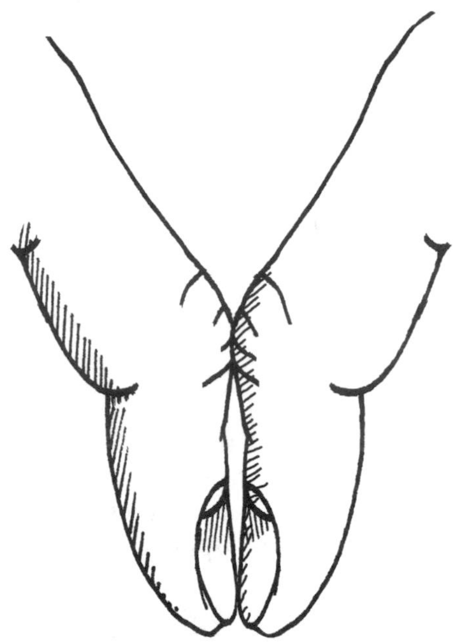

A. phalangeal depth ratio.
B. hyponychial angle.
C. Schamroth's window.
D. the "diamond" test.

10–91 *What is the normal respiratory rate of an 18-month-old child while awake?*

A. 58–75 breaths per minute
B. 30–40 breaths per minute
C. 23–42 breaths per minute
D. 19–36 breaths per minute

10–92 *A definitive test for cystic fibrosis is:*

A. the sweat test.
B. a sputum culture.
C. a fecal fat test.
D. a Chymex test for pancreatic insufficiency.

10–93 *What is the most common cause of sudden and unexpected death in infants, accounting for 80% of postneonatal infant mortality with a peak incidence at 6 months?*

A. Choking
B. Shaken baby syndrome
C. Infantile pneumonia
D. Sudden infant death syndrome (SIDS)

10–94 *The two most predominant organisms constituting the normal flora of the oropharynx are:*

A. streptococci and staphylococci.
B. streptococci and *Moraxella catarrhalis*.
C. staphylococci and *Candida albicans*.
D. various protozoa and staphylococci.

10–95 *What early acid-base disturbance occurs in a teenager admitted for an aspirin overdose?*

A. Respiratory acidosis
B. Respiratory alkalosis
C. Metabolic acidosis
D. Metabolic alkalosis

10–96 *Which of the following statements regarding the respiratory status of the pregnant woman are false?*

A. The thoracic cage may appear wider.
B. The costal angle may feel wider.
C. Respirations may be deeper.
D. Oxygenation is decreased.

10–97 *Which shape of the thorax is normal in an adult?*

A. Elliptical
B. Funnel
C. Pectus carinatum
D. Barrel

10–98 *Which of the following workers is at risk for developing pneumoconiosis?*

A. Farmers
B. Coal miners
C. Construction workers
D. Potters

10–99 *Cough and congestion result when breathing:*

A. carbon monoxide.
B. sulfur dioxide.
C. tear gas.
D. carbon dioxide.

10–100 *A cough caused by a postnasal drip related to sinusitis is more prevalent at what time of day?*

A. Continuously throughout the day
B. In the early morning
C. In the afternoon and evening
D. At night

Answers

10–1 Answer C

The treatment of viral croup is supportive. Mist therapy, oral hydration, and minimal handling are recommended. The presence of stridor at rest requires hospitalization. Antibiotic therapy is not indicated because this condition is viral. The use of corticosteroids remains controversial in this instance. A short course may be tried if the client is unresponsive to epinephrine, but the corticosteroid is given orally or parentally. Nebulized steroids may also be effective, but are not available in the United States.

10–2 Answer A

Respiratory acidosis results when the serum $PaCO_2$ exceeds 45 mm Hg and the serum pH is less than 7.35. It occurs when there is a reduction in the rate of alveolar ventilation in relation to the rate of carbon dioxide production. The end result is an accumulation of dissolved carbon dioxide or carbonic acid. Mr. Marks' chronic obstructive pulmonary disease leads to alveolar hypoventilation with an acute retention of carbon dioxide, resulting in acute respiratory acidosis. With respiratory alkalosis, hyperventilation is usually evident, the $PaCO_2$ is less than 35 mm Hg, and the pH greater than 7.45. In metabolic acidosis, the HCO_3 is less than 22 mEq/L and the pH less than 7.35. In metabolic alkalosis, the HCO_3 is more than 26 mEq/L and the pH is greater than 7.45.

10–3 Answer C

Daily performance of chest physiotherapy with postural drainage, percussion, and vibration to remove the abnormally viscous mucus is essential for the client with cystic fibrosis. With cystic fibrosis, the problem lies at the level of the epithelial cells of the small airways, not the bronchia; therefore bronchodilators do not help. Antibiotics should be administered during an infectious process, not prophylactically. Oxygen therapy may be required for hypoxemia, but not continuously.

10–4 Answer B

Alcohol intake does not predispose a woman to pulmonary embolism. A large prospective study in women showed that obesity, cigarette smoking, and hypertension increased their risk for pulmonary embolism.

10–5 Answer B

The normal anteroposterior diameter of the chest as compared to the transverse diameter is approximately 1:2. An anteroposterior measurement that equals the transverse measurement is defined as a barrel chest, which usually indicates some obstructive lung disease.

10–6 Answer B

Clients with chronic obstructive pulmonary disease often sit in a tripod position: leaning forward with their arms braced against their knees, a chair, or a bed. This provides clients with leverage, so that their rectus abdominal, intercostal, and accessory neck muscles can all assist with expiration.

10–7 Answer B

Increased tactile fremitus occurs with compression or consolidation of lung tissue, such as occurs in conditions like lobar pneumonia. Decreased tactile fremitus occurs when anything obstructs the transmission of vibrations, such as occurs in conditions like pleural effusion, pneumothorax, or emphysema, or with an obstructed bronchus.

10–8 Answer A

Hyperresonance on percussion of the chest is found when too much air is present, such as occurs with emphysema or a pneumothorax. A dull sound on percussion indicates an abnormal density in the lungs, such as occurs with pneumonia, pleural effusion, a lung tumor, or atelectasis.

10–9 Answer B

With bronchovesicular breath sounds, the inspiratory rate equals the expiratory rate. With bronchial or tracheal breath sounds, the inspiratory rate is shorter than the expiratory rate, and with vesicular breath sounds, the inspiratory rate is greater than the expiratory rate.

10–10 Answer B

With egophony, you normally hear a muffled (and sometimes nondistinct) "eeee" through the stethoscope if you auscultate the chest when the client says "eeee." When consolidation is present, the "eeee" sound changes to an "aaaaa" sound. With bronchophony, when the client repeats "99-99-99," normally you can hear a soft, muffled, indistinct sound, but cannot distinguish what is being said. With whispered pectoriloquy, when the client whispers "1 2 3," a normal response is faint, muffled, and almost inaudible. Tonometry measures intraocular pressure.

10–11 Answer D

Harrison's groove is the name of the horizontal groove in the rib cage at the level of the diaphragm, extending from the sternum to the midaxillary line. It occurs normally in some children and also occurs in children with rickets.

10–12 Answer A

A 1-minute Apgar score of 7–10 indicates that the newborn is in good condition, needing only suctioning of the nose and mouth and otherwise routine care. A 1-minute Apgar score of 3–6 indicates a moderately depressed newborn requiring more resuscitation and close monitoring. A 1-minute Apgar score of 0–2 indicates a severely depressed newborn requiring full resuscitation, ventilator support, and intensive care.

10–13 Answer A

Retractions occur more often in the newborn and infant than other ages because the intercostal tissues are weak and underdeveloped. Supraclavicular or suprasternal retractions suggest upper airway obstruction, and retraction of intercostals or subcostal muscles suggest lower airway obstruction.

10–14 Answer C

An infant who has periodic breathing with persistent or prolonged apnea (greater than 20 seconds) may have an increased risk of sudden infant death syndrome. Rapid respiratory rates accompany pneumonia, anemia, fever, pain, and heart disease. Tachypnea (a respiratory rate of 50–100 breaths per minute) during sleep may be an early sign of left-sided congestive heart failure.

10–15 Answer D

Stridor, a high-pitched inspiratory crowing sound, can be heard on auscultation when a client has acute epiglottitis or croup. Persistent fine crackles can be heard with atelectasis, expiratory wheezes with asthma, and persistent peristaltic sounds with diminished breath sounds on the same side with a diaphragmatic hernia.

10–16 Answer A

The nursing diagnosis of "impaired gas exchange" may be demonstrated by clubbing of the fingers. Nasal flaring and cough are present if the client has a nursing diagnosis of "ineffective airway clearance" or "ineffective breathing pattern." The use of accessory muscles to assist breathing may indicate a nursing diagnosis of "ineffective breathing pattern."

10–17 Answer B

Biot's respirations is the term for an irregular respiratory pattern of a series of three to four normal respirations followed by a period of apnea. It is seen with head trauma, brain abscess, heat stroke, spinal meningitis, and encephalitis. Cheyne-Stokes respirations are similar, except that the pattern is regular. The most common cause of Cheyne-Stokes respirations is severe congestive heart failure followed by renal failure, meningitis, drug overdose, and increased intracranial pressure. This regular pattern occurs normally in infants and older adults during sleep. Kussmaul's respiration is hyperventilation with an increase in both the rate and depth of the breaths. Hypoventilation is a reduced rate and depth of breathing that causes an increase in carbon dioxide in the bloodstream.

10–18 Answer B

The definition of the spirometric assessment of residual volume is the amount of gas left in the lung after exhaling all that is physically possible. This measurement is expressed as a ratio of total lung capacity to vital capacity. The total lung capacity is the sum of the vital capacity and the residual volume. The expiratory reserve volume is the volume that can be maximally exhaled after a passive exhalation. The peak flow is the measurement of the maximum flow rate achieved during the forced vital capacity maneuver.

10–19 Answer A

Asthma is characterized by intermittent episodes of airway obstruction caused by bronchospasm, excessive bronchial secretion, or edema of bronchial mucosa. Atelectasis is a collapse of alveolar lung tissue and findings reflect the presence of a small, airless lung. It is caused by complete obstruction of a draining bronchus by a tumor, thick secretions, or an aspirated foreign body. Acute bronchitis is an inflammation of the bronchial tree characterized by partial bronchial obstruction and secretions or constrictions. It results in abnormally deflated portions of the lung. Emphysema is a permanent hyperinflation of lung beyond the terminal bronchioles with destruction of the alveolar walls.

10–20 Answer B

In acute bronchitis, the breath sounds are vesicular, vocal resonance is moderate, and the adventitious sounds are localized crackles with sibilant wheezes. In bronchiectasis, the breath sounds are usually vesicular, vocal resonance is usually muffled, and crackles are the adventitious sounds. In emphysema, the breath sounds are of decreased intensity and often with prolonged expiration, vocal resonance is muffled or decreased, and the adventitious sounds are occasional wheezes and often fine crackles in late inspiration. In asthma, the breath sounds are distant, vocal resonance is decreased, and wheezes are the adventitious sounds.

10–21 Answer A

With pleural effusion and thickening, the trachea would be deviated toward the normal side because of fluid displacing the pleural space. The trachea is usually not displaced with pneumonia. With bronchiectasis, the trachea is midline or deviated toward the affected side, and with pulmonary fibrosis, the trachea is deviated to the most affected side.

10–22 Answer C

The sympathomimetic agents that are the first-line drugs of choice for hyperreactive airway disease (asthma) are the $beta_2$ agonists. There are different adrenergic receptors in different tissues. $Beta_2$-adrenergic agents (agonists) are more specific in their action to promote bronchodilation and less likely to be associated with side effects. In addition to promoting bronchodilation, these agents also increase secretion of electrolytes by the airways and enhance mucociliary activity. Protein kinase A levels increase within the smooth muscle cells, resulting in inhibition of myosin phosphorylation and smooth muscle cell relaxation. Alpha agonists cause vasoconstriction and $beta_1$-adrenergic agents (agonists) increase cardiac contractility and heart rate, effects that are undesirable in clients with asthma. Alpha antagonist is not a drug class.

10–23 Answer B

If a client develops moderate asthma, defined as more than two episodes per week, an inhaled steroid should be prescribed and used in conjunction with the beta$_2$-adrenergic metered-dose inhaler. With no improvement, a longer-acting bronchodilator, such as salmeterol xinafoate (Serevent), may be added. If the asthma worsens, then a short course of oral steroids may be tried. Theophylline is no longer used except in extremely resistant cases.

10–24 Answer A

Streptococcus pneumoniae causes 30–75% of all community-acquired bacterial pneumonia, followed by *Mycoplasma pneumoniae* (5–35%); *Haemophilus influenzae* (6–12%), and *Staphylococcus aureus* (3–10%).

10–25 Answer C

The antibiotic of choice for the treatment of *Streptococcus pneumoniae* pneumonia is penicillin. Alternative choices are erythromycin and clindamycin. Dicloxacillin is the antibiotic of choice for *Staphylococcus aureus;* erythromycin is the antibiotic of choice for *Mycoplasma pneumoniae;* and ampicillin-clavulanate is the antibiotic of choice for *Moraxella catarrhalis*.

Once therapy has been started, the client's respiratory and cardiovascular status should be monitored, along with his or her general overall status, including level of energy, appetite, and temperature. Most clients on the appropriate antibiotic therapy improve within 48–72 hours. Fever that continues more than 24 hours after initiating therapy usually does not indicate failure of the antibiotic; rather, the usual response to therapy is a gradual reduction in the maximum daily temperature.

10–26 Answer A

If a client has pneumonia, the following are indications for hospitalization: inability to take oral medications; multilobar involvement on chest x ray; acute mental status changes; a severe vital sign abnormality (pulse rate greater than 140 per minute, systolic blood pressure less than 90 mm Hg, or a respiratory rate greater than 30 per minute); a secondary suppurative infection such as empyema, meningitis, or endocarditis; or a severe acute electrolyte, hematologic, or metabolic abnormality.

10–27 Answer D

In the client with pulmonary tuberculosis, night sweats are often noted as a manifestation of fever. With pulmonary tuberculosis, systemic manifestations are usually present; they are not confined to the respiratory system. Fever occurs in 50–80% of cases and symptoms such as malaise and weight loss are frequent. Dyspnea, an ominous feature, usually occurs with widespread advanced disease. Crackles and bronchial breath sounds may be present, but more often there are no abnormal findings, even in well-developed pulmonary disease.

10–28 Answer D

Groups at high risk for tuberculosis include racial and ethnic minorities (70% of all reported cases in the United States); foreign-born individuals (24% of all cases in the United States); substance abusers (5–20 times normal); individuals with human immunodeficiency virus infection (40–100 times normal); and residents of prisons, nursing homes, and shelters (2–10 times normal).

10–29 Answer D

Individuals predisposed to have a false-negative reaction to the Mantoux test include newborns and those over age 60; those in an immunosuppressive state, such as persons taking corticosteroids and anticancer agents or those with human immunodeficiency virus infection or chronic renal failure; persons with a neoplasm, especially lymphoid leukemia and lymphomas; and persons with an acute infection, such as measles, mumps, chickenpox, typhoid fever, brucellosis, typhus, and pertussis. Tuberculosis had been close to eradication until HIV appeared. Coughing alone is not predictive of TB.

10–30 Answer D

Tuberculosis is a reportable disease. Every potential case must be reported to the local health department. This includes when the client's Mantoux test shows an induration of 15 mm; when a case of tuberculosis is merely suspected; and when an asymptomatic client has a positive chest x ray for pulmonary tuberculosis. Screening tests in higher risk areas with suspected infection that do not have a positive reaction do not need to be reported. These include the appearance of a red area with an induration of less than 10 mm on the first test (less than 5 mm on employees with a yearly screen).

10–31 Answer C

Treatment of tuberculosis in pregnant women is essential and should not be delayed; therefore Marisa's treatment should begin now. The preferred initial treatment is isoniazid (Nydrazid), rifampin (Rimactane), and ethambutol (Myambutol). The teratogenicity of pyrazinamide is undetermined, so it is not wise to use this drug unless resistance to the other drugs is demonstrated or is likely. Streptomycin is ototoxic to the fetus and should not be administered unless lack of other options demands it.

10–32 Answer A

The prevalence of chronic obstructive pulmonary disease (COPD) is directly related to increasing age. Men are affected much more often than women because the percentage of men who smoke is greater than that of women. The risk of developing COPD is related to the number of cigarettes smoked and the duration of smoking. Cigar or pipe smoking also increases the risk of developing COPD, but to a lesser extent than does cigarette smoking. The usual client with COPD is one who is over age 50 and has smoked one pack of cigarettes per day for more than 20 years.

10–33 Answer D

Theophylline, a methylxanthine derivative, acts as a bronchodilator, decreases dyspnea, improves mucociliary clearance, improves gas exchange, enhances respiratory muscle performance, increases neuroinspiratory drive, and has a positive inotropic effect. The decision to institute theophylline therapy must be individualized and should not be universally made in all clients with chronic obstructive pulmonary disease. It should be added to the treatment plan in clients who have not achieved an optimal clinical response to beta agonists and ipratropium (Atrovent) metered-dose inhalers.

10–34 Answer D

The major bacterial pathogens causing infectious exacerbations in clients with chronic obstructive pulmonary disease (COPD) are *Streptococcus pneumoniae, Haemophilus influenzae,* and *Branhamella catarrhalis*. Antibiotics are frequently prescribed to clients with COPD as therapy or to prevent an acute infectious exacerbation. These exacerbations are characterized by worsening dyspnea; increased cough, sputum production, and sputum purulence; and worsened pulmonary function during the infection.

10–35 Answer D

A primary spontaneous pneumothorax usually occurs in healthy individuals without pre-existing lung disease; occurs more commonly in young, tall, asthenic men; and is an accumulation of air in the normally airless pleural space between the lung and chest wall. Persons with Marfan's syndrome are more prone to aortic aneurysms.

10–36 Answer D

The following contribute to the incidence of carcinoma of the lung: cigarette smoking; exposure to materials such as asbestos, uranium, and radon; and chronic interstitial lung diseases such as pulmonary fibrosis arising from scleroderma. It is estimated that approximately 2 million persons will develop carcinoma of the lung in each of the next several years; 85% of all lung carcinomas are secondary to cigarette use.

10–37 Answer A

A T1SN1M1 indicates that the lung carcinoma is in situ, has metastasis to the lymph nodes in the peribronchial or the ipsilateral hilar region, and has distant metastasis to the spine. Although the TNM system is generalized for all solid tumors, it is often adapted for specific types of cancers. T is for the relative tumor size, N indicates the presence and extent of lymph node involvement, and M denotes distant metastases. For specific lung cancer staging, the T may range from 0, with no evidence of primary tumor, to 4, which indicates that the tumor has invaded the mediastinum or involves the heart, great vessels, trachea, esophagus, vertebral body, or carina and there is presence of malignant pleural effusion. The N may range from 0, indicating no regional lymph node metastasis, to 3, indicating metastasis to the contralateral, mediastinal, scalene, or supraclavicular nodes. The M may range from X, indicating that the presence of distant metastasis cannot be assessed, to 1, meaning that distant metastasis is present.

10–38 Answer C

With the use of multiple drug therapy for tuberculosis, the duration of the therapy has shortened from 1 year to a standard of 6–9 months. If the client has a drug-resistant organism or is immunodeficient, the precise duration of therapy is uncertain, but may extend from 1–2 years in some cases.

10–39 Answer C

Current recommendations for well individuals suggest screening for tuberculosis (TB) using an intradermal or multipuncture skin test at age 1 year, then again at entry to preschool or kindergarten, and then at some point during adolescence. TB testing should be considered for all new immigrants, as well as young people planning to study or travel extensively in areas where TB is endemic.

10–40 Answer D

The changes in the lungs that account for decreased cough effectiveness in older adults include a decrease in vital capacity, an increase in residual volume, and less lung elasticity.

10–41 Answer D

Clinical manifestations of cancer of the larynx include earache, halitosis, hoarseness, change in the voice, painful swallowing, dyspnea, and a palpable lump in the neck. The most notable manifestation of glottic cancer is hoarseness or a change in the voice because the tumor prevents complete closure of the glottis during speech.

10–42 Answer A

After a total laryngectomy for laryngeal cancer, the client will have a permanent tracheostomy, because no connection exists between the trachea and the esophagus.

10–43 Answer B

If a client has a dry cough, dyspnea, chills, fever, general malaise, headache, confusion, anorexia, diarrhea, myalgias, and arthralgias, suspect Legionnaires' disease. Legionnaires' disease also has a gradual onset. Bronchopneumonia has a gradual onset with a cough, scattered crackles, minimal dyspnea and respiratory distress, and a low-grade fever. Primary atypical pneumonia has a gradual onset with a dry, hacking, nonproductive cough; fever; headache; myalgias; and arthralgias. *Pneumocystis carinii* pneumonia occurs in clients with AIDS. It has an abrupt onset with a dry cough, tachypnea, shortness of breath, significant respiratory distress, and fever.

10–44 Answer C

In trying to differentiate between chronic bronchitis and emphysema, chronic bronchitis presents with adventitious sounds, wheezing and rhonchi, and a normal percussion note. Chronic bronchitis usually occurs after age 35, with recurrent respiratory infections. There is usually a persistent, productive cough of copious mucopurulent sputum; pulmonary function studies show normal or decreased total lung capacity with a moderately increased residual volume. In a client with emphysema, the onset is usually after age 50. There is an insidious progressive dyspnea and the cough is usually absent or mild with scant clear sputum, if any. There are also distant or diminished breath sounds and a hyperresonant percussion note. The pulmonary function studies show an increased total lung capacity with a markedly increased residual volume.

10–45 Answer D

Coccidioidomycosis is the southwestern United States' leading mycotic infection, with an annual morbidity estimated at 35,000 cases. Although the majority of those infected spontaneously recover without antibiotic intervention, for immunocompromised persons, the disseminated disease can lead to high morbidity and a greater than 50% mortality rate. Providers should suspect coccidioidomycosis in clients presenting with pulmonary complaints, particularly those who may have recently visited an endemic area. An influenza-like syndrome appears 7–28 days after inhalation of *Coccidioides immitis* in fewer than half of clients infected. Symptoms, in descending order of frequency, include fever, cough, chest pain, chills, sputum production, sore throat, and hemoptysis. Cutaneous manifestations occur in 10% of clients, particularly younger ones, and present as generalized maculopapular erythematous eruptions. Coccidioidomycosis is readily treatable if recognized at an early stage. For the majority of infected individuals, the prognosis is excellent even without therapy. Systemic antifungal therapy should be considered in infants, older adults, debilitated persons, those with prolonged primary disease, and populations at high risk of dissemination. Intravenous amphotericin B is the mainstay of therapy.

10–46 Answer C

In a study of 476 children from an inner-city study, researchers determined that the combination of cockroach allergy and exposure to the insects is an important cause of asthma-related illness and hospitalizations among that group of children. Levels of cockroach, dust mite, and cat allergens in the children's homes were measured and allergy skin tests were performed on the children. Of these children, 37% were allergic to cockroaches, 35% to dust mites, and 23% to cats. They then assessed the severity of the children's asthma over 12 months and found that children who were both allergic to cockroaches and exposed to high cockroach allergen levels were hospitalized for their asthma 3.3 times more often than children who were allergic but not exposed to high levels of cockroach allergen, or children who were exposed to high levels of cockroach allergen but who were not allergic.

10–47 Answer C

Jill has daily symptoms of asthma. She uses her inhaled short-acting $beta_2$ agonist daily. Her exacerbations affect her activities and they occur at least twice weekly and may last for days. She is affected more than once weekly during the night with an exacerbation. Jill is in the step 3 (moderate persistent) category of asthma severity. This is because she has daily symptoms along with exacerbations affecting her activity, and nocturnal symptoms that occur more than once per week. In step 1 (mild intermittent) asthma, symptoms are no more frequent than twice weekly and nocturnal symptoms are no more frequent than twice per month. In step 2 (mild persistent) asthma, symptoms are more frequent than twice weekly but less than once a day, exacerbations may affect activity, and nocturnal symptoms are more frequent than twice per month. In step 4 (severe persistent) asthma, the client has continous symptoms with limited physical activity, frequent exacerbations, and frequent nocturnal symptoms.

10–48 Answer A

Occupational asthma should be considered in all clients with adult-onset asthma or in clients with asthma that worsens in adulthood. As many as one in five cases of asthma may be a result of exposure to chemicals in the workplace. Roughly 250 chemicals have been found to cause occupational asthma symptoms, which usually appear soon after a worker is first exposed to the asthma-inducing chemical, but sometimes may appear months to years later.

10–49 Answer C

Symptoms in about one-third of pregnant women with asthma will improve during pregnancy; about one-third will be unchanged; and about one-third will worsen. Pregnancy is associated with changes in lung volume. There is an increase in tidal volume and a

20–50% increase in minute ventilation. The clinical course of asthma during pregnancy may be predicted by the course during the first trimester, and most clients have the same pattern of response with repeated pregnancies. The treatment of asthma during pregnancy follows the same principles as with other clients. Medications not specifically required should not be given in the first trimester, and all medications should be given at their minimal effective dose and frequency.

10–50 Answer D

Associated pathophysiology in clients with chronic bronchitis include dysfunctional cilia, increased numbers and altered immune response of neu-trophils and macrophages, increased permeability of the pulmonary epithelium, bacterial colonization, chronic inflammation, increased concentration of goblet cells, and increased volume and viscosity of sputum. There is hyperplasia of the mucus glands in the bronchial wall.

10–51 Answer D

The most common bacterial organisms associated with bronchitis include *Streptococcus pneumoniae* and *Haemophilus influenzae*. The viral pathogens common in exacerbations of chronic bronchitis include influenza virus, rhinovirus, coronavirus, and respiratory syncytial virus. Bacterial and viral exacerbations are common in clients who have chronic bronchitis. About 70% of clients have bacterial colonization, whereas about 30% have viral infections. These infections tend to be seasonal and are more common in the winter and in certain parts of the United States. Frequent viral infections predispose clients to secondary bacterial colonization and infection.

10–52 Answer D

A rescue course of prednisolone should be initiated for an attack of asthma whenever the client needs it, at any time and at any step. Attempts should be made to use systemic corticosteroids in an acute or rescue fashion: a short burst followed by tapering to the lowest dose possible and preferably discontinued, with inhaled steroids prescribed for chronic or maintenance therapy.

10–53 Answer C

Shawna should perform a peak expiratory flow meter reading daily during a 2-week period when she feels well. The highest number recorded during this period is her "personal best." A green zone (80-100% of her personal best) is when no asthma symptoms are present and she should continue with her normal medication regimen. A yellow zone (50-80% of her personal best) occurs when asthma symptoms may be starting and signals caution. A red zone (below 50% of her personal best) indicates when Shawna should take her inhaled beta 2-agonist and repeat the peak flow assessment as it indicates an asthma attack is happening. There is no white zone.

10–54 Answer B

Despite widespread endorsement by numerous medical and nursing organizations, the pneumococcal polysaccharide vaccine is administered to only 30% of individuals for whom it is indicated. Experts from the Advisory Committee on Immunization Practices estimate that as many as 90% of deaths attributed to *Streptococcus pneumoniae* could be prevented if use of the currently available vaccine were more common. Pneumococci account for more deaths than any other vaccine-preventable disease.

10–55 Answer A

Of the nearly 46 million adults who smoke, 34% try to quit each year, but only 2.5% succeed. Although the overall success rate of smoking cessation is disappointing, smoking cessation programs have been extremely helpful. Motivation is the key to a successful effort, along with making every clinical encounter an opportunity to discuss the topic. At the very least, every client should be asked about his or her smoking history. Clinicians should advise smokers to quit, assist them by setting a quitting date, provide self-help materials, and evaluate them for nicotine replacement therapy (patches, nasal spray, or gum) or pharmacological therapies.

10–56 Answer B

The first-line bronchodilator therapy for chronic obstructive pulmonary disease (COPD) is inhaled ipratropium (Atrovent). Ipratropium has a superior bronchodilatory activity in the tolerated dosage range, a long duration of action, and a slow onset of action. Although beta agonists produce rapid bronchodilatation, their effectiveness in managing COPD is limited by two factors: the density of $beta_2$ receptors in the airways decreases with age; and despite the relative selectivity of some of these agents for the $beta_2$ receptor, cross-reactivity with $beta_1$ receptors in the heart may induce tachycardia. Tachycardia is particularly problematic in the COPD-afflicted population, which consists largely of older adults and current or former smokers, many of whom may have coexisting coronary artery disease. Thus, an alternative to beta agonists is desirable.

10–57 Answer D

For a diagnosis of asthma to be made, three components must be demonstrated: the client must demonstrate episodic symptoms of airflow obstruction; show evidence that the airflow obstruction is at least partly reversible; and have other conditions excluded from the differential diagnosis. A careful medical history and physical examination, with special attention to the upper respiratory tract, chest, and skin, is also an essential component of the diagnostic process. It may reveal significant symptoms, identify precipitating factors such as allergy, or suggest another diagnosis. Proventil is a treatment for asthma, not a diagnosis indicator.

10–58 Answer B

Daily peak flow monitoring has long been recommended for clients with asthma. The new guidelines from the National Asthma Education and Prevention Program of the National Heart, Lung, and Blood Institute increase the flexibility of this recommendation and suggest that the use of peak flow measurements be individualized. The guidelines recommend that all clients with persistent asthma assess peak flow each morning. Subsequent assessments are necessary during the day when the morning measurement is less than 80% of the client's personal best peak expiratory flow (PEF) measurement. The goal of daily PEF monitoring is to recognize early signs of deterioration in airway function so that corrective steps can be initiated.

10–59 Answer D

To control the common asthma trigger of dust mites, the following measures are recommended: cover the mattress and pillows in airtight, dustproof covers; wash the bedding weekly and dry it on a hot setting for 20 minutes; avoid sleeping on natural fibers such as wool or down; remove all carpeting from bedrooms; and reduce indoor humidity to less than 50%. Opening the windows daily would allow allergens to enter.

10–60 Answer D

There are both diagnostic and therapeutic indications for a bronchoscopy. Diagnostic uses include evaluation of indeterminate lung lesions (abnormal chest film); preoperative staging of cancer; determination of the extent of injury secondary to burns, inhalation, or other trauma; assessment of airway patency, including problems associated with endotracheal tubes, wheeze, and stridor; investigation of unexplained symptoms (cough, hemoptysis, stridor, etc.) or unexplained findings (recurrent laryngeal nerve paralysis, recent diaphragmatic paralysis); evaluation of suspicious or malignant sputum cytology; bronchoalveolar lavage for interstitial lung disease; and specimen collection for selective cultures or suspected infection. The therapeutic uses include removal of mucous plugs, secretions, and foreign bodies; assistance with difficult endotracheal intubations; and treatment of endobronchial neoplasms. A bronchoscopy is not used in patients with severe tracheal stenosis as it is difficult to pass the scope.

10–61 Answer C

Recurrence rates for both primary and secondary spontaneous pneumothorax are similar. Recurrence rates range from 10–50%, and about 60% of those clients will have a third recurrence. After three episodes, the recurrence rate exceeds 85%. Repeated spontaneous pneumothorax should be treated by pleurodesis or surgical intervention, including parietal pleurectomy.

10–62 Answer D

Lung diseases that may cause a secondary spontaneous pneumothorax include chronic obstructive pulmonary disease, lung abscess, cystic fibrosis, asthma, adult respiratory distress syndrome, neoplasm, Marfan's syndrome, sarcoidosis, tuberculosis, and eosinophilic granuloma.

10–63 Answer B

Hamman's sign, named after the American physician Louis Hamman, is an auscultation sound at the mediastinum in the presence of a mediastinal "crunch" that coincides with cardiac systole and diastole. It is present with spontaneous mediastinal emphysema or pneumomediastinum.

10–64 Answer A

The community-acquired pneumonia seen more often in the client with or without an alcohol problem is pneumococcal. Although they are at risk for the usual pathogens, alcoholics have a higher incidence of pneumonia caused by gram-negative organisms (including *Klebsiella pneumoniae* and *Haemophilus influenzae*) and anaerobic pneumonia secondary to aspiration.

10–65 Answer D

Risk factors predisposing clients to the development of nosocomial (hospital-acquired) pneumonia include increased severity of the underlying illness; presence of an indwelling urethral catheter; use of broad-spectrum antibiotics (which increase the risk of superinfection); previous hospitalization, presence of intravascular catheters, intubation (especially prolonged intubation), and recent thoracic or upper abdominal surgery.

10–66 Answer C

Nosocomial pneumonia, a pneumonia occurring within 48 hours after admission, is most commonly caused by gram-negative organisms, including *Pseudomonas aeruginosa, Klebsiella pneumoniae, Escherichia coli,* and *Enterobacter* species. *Staphylococcus aureus*, including methicillin-resistant organisms, *Streptococcus pneumoniae*, anaerobes, *Candida,* and polymicrobial infections are also common. Mortality from nosocomial pneumonia remains high (30–50%) despite antimicrobial therapy.

10–67 Answer A

Although all of these tests might be indicated, the first test that should be ordered for a client presenting with productive cough, weight loss, weakness, anorexia, night sweats, and generalized malaise for 8 weeks' duration would be a Mantoux skin test for tuberculosis (TB). The client is at high risk for developing TB because of his residence in a shelter and his low socioeconomic status.

10–68 Answer A

Cigarette smoking increases the clearance rate of theophylline and may result in the need for a larger dose. Hepatic insufficiency, allopurinol (Zyloprim), and cimetidine (Tagamet) all decrease the clearance rate of theophylline and may result in the need for a smaller dose.

10–69 Answer C

Sarcoidosis is a multisystem disorder of unknown cause that has a prevalence of about 20 cases in 10,000. It usually occurs in clients age 20–40, but can occur at any age. Sarcoidosis occurs more frequently in women than in men, and in the United States, it is more common in blacks than in whites (about 10:1). Although many organs may be involved, the most involved organ is the lung (90%).

10–70 Answer A

For adolescents, as well as all clients, with step 1 (mild intermittent) asthma, no long-term control therapy is indicated. Clients with step 1 asthma only need quick relief with a $beta_2$ agonist as needed. There is no indication for long-term control until they approach step 2 (mild persistent) asthma.

10–71 Answer B

The most common cause of a persistent cough in children of all ages is recurrent viral bronchitis. Recurrent viral bronchitis is most prevalent in preschool and young school-age children, and there may be a genetically determined host susceptibility to frequently recurring bronchitis. The key words are persistent cough. Young clients with recurrent cough often have asthma, but it is not usually persistent. Providers should be suspicious of underlying asthma contributing to a recurrent cough when there is a family history of allergies, atopy, or asthma. Similarly, allergies and an upper respiratory infection do not present with a persistent cough; rather, they present with an intermittent one.

10–72 Answer D

Chronic cough in children frequently is caused by allergic rhinitis, chronic sinusitis, or enlarged adenoids. Although rare, chronic cough in children under age 1 should suggest congenital malformations or neonatal infections, including viral and chlamydial pneumonias. Other relatively rare causes of chronic cough in young infants include recurrent aspiration of milk, saliva, or gastric contents and cystic fibrosis. A chronic cough in children age 1–5 years should suggest bronchiectasis or cystic fibrosis after the more common causes have been ruled out.

10–73 Answer C

Unexplained nocturnal cough in an older adult should suggest congestive heart failure. Older adults, whose physical activity may be restricted by arthritis or other associated diseases, may not present with the usual symptom of dyspnea on exertion. The main complaint instead may be a chronic unexplained cough that may occur only at night while the client is recumbent or a cough that may worsen at night.

10–74 Answer D

Dyspnea can be caused by increased rigidity of lung tissue, increased airway resistance, enhanced ventilation during exercise, or any combination of these. Determining the cause of dyspnea is assisted by first classifying it into different types, such as wheezing dyspnea, dyspnea on exertion, paroxysmal nocturnal dyspnea, hyperventilation, and dyspnea of cerebral origin. An easier classification is acute, chronic, or recurrent. The most common causes of dyspnea include chronic obstructive pulmonary disease, asthma, congestive heart failure, anxiety, obesity, and poor physical condition.

10–75 Answer B

When trying to differentiate pulmonary from cardiac causes of dyspnea on exertion, it is important to remember that clients with dyspnea from cardiac causes remain dyspneic much longer after cessation of exercise. The heart rate also takes longer to return to pre-exercise levels. When the cause is pulmonary, the rate of recovery to normal respiration is fast and the dyspnea is gone a few minutes after the cessation of exercise. Clients with pulmonary dyspnea usually do not have dyspnea at rest. Clients with severe cardiac dyspnea demonstrate a volume of respiration that is greater than normal at every level of exercise and they experience the dyspnea sooner after beginning the exertion.

10–76 Answer C

If a client presents with an acute onset of dyspnea with associated symptoms of chest pain, faintness, tachypnea, peripheral cyanosis, low blood pressure, crackles, and some wheezes, and has a history of taking birth control pills and smoking, suspect pulmonary emboli. Other signs and symptoms associated with pulmonary emboli include loss of consciousness and a pleural friction rub. Precipitating and aggravating factors include the use of oral contraceptives and prolonged recumbency. Acute dyspnea would also occur with asthma, but the physical findings would include bilateral wheezing; sibilant, whistling sounds; and prolonged expiration. With bronchitis, dyspnea is not necessarily the presenting symptom. A cough precedes the dyspnea and there would be rhonchi present on auscultation. With a pneumothorax, there is an acute onset of dyspnea and the physical findings would include decreased or absent breath sounds with a tracheal shift.

10–77 Answer B

Of persons who smoke one pack of cigarettes per day or more, 40–60% have a cough. It is defined as chronic bronchitis if the cough has been productive for at least 3 months during each of 2 consecutive years.

10–78 Answer B

The most common reason for a chronic cough in children is a postinfection. The other reasons, in order of frequency, are asthma, a postnasal drip, and irritants. Uncommon causes include other respiratory infections, pertussis, a foreign body, cystic fibrosis, congenital abnormalities, and psychogenic reasons.

10–79 Answer A

A pulmonary function test, such as spirometry, is helpful in the diagnosis of obstructive lung disease (including chronic bronchitis and asthma) and restrictive lung disease. Clients with postinfectious or cough-variant asthma may show mild obstruction, but they often have normal spirometry. A chest x ray confirms the diagnosis of pneumonia. While spirometry may show a decrease in lung capacity with advanced lung cancer, it is not diagnostic.

10–80 Answer C

Although weather changes may affect and even precipitate an asthma attack, they are not one of the three principal triggers for an exacerbation of asthma. Allergens, infections, and psychological factors are the three principal triggers. Allergens include inhaled substances, such as molds, pollens, dust, animal dander, tobacco smoke, and medications, especially beta blockers and aspirin. Viral upper respiratory infections (URIs) are particularly problematic. In children, it is common for an asthma attack to follow a URI. Psychological factors play a significant role and may not be readily recognized.

10–81 Answer D

To decrease mortality in clients with chronic obstructive pulmonary disease whose oxygen saturations are less than 89%, oxygen must be used at least 18 hours per day to be of more than symptomatic benefit. The oxygen can be either a specific concentration delivered by mask or a flow rate administered through a nasal cannula. It is needed to maintain adequate oxygenation levels during both activity and rest.

10–82 Answer D

Currently, there is no accepted mass screening test for lung cancer. Because of cost, mass screening for lung cancer in healthy individuals with no risk factors is not recommended. Individuals who are at high risk (those who are cigarette smokers, have been exposed to radon or asbestos, and have a strong family history) should be periodically screened through the use of an annual physical examination, chest x ray, and possibly sputum cytology. Suspicious chest x rays should be followed by further diagnostic tests.

10–83 Answer D

Chest physiotherapy is effective in the treatment of pneumonia, atelectasis, and diseases resulting in weak or ineffective coughing, such as cystic fibrosis. This technique uses percussion and postural drainage along with coughing and deep breathing exercises. It is performed by positioning the client so the involved lobes of the lung are placed in a dependent drainage position and then using a cupped hand or vibrator to percuss the chest wall. Nasotracheal suctioning is quite uncomfortable but still useful in the appropriate clinical setting in the absence of significant coagulopathy.

10–84 Answer D

The following medical conditions are known to substantially increase the risk of tuberculosis: human immunodeficiency virus infection, jejunoileal bypass, chronic renal failure, silicosis, gastrectomy, weight 10% or more below ideal weight, diabetes mellitus, conditions requiring prolonged high-dose corticosteroid therapy or other immunosuppressive therapy, some hematologic disorders such as leukemia and lymphomas, and other malignancies.

10–85 Answer D

Smokers weigh 5–10 lb less than nonsmokers of comparable age and height. When smokers quit, 80% of them gain weight; the average weight gain is 5 lb, although of that 80% about 10% gain more than 25 lb. Women gain more weight than men: 8 lb as compared to 5 lb. Heavy smokers (those who smoke two packs per day or more) gain more weight than light smokers. This weight gain is caused by replacing the habit of smoking cigarettes with eating to satisfy the need for oral gratification.

10–86 Answer B

When teaching smokers about using nicotine gum to aid in smoking cessation, tell them to discard the gum after 30 minutes. The gum should not be chewed like regular gum. A piece is chewed only long enough to release the nicotine, which produces a peppery taste, then "parked" between the gums and buccal mucosa to allow for nicotine absorption. Drinking liquids while the gum is in the mouth should be avoided. Acidic beverages such as coffee should be avoided for 1–2 hours before the use of the gum. The smoker should be instructed to chew 9–12 pieces daily to help prevent nicotine withdrawal.

10–87 Answer B

The peripharyngeal upper respiratory tract infection that occurs most often in children age 2–5 years is epiglottitis. Peritonsillar abscess occurs more frequently during the teenage years; laryngotracheobronchitis (croup) in children age 3 months to 3 years; and bacterial tracheitis in children age 3–10 years.

10–88 Answer A

If a cough characteristically occurs all day long but never during sleep, suspect that it is a psychogenic cough (or habit). Allergic rhinitis results in a cough that is seasonal; pertussis in a cough that is followed by a "whoop"; and a postnasal drip results in a throat-clearing cough.

10–89 Answer D

Cholinesterase inhibitors cause a cough by inducing mucus production (bronchorrhea). Tobacco and marijuana cause a cough by being direct irritants. Beta-adrenergic blockers, aspirin, and nonsteroidal anti-inflammatory drugs cause a cough by potentiating reactive airway disease.

10–90 Answer C

Schamroth's window is useful as a quick method of assessing for digital clubbing. The dorsal surfaces of the terminal phalanges of similar fingers are placed together. With clubbing, the normal diamond-shaped window at the bases of the nail beds disappears and a prominent distal angle forms between the end of the nails. Normally, this angle is minimal or nonexistent. The phalangeal depth ratio measures the ratio of the distal phalangeal depth to the interphalangeal depth. It is normally less than 1 but increases to more than 1 with finger clubbing. It can be measured with calipers or more accurately with finger casts.

10–91 Answer B

The normal respiratory rate of an 18-month-old child (age 1–2 years) while awake is 30–40 breaths per minute. Between ages 6 and 12 months, the awake child breathes between 58 and 75 times per minute. An awake child age 2–4 years breathes between 23 and 42 times per minute; and a child age 4–6 years breathes between 19 and 36 times per minute.

10–92 Answer A

The definitive tests for cystic fibrosis (CF) are the sweat test and DNA analysis. A sputum or throat culture positive for mucoid *Pseudomonas aeruginosa* is suggestive of CF. An abnormal Chymex test for pancreatic insufficiency is a supportive laboratory test to diagnosis CF. A fecal fat test, while reliable, is not specific to CF. Any condition affected by malabsorption or maldigestion will be associated with increased fecal fat. Early diagnosis improves the poor prognosis for untreated CF. If untreated, most clients die by age 1–2 years. With current care, median survival is to age 29. The diagnosis is confirmed by a positive sweat test or confirming the presence of two of the recognized CF mutations in DNA, one each on the maternally and paternally derived chromosome 7. Sweat testing can be performed at any age; newborns in the first few weeks of life may not produce a large enough volume of sweat to analyze, but in those who do, the results will be accurate. Immunoreactive trypsinogen (IRT) levels in CF infants are elevated in most infants with CF for the first several weeks of life; however, this test has relatively poor specificity because as many as 90% of the positives on the initial screen are false positives.

10–93 Answer D

Sudden infant death syndrome (SIDS) is the most common cause of sudden and unexpected death in infants; 40–50% of postneonatal infant mortality is caused by SIDS. The peak incidence of SIDS is at age 2–4 months; 95% of all SIDS deaths occur by age 6 months.

10–94 Answer A

Viridans (streptococci) and staphylococci are the two most predominant organisms constituting the normal flora of the oropharynx. They are followed by *Streptococcus pyogenes, Streptococcus pneumoniae, Moraxella catarrhalis, Neisseria* species, and lactobacilli.

10–95 Answer B

Respiratory alkalosis is the early acid-base disturbance that occurs in an aspirin overdose (salicylate intoxication). It results from direct stimulation of the respiratory center in the medulla, which causes an increase in pH and a decrease in $PaCO_2$. This leads to metabolic acidosis as the body compensates by renal excretion of bicarbonate to normalize the pH.

10–96 Answer D

In the pregnant woman, the thoracic cage may appear wider and the costal angle may feel wider than in the nonpregnant state. Respirations may be deeper, although this can be quantified only with pulmonary function tests.

10–97 Answer A

The normal adult has a thorax that has an elliptical shape with an anteroposterior:transverse diameter ratio of 1:2 or 5:7. Pectus excavatum (funnel breast) is a markedly sunken sternum and adjacent cartilages. It is congenital and usually not symptomatic. Pectus carinatum (pigeon breast) is a forward protrusion of the sternum with ribs sloping back at either side and vertical depressions along the costochondral junctions. It is less common than pectus excavatum and requires no treatment. A barrel-shaped chest is where the anteroposterior and transverse diameters of the chest are equal and the ribs are horizontal instead of in the normal downward slope. It is associated with normal aging and with chronic emphysema and asthma caused by hyperinflation of the lungs.

10–98 Answer B

Coal miners are at risk for developing pneumoconiosis. Pneumoconiosis is caused by the inhalation of dust particles and is an occupational hazard in mining and stone cutting. Farmers may be at risk for grain and/or pesticide inhalation. Certain areas of North America have a risk of histoplasmosis exposure. Potters, stonecutters, and miners are at risk for silicosis. Construction workers handling asbestos may develop asbestosis.

10–99 Answer B

Cough and congestion result when breathing sulfur dioxide. Carbon monoxide produces dizziness, headache, and fatigue. Tear gas irritates the conjunctiva and produces a flow of tears. Carbon dioxide produces sleepiness.

10–100 Answer D

Some conditions have a characteristic timing of a cough. A cough caused by a postnasal drip related to sinusitis is more prevalent at night. A cough associated with an acute illness, such as a respiratory infection, is continuous throughout the day. A cough in the early morning is usually caused by chronic bronchial inflammation from habitual smoking. A cough in the afternoon and/or evening may reflect exposure to irritants at work.

Bibliography

Blitz, BK: Smoking cessation programs: Making them work. Clin Rev (suppl), Nov 4, 1997.

Dillon, PD: Nursing Health Assessment. FA Davis, Philadelphia, 2003.

Dunphy, LM, and Winland-Brown, J: Primary Care: The Art and Science of Advanced Practice Nursing. FA Davis, Philadelphia, 2004.

Dunphy, LM: Management Guidelines for Nurse Practitioners Working with Adults, ed 2. FA Davis, Philadelphia, 2004.

Ferguson, GT: Asthma: Recognition and management. Clinical Advisor 1(1):29, 1998.

Gales, M, and Phillips, CM: Coccidioidomycosis: A mycotic infection on the rise. Clin Rev 7(4):71, 1997.

Hafner, JP, and Ferro, TJ: Recent developments in the management of COPD. Hosp Med 34(1):29, 1998.

Higgins, B, and Barrow, S: Asthma in adolescents. Adv Nurse Pract 6(2):28, 1998.

Kaptein, A: The human factor in effective COPD management. Strategic Med 1(2):22, 1997.

Lemanske, RF, and Busse, WW: Asthma. JAMA 278(22):1855, 1997.

Richman, E: Asthma diagnosis and management: New severity classifications and therapy alternatives. Clin Rev 7(8):76, 1997.

Rigotti, NA: Smoking. In Feldman, MD, and Christensen, JF (eds): Behavioral Medicine in Primary Care: A Practical Guide. Appleton & Lange, Norwalk, CT, 1997.

Rosenstreich, DL, et al: The role of cockroach allergy and exposure to cockroach allergen in causing morbidity among inner-city children with asthma. N Engl J Med 336:1356, 1997.

Schworer, PB: Chronic bronchitis: An approach to antimicrobial therapy. Fam Pract Recertification 19(7):14, 1997.

Venables, KM: Occupational asthma. Lancet 349:1465, 1997.

HOW WELL DID YOU DO?

85% AND ABOVE CONGRATULATIONS! THIS SCORE SHOWS APPLICATION OF TEST-TAKING PRINCIPLES AND ADEQUATE CONTENT KNOWLEDGE.

75–85% KEEP WORKING! REVIEW TEST-TAKING PRINCIPLES AND TRY AGAIN.

65–75% HANG IN THERE! SPEND SOME TIME REVIEWING CONCEPTS AND TEST-TAKING PRINCIPLES AND TRY THE TEST AGAIN.

Cardiovascular Problems 11

SUSAN ELAINE SLOAN,
JILL E. WINLAND-BROWN,
and
GRETCHEN HOPE MILLER HEERY

11–1 *Which of the following statements regarding the JNC 7 category about prehypertension is true?*

A. Patients with prehypertension usually remain in that category forever.
B. Patients with a blood pressure (BP) in the range of 130/80 to 139/89 mm Hg are twice as likely to develop hypertension as those with lower values.
C. All patients in this category should be started on diuretics immediately to avoid future end-organ disease.
D. Diastolic BP control should be the focus of treatment.

11–2 *Which of the following conditions is the least frequent cause of heart failure?*

A. Hypertension
B. Aortic stenosis
C. Ischemic cardiomyopathy
D. Valvular heart disease (mitral and tricuspid)

11–3 *Mr. Michaels has a long-standing cardiac problem. His electrocardiogram rhythm strip is shown below. Which medication would he be taking to prevent a pulmonary or cerebral problem?*

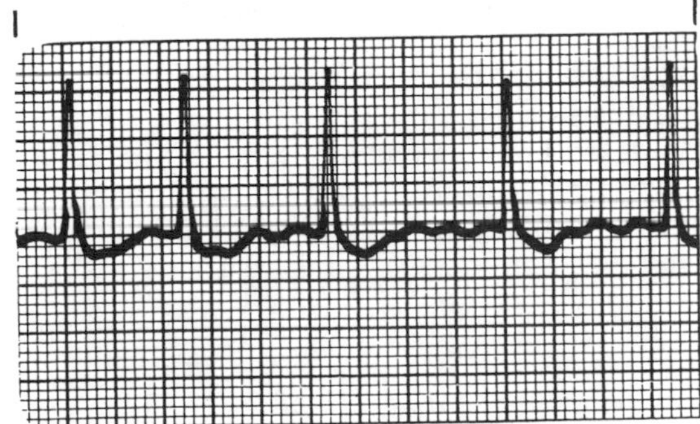

Lead II

A. An angiotensin-converting enzyme (ACE) inhibitor, such as enalapril (Vasotec)
B. An antiarrhythmic agent, such as procainamide (Procan-SR)
C. An anticoagulant, such as warfarin (Coumadin)
D. An anticonvulsant, such as phenytoin (Dilantin)

11–4 *While you are examining Jack, age 69, during an office visit, you suspect that he is having an acute myocardial infarction. Indications that he is a candidate for thrombolysis include all of the following* ***except:***

A. 12-lead electrocardiogram findings indicating an acute left bundle branch block.
B. ST segment elevation.
C. symptoms of ischemia.
D. a history of a recent hypertensive crisis.

11–5 *To reduce the progression of atherosclerotic lesions and occlusions in post-coronary artery bypass graft clients, it is recommended that the low-density lipoprotein cholesterol level be aggressively reduced to:*

A. 100 mg/dL or less.
B. 101–120 mg/dL.
C. 121–140 mg/dL.
D. 141–160 mg/dL.

11–6 *Greg has just been given a diagnosis of congestive heart failure. Which of his medications should be discontinued?*

A. Nifedipine (Procardia XL) for long-term management of his chronic stable angina
B. Hydrochlorothiazide (Hydrodiuril) for his hypertension
C. Enalapril (Vasotec) for his hypertension
D. Butalbital (Esgic) for his headaches

11–7 *Mary Lou, age 56, underwent lipid testing at a health fair and learned that her total cholesterol measurement was 248 mg/dL. She then came to the clinic for further evaluation. Mary Lou states that she feels well, but has a history of hypertension and asthma and has been postmenopausal for 6 years. She has smoked half a pack of cigarettes a day for the past 40 years and denies any alcohol use. Her current medications include hydrochlorothiazide (Hydrodiuril) 50 mg once a day and an occasional ibuprofen (Advil) for minor pain. Her vital signs are: blood pressure, 162/90; heart rate, 63; and respiration 16. She is 5 feet 3 inches tall and weighs 110 lb. Current laboratory studies show Na^+ 141; K^+ 4.0; Cl^- 103; CO_2 25; BUN 12; Cr 0.9; and fasting blood sugar, 98. Her fasting cholesterol profile includes total cholesterol, 245; triglycerides, 175; high-density lipoprotein, 40; and calculated low-density lipoprotein, 170. Risk factors for coronary artery disease in this client include all of the following* ***except:***

A. hypertension.
B. asthma.
C. an elevated low-density lipoprotein cholesterol level.
D. postmenopausal status.

11–8 *Mary, age 60, tells you that she has been taking Prempro for years because, when it was prescribed, you told her that it was cardioprotective. She says that recently she has been told otherwise. How do you respond?*

A. "Yes, when I prescribed it for you 6 years ago, it was thought to be cardioprotective. Because you've had no problems, you can continue with it."
B. "Because you have no cardiac risk factors, continue with the same dosage."
C. "Let's stop it now; you probably don't have any more hot flashes."
D. "Continue with it; you need it for the osteoporosis benefit."

11–9 *Sarah, who is postmenopausal, has asthma and hypertension and smokes cigarettes. She has a low-density lipoprotein (LDL) cholesterol level of 170 mg/dL and a high-density lipoprotein (HDL) cholesterol level of 40 mg/dL. To reduce Sarah's risk of a coronary event, the treatment plan would focus on:*

A. lowering her LDL cholesterol level.
B. lowering her HDL cholesterol level.
C. aggressively treating and controlling her hypertension and asthma.
D. all of the above.

11–10 *For a postmenopausal client who smokes cigarettes, has hypertension, and has a low-density lipoprotein cholesterol level of 170 mg/dL, the initial treatment plan would include all of the following* ***except:***

A. modifying risks through step II diet counseling and smoking cessation.
B. initiating hormone replacement therapy.
C. switching to a different class of antihypertensive agent.
D. initiating hypolipidemic pharmacologic therapy.

11–11 *To reduce the incidence of coronary events in an individual without coronary artery disease who has two or more risk factors, the goal serum low-density lipoprotein cholesterol level should be:*

A. 170–190 mg/dL.
B. 150–170 mg/dL.
C. 130–150 mg/dL.
D. less than 130 mg/dL.

11–12 *The cholesterol component(s) considered most responsible for atherosclerotic plaque formation is (are):*

A. total cholesterol.
B. low-density lipoprotein cholesterol.
C. high-density lipoprotein cholesterol.
D. phospholipids.

11–13 *The leading cause of death in women in the United States is:*

A. trauma.
B. cardiovascular disease.
C. diabetes.
D. cancer.

11–14 *For clients with known coronary artery disease, it is recommended that the low-density lipoprotein cholesterol be:*

A. 200 mg/dL or more.
B. 100 mg/dL or less.
C. 101–130 mg/dL.
D. 131–200 mg/dL.

11–15 *Nicotinic acid is an inexpensive drug used to treat serum hyperlipidemia. All of the following are true about nicotinic acid* ***except:***

A. Nicotinic acid lowers low-density lipoprotein cholesterol levels, raises high-density lipoprotein cholesterol levels, and decreases triglyceride levels.
B. Nicotinic acid is the drug of choice for individuals with diabetes.
C. Nicotinic acid may potentiate the effect of some antihypertensive agents.
D. Common adverse reactions of nicotinic acid include flushing, pruritus, and gastrointestinal upset.

11–16 *Which statement is true of hydroxymethylglutaryl-coenzyme A reductase inhibitors (statins)?*

A. They are the first drugs of choice for men under age 45.
B. They should be given in the morning after breakfast.
C. They may cause myopathies, especially at higher dosages or in combination with certain drugs.
D. They are contraindicated in clients taking Coumadin.

11–17 *Liver function tests should be monitored routinely every 4 months in the client on maintenance therapy with all hypolipidemic drugs* ***except:***

A. bile acid sequestrants (Questran, Colestid).
B. hydroxymethylglutaryl-coenzyme A reductase inhibitors (statins).
C. nicotinic acid (niacin).
D. fibric acid derivatives (Gemfibrozil).

11–18 *Symptoms of digitalis toxicity include all of the following* ***except:***

A. anorexia.
B. tingling of the extremities.
C. nausea and vomiting.
D. headache.

11–19 *Which statement regarding rheumatic fever in children is true?*

A. The peak period of risk is ages 1–5 years.
B. The disease is more common in boys.
C. The disease is more common in whites.
D. The environmental trigger is group A beta-hemolytic streptococcal infection of the upper respiratory tract.

11–20 *The cardinal sign of right-sided heart failure in infants and children is:*

A. hepatomegaly.
B. edema of the lower extremities.
C. tachypnea.
D. cyanosis.

11–21 *Rick is modifying his diet to try to lose weight, but after 3 months, he has not lost any weight, even though he has complied with his diet plan. A follow-up lipid profile reveals the following: total cholesterol, 238 mg/dL; triglycerides, 100 mg/dL; high-density lipoprotein cholesterol, 28 mg/dL; and low-density lipoprotein cholesterol, 190 mg/dL. What would you recommend?*

A. Continuing the diet plan for another month
B. Starting an exercise program with a goal of uninterrupted aerobic exercise for 30 minutes 2 days a week
C. Stopping his current diet plan and trying another
D. Starting hypolipidemic drug therapy

11–22 *When evaluating a client's risk factors for hyperlipidemia, what other cause(s) should be considered?*

A. Endocrine dysfunction
B. Renal insufficiency
C. Drug interactions
D. All of the above

11–23 *The most common cause of elevated total and low-density lipoprotein cholesterol levels in the United States is:*

A. heredity.
B. hypothyroidism.
C. diabetes.
D. a diet high in saturated fat.

11–24 *Individuals with clinical evidence of chronic ischemic heart disease (abnormal electrocardiogram, chest pain syndrome, unusual dyspnea, or fatigue) should have a full evaluation done to evaluate their risk for myocardial infarction or sudden death. The initial data for this risk stratification is obtained from all* ***except:***

A. careful history and physical examination.
B. exercise stress testing with or without nuclide imaging.
C. cardiac catheterization.
D. chest x ray.

11–25 *Exercise stress testing is used for all* ***except:***

A. assisting in the diagnosis of suspected coronary artery disease.
B. identifying clients with possible exercise-induced arrhythmias.
C. determining the success or failure of coronary artery bypass graft surgery or angioplasty.
D. Identifying clients with the potential for having a myocardial infarction.

11–26 *All of the following statements are true about chronic stable angina* ***except:***

A. It always presents as generalized discomfort in the chest or referred areas such as the neck, jaw, or arms.
B. It results from an imbalance between myocardial oxygen demand and supply.
C. It may be caused by a fixed atherosclerotic narrowing of the coronary vessels.
D. It may be caused by reduced oxygen supply from transient changes in coronary vascular tone (vasospasm) or coronary artery anomalies.

11–27 *Charles has chronic ischemic heart disease and is taking a beta blocker, which causes:*

A. an added benefit of an increase in high-density lipoprotein cholesterol.
B. a reduced heart rate.
C. a decreased diastolic filling time.
D. increased sexual desire.

11–28 *Mort is hypertensive. Which of the following factors influenced your choice of using an alpha blocker as the antihypertensive medication?*

A. Mort is black.
B. Mort also has congestive heart failure.
C. Mort has benign prostatic hyperplasia (BPH).
D. Mort has frequent migraine headaches.

11–29 *Management of chronic stable angina or new-onset angina includes all of the following* ***except:***

A. prescribing aspirin, nitrates, beta blockers, and/or calcium channel blockers.
B. correcting risk factors.
C. markedly limiting all activities to reduce oxygen requirements.
D. counseling regarding changes in lifestyle.

11–30 *Sexual activity is a major concern for clients with chronic ischemic heart disease. All the following statements are true* ***except:***

A. The sexual partner should be included in the education process.
B. The physical stress of sexual intercourse is equivalent to running a half a mile.
C. Antianginal medication taken before sexual activity can help prevent symptoms.
D. Sexual activity should be attempted when the client is well rested.

11–31 *Before counseling partners about sexual activity following a myocardial infarction, what factor(s) should the provider consider?*

A. Most clients do not want to know how their condition affects their sex life.
B. Spouses are knowledgeable about their partner's condition; therefore, they do not need counseling.
C. Most clients return to the same frequency of sexual intercourse after they have regained their physical strength.
D. Depression, loss of interest, spousal reluctance, and anxiety may interfere with a client's resumption of sexual activities.

11–32 *Marvin, age 56, is a smoker with diabetes mellitus. He has just been diagnosed as hypertensive. Which classification of drug would you not prescribe?*

A. Angiotensin-converting enzyme (ACE) inhibitors
B. Beta blockers
C. Calcium channel blockers
D. Diuretics

11–33 *Which statement regarding unstable angina is false?*

A. It is a clinical syndrome that falls between stable angina and acute myocardial infarction.
B. It does not present greater risks for adverse outcomes than chronic angina.
C. It occurs from disruption of plaque covering, frequent thrombus formation, and vasoconstriction of coronary vessels.
D. It may occur as an initial presentation.

11–34 *Harry comes to your office with waxing and waning ischemic symptoms over a period of days and weeks, an increase in angina while at rest, and transient ST changes on his electrocardiogram. This presentation leads you to believe that he is experiencing:*

A. a stroke.
B. a myocardial infarction.
C. stable angina.
D. unstable angina.

11–35 *Jamie, age 49, who has a history of hyperlipidemia, has symptoms that lead you to suspect unstable angina. Your next action would be to:*

A. start aspirin therapy and schedule an exercise stress test at the client's convenience.
B. initiate lipid-lowering agents.
C. hospitalize the client in a monitored setting with pharmacologic control of ischemia, arrhythmias, and thrombosis as appropriate.
D. Prescribe a Holter monitor and start her on a beta blocker.

11–36 *Long-term secondary prevention of chronic ischemic heart disease includes all of the following* ***except:***

A. use of aspirin.
B. use of beta blockers, calcium channel blockers, and nitrates.
C. risk factor and lifestyle modification.
D. periodic coronary angiography to evaluate progression of the disease.

11–37 *Jim, age 72, has a history of non–insulin-dependent diabetes mellitus (NIDDM) that has been controlled by diet. He has come for a routine examination and reports feeling more tired than usual. On his electrocardiogram (ECG), you notice Q waves in leads II, III, and aVF that were not present on his previous ECGs. What do you do?*

A. Immediately hospitalize Jim and order a cardiology consultation, start intravenous administration of an anticoagulant and nitrates, and run serial cardiac enzyme tests.
B. Nothing, because you know the normal progression of NIDDM in older adults includes changes in their ECG because of neuropathy involving the transmission of electrical impulses.
C. Initiate aspirin therapy and refer Jim to a cardiologist for evaluation of occult ischemic heart disease and left ventricular function as soon as possible.
D. Initiate lipid-lowering therapy because Jim may have had an acute myocardial infarction.

11–38 *The mechanism(s) that lead(s) to coronary artery disease and acute coronary syndrome include:*

A. injury to the endothelium with accumulation of lipids and macrophages.
B. disruption of lipid fibrous capsules resulting in hemorrhage and thrombus formation.
C. changes in endothelial vascular reactivity leading to diminished vasodilatation and exaggerated vasoconstrictor response.
D. all of the above.

11–39 *The classic 12-lead electrocardiogram change(s) that indicate(s) myocardial ischemia is (are):*

A. ST-segment elevation.
B. ST-segment depression or T-wave inversion.
C. flipped P waves with a prolonged PR interval.
D. deep Q waves.

11–40 *The classic 12-lead electrocardiogram change(s) that indicate(s) an acute myocardial infarction is(are):*

A. ST-segment elevation.
B. T-wave inversion.
C. flipped P waves with a prolonged PR interval.
D. deep Q waves.

11–41 *Janice, age 64, arrives at the office this morning without an appointment. She appears quite anxious and pale and is complaining of an intermittent aching across her sternum and into her jaw and left arm that started about an hour ago and woke her out of a sound sleep. She took an antacid and acetaminophen (Tylenol), but they did not seem to help. Her blood pressure is 160/90 and heart rate is 98. An electrocardiogram shows normal sinus rhythm with 2-mm ST-segment elevations in leads II, III, and aVF. What do you suspect?*

A. An acute anterior wall myocardial infarction (MI)
B. An acute inferior wall MI
C. Severe gastrointestinal reflux
D. An anxiety attack

11–42 *Bob is being seen in the office and you suspect an acute ischemic syndrome and an acute myocardial infarction. His treatment would include all of the following* ***except:***

A. prompt admission to a monitored bed with cardiology consultation.
B. initiation of aspirin, intravenous heparin, and anti-ischemic therapy with nitrates or beta blockers.
C. measurement of serum lipid levels to determine risk factors of hyperlipidemia.
D. evaluation for possible angiography with rescue percutaneous transluminal coronary angioplasty or thrombolytic therapy.

11–43 *An anterior wall myocardial infarction most likely occurs from occlusion of the:*

A. left circumflex artery.
B. left main artery.
C. right coronary artery.
D. left anterior descending artery.

11–44 *The lactic dehydrogenase flip ("LDH flip"), in which LDH_1 concentration exceeds LDH_2 concentration:*

A. is helpful in differentiating an anterior wall myocardial infarction (MI) from an inferior wall MI.
B. is helpful in dentifying Prinzmetal's angina from an acute MI.
C. is helpful in determining the occurrence of an acute MI in clients who present 2–3 days after the event.
D. has no significance at all.

11–45 *Besides electrocardiographic findings, diagnostic tests that can confirm an acute myocardial infarction (MI) include:*

A. serum markers such as myoglobin or creatine kinase-MB.
B. radionuclide imaging.
C. two-dimensional echocardiography.
D. all of the above.

11–46 *A blood pressure of 160/100 is classified as:*

A. prehypertension.
B. stage 1 hypertension.
C. stage 2 hypertension.
D. stage 3 hypertension.

11–47 *Ted, age 18, is to have a cardiac screening examination to determine if he can play college basketball. The diagnostic test of choice for detecting hypertrophic cardiomyopathy or idiopathic left ventricular hypertrophy is a(n):*

A. echocardiogram.
B. electrocardiogram.
C. arteriogram.
D. stress test.

11–48 *Management of a client who has documented hypertension (blood pressure of 140/92 mm Hg confirmed on multiple visits) and no other medical history includes all the following* ***except:***

A. immediate initiation of antihypertensive drug therapy to prevent any complications.
B. identification of known causes of hypertension.
C. assessment of the presence or absence of target organ damage and the extent of the disease.
D. identification of clinical cardiovascular disease (CVD) and risk factors, as well as other concomitant disorders that may guide prognosis and treatment.

11–49 *Rona, age 69, has hypertension (HTN), drinks 1 glass of white wine per day, and is slightly overweight. She asks you if making changes in her life at this age will make any difference. You tell her that lifestyle modifications for the control of HTN:*

A. are not as effective in older adults because HTN is an inevitable consequence of aging.
B. require a marked reduction in weight and a very limited choice of foods to achieve any benefit.
C. should include at least three glasses of red wine every day because it improves high-density lipoprotein cholesterol levels, a known cardiovascular risk factor, which may be worsened by HTN.
D. may prevent HTN, lower elevated blood pressure, and may reduce the number and dosage of antihypertensive medications needed to manage a condition.

11–50 *The decision to initiate pharmacologic treatment for a client with hypertension requires consideration of all of the following* **except:**

A. the client's belief that the medication will work.
B. the managed-care program in which the client is enrolled.
C. the degree of blood pressure elevation.
D. the presence of other cardiovascular disease, concurrent diseases, target organ disease, or other risk factors.

11–51 *General guidelines to follow when prescribing antihypertensive medications include using a stepped approach, beginning with the lowest dosage and titrating upward; considering low-dosage combination therapy if moderate-dose monotherapy does not work; and choosing all* **except:**

A. diuretic or aspirin.
B. beta blockers or calcium channel blockers.
C. angiotension-converting enzyme or angiotension receptor blockers.
D. digoxin or procardia.

11–52 *Martin, age 56, has hypertension and has been taking antihypertensive medication for about 10 years. He has been very stable. You have not seen him in about 6 months. His examination today should specifically:*

A. include a blood pressure measurement with the client seated comfortably.
B. include a fundoscopic examination.
C. be a focused examination limited to the respiratory and cardiovascular systems.
D. include a discussion of weaning him off his medication.

11–53 *Shirley, age 56, presents with a blood pressure of 156/94 mm Hg. Your history taking should:*

A. focus on symptoms suggesting causes of hypertension.
B. include an evaluation of lifestyle, dietary intake and physical activity.
C. include an evaluation of all over-the-counter drugs, herbal remedies, and illicit drug use.
D. include all of the above.

11–54 *To determine the presence of target organ damage and other risk factors in the client with hypertension, basic diagnostic tests that should be ordered include:*

A. chest x ray, electrocardiogram, urinalysis, complete blood count, chemistry profile, lipid profile, and thyroid-stimulating hormone level.
B. renal arteriogram.
C. plasma renin activity and 24-hour urinary sodium.
D. echocardiogram.

11–55 *Which of the following statements about hypertension is true?*

A. It is frequently caused by pheochromocytoma.
B. It is usually the result of an underlying correctable problem.
C. The cause is unknown in approximately 95% of cases.
D. It has a higher incidence among adult white men than any other group.

11–56 *Terry, a 42-year-old black man who just moved into the area, comes into the clinic for a new-client visit. He brings his medical records from his previous healthcare provider, which show a blood pressure of 140/104 mm Hg on two separate occasions. Recent laboratory tests (complete blood count, chemistry profile, urinalysis, and thyroid-stimulating hormone) are normal. A recent electrocardiogram shows normal sinus rhythm with left ventricular hypertrophy. He denies any medical problems and tells you he has never been diagnosed with hypertension. He is not taking any medications, does not smoke, and drinks about two beers a day. He is currently unemployed. His blood pressure today is 150/110 mm Hg. Your next step would be to:*

A. obtain plasma and urine catecholamine measurements.
B. have him keep a food diary for 1 week, then return for a repeat blood pressure reading.
C. begin drug therapy with hydrochlorothiazide (Hydrodiuril), 25 mg once a day.
D. Start him on metapropol (Lopressor) 100 mg twice a day.

11–57 *When teaching a client with hypertension about restricting dietary sodium, you would include the following instruction:*

A. Sodium restriction can cause serious adverse effects.
B. Diets with markedly reduced intake of sodium may be associated with other beneficial effects beyond blood pressure control.

C. Seventy-five percent of sodium intake is derived from processed food.
D. A goal of 3 g of sodium chloride or 1.2 g of sodium per day is easily achievable.

11–58 *All of the following statements are true about hypertension during pregnancy* ***except:***

A. Methyldopa (Aldomet) is the drug of choice for women first diagnosed with hypertension during pregnancy.
B. Beta blockers are safe in the first trimester of pregnancy.
C. Angiotensin-converting enzyme (ACE) inhibitors (I and II) have been associated with serious fetal abnormalities.
D. Beta blockers are safe in the latter part of pregnancy.

11–59 *Which of the following drugs should be considered as first-line therapy for a client with hypertension and heart failure?*

A. Enalapril (Vasotec)
B. Diltiazem (Cardizem)
C. Atenolol (Tenormin)
D. Metoprolol (Lopressor)

11–60 *Which of the following statements is true regarding bacterial endocarditis protection in clients with mitral value prolapse?*

A. Antibiotic prophylaxis is indicated in clients with mitral valve prolapse without regurgitation.
B. Prophylaxis should be given 4 hours after an invasive procedure.
C. Prophylaxis with penicillin is indicated for genitourinary and gastrointestinal procedures.
D. Antimicrobial prophylaxis within 1 hour before a procedure will provide effective protection.

11–61 *When evaluating a client's need for bacterial endocarditis prophylaxis, all the following should be considered* ***except:***

A. the degree of risk for endocarditis because of the client's underlying heart disease.
B. the age of the client.
C. the risk of bacteremia for the given procedure.
D. the potential for adverse reactions for the antibiotic prophylaxis.

11–62 *Procedures for which endocarditis prophylaxis is recommended include:*

A. vaginal or cesarean deliveries.
B. insertion or removal of intrauterine devices.
C. dental procedures or extractions.
D. body piercings.

11–63 *Endocarditis prophylaxis is not recommended for clients with:*

A. a prosthetic cardiac valve.
B. previous bacterial endocarditis.
C. mitral valve prolapse with regurgitation or valvular dysfunction.
D. a pacemaker or internal defibrillator.

11–64 *An active 68-year-old man under your care has known acquired valvular aortic stenosis and mitral regurgitation. He also has a past history of infectious endocarditis. He has recently been told he needs elective replacement of his aortic valve. When he comes in, you discover that he has 10 remaining teeth in poor repair. Your recommendation would be to:*

A. defer any further dental work until his valve replacement is completed.
B. instruct the client to have dental extraction done cautiously, having no more than two teeth per visit removed.
C. suggest that he consult with his oral surgeon about removing all the teeth at once and receiving appropriate antibiotic prophylaxis.
D. coordinate with his cardiac and oral surgeons to have the tooth extraction and valve replacement done at the same time to reduce the risk of anesthetic complications.

11–65 *All of the following statements are true of auscultation of the aortic valve* ***except:***

A. It is best performed using the diaphragm of the stethoscope.
B. It is best heard at the second right intercostal space.
C. It should include auscultation at other locations such as neck, apex, and right parasternal region.
D. It is best performed using the bell of your stethoscope.

11–66 *Aortic stenosis (AS), which may be congenital or acquired, results in reduction in the opening of the valve area, a diminished stroke volume, and gradual increase in the size of the left ventricle. Cardinal signs and symptoms of AS include all* ***except:***

A. dyspnea.
B. angina.
C. syncope.
D. hyperactivity.

11–67 *All of the following statements are true concerning auscultation of the typical murmur associated with aortic stenosis* ***except:***

A. It is a harsh, crescendo-decrescendo ejection type that often radiates to the carotid arteries.
B. It is a diastolic murmur.
C. It is best heard at the base of the heart.
D. The loudness of the murmur does not reflect the severity of the lesion.

11–68 *Management of the client with aortic stenosis includes all the following* ***except:***

A. prophylaxis for endocarditis.
B. treatment of associated hypertension, arrhythmias, and heart failure.
C. the use of diuretics and nitrates.
D. routine Doppler echocardiography to evaluate the progression of the valve lesion.

11–69 *Which classification of antihypertensive drugs is the first-choice therapy for treating hypertension and angina in clients with known coronary artery disease?*

A. Diuretics
B. Beta blockers
C. Calcium channel blockers
D. Angiotensin-converting enzyme inhibitors

11–70 *Which classification of antihypertensive drugs is the most effective for treating hypertension in black clients and older adults?*

A. Diuretics
B. Angiotensin-converting enzyme (ACE) inhibitors
C. Beta blockers
D. Alpha-adrenergic blockers

11–71 *Which drugs are used to lower blood pressure in a client with coexisting benign prostatic hypertrophy?*

A. Beta blockers
B. Angiotensin-converting enzyme inhibitors
C. Alpha-adrenergic blockers
D. Calcium channel blockers

11–72 *Which of the following findings are suggestive of renovascular hypertension?*

A. Bilateral flank pain on percussion
B. Renal arterial bruits in the abdomen, flanks, or back
C. A palpable mass in the right lower quadrant
D. Decreased urine output

11–73 *Cough, loss of taste, and rash are adverse effects associated with which class of antihypertensive agents?*

A. Diuretics
B. Beta blockers
C. Angiotensin-converting enzyme inhibitors
D. Calcium channel blockers

11–74 *Headache, flushing, tachycardia, and peripheral edema are adverse effects associated with which class of antihypertensive agents?*

A. Beta blockers
B. Calcium channel blockers
C. Angiotensin-converting enzyme inhibitors
D. Diuretics

11–75 *Which of the following antihypertensive agents would most likely produce a rebound hypertensive crisis following its abrupt withdrawal?*

A. Doxazosin (Cardura)
B. Lisinopril (Prinivil)
C. Losartan (Cozaar)
D. Clonidine (Catapres)

11–76 *When auscultating a patient's heart, you note a short, high-frequency click (opening snap) after S2 during the beginning of diastole. What could this indicate?*

A. Aortic regurgitation
B. Mitral stenosis
C. Mitral regurgitation
D. Nothing; this is normal

11–77 *Joanne has mitral stenosis. When she asks you what is causing her symptoms (dyspnea on exertion, fatigue and weakness, orthopnea, and paroxysmal nocturnal dyspnea), you tell her they are most likely related to all but:*

A. increased left atrial pressures and volumes that are reflected backward into the pulmonary vasculature.
B. elevated pulmonary pressures resulting in pulmonary hypertension.
C. reduction of the size of the mitral valve orifice by more than 50%.
D. lung cancer.

11–78 *Which of the following statements is true of mitral regurgitation?*

A. It may be noted as a holosystolic murmur.
B. It is caused by stiff, noncompliant leaflets that limit flow from the left atrium to the left ventricle.
C. It occurs only as the result of congenital malformation of the mitral valve, which inhibits contact and closure of the cusps.
D. It results in a prolonged PR interval on electrocardiogram.

11–79 *Mitral valve prolapse is characterized by:*

A. elongation of the chordae tendineae and enlarged valve leaflets.
B. ballooning (prolapse) of the cusps into the ventricle during diastole.
C. an early diastolic murmur.
D. an early systolic murmur.

11–80 *Clinical findings of mitral valve prolapse may include all the following* ***except:***

A. palpitations, postural hypotension, and chest pain.
B. atrial and ventricular arrhythmias.
C. a shortened PR interval on the client's electrocardiogram.
D. fatigue.

11–81 *Treatment considerations for clients with mitral valve prolapse (MVP) include all of the following* ***except:***

A. These clients have an increased risk of infective endocarditis.
B. A follow-up echocardiography is usually recommended every 1–4 years depending on the client's symptoms.
C. Antibiotic prophylaxis is recommended for all clients with MVP.
D. Beta blockers are used if the client has supraventricular or ventricular arrhythmias.

11–82 *When counseling a client with symptomatic mitral valve prolapse, your teaching should include advising the client to do all* ***except:***

A. increase fluids, eliminate caffeine, and lower sugar and fat intake.
B. start an exercise program using moderate aerobic activity
C. use stress reduction techniques such as biofeedback, imagery, and meditation.
D. isometric exercises.

11–83 *Clinical findings associated with aortic regurgitation include:*

A. pulsus paradoxus.
B. waterhammer pulses.
C. pulsus alternans.
D. weak, thready pulses.

11–84 *Murmurs are graded according to their intensity (loudness). A murmur that is audible with the stethoscope off the chest is a:*

A. grade III murmur.
B. grade IV murmur.
C. grade V murmur.
D. grade VI murmur.

11–85 *Pharmacologic therapy for mitral valve disease includes:*

A. treatment of dyspnea with diuretics to relieve congestion.
B. reduction of fast ventricular rates with digoxin, beta blockers, or calcium channel blockers.
C. preload reduction with antihypertensive agents to decrease regurgitant flow.
D. daily antibiotic use to ward off bacterial infections.

11–86 *Signs of right-sided heart failure include:*

A. a low cardiac output.
B. signs of fluid retention.
C. dyspnea.
D. elevated pulmonary venous pressure.

11–87 *Martha, age 36, presents with a complaint of increasing shortness of breath and fatigue over the past 6 months. She has been trying to lose weight, has been on a walking exercise program for over a year, and had taken the fenfluramine-phentermine (Fen-Phen) combination several years ago but stopped when its adverse effects were reported. Your examination reveals a grade II/VI systolic murmur along the apex. What do you do?*

A. Obtain pulmonary function tests.
B. Instruct the client about other exercise activities that may not produce her symptoms.
C. Refer the client to a cardiologist for an echocardiogram and cardiovascular workup.
D. Start endocarditis prophylaxis.

11–88 *Sheila, age 78, presents with a chief complaint of waking up during the night coughing. You examine her and find an S_3 heart sound, pulmonary crackles (rales) that do not clear with coughing, and peripheral edema. What do you suspect?*

A. Asthma
B. Nocturnal allergies
C. Heart failure
D. Valvular disease

11–89 *Which of the following is usually the earliest sign or symptom of chronic occlusive arterial disease in the extremities?*

A. Loss of hair over the lower extremity
B. Intermittent claudication
C. Painful ulcerations of the toes of the affected extremity
D. Muscle atrophy

11–90 *Discriminating between symptoms of occlusive arterial disease and other disorders (such as musculoskeletal or neurological disorders) requires a careful history. All of the following symptoms are noted with occlusive arterial disease* ***except:***

A. pain occurring in the calves or thighs when walking, with relief obtained when standing still.
B. pain when standing as well as walking that is relieved by sitting or lying down.
C. severe pain at rest that requires the client to hang the leg over the side of the bed to obtain relief.
D. pallor or mottling with collapsed superficial veins.

11–91 *Management of the client with intermittent claudication may include all of the following* ***except:***

A. controlling risk factors such as smoking and lipid reduction.
B. initiating an exercise program.
C. recommending open shoes to protect the feet from pressure.
D. ordering pentoxifylline (Trental) 400 mg tid.

11–92 *Characteristics of ischemic arterial ulcers include:*

A. an irregularly shaped border with crusting or scaling at the edges.
B. severe pain.
C. a location anywhere on the leg.
D. a moist ulcer base with ill-defined borders.

11–93 *Management of ischemic arterial ulcers may include all the following* ***except:***

A. use of hyperbaric oxygen therapy.
B. revascularization of the lower extremities.
C. use of medications such as aspirin, pentoxifylline (Trental), or an anticoagulant.
D. immediate debridement of dry, uninfected necrotic areas (eschar).

11–94 *Dana has ischemic arterial ulcers. When counseling her, you recommend that she do three things to decrease her risk of further damage. They include all of the following* ***except:***

A. reducing risk factors such as stopping smoking and reducing fat (lipid) intake.
B. avoiding restrictive garments and trauma (mechanical, chemical, and thermal).
C. maintaining adequate hydration but avoiding drinks containing caffeine.
D. begin an intense aerobic program.

11–95 *Selma has acute peripheral arterial occlusion of a lower extremity. Before you begin your examination, you know that it:*

A. may present with only complaints of coldness or paresthesia of the extremity.
B. may present as the only disease.
C. always occurs in the lower extremities.
D. will result in an extremity that appears "blue."

11–96 *Nathan, age 63, comes for his annual physical. He has a history of mild hypertension and hyperlipidemia that he has not been successful in treating by diet and weight loss. His only complaint is a problem with impotence. On physical examination, you note a palpable, pulsatile abdominal mass in the umbilical region; a bruit above the umbilical region; and diminished femoral pulses. You suspect:*

A. renal artery stenosis.
B. an abdominal aortic aneurysm.
C. a cardiac tumor.
D. a thoracic aortic aneurysm.

11–97 *Management of a client with hypertension with an abdominal aortic aneurysm would not include:*

A. an abdominal aortic ultrasound or computed tomography scan with contrast.
B. aggressive management of the client's hypertension.
C. referral to a cardiologist.
D. immediate cardiac catheterization.

11–98 *Deep-vein thrombosis may result in:*

A. generalized edema of the involved extremity.
B. atrophy of leg muscles.
C. loss of sensation in the affected extremity.
D. the release of fat emboli.

11–99 *Pathological mechanisms that contribute to thrombosis include all the following* ***except:***

A. bradycardia.
B. stasis of blood flow.
C. hypercoagulability of blood.
D. injury to the endothelial layers of the vascular system.

11–100 *Judy has a deep venous thrombosis of her right popliteal vein. Management includes all of the following* ***except:***

A. intravenous heparin therapy followed by oral anticoagulation therapy for 3–6 months.
B. bedrest with the extremity elevated until signs and symptoms have resolved.
C. early ambulation to prevent stasis of blood flow and prevent further thrombus development.
D. progressive ambulation with external compression stockings after signs and symptoms subside.

Answers

11–1 Answer B

The Seventh Report of the Joint National Committee on Prevention, Detection, Evaluation, and Treatment of High Blood Pressure (JNC 7) includes a new category designated as prehypertension. The range for the systolic pressure is 120 to 139 and that for diastolic pressure 80 to 89. Patients with prehypertension are at an increased risk for progression to hypertension. Patients in the 130/80 to 139/89 mm Hg blood pressure (BP) range have twice the risk of developing hypertension as those with lower values. The report also states that systolic BP control should be the focus of treatment.

11–2 Answer D

Valvular heart disease (mitral and tricuspid) has become the least common cause of heart failure of the conditions listed because of the declining incidence and severity of rheumatic fever. On the other hand, aortic stenosis occurs frequently and is reversible. The most common cause of heart failure is ischemic cardiomyopathy. Systemic hypertension remains a common cause of congestive heart failure.

11–3 Answer C

Mr. Michaels's electrocardiogram rhythm strip shows atrial fibrillation. To prevent continuous release of microemboli into the circulation, resulting in a pulmonary embolism or cerebrovascular accident, Mr. Michaels will probably be taking warfarin (Coumadin). In addition, digitalis (Digoxin) is usually ordered, sometimes in combination with either a beta blocker or calcium channel blocker. Procainamide (Procan-SR) is used for ventricular arrhythmias. Anticonvulsants are not indicated.

11–4 Answer D

Indications that Jack is a candidate for thrombolysis after an acute myocardial infarction include 12-lead electrocardiogram (ECG) findings indicating an acute left bundle branch block; symptoms of ischemia; and ST-segment elevation of at least 1 mm in at least two contiguous ECG leads. Contraindications for thrombolysis include a history of a recent hypertensive crisis; active gastrointestinal or genitourinary bleeding (excluding menses); abdominal or thoracic surgery within the past month; head trauma; recent cerebrovascular accident; aortic dissection; and pancreatitis.

11–5 Answer A

A study by the Post Coronary Artery Bypass Graft Trial investigators found that aggressively lowering the low-density lipoprotein cholesterol level to 100 mg/dL or less in clients who had previously undergone bypass surgery was more effective in reducing the progression of atherosclerotic lesions and occlusions than any other moderate treatment.

11–6 Answer A

Nifedipine (Procardia XL), a calcium channel blocker, should be discontinued, along with antiarrhythmic agents, when a client develops congestive heart failure (CHF) because both of these medications are important causes of worsening heart failure. Diuretics are the most effective means of providing symptomatic relief in clients with CHF, so Greg should stay on his hydrochlorothiazide (Hydrodiuril). Angiotensin-converting enzyme inhibitors should be the initial treatment, along with diuretics in most symptomatic clients, so Greg can also continue taking his enalapril (Vasotec). Butalbital (Esgic) is not contraindicated in clients with CHF.

11–7 Answer B

Asthma is not a risk factor for the development of coronary artery disease (CAD). Risk factors for CAD include hypertension, cigarette use, postmenopausal status for women, and low-density lipoprotein cholesterol levels greater than 130 mg/dL (in individuals without evidence of CAD but with two or more risk factors).

11–8 Answer C

Because Prempro has been found not to be cardioprotective, as once thought, it should be stopped if ordered for that reason. Women have been shown to have a 29% increase for nonfatal myocardial infarctions when taking estrogen plus progestin. Stroke rates are also increased by 41% in this group (women taking estrogen plus progestin), and there is a twofold greater rate of venous thromboembolism. Total cardiovascular disease was increased by 22%, so Mary's Prempro should be stopped. A bone density study should be done to determine if she needs to take something for osteoporosis.

11–9 Answer A

According to the National Cholesterol Education Program (NCEP) expert panel, Sarah's treatment should focus on lowering her low-density lipoprotein cholesterol to less than 130 mg/dL because she has at least two risk factors for coronary artery disease.

11–10 Answer D

For a postmenopausal client who smokes cigarettes, has hypertension, and has a low-density lipoprotein cholesterol (LDL-C) level of 170 mg/dL, the initial treatment plan would include all of the options except initiating hypolipidemic pharmacologic therapy. Modifying risks through step II diet counseling and smoking cessation, initiating hormone replacement therapy (HRT), and switching to a different class of antihypertensive agent should be tried before initiating pharmacologic therapy for hyperlipidemia. Although a first-line drug for primary prevention could be considered because the National Cholesterol Education Program (NCEP) guidelines recommend treatment for individuals without coronary artery disease, but with two or more risk factors and an LDL-C level above 160 mg/dL, a decision to try risk modification, especially smoking cessation and HRT, should be done first. If the client does not stop smoking or the other measures do not help the client, hypolipidemic drug therapy should be initiated.

11–11 Answer D

The National Cholesterol Education Program (NCEP) guidelines recommend a goal serum low-density lipoprotein cholesterol level of less than 130 mg/dL for individuals without coronary artery disease but with two or more risk factors.

11–12 Answer B

The cholesterol component considered most responsible for atherosclerotic plaque formation is an elevated low-density lipoprotein cholesterol level.

11–13 Answer B

The leading cause of death for women in the United States is cardiovascular disease, including heart and cerebrovascular disease. Although the incidence of cardiovascular disease is lower in younger women, it dramatically increases in women over age 45 and is a major cause of chronic illness and disability in these women.

11–14 Answer B

According to the National Cholesterol Education Program guidelines, for clients with known coronary artery disease (CAD), it is recommended that the low-density lipoprotein cholesterol level be 100 mg/dL or less. Studies, including the Scandinavian Simvastatin Survival Study and the West of Scotland Coronary Prevention Group Study, reported that lowering LDL-C levels resulted in a significant reduction of vascular events such as myocardial infarction or cerebrovascular accident in individuals with and without CAD.

11–15 Answer B

Nicotinic acid is not the drug of choice for individuals with diabetes. A potential adverse effect of nicotinic acid is impairment of glucose intolerance; therefore, it should be used with caution in clients with diabetes. If instituted, serum glucose and liver function tests should be closely monitored. Nicotinic acid lowers low-density lipoprotein cholesterol levels, raises high-density lipoprotein cholesterol levels, and decreases triglyceride levels; may potentiate the effect of some antihypertensive agents; and may cause adverse reactions including flushing, pruritus, and gastrointestinal upset.

11–16 Answer C

Although rare, hydroxymethylglutaryl-coenzyme A reductase inhibitors (statins) may cause myopathies, especially at higher dosages or in combination with certain drugs, such as gemfibrozil (Lopid), nicotinic acid (Nicobid), or erythromycin (E-Mycin). Any reports of muscle pain and weakness should be evaluated. According to National Cholesterol Education Program guidelines, bile acid sequestrants are preferred to statins for primary prevention of coronary events in men under age 45 and women under age 55 unless hypercholesteremia is severe or other contraindications exist. The liver is more active in the production of cholesterol during the evening hours; therefore, the recommendations for all statins (except atorvastatin [Lipitor], which has a longer half-life) is for dosing to be done in the evening or at bedtime. Statins may increase the international normalized ratio and require an adjustment of Coumadin dosage; however, Coumadin use is not a contraindication to use of statins.

11–17 Answer A

Bile acid sequestrants (Questran, Colestid) are not absorbed from the gastrointestinal tract and lack systemic toxicity; therefore, liver function tests do not need to be monitored in clients taking these drugs. Hepatotoxicity is a serious adverse effect of hydroxymethylglutaryl-coenzyme A reductase inhibitors (statins), nicotinic acid (niacin), and fibric acid derivatives such as gemfibrozil; therefore, liver function tests should be routinely monitored in clients taking these drugs.

11–18 Answer B

Symptoms of digitalis toxicity include anorexia, nausea and vomiting, headache, disorientation, xanthopsia, and verdopsia. The symptoms usually occur before any cardiotoxic effects take place and are warning signs that the dosage needs to be adjusted. Tingling of the extremities is not a symptom of digitalis toxicity.

11–19 Answer D

Group A beta-hemolytic streptococcal infections of the upper respiratory tract remain the primary environmental trigger that acts on predisposed children to cause rheumatic fever and subsequent cardiovascular disease. Although the incidence of the disease has significantly declined over the past half century, there has been a resurgence in several regions of the United States since the mid-1980s. Children between the ages of 5 and 15 are at most risk; blacks are slightly more at risk than whites, and girls more at risk than boys.

11–20 Answer A

Hepatomegaly is the cardinal sign of right-sided heart failure in infants and children. Edema of the lower extremities is indicative of right ventricular heart failure in older children and adults. Tachypnea is the cardinal sign of left-sided congestive heart failure in children. Cyanosis is a clue to the presence of heart disease, but not specifically a sign of right-sided heart failure.

11–21 Answer D

Because dietary therapy has not resulted in any significant reduction of Rick's low-density lipoprotein cholesterol (LDL-C) level, starting him on hypolipidemic drug therapy is strongly recommended to help him achieve an LDL-C goal of less than 130 mg/dL. To further help reduce the risk of heart disease, regular physical activity of moderate intensity (the minimal goal is 30 minutes, 5 times a week), along with lowering blood pressure and reducing weight, is important. No further diagnostic intervention is indicated unless the client begins to complain of symptoms of ischemia such as chest pain, increasing fatigue, or dyspnea.

11–22 Answer D

Hyperlipidemia may be secondary to underlying conditions such as endocrine dysfunction (diabetes, myxedema), renal insufficiency, nephrotic syndrome, and dysproteinemia. Drug interactions may also cause hyperlipidemia. Commonly used medications that alter lipid profiles include diuretics and beta blockers.

11–23 Answer D

Although heredity, hypothyroidism, and diabetes contribute to abnormal serum lipid levels, a diet high in saturated fat is the most common cause of elevated total and low-density lipoprotein cholesterol in the United States.

11–24 Answer C

Cardiac catheterization is not generally performed during initial data collection. Selected individuals may require catheterization for severe or extremely unstable symptoms; however, angiography is generally reserved for those with positive exercise stress tests. The initial history and physical exam should explore severity of symptoms, functional disability, quality of life, and cardiac risk factors. This assists the provider in identifying high-risk individuals who would benefit from further diagnostic testing. Electrocardiographic stress testing has a high false positive rate. The use of thallium or sestamibi agents with exercise testing has a lower frequency of false positive results. Nuclide imaging may be used for initial evaluation of clients or to confirm those with a questionable history and a positive exercise stress test. A chest x ray can identify any structural abnormalities such as cardiomegaly or aortic aneurysm that suggest underlying cardiovascular pathology.

11–25 Answer D

Exercise stress testing, with or without the use of thallium or sestamibi agents, is used to assist in the diagnosis of suspected coronary artery disease as well as to predict its severity and prognosis; identify clients with possible exercise-induced arrhythmias; and determine the success or failure of coronary artery bypass graft surgery or angioplasty by evaluating the patency of revascularized vessels.

11–26 Answer A

Clients with chronic stable angina do not always have generalized discomfort in the chest or referred areas such as the neck, jaw, or arms. Although the majority of clients do have these complaints, a number of clients complain of symptoms which are "anginal equivalents," such as dyspnea, fatigue, breathlessness, indigestion, and faintness. Chronic stable angina results from an imbalance between myocardial oxygen demand and supply. It may be caused by a fixed atherosclerotic narrowing of the coronary vessels, by reduced oxygen supply from transient changes in coronary vascular tone (vasospasm), or by coronary artery anomalies.

11–27 Answer B

Beta blockers reduce the heart rate, which results in a decrease in oxygen demand and an increase in coronary blood flow from the increased diastolic filling time. Studies have also shown that beta blockers reduce mortality in clients who have had acute myocardial infarctions and reinfarction. Adverse effects of all beta blockers include a decrease in high-density lipoprotein cholesterol, bronchospasm, fatigue, sleep disturbance, worsening of congestive heart failure, gastrointestinal disturbances, and impotence.

11–28 Answer C

An alpha blocker is the antihypertensive agent of choice because Mort has benign prostatic hyperplasia (BPH). In addition to lowering the client's blood pressure, it will provide symptomatic relief of his BPH. Calcium channel blockers or diuretics are effective antihypertensive agents in blacks, whereas a beta blocker would be the drug of choice if Mort had migraine headaches in addition to his BPH. Diuretics and angiotensin-converting enzyme inhibitors are the drugs of choice for treating congestive heart failure with accompanying hypertension.

11–29 Answer C

Management of chronic stable angina or new-onset angina includes prescribing aspirin, nitrates, beta blockers, or calcium channel blockers; correcting risk factors; and counseling regarding changes in lifestyle. Markedly limiting all activities to reduce oxygen requirements is not part of the management because you do not want to turn clients into "cardiac cripples" by curtailing all or most of their activities.

11–30 Answer B

The physical stress of sexual intercourse is usually equivalent to that of climbing one flight of stairs at a normal pace, or any other activity that induces a heart rate of 120 beats per minute. Clients should be reassured that if they can carry out these activities without symptoms, they can probably engage in sexual activity without symptoms. If symptoms occur, they may be managed with proper precautions such as timing activities more than 2 hours after meals, taking an extra dose of a short-acting beta blocker 1 hour before intercourse, or taking nitroglycerin 15 minutes before intercourse. True statements concerning sexual activity for clients with chronic ischemic heart disease include that the sexual partner should be included in the education process, that antianginal medication taken before sexual activity can help prevent symptoms, and that sexual activity should be attempted when the client is well rested, although morning hours may not always be best. Chronic angina exhibits a circadian rhythm characterized by a propensity toward transient ischemic episodes in the morning hours.

11–31 Answer D

Before counseling partners about sexual activity following a myocardial infarction (MI), the provider should consider that depression, loss of interest, spousal reluctance, and anxiety may interfere with a client's resumption of sexual activities. The diagnosis of heart disease affects the spouse as well as the client. Spouses may display anxiety and depression, yet often are not included in the assessment, counseling, and treatment processes. The level of sexual activity reported 1 year after an MI is only about 60% of the level before illness.

11–32 Answer B

Beta blockers should not be ordered for Marvin for two reasons: he smokes and he is a diabetic. The adverse effects of all beta blockers include the potential for developing bronchial asthma and inhibiting gluconeogenesis, and therefore they may prolong hypoglycemic episodes.

11–33 Answer B

Unstable angina does present greater risks for adverse outcomes than chronic angina. It increases the risk of continuing angina, acute myocardial infarction, and death. Unstable angina is a clinical syndrome that falls between stable angina and acute myocardial infarction; is caused by disruption of plaque covering, frequent thrombus formation, and vasoconstriction of coronary vessels; and may occur as an initial presentation without any other warning signs.

11–34 Answer D

The clinical presentation of unstable angina may include waxing and waning of ischemic symptoms over a period of days or weeks; often involves a progressive increase in symptoms in those with stable angina, including rest angina; and may include transient ST changes on the electrocardiogram.

11–35 Answer C

According to the Agency for Healthcare Policy and Research clinical practice guidelines, clients with angina at rest, postinfarction angina, or rapidly progressive angina with electrocardiogram changes should be managed with hospitalization in a monitored setting, bedrest, control of precipitating factors, and initiation of medical therapy.

11–36 Answer D

Long-term secondary prevention for chronic ischemic heart disease includes the use of aspirin, beta blockers, calcium channel blockers, or nitrates and risk factor and lifestyle modification. To evaluate the progression of the disease, periodic testing should include noninvasive procedures such as exercise stress testing and coronary angiography. Invasive testing should be reserved for clients who have markedly positive stress tests or angina that is refractory to medical treatment.

11–37 Answer C

Older adults and clients with diabetes frequently demonstrate defective anginal warning systems—a result of altered cardiac neural pathways (older age, diabetics), physical interruption of nerve pathways (cardiac transplant or bypass surgery), an abnormally high pain perception threshold, or milder degrees of ischemia. Because Jim is an older adult with diabetes, he may have had a silent myocardial infarction (MI) as well as silent ischemia. Neither his electrocardiogram nor his clinical presentation suggest an acute MI, so hospitalization is not indicated. However, aspirin therapy (unless contraindicated for other reasons) is indicated because it has been shown to be an independent factor in reducing the risk of subsequent MI. Workup for a possible silent MI should include exercise stress testing with thallium imaging to determine ischemic burden and changes indicative of MI. Evaluation for left ventricular wall motion abnormalities and ejection fraction with echocardiography may also confirm previous MI or the presence of ischemia.

11–38 Answer D

The mechanisms that lead to coronary artery disease and acute coronary syndrome include injury to the endothelium with accumulation of lipids and macrophages; disruption of lipid fibrous capsules resulting in hemorrhage and thrombus formation; and changes in endothelial vascular reactivity leading to diminished vasodilatation and exaggerated vasoconstrictor response.

11–39 Answer B

The classic 12-lead electrocardiogram changes that indicate myocardial ischemia are ST-segment depression and T-wave inversion.

11–40 Answer A

The classic 12-lead electrocardiogram (ECG) change that indicates an acute myocardial infarction (MI) is ST-segment elevation. Q waves may evolve subsequent to the initial event and persist over time. Not all clients show this classic ECG evolution, however. Up to one-third of those with a diagnosis of an acute MI do not develop Q waves and nearly one-half of nontransmural infarctions produce Q waves. As a result, use of the terms "Q-wave" and "non-Q-wave" infarction is favored over the terms "transmural" and "nontransmural" MI.

11–41 Answer B

A 12-lead electrocardiogram (ECG) showing 2-mm ST-segment elevations in leads II, III, and aVF indicate an acute inferior wall myocardial infarction (MI). Ischemic syndromes often follow a circadian rhythm, with an MI occurring more frequently in the morning hours between 8 AM and 12 noon. Ischemic heart disease should always be a consideration in female clients because it causes 23% of all deaths in women and is the leading cause of death in women over age 50. In anterior wall MIs, the site of the block is distal, below the atrioventricular (AV) node, so some evidence of an intraventricular conduction defect would probably be evident on the ECG. Gastrointestinal reflux may produce pain suggestive of angina, but is usually related to a heavy meal, occurs in recumbency or bending over, and is usually relieved by antacids, which Janice's was not. Anxiety attacks do not usually wake someone up out of a sound sleep, and would not produce an abnormal ECG except for tachycardia.

11–42 Answer C

Regardless of the client's risk factors, individuals demonstrating acute ischemic changes require immediate treatment of symptoms. It is also essential to identify and treat the underlying cause of disruption of blood flow in order to salvage or reduce the size of injury to the myocardium. Evaluating serum lipid levels during an acute event may lead to false results. Serum cholesterol responds to acute stress events with a decrease in both low-density lipoprotein cholesterol (LDL-C) and high-density lipoprotein cholesterol (HDL-C), as well as an increase in triglyceride levels. This change can persist for up to 6 weeks. Lipid profiles drawn during an acute myocardial infarction will generally demonstrate lower total, LDL-C, and HDL-C cholesterol levels, resulting in an underestimation of this risk factor.

11–43 Answer D

Occlusion of the left anterior descending artery results in damage to the anterior wall of the left ventricle as well as the septum. Occlusion of the right coronary artery usually results in damage to the inferior wall of the left ventricle. However, for some clients, the left circumflex artery (LCX) is the dominant vessel and can be responsible for damage to the inferior wall of the left ventricle. The LCX normally supplies the lateral wall of the left ventricle as well as the posterior wall.

11–44 Answer C

The "LDH flip," in which LDH_1 exceeds LDH_2, is helpful in determining the occurrence of an acute myocardial infarction (MI) in clients who present 2–3 days after the event. The two isoenzymes most helpful in the diagnosis of an acute MI are creatine kinase-MB (CK-MB) and LDH_1 and LDH_2, because they are specifically concentrated in cardiac muscle. The CK-MB level rises first after an acute MI, but returns to normal in 48–72 hours. LDH rises later than CK-MB, so it is useful when CK-MB was not measured within the first 24 hours of an acute MI. Normally, levels of LDH_2 are greater than LDH_1. However, after an acute MI, the ratio reverses, producing the LDH flip.

11–45 Answer D

Besides electrocardiographic (ECG) findings, diagnostic tests that can confirm an acute myocardial infarction (MI) include serum markers such as myoglobin or creatine kinase-MB (CK-MB), radionuclide imaging, and two-dimensional echocardiography.

11–46 Answer C

In the new JNC 7 guidelines, hypertension stages 2 and 3 have been combined. A blood pressure of 160 or greater systolic and 100 or greater diastolic is now considered to be stage 2 hypertension. Pharmacologic therapy is definitely indicated. Several drugs are usually required for management of this stage. Hypertensive patients should have a goal BP of <140/90, or <130/80 if they have diabetes or chronic kidney disease.

11–47 Answer A

In athletes under age 30, the three most common causes of sudden death are hypertrophic cardiomyopathy, idiopathic left ventricular hypertrophy, and coronary artery anomalies. The diagnostic test that should be employed to detect a potential problem when Ted plays a strenuous sport is an echocardiogram, which many colleges are now instituting as part of their screening criteria for athletes. The echocardiogram will detect hypertrophic cardiomy opathy and idiopathic left ventricular hypertrophy. The arteriogram is the only reliable test available to detect coronary artery anomalies. An electrocardiogram will diagnose rhythm disturbances. A stress test will record the effects of stress on the heart.

11–48 Answer A

Treatment of hypertension is dependent on risk stratification. Full evaluation of the client is needed to determine the presence of target organ damage (TOD), cardiovascular disease (CVD), and major risk factors. Also, those with identifiable causes should have the underlying problem addressed.
If the client has no risk factors (except diabetes) and no TOD or CVD, the client would initially be started on lifestyle modification. The Joint National Committee on Prevention, Detection, Evaluation, and Treatment of High Blood Pressure recommends that individuals who have high-normal blood pressure as well as known renal insufficiency, heart failure, or diabetes mellitus should be considered for prompt pharmacologic therapy as well as lifestyle modification.

11–49 Answer D

Lifestyle modifications are essential for the control of hypertension (HTN). Weight reduction of as little as 4.5 kg (10 lb) reduces blood pressure in a large proportion of overweight persons with HTN. It can also enhance the blood pressure-lowering effect of concurrent antihypertensive agents and reduce cardiovascular risk factors. The Dietary Approaches to Stop Hypertension recommendations allow a combination of foods rich in fruits, vegetables, and low-fat dairy products and is not based on excessive calorie restriction. Elevated blood pressure is not an inevitable consequence of aging. Excessive alcohol intake is an important risk factor for HTN because it can cause resistance to antihypertensive therapy. Individuals who drink should be counseled to limit their daily intake to no more than 1 oz of ethanol for average-size men and 0.5 oz of ethanol for women or lighter-weight individuals. (1 oz of ethanol equals 2 oz of whiskey, 24 oz of beer, or 10 oz of wine).

11–50 Answer B

The decision to initiate pharmacological treatment of a client with hypertension does not depend on the managed-care program in which the client is enrolled. It might determine the exact medication on the formulary that the plan will pay for, but not the decision to start an antihypertensive agent.

11–51 Answer D

General guidelines to follow when prescribing antihypertensive medications include using a stepped approach, beginning with the lowest dosage and titrating upward; choosing a diuretic, calcium channel blocker, angiotensin-converting enzyme inhibitor, angiotensin receptor blocker, or beta blocker if the client has uncomplicated hypertension; and considering low-dosage combination therapy if monotherapy does not work. In general, diuretics, beta blockers, angiotensin-converting enzyme inhibitors, angiotensin receptor blockers, and calcium channel blockers may all be considered as first-line therapy. Combinations of low doses of two agents from different classes have been shown to provide additional antihypertensive efficacy, thereby reducing the possibility of dose-dependent adverse effects. An effort to decrease the dosage and number of antihypertensive drugs (unless they are also treating a concurrent chronic condition) should be considered after hypertension has been effectively controlled for at least 1 year. Step-down therapy is more often successful in clients who have made lifestyle modifications.

11–52 Answer B

Fundoscopic examination for hypertensive retinopathy (arteriovenous nicking, arteriole narrowing, hemorrhages, exudates, and disc edema) should be included in the physical exam of a client with hypertension (HTN). When examining the client with HTN, at least two blood pressure measurements separated by 2 minutes, should be performed with the client seated. An additional blood pressure reading taken with the client standing should also be included. A full examination is necessary to evaluate the client for possible causes of HTN (such as an enlarged thyroid or truncal obesity with purple striae in Cushing's syndrome) and to note possible target organ damage.

11–53 Answer D

There are multifactorial causes of hypertension, as well as factors that affect the response to treatment. The clinician needs not only to focus on the physical review of systems, but must thoroughly investigate other factors that may contribute to the client's hypertension or response to treatment, such as an evaluation of dietary intake and physical activity; evaluation of all over-the-counter drugs, herbal remedies, or illicit drugs used; and any stressors that the client may be encountering that may affect the blood pressure.

11–54 Answer A

To determine the presence of target organ damage and other risk factors in the client with hypertension, basic diagnostic tests that should be ordered include a chest x ray, electrocardiogram, urinalysis, complete blood count, chemistry profile, lipid profile, and thyroid stimulating hormone level. Renal arteriogram, plasma renin activity, 24-hour urinary sodium, and echocardiogram are more expensive tests. They are indicated when hypertension is severe or refractory to treatment, or when underlying renal pathology is suspected.

11–55 Answer C

The cause of hypertension is unknown (idiopathic) in approximately 95% of cases. This form of hypertension is known as primary or essential hypertension. The remaining 5% of cases are secondary to other underlying disease processes such as renal disease or pheochromocytoma. The incidence of hypertension is greatest in adult black men and women.

11–56 Answer C

Pharmacologic therapy is indicated for Terry because his blood pressure has been elevated on three separate occasions. Target organ damage to the heart is suggested by the left ventricular hypertrophy noted on his electrocardiogram. Diuretics such as hydrochlorothiazide (Hydrodiuril) have been proven to reduce hypertensive morbidity and mortality in blacks and should be the first drug of choice. In addition to being inexpensive, diuretics, when used as antihypertensive agents in blacks who have low plasma renin activity, are more potent than other antihypertensive drugs. Calcium channel blockers are also effective for this population, whereas beta blockers and angiotensin-converting enzyme inhibitors are less effective. The client does not report symptoms suggesting pheochromocytoma, and its occurrence is rare, so plasma and urine catecholamine level tests are not indicated at this time. Analyzing the client's food diary will allow the practitioner to make recommendations for limiting salt intake as well as improving dietary choices; however, a diary of 3 days in length would be sufficient. In addition, hypertension in black clients is often responsive to a reduction in salt intake.

11–57 Answer C

When teaching a client with hypertension about restricting dietary sodium, it is important to stress that 75% of sodium intake is derived from processed food. Although concern about severe sodium restriction has been raised, there is no evidence that lower levels of sodium intake cause any hazards. A sodium reduction to approximately 6 g of sodium chloride or 2.4 g of sodium a day is recommended for most clients and is easily achievable.

11–58 Answer B

Beta blockers are considered safe for the treatment of hypertension in the latter part of pregnancy; their use in early pregnancy may be associated with growth retardation of the fetus. Methyldopa (Aldomet) is the drug of choice for women first diagnosed with hypertension during pregnancy. Angiotensin-converting enzyme inhibitors (I and II) have been associated with serious fetal abnormalities.

11–59 Answer A

Enalapril (Vasotec), an angiotensin-converting enzyme (ACE) inhibitor, should be considered as first-line therapy for a client with hypertension (HTN) and heart failure. Reports from the Framingham Heart Study demonstrated that HTN continues to be the major cause of left ventricular failure in the United States. In treating heart failure, ACE inhibitors alone or with digoxin or a diuretic are effective in reducing morbidity and mortality. The dihydropyridine calcium channel blockers amlodipine and felodipine have been shown to be safe in treating angina and hypertension in clients with heart failure when used along with ACE inhibitors. Other calcium channel blockers, such as diltiazem (Cardizem), are not recommended. Beta blockers, such as atenolol (Tenormin), are contraindicated in clients with congestive heart failure. Their adverse effects include atrioventricular conduction defects and left ventricular failure.

11–60 Answer D

Only a few individuals with mitral valve prolapse (MVP) develop complications at any age. When prolapsed valves do not leak and there is no evidence of regurgitation by a Doppler echocardiogram, the risk of endocarditis is not increased, and prophylaxis is not indicated. Clients with leaking prolapsed valves should receive prophylaxis. Recommendations are for a dosage to be given 30 minutes to 1 hour before the anticipated procedure. With procedures involving genitourinary or gastrointestinal instrumentation, the most common organism to cause endocarditis is *Enterococcus faecalis*. For clients at high risk of endocarditis, ampicillin (50 mg/kg) and gentamycin (1.5 mg/kg) should be given intravenously within 30 minutes of starting the procedure, and an additional dose of ampicillin IV or amoxicillin PO (25 mg/kg) should be given 6 hours after the first dosage. Although these recommendations only require prophylactic therapy for clients with MVP with regurgitation, many dentists request that all clients with MVP be treated before procedures.

11–61 Answer B

Various factors are taken into consideration in determining the need for antibiotic prophylaxis against bacterial endocarditis, such as the degree of risk for endocarditis because of the client's underlying heart disease; the risk of bacteremia for the given procedure; and the potential for adverse reactions to the antibiotic prophylaxis. The age of the client is not a determinant.

11–62 Answer C

Dental procedures and extractions require antibiotic prophylaxis against bacterial endocarditis. The recommendations from cardiologists reflect an analysis of relevant literature regarding procedure-related endocarditis. The recommendations serve only as guidelines. Because endocarditis may occur even with appropriate use of antimicrobials, one must be concerned if fever, night chills, weakness, myalgia, or malaise are reported after these procedures.

11–63 Answer D

Clients with a pacemaker or internal defibrillator, as well as those with mitral valve prolapse without regurgitation, are not at a greater risk than the general population for bacterial endocarditis and do not require antibiotic prophylaxis. Clients with a prosthetic cardiac valve, previous bacterial endocarditis, and mitral valve prolapse with regurgitation or valvular dysfunction are all considered high-risk individuals and should receive antibiotic prophylaxis according to high-risk categories.

11–64 Answer C

The client's poor dental status is a probable source of endocarditis. Proper management of his dental work is essential before valve replacement, because that will lower the risk for endocarditis. Removing the teeth in a single procedure reduces the repetitive risks of extraction-related bacteremia as well as the possibility of developing antibiotic resistance from repeating prophylaxis regimens. Performing the extraction concurrently with valve surgery will add stress and risk of bacteremia to the procedure.

11–65 Answer D

Auscultation of the aortic valve (the second heart sound [S_2], which signifies closure of the aortic and pulmonic valves) is best performed using the diaphragm of the stethoscope because it is a high-pitched sound and is best heard at the second right intercostal space. It should also include auscultation at other locations such as neck, apex, and right parasternal region because important findings are sometimes present in other locations.

11–66 Answer D

Cardinal signs of aortic stenosis include dyspnea, angina, and syncope. In adults, manifestations of reduced cardiac output are usually not present until late in the course of the disease and typically occur between ages 60 and 70. Once symptoms appear, life expectancy without surgery is between 2 and 5 years.

11–67 Answer B

Auscultation of the typical murmur associated with aortic stenosis usually reveals the following: it is a systolic murmur, best heard at the base of the heart, of a harsh, crescendo-decrescendo ejection type. It often radiates to the carotid arteries. In clients with a calcified aortic valve, the murmur is harsh and rasping at the base. As the client's left ventricular dysfunction worsens, the typical harsh murmur becomes less loud and resembles the murmur of mitral regurgitation. The loudness of the murmur does not reflect the severity of the lesion.

11–68 Answer C

Management of the client with aortic stenosis includes antibiotic prophylaxis before surgical or dental procedures for bacterial endocarditis and treatment of associated conditions such as hypertension, arrhythmias, and heart failure. Therapy has limited effectiveness in terms of improving the functional status of the lesion; therefore routine, such as yearly, Doppler echocardiography to evaluate the progression of the valve lesion is recommended. Clients should avoid overuse of diuretics and nitrates because they can reduce preload and result in orthostatic hypotension and syncope. They should also avoid beta blockers and calcium channel blockers because they may further depress left ventricular function and precipitate failure.

11–69 Answer B

Beta blockers are the first-choice therapy for treating hypertension and angina in clients with known coronary artery disease because they control angina by decreasing myocardial demand through reduction of heart rate, systolic blood pressure, and contractility. Beta blockers have also been shown to reduce the risk of subsequent myocardial infarctions (MIs) and sudden cardiac death in clients who have had a previous MI.

11–70 Answer A

Diuretics are effective in lowering blood pressure in all clients, especially blacks and older adults. Numerous studies have shown reductions in morbidity and mortality with these agents. Relative to beta blockers and angiotensin-converting enzyme inhibitors, diuretics are more potent in blacks, older adults, obese clients, and other subgroups who exhibit increased plasma volume or low plasma renin activity. Alpha-adrenergic blockers may be used effectively if the client has coexisting prostatism.

11–71 Answer C

Alpha-adrenergic blockers are used both to lower blood pressure and to relieve some of the symptoms associated with benign prostatic hypertrophy. They decrease the resistance along the prostatic urethra by relaxing the smooth muscle component of the prostate. Alpha-adrenergic blockers can cause postural hypotension during the initial doses of therapy; therefore the dosage should "start low and go slow" and then gradually increase depending on the effectiveness.

11–72 Answer B

Renal artery bruits, which indicate renal artery stenosis, particularly those of diastolic timing, are a suggestive sign of renovascular hypertension. They are often heard or palpated (as a thrill) in the abdomen, flanks, or back. Systolic bruits are commonly detected, especially in older adults, and may not be associated with renal artery stenosis.

11–73 Answer C

A cough, loss of taste, and a rash are all adverse effects of angiotensin-converting enzyme (ACE) inhibitors. They all disappear with discontinuance of the medication and may or may not reappear if therapy is resumed with another ACE inhibitor. Some diuretics may cause electrolyte disturbances, fatigue, and, depending on the type, rash and impotence. Beta blockers may cause bronchospasm, increase plasma triglyceride levels, and result in central nervous system disturbances. Calcium channel blockers may cause adverse vasodilatory effects such as headache, flushing, palpitation, and ankle edema.

11–74 Answer B

Headache, flushing, tachycardia, and peripheral edema are adverse effects associated with calcium channel blockers. Calcium channel blockers may antagonize any of several cell membrane calcium entry channel receptors. As a result, some of these agents can express different effects on regional circulation. Although verapamil (Calan) and diltiazem (Cardizem) may reduce sinus rate, dihydropyridine calcium channel blockers may cause more potent peripheral vasodilatation and can also cause headache, flushing, and tachycardia. Calcium channel blockers may also cause peripheral edema from reflex postcapillary constriction, which causes an increase in capillary hydrostatic pressure. This leads to movement of intravascular fluid to peripheral tissues and edema that is unassociated with weight gain.

11–75 Answer D

Abrupt withdrawal of clonidine (Catapres), a central alpha agonist, will most likely produce a rebound hypertensive crisis. Blood pressure may return to or even exceed pretreatment levels after withdrawal of clonidine. This is rarely seen following withdrawal of beta blockers, diuretics, angiotensin-converting enzyme inhibitors, or calcium channel blockers. The most noticeable symptoms include sweating, palpitations, nervousness, headache, abdominal cramping, and nausea along with elevated blood pressure. The mechanism for clonidine withdrawal is thought to be catecholamine overproduction.

11–76 Answer B

When auscultating the heart, if you note a short, high-frequency click (opening snap) after S_2 during the beginning of diastole, suspect mitral stenosis. Mitral stenosis occurs with a stiff stenotic valve. The valve opening becomes restricted, impeding forward flow. The stenosis generates increased left atrial pressures, which are necessary to overcome the increased resistance to flow. The "snap" is created when the mitral valve leaflet is rapidly reversed toward the left ventricle in early diastole (as left ventricular pressures are reduced) by the high left atrial pressures.

11–77 Answer D

Mitral stenosis causes symptoms of dyspnea on exertion; fatigue and weakness; orthopnea; and paroxysmal nocturnal dyspnea. These symptoms are caused by increased left atrial pressures and volumes, which are reflected backward into the pulmonary vasculature; elevated pulmonary pressures resulting in pulmonary hypertension; and reduction of the size of the mitral valve orifice by more than 50%. In mitral stenosis, the left atrial musculature enlarges (hypertrophies) to increase its pumping force and dilates to accommodate the greater volume. The increased pressure and volume are transmitted backward into the pulmonary vasculature, resulting in elevated pulmonary artery pressures. This adaptive response is essential to ensure an adequate pressure gradient for blood to flow through the pulmonary artery and vein. These increased pressures result in pulmonary congestion, causing dyspnea. Weakness and fatigue are the result of the fixed and eventually diminished cardiac output.

11–78 Answer A

Mitral regurgitation may be noted as a holosystolic murmur. Because ventricular pressure exceeds atrial pressure at the beginning of systole, regurgitant backflow begins with the first heart sound (S_1). The ensuing regurgitant murmur persists up to the second heart sound (S_2), provided that the ventricular pressure at the end of systole still exceeds the atrial pressure. The direction of regurgitant flow (intra-arterial jet) may be noted on auscultation. If the direction of the jet is medial against the atrial septum near the base of the aorta, the murmur radiates from the apex to the second left intercostal space and even into the neck. If the jet is directed posterolaterally within the left atrial cavity, the murmur can be noted into the axilla, to the left scapula, and occasionally to the vertebral column. Mitral regurgitation is caused by shrunken, deformed cusps or shortened, fused chordae tendinae, which prevent closure of the leaflets.

11–79 Answer A

Mitral valve prolapse (MVP) is a congenital syndrome characterized by elongation of the chordae tendinae and enlarged valve leaflets. Ballooning of the cusps (prolapse) into the atrium occurs to varying degrees during ventricular systole. MVP is characterized by a midsystolic click and late systolic murmur.

11–80 Answer C

Although many clients with mitral valve prolapse (MVP) are asymptomatic, clients may appear with a variety of symptoms, including what some have described as "MVP syndrome": a characteristic click, fatigue, palpitations, postural hypotension, chest pain, atrial and ventricular arrhythmias, anxiety, and symptoms of autonomic dysfunction (excessive secretion of catecholamines causing vasoconstriction and orthostatic tachycardia).

11–81 Answer C

Treatment considerations for clients with mitral valve prolapse (MVP) include the following: These clients have an increased risk of infective endocarditis; a follow-up echocardiogram is usually recommended every 1–4 years depending on the client's symptoms; beta blockers are indicated if the client has supraventricular or ventricular arrhythmias. Antibiotic prophylaxis is not recommended for all clients with MVP. It is only recommended for clients with mitral regurgitation or the presence of a mitral regurgitation murmur.

11–82 Answer D

When counseling a client with symptomatic mitral valve prolapse, your teaching should include advising the client to increase fluids; eliminate caffeine; lower sugar and fat intake; start an exercise program using moderate aerobic activity, but avoid heavy weight lifting or isometric exercise; and use stress-reduction techniques such as biofeedback, imagery, and meditation.

11–83 Answer B

Waterhammer pulses (Corrigan's pulses) are present in a client with aortic regurgitation or aortic insufficiency. The forceful, high-volume left ventricular ejection of blood into the aorta during systole is accompanied by a reflux of blood back into the left ventricle during diastole. Usually, the peripheral vascular resistance is low in aortic regurgitation; this maximizes the forward flow of blood into the periphery. As a result of this forceful movement of blood and subsequent backflow, the waveform of peripheral pulses is characterized by a rapid rise and collapse. Other findings resulting from this phenomenon include pistol-shot pulses (Diroziez's murmur), which are audible on auscultation of the femoral artery; alternating flushing and paling of the nailbed capillaries (Quincke's capillary pulsation); and systolic head bobbing as the collapsed neck vessel fills rapidly (Musset's sign).

11–84 Answer D

The intensity of a murmur is determined by the quantity and velocity of blood flow across the sound-producing area, its distance from the stethoscope, and the type of tissue between the murmur and the stethoscope. A murmur that is audible with the stethoscope off the chest is a grade VI murmur. A grade I murmur is barely heard; grade II is quietly heard; grade III is loudly heard; grade IV is loud; grade V is very loud; and grade VI is the loudest. A thrill may accompany murmurs of grades IV, V, and VI.

11–85 Answer A

Pharmacologic therapy for mitral valve disease includes treatment of dyspnea with diuretics to relieve congestion. It also consists of afterload (not preload) reduction with antihypertensive agents to decrease regurgitant flow. Other therapies may include antiarrhythmics for atrial fibrillation, because this can exacerbate symptoms as a result of ventricular filling, and antibiotic prophylaxis when indicated.

11–86 Answer B

Signs of right-sided heart failure focus on fluid retention with edema, hepatic congestion, and occasionally ascites. Signs of left-sided heart failure focus on a low cardiac output and an elevated pulmonary venous pressure, with dyspnea being the cardinal feature.

11–87 Answer C

Martha should be referred to a cardiologist for an echocardiogram and cardiovascular workup because she has taken the fenfluramine-phentermine (Fen-Phen) combination. The United States Department of Health and Human Services issued the following recommendations for individuals who took fenfluramine and dexfenfluramine: (1) Persons who have had the drugs should undergo a careful history and cardiovascular examination by their healthcare provider; (2) Individuals with signs or symptoms suggesting valvular disease should have an echocardiogram; and (3) An echocardiogram should be strongly considered for those (even without signs or symptoms) who are about to undergo a procedure for which endocarditis prophylaxis is recommended.

11–88 Answer C

The greater the number of symptoms in a client, the more reliable is the diagnosis of heart failure. One of the classic symptoms that Sheila has is a nocturnal cough that wakes her up. Other findings indicative of heart failure include an elevated jugular venous pressure, an S_3 heart sound, a laterally displaced apical impulse, pulmonary crackles (rales) that do not clear with coughing, and peripheral edema that is not caused by venous insufficiency. A persistent night cough is often the only symptom seen with some types of asthma, but the cough is dry without any of the other symptoms that Sheila has. Allergies may present as a dry cough at night with postnasal drip. Valvular heart disease may present with dyspnea, orthopnea, and paroxysmal nocturnal dyspnea, but not a cough with crackles (rales).

11–89 Answer B

The clinical symptoms of chronic occlusive arterial disease occur slowly over a period of years and result primarily from tissue underperfusion and ischemia. Usually, the earliest symptom is intermittent claudication. Latter signs and symptoms of chronic occlusive arterial disease in the lower extremities include changes in skin texture, loss of hair, muscle wasting, reduced muscle strength and sensation, and the development of ulcers on the toes or heels.

11–90 Answer B

Symptoms of occlusive arterial disease include pain occurring in the calves or thighs when walking, with relief obtained when standing still; and severe pain at rest that requires the client to hang the leg over the side of the bed to obtain relief. True intermittent claudication occurs with walking and is relieved by standing. With the progression of occlusive disease, ischemic symptoms worsen. Pain, usually in the foot or toes, can occur at rest, and is typically worse at night. Assuming a dependent position with the extremity off the side of the bed can afford some relief. (Rest pain indicates 90% occlusion.) Pseudoclaudication may be caused by lumbar spinal stenosis, which causes lower-extremity symptoms with any erect posture (standing as well as walking) and is not relieved by standing still. Instead, the client must sit or lie down to obtain relief of symptoms. Pallor or mottling of the extremities due to collapsed superficial veins may also occur with occlusive arterial disease.

11–91 Answer C

Management of the client with intermittent claudication may include controlling risk factors such as smoking and lipid reduction; initiating an exercise program (such as a walking program, which encourages the development of collateral circulation); and ordering pentoxifylline (Trental) 400 mg tid to improve microcirculation. It is essential to instruct clients how to protect their extremities from all trauma because the ability to heal is reduced by the arterial insufficiency. The client should wear well-fitted, closed shoes (not open shoes) to avoid external injury.

11–92 Answer B

Characteristics of ischemic arterial ulcers include severe pain and a discrete border (which may have a "punched-out" appearance) with a pale, dry ulcer base and a slightly inflamed "halo" around the border if infected, They are typically located distally and are usually a result of trauma.

11–93 Answer D

Management of ischemic arterial ulcers may include the use of hyperbaric oxygen therapy, revascularization of the lower extremities, and use of medications such as aspirin, pentoxifylline (Trental), or an anticoagulant. Débridement of dry, uninfected necrotic wounds is contraindicated until perfusion or blood flow has been evaluated to be adequate for wound healing. If there are no signs of infection, the eschar serves as a barrier to bacterial invasion, and its removal may result in overwhelming infection. If the wound is infected, débridement is required; however, a surgical consultation is necessary.

11–94 Answer D

The first priority for managing ischemic arterial ulcers is to improve tissue perfusion. When counseling clients, tell them to decrease their risk of further damage by reducing risk factors. Ways to reduce risk factors include stopping smoking; reducing fat (lipid) intake; avoiding restrictive garments and trauma (mechanical, chemical, and thermal); maintaining adequate hydration; and avoiding caffeinated drinks. Smoking and caffeine can cause vasoconstriction and reduce blood flow. Lipid lowering can restore some of the arterial vessels' ability to vasodilate and "self-regulate" blood flow in response to tissue needs. Adequate hydration reduces blood viscosity, improves blood flow, and reduces chances for microemboli formation. Although an intense aerobics program should not be initiated, Buerger-Allen exercises should be done three to four times per day. The client raises and lowers the extremities, with each of 5 repetitions taking about 2 minutes. The legs should be raised to a 45-degree angle, then lowered again to the supine position. The changes in position cause the arteries of the legs to refill by gravity.

11–95 Answer A

The manifestation of acute peripheral arterial occlusion is classically a dramatic one with sudden pain, pallor, paresthesia, paralysis, and pulselessness. However, it may also be more gradual and less dramatic, presenting with only complaints of coldness or paresthesia of the extremity. The occlusion may be caused by previously unknown cardiac disease, a vascular lesion, or an occult systemic disease, such as connective tissue diseases or arteritis, and should serve as a clue to look for other conditions because it rarely occurs by itself. Occlusions can occur in upper or lower extremities.

11–96 Answer B

A pulsating abdominal mass in the region of the umbilicus is suggestive of an abdominal aortic aneurysm. Abdominal aortic aneurysms may be asymptomatic or may cause abdominal or back pain, as well as impotence or difficulties with digestion. Thoracic aneurysms must be quite large to produce symptoms and consequently may be discovered incidentally by chest x ray. The symptoms are caused by expansion and compression of adjacent thoracic structures and may include dysphagia, hoarseness, and edema of the head and arms. Abdominal aortic aneurysms can also cause chest pain. Aneurysm rupture is catastrophic and may present with severe chest, abdominal, or back pain; paralysis; or shock. Renal artery stenosis is a common cause of secondary hypertension and presents in the same manner as essential hypertension. Primary cardiac tumors are rare and are usually atrial myxomas. Metastases to the heart from malignant tumors elsewhere in the body are more frequent. The client usually presents with fever, malaise, weight loss, leukocytosis, an elevated erythrocyte sedimentation rate, and peripheral or pulmonary emboli.

11–97 Answer D

Management of a client with hypertension who also has an abdominal aortic aneurysm would include an abdominal aortic ultrasound or computed tomography (CT) scan with contrast; aggressive management of the client's hypertension; and referral to a cardiologist. Because most arterial aneurysms are atherosclerotic in origin, coronary artery disease (CAD) and arterial disease are frequent comorbid conditions. The client should be evaluated for occult CAD. Determining the size of the aneurysm is essential so that decisions can be made about whether to treat medically with close monitoring or to refer for surgical intervention. In a good-risk client, elective surgical treatment of abdominal aortic aneurysm is advisable for those in the range of 4.5–5 cm. Serial observation with ultrasound every 3–4 months is appropriate for asymptomatic abdominal aortic aneurysms smaller than 4.5 cm, or for larger asymptomatic aneurysms in poor-risk clients. If the aneurysm becomes symptomatic or enlarges, then elective surgery is appropriate. Control of hypertension is essential to reduce stress on the aneurysm and slow its progression. A cardiac catheterization will show the size/condition of the cardiac arteries, not the abdominal arteries.

11–98 Answer A

Deep vein thrombosis (DVT) may result in generalized edema of the involved extremity. DVT usually originates in the pelvis and lower extremities. It is typically asymptomatic. Pulmonary embolus may be the first indication of thrombosis. Thrombus formation may not be clinically apparent because of the large capacity of the venous system and development of collateral circulation around obstructions. Pain is the most common symptom and may be aching or throbbing. Most pulmonary emboli are caused by DVT. There is no atrophy of the leg muscles, and although there is pain, there is not a loss of sensation. DVT may result in a thromboembolism. Other emboli include tumors that have invaded the venous circulation (tumor emboli), amniotic fluid, air, fat, bone marrow, or foreign intravenous material.

11–99 Answer A

The precise mechanisms that initiate thrombosis are not well-defined; however, three factors, referred to as Virchow's triad, are generally recognized as contributing to formation of thrombus: stasis of blood flow, hypercoagulability of blood, and injury to the endothelial layers of the vascular system.

11–100 Answer C

Although early ambulation after surgical procedures is recognized as minimizing the risk of venous stasis, it is not used in the presence of established deep venous thrombosis (DVT). The goal of therapy for the client with DVT is to prevent thrombus extension, formation of new thrombi, and embolization. Management includes intravenous heparin therapy followed by oral anticoagulation therapy for 36 months; bedrest with the extremity elevated until signs and symptoms have resolved (this allows time for clot organization and adherence to the vessel wall); and progressive ambulation with external compression stockings after signs and symptoms subside.

Bibliography

AHA Science Advisory: Guide to primary prevention of cardiovascular diseases: A statement for healthcare professionals from the task force on risk reduction. Circulation 95, 1997.

Chobanian, AV, et al: The seventh report of the Joint National Committee on Prevention, Detection, Evaluation, and Treatment of High Blood Pressure—The JNC 7 Report. JAMA 289:2560–2570, 2003.

Dejani, AS, et al for the American Heart Association: Prevention of bacterial endocarditis. JAMA 277, 1997.

Dunphy, LM, and Winland-Brown, JE: Primary Care: The Art and Science of Advanced Practice Nursing. FA Davis, Philadelphia, 2001.

Editorial: Reducing atherosclerotic changes in bypass grafts. Emerg Med 29:9, 1997.

Elliot, W: Prevention of bacterial endocarditis. Physician's Therapeutics Drug Alert 2:5, 1997.

Kottke, TE, Stroebel, RJ, and Hoffman, RS: JNC 7—It's more than high blood pressure. JAMA 289:2573–2574, 2003.

Messerli, FH: Salt: A perpetrator of hypertensive target organ disease? Arch of Int Med 157, 1997.

National Cholesterol Education Program: The second report of the expert panel on detection, evaluation, and treatment of high blood cholesterol in adults (adult treatment panel II):National Institutes of Health: National Heart, Lung, and Blood Institute, Bethesda, MD, 1993.

Sacks, FM, et al. for the Cholesterol and Recurrent Events Trial Investigators: The effect of pravastatin on coronary events after myocardial infarction in patients with average cholesterol levels. N Engl J Med, 335, 1996.

Shannon, CK: Drugs and the prolonged QT interval: Knowing what to look for. Fam Pract Recertification 19:7, 1997.

United States Department of Health and Human Services: Healthy People 2010: Understanding and Improving Health. United States Department of Health and Human Services, 2000.

United States Department of Health and Human Services, Centers for Disease Control: Cardiac valvulopathy associated with exposure to fenfluramine or dexfenfluramine: US Department of Health and Human Services interim public health recommendations. Morbidity and Mortality Weekly Report 46, November 14, 1997.

HOW WELL DID YOU DO?

85% AND ABOVE CONGRATULATIONS! THIS SCORE SHOWS APPLICATION OF TEST-TAKING PRINCIPLES AND ADEQUATE CONTENT KNOWLEDGE.

75–85% KEEP WORKING! REVIEW TEST-TAKING PRINCIPLES AND TRY AGAIN.

65–75% HANG IN THERE! SPEND SOME TIME REVIEWING CONCEPTS AND TEST-TAKING PRINCIPLES AND TRY THE TEST AGAIN.

Abdominal Problems 12

JILL E. WINLAND-BROWN

12–1 *Which of the following treatments for ulcerative colitis is contraindicated?*

A. A high-calorie, nonspicy, caffeine-free diet that is low in high-residue foods and milk products
B. Corticosteroids in the acute phase
C. Antidiarrheal agents
D. Colectomy with permanent ileostomy in severe cases

12–2 *In a 2-month-old infant with vomiting and diarrhea, the most effective way of determining a fluid deficit is to check for:*

A. decreased peripheral perfusion.
B. hyperventilation.
C. irritability.
D. hyperthermia.

12–3 *You suspect that Harry has a peptic ulcer and tell him that it has been found to be strongly associated with:*

A. anxiety and panic attacks.
B. long-term use of nonsteroidal anti-inflammatory drugs.
C. infection by *Helicobacter pylori*.
D. a family history of peptic ulcers.

12–4 *The American Cancer Society recommends a sigmoidoscopy for colon cancer screening in persons at average risk every:*

A. year, beginning at age 50 for 2 years, then every 3–5 years thereafter.
B. 3 years, beginning at age 40.
C. other year for clients with a family history of colon cancer.
D. 2 years, beginning at age 45.

12–5 *A false positive result with the fecal occult blood test can result from:*

A. ingestion of large amounts of vitamin C.
B. a high dietary intake of rare-cooked beef.
C. a colonic neoplasm that is not bleeding.
D. stool that has been stored before testing.

12–6 *Which area(s) of Jill's gastrointestinal tract may be affected by her Crohn's disease?*

A. All areas from the mouth to the anus
B. The colon
C. The sigmoid colon
D. The small intestine

12–7 *Harvey just came back from Mexico. Which pathogen do you suspect is responsible for his diarrhea?*

A. Enterococci
B. *Escherichia coli*
C. *Klebsiella*
D. Staphylococci

12–8 *The most common causes of upper gastrointestinal hemorrhage are:*

A. esophagitis and carcinomas.
B. erosive gastritis and peptic ulcer disease.
C. peptic ulcer disease and esophageal varices.
D. carcinomas and arteriovenous malformations.

12–9 *Sigrid, age 82, has irritable bowel, chronic constipation, and diverticulitis. Which pharmacological agent do you recommend?*

A. Bulking agents
B. Stool softeners
C. Laxatives
D. Lubricants

12–10 *The metabolism of which drug is not affected in Marsha, age 74?*

A. Alcohol
B. Anticonvulsants
C. Psychotropics
D. Oral anticoagulants

12–11 *The proper order of assessing the abdomen is:*

A. palpation, percussion, auscultation, inspection.
B. inspection, palpation, auscultation, percussion.
C. inspection, auscultation, percussion, palpation.
D. percussion, auscultation, inspection, palpation.

12–12 *You assess for Cullen's sign in Dan, age 62, after surgery. Cullen's sign may indicate:*

A. intra-abdominal bleeding.
B. a ventral hernia.
C. appendicitis.
D. jaundice.

12–13 *Striae may occur with all the following* ***except:***

A. pregnancy.
B. excessive weight gain.
C. diabetes.
D. ascites.

12–14 *When percussing the abdomen, hyperresonance is present:*

A. when there is gaseous distention.
B. over a distended bladder.
C. over adipose tissue.
D. over fluid or a mass.

12–15 *You elicit costovertebral angle tenderness in Gordon, age 29. Which condition do you suspect?*

A. Cirrhosis
B. Inflammation of the kidney
C. Inflammation of the spleen
D. Peritonitis

12–16 *A positive fluid wave test may occur with all of the following conditions* ***except:***

A. congestive heart failure.
B. portal hypertension.
C. inflammation of the spleen.
D. cirrhosis.

12–17 *Rebound tenderness may indicate:*

A. peritoneal inflammation.
B. a ventral hernia.
C. portal hypertension.
D. Crohn's disease.

12–18 *How do you respond when Andrea, who is taking her newborn home from the hospital, asks you when her baby's umbilical cord stump will fall off?*

A. "Within 7 days."
B. "In 10–14 days."
C. "In 14–21 days."
D. "In 21–30 days."

12–19 *By what age do abdominal respirations cease?*

A. 2 years
B. 5 years
C. 7 years
D. 13 years

12–20 *Hyperactive bowel sounds (borborygmi) are present in all of the following conditions* ***except:***

A. cirrhosis.
B. laxative use.
C. early mechanical bowel obstruction.
D. gastroenteritis.

12–21 *You auscultate Julie's abdomen and hear a peritoneal friction rub. Which condition do you rule out?*

A. Peritonitis
B. A liver or spleen abscess
C. A liver or spleen metastatic tumor
D. Irritable bowel syndrome

12–22 *Lipids are broken down in which area of the gastrointestinal tract?*

A. Duodenum
B. Stomach
C. Small intestine
D. Large intestine

12–23 *When George tells you that his feces are foul-smelling, you may suspect all of the following* ***except:***

A. blood in the stool.
B. ingestion of a high-fat diet.
C. colon cancer.
D. appendicitis.

12–24 *Simon states that he is worried because he has a bowel movement only every third day. You respond:*

A. "You should have 2 to 3 stools per day."
B. "You should defecate once a day."

C. "You should have at least 3 stools per week."
D. "There is no such thing as a 'normal' pattern of defecation."

12–25 *Anson tells you that he thinks his antacids are causing his diarrhea. You respond:*

A. "Antacids contain fructose that may not be totally absorbed and results in fluid being drawn into the bowel."
B. "Antacids contain sorbitol or mannitol, sugars that aren't absorbed and can cause fluid to be drawn into the bowel."
C. "Antacids contain caffeine, which decreases bowel transit time."
D. "Antacids may contain magnesium, which decreases bowel transit time and may contain poorly absorbed salts that draw fluid into the bowel."

12–26 *How do diphenoxylate (Lomotil) and loperamide (Imodium) help relieve diarrhea?*

A. They reduce bowel spasticity and acid secretion in the stomach.
B. They decrease the motility of the ileum and colon, slowing the transit time and promoting more water absorption.
C. They increase motility to assist in removing all of the stool.
D. By decreasing the sensations of the gastric nerves, they send a message to the brain to slow down peristalsis.

12–27 *Sara is taking polyethylene glycol (GoLYTELY) in preparation for a barium enema. What do you teach her about the medication?*

A. Drink the solution at room temperature.
B. Take the medication with food so that it will be absorbed better.
C. Take the medication in the early evening so as not to interfere with sleep.
D. Drink all of the solution in one sitting.

12–28 *Which laxative is safe for long-term use?*

A. Mineral oil
B. Bisacodyl (Dulcolax)
C. Methylcellulose (Citrucel)
D. Magnesium hydroxide (milk of magnesia)

12–29 *Steve, age 79, has GERD. When teaching him how to reduce his lower esophageal sphincter pressure, which substances do you recommend that he avoid?*

A. Apples
B. Peppermint
C. Cucumbers
D. Popsicles

12–30 *Rebound tenderness at McBurney's point would alert you to:*

A. appendicitis.
B. peritonitis.
C. a spleen injury.
D. irritable bowel syndrome.

12–31 *Marcie just returned from Central America with traveler's diarrhea. Which antibiotic do you order?*

A. Ampicillin (Polycillin)
B. Tetracycline (Achromycin)
C. Ciprofloxacin (Cipro)
D. Azithromycin (Zithromax)

12–32 *Which protozoal infection is the most common intestinal infection in the United States that also occurs worldwide?*

A. Salmonellosis
B. Giardiasis
C. Botulism
D. Shigellosis

12–33 *Which laboratory value would you expect to be increased in the presence of significant diarrhea?*

A. Serum potassium
B. Serum sodium
C. Serum chloride
D. Bicarbonate

12–34 *Martina, age 34, has AIDS and currently suffers from diarrhea. You suspect that she has which protozoal infection of the bowel?*

A. Giardiasis
B. Amebiasis
C. Cryptosporidiosis
D. *Escherichia coli*

12–35 *Cydney has been given a diagnosis of ascariasis. Which symptoms would you expect to see?*

A. Low-grade fever, productive cough with blood-tinged sputum, wheezing, and dyspnea
B. Nocturnal perianal and perineal pruritus
C. Diarrhea, cramps, and malaise
D. Ascites and facial and extremity edema

12–36 *Sam has ulcerative colitis and is on a low-residue diet. Which foods do you recommend that Sam should avoid?*

A. Potato skins, potato chips, and brown rice
B. Vegetable juices and cooked and canned vegetables
C. Ground beef, veal, pork, and lamb
D. White rice and pasta

12–37 *After Martin has had an ileostomy for ulcerative colitis, which self-care measures do you teach him to relieve food blockage?*

A. Lie in a supine position.
B. Massage the peristomal area.
C. Take a hot shower or tub bath.
D. Drink cold fluids.

12–38 *Olive has an acute exacerbation of Crohn's disease. Which laboratory test value(s) would you expect to be decreased?*

A. Sedimentation rate
B. Liver enzyme levels
C. Vitamins A, B complex, and C levels
D. Bilirubin level

12–39 *Clients with sprue usually have:*

A. a large-in-stature appearance.
B. accelerated maturity.
C. polycythemia.
D. steatorrhea.

12–40 *Sandra has celiac disease. You place her on which diet?*

A. A low-fat diet
B. A low-residue diet
C. A gluten-free diet
D. A high-protein diet

12–41 *Deena asks you what it meant when her husband came back from his oncologist with a classification of T1N2MX of his colorectal cancer. How do you respond?*

A. "The cancer is invading the submucosa, there are two lymph nodes involved, but there is no distant metastasis."
B. "The tumor is invading the submucosa, there is metastasis in four or more lymph nodes, and the presence of distant metastasis can't be assessed."
C. "The cancer is in situ, two lymph nodes are not affected, and there is no metastasis."
D. "The tumor has perforated the surrounding area, there are more than two lymph nodes affected, and there is no metastasis."

12–42 *Ruby has a colostomy and complains that her stools are too loose. What food(s) do you suggest to help thicken the stools?*

A. Cheese
B. Leafy green vegetables
C. Raw fruits and vegetables
D. Dried beans

12–43 *All of the following may contribute to the development of an umbilical hernia* ***except:***

A. pregnancy.
B. obesity.
C. ascites.
D. previous surgery.

12–44 *Rose has gastroesophageal reflux disease. She asks you what she can do to help alleviate the problem. You suggest all the following* ***except:***

A. avoiding coffee, alcohol, chocolate, peppermint, and spicy foods.
B. eating smaller meals.
C. having a snack before retiring so that the esophagus and stomach are not empty at bedtime.
D. stopping smoking.

12–45 *Rose, your client with gastroesophageal reflux disease, has many other concurrent conditions. She wants to know if there are any medications she should not take. You tell her to avoid:*

A. antibiotics.
B. nonsteroidal anti-inflammatory drugs.
C. oral contraceptives.
D. antifungals.

12–46 *Treatment for achalasia may include:*

A. balloon dilation of the lower esophageal sphincter.
B. beta blockers.
C. a fundoplication.
D. an esophagogastrectomy.

12–47 *Matt, aged 26, recently returned from a camping trip and has gastroenteritis. He says that he has been eating only canned food. Which of the following pathogens do you suspect?*

A. *Campylobacter jejuni*
B. *Clostridium botulinum*
C. *Clostridium perfringens*
D. *Staphylococcus*

12–48 *Duodenal and gastric ulcers have many of the same manifestations. Which is more common with gastric ulcers rather than duodenal ulcers?*

A. Epigastric or abdominal pain
B. Vomiting
C. Possibility of perforation
D. Obstruction of the gastrointestinal tract

12–49 *Martha has a Cushing's ulcer. What might have precipitated this?*

A. Her house burned down when she was not at home.
B. She was in a bad auto accident in which she sustained a head injury.
C. She spent the weekend deep-sea diving.
D. She was on an overseas airline flight that lasted over 24 hours.

12–50 *Which procedure enlarges the opening between the stomach and duodenum to improve gastric emptying?*

A. Billroth I
B. Total gastrectomy

C. Pyloroplasty
D. Vagotomy

12–51 *Timothy, age 68, complains of an abrupt change in his defecation pattern. You evaluate him for:*

A. constipation.
B. colorectal cancer.
C. irritable bowel syndrome.
D. acute appendicitis.

12–52 *After being treated for* Helicobacter pylori *infection, Sue would like a test to see if it has been cured. What do you recommend as the easiest, yet still reliable, test?*

A. An enzyme-linked immunosorbent assay titer
B. A urea breath test
C. A rapid urease test (*Campylobacter*-like organism)
D. A repeat endoscopy

12–53 *Marian, age 52, is obese. She complains of a rapid onset of severe right upper quadrant abdominal cramping pain, nausea, and vomiting. Your differential diagnosis might be:*

A. appendicitis.
B. irritable bowel syndrome.
C. cholecystitis.
D. Crohn's disease.

12–54 *Which oral medication might be used to treat a client with chronic cholelithiasis who is a poor candidate for surgery?*

A. Ursodiol (Actigall)
B. Ibuprofen (Advil)
C. Prednisone (Deltasone)
D. Methylterthutyl ether

12–55 *The most common cause of elevated liver function tests is:*

A. hepatitis.
B. biliary tract obstruction.
C. chronic alcohol abuse.
D. a drug-induced injury.

12–56 *All of the following are current recommendations to aid in preventing colorectal cancer* ***except:***

A. decreased fat intake.
B. increased fiber intake.
C. daily use of aspirin.
D. increasing fluid intake.

12–57 *Lucy, age 49, has left upper quadrant pain. This might lead you to suspect all the following* ***except:***

A. a gastric ulcer.
B. gastritis.
C. pelvic inflammatory disease.
D. pancreatitis.

12–58 *Which of the following antibiotics causes more episodes of nausea and/or vomiting than the others?*

A. Azithromycin (Zithromax)
B. Erythromycin (E-Mycin)
C. Penicillin (Pen-Vee K)
D. Tetracycline (Achromycin)

12–59 *All of the following medications are used for the control of nausea and vomiting. Which medication works by affecting the chemoreceptor trigger zone, thereby stimulating upper gastrointestinal motility and increasing lower esophageal sphincter pressure?*

A. Anticholinergics such as scopolamine (Donnatal)
B. Antidopaminergic agents such as prochlorperazine (Compazine)
C. Antidopaminergic and cholinergic agents such as metoclopramide (Reglan)
D. Tetrahydrocannabinols such as dronabinol (Marinol)

12–60 *To differentiate among the different diagnoses of inflammatory bowel diseases, you look at the client's histologic, culture, and radiologic features. Mary has transmural inflammation, granulomas, focal involvement of the colon with some skipped areas, and sparing of the rectal mucosa. What do you suspect?*

A. Crohn's disease
B. Ulcerative colitis
C. Infectious colitis
D. Ischemic colitis

12–61 *Which of the following signs or symptoms indicates biliary obstruction with liver disease?*

A. Pruritus
B. Increased abdominal girth
C. Right upper quadrant pain
D. Easy bruising

12–62 *Sally had an ileostomy performed for inflammatory bowel disease. What type of fecal output can Sally* ***expect?***

A. Hard, formed stool
B. Semisoft stool
C. Semisoft to very soft stool
D. A continuous soft to watery effluent

12–63 *Shelby has recently been diagnosed with pancreatitis. Which of the following objective findings, also known as Grey Turner's sign, can result from the pancreatic inflammatory process that you might find on a rare occasion?*

A. Left-sided pleural effusion
B. Bluish discoloration over the flanks
C. Bluish discoloration over the umbilicus
D. Jaundice

12–64 *All of the following are common signs of gastric cancer* ***except:***

A. weight loss.
B. dysphagia.
C. hematemesis.
D. gastrointestinal bleeding.

12–65 *Once gastric cancer has been diagnosed, which test should be ordered to accurately determine the correct staging?*

A. Computed tomography
B. Magnetic resonance imaging
C. Endoscopic ultrasound
D. Ranson's test

12–66 *Margie, age 52, has an extremely stressful job and was just given a diagnosis of gastric ulcer. She tells you that she is sure that it is going to be malignant. How do you respond?*

A. "Don't worry, gastric ulcers are not gastric cancer."
B. "About 95% of gastric ulcers are benign."
C. "You have about a 50/50 chance of having gastric cancer from your ulcer."
D. "Even if it is cancer, surgery is 100% successful."

12–67 *Jonas, age 34, had a Billroth II (hemigastrectomy and gastrojejunostomy with vagotomy) performed 1 week ago and just started eating a bland diet. What do you suspect when he complains of epigastric fullness, distention, discomfort, abdominal cramping, nausea, and flatus after eating?*

A. Obstruction
B. Dumping syndrome
C. Metabolic acidosis
D. Infectious colitis

12–68 *When Sammy asks you what he can do to help his wife, who has dumping syndrome, what do you suggest he tell her to do?*

A. Eat foods higher in carbohydrates.
B. Eat three large meals plus three snacks per day.
C. Eat foods with a moderate fat and protein content.
D. Drink fluids with each meal.

12–69 *Marvin, a known alcoholic, has alcoholic cirrhosis, is frequently admitted for coagulopathies, and occasionally receives blood transfusions. His wife asks you why he has bleeding problems. How do you respond?*

A. "Occasionally he accumulates blood in the gut."
B. "There is an interruption of the normal clotting mechanisms."
C. "Long-term alcohol abuse has made his vessels very friable."
D. "His bone marrow has been affected."

12–70 *Your client's 2-month-old daughter is admitted with gastroenteritis with dehydration after 2 days of vomiting and diarrhea. When she asks you what is causing the diarrhea, how do you respond?*

A. "She must be lactose intolerant from the formula, and this alters the fluid balance."
B. "Her body's telling you that it's time to initiate some solids into her system."
C. "The virus is causing irritation of the gastrointestinal lining, which causes an increase in gastrointestinal motility."
D. "The infectious agent invaded the gastrointestinal mucosa and affected the balance of water and electrolytes."

12–71 *Marisa, age 42, has celiac disease. She is prone to osteopenic bone disease as a result of impaired calcium absorption because of:*

A. increased calcium absorption by the small intestine.
B. increased absorption of the fat-soluble vitamin D.
C. the binding of calcium and magnesium in the intestinal lumen by unabsorbed dietary fatty acids.
D. decreased magnesium absorption.

12–72 *The most important diagnostic test for celiac disease is:*

A. confirming malabsorption by laboratory tests.
B. a barium enema.
C. a peroral biopsy of the duodenum.
D. a gluten-free diet trial with an accompanying improvement in mucosal histologic response.

12–73 *Dottie brings in her infant who has gastrointestinal reflux. What do you tell her about positioning her infant?*

A. Always position infants on their back to prevent sudden infant death syndrome.
B. Rotate your infant between lying on the back and on the stomach.
C. The infant should be placed on the left side.
D. Place the infant in whatever position the infant remains quiet.

12–74 *Which of the following findings is not associated with diverticulitis?*

A. Left lower quadrant abdominal pain
B. A history of irritable bowel syndrome
C. A tender mass in the left lower quadrant
D. An elevated temperature

12–75 *A common complication of viral gastroenteritis in children is:*

A. dehydration.
B. gastrointestinal bleeding.
C. peritonitis.
D. bacterial sepsis.

12–76 *Tenesmus refers to:*

A. projectile vomiting.
B. severe lower abdominal pain.
C. constipation.
D. a persistent desire to empty the bowel or bladder.

12–77 *Lillian, who is lactose intolerant, asks you what foods she should avoid. You tell her to avoid:*

A. yogurt.
B. foods containing whey.
C. prehydrolyzed milk.
D. oranges.

12–78 *All of the following may contribute to a malignant neoplasm of the stomach* **except:**

A. alcohol intake of one to two drinks per day.
B. a diet low in fruits and vegetables.
C. a diet high in foods with additives, such as smoked, pickled, or salted foods.
D. highly spiced foods.

12–79 *While you are obtaining Henry's history, he tells you that he had a portacaval shunt done in the past. What does this imply?*

A. A history of liver cancer
B. A history of alcohol abuse
C. A congenital biliary problem
D. Heavy tobacco use

12–80 *Samantha is 100 lb overweight and wants to have a gastroplasty performed. In discussing this with her, you explain that by having this procedure she may:*

A. develop diarrhea.
B. lose too much weight.
C. develop hemorrhoids.
D. vomit after she eats.

12–81 *Sidney has ulcerative colitis and asks you about a Koch pouch. You respond:*

A. "It's a method of bowel training for clients with chronic diarrhea."
B. "It's a name for a continent ileostomy."
C. "It's a packet of daily pills to take to relieve diarrhea."
D. "It's like a sanitary pad and it's used to contain any rectal leakage."

12–82 *Stacy, a nursing student, is to begin her series of hepatitis B vaccinations. You test her for a serologic marker and the results show hepatitis B surface antibodies (HbsAb). You tell Stacy that she:*

A. needs to begin the hepatitis B series as soon as possible.
B. needs to be tested again because one reading is not indicative of immunity.
C. is permanently immune to hepatitis B.
D. has an acute hepatitis B infection.

12–83 *Maura had a less than 7% value on her Schilling test. What medication do you anticipate that Maura might need?*

A. Folic acid
B. Vitamin B_{12}
C. Thyroid medication
D. Hormone replacement therapy

12–84 *Tina has a chronic hepatitis C infection. She asks you how to prevent its transmission. You respond:*

A. "Do not donate blood until 1 year after diagnosis."
B. "A vaccine is available to prevent transmission."
C. "There is no possibility of transmission through razors or toothbrushes."
D. "Abstain from sex during your period."

12–85 *You suspect that Nikki has a gastroduodenal ulcer caused by* Helicobacter pylori *and plan to treat her empirically. What medications should you order?*

A. Bismuth subsalicylate (Pepto-Bismol), tetracycline (Achromycin) or amoxicillin (Amoxil), and metronidazole (Flagyl)
B. Bismuth subsalicylate (Pepto-Bismol) and omeprazole (Prilosec)
C. Amoxicillin (Amoxil) and omeprazole (Prilosec)
D. Clarithromycin (Biaxin) and metronidazole (Flagyl)

12–86 *Nausea is difficult to discern in a young child. What question might you ask to determine if the child has nausea?*

A. "Are you sick to your tummy?"
B. "Are you hungry?"
C. "Are you eating the way you normally eat?"
D. "Are you nauseous?"

12–87 *A mother is bringing in her 4-year-old child, who she states has acute abdominal pain and a rash. Which of the following do you initially rule out?*

A. Rocky Mountain spotted fever
B. Measles
C. Appendicitis
D. A food allergy

12–88 *Bobby, age 6, has constant periumbilical pain shifting to the right lower quadrant, vomiting, a small volume of diarrhea, absence of headache, a* *mild elevation of the white blood cell count with an early left shift, and white blood cells in the urine. You suspect:*

A. appendicitis.
B. gastroenteritis.
C. acute pancreatitis.
D. Rocky Mountain spotted fever.

12–89 *The most common viral infection causing diarrhea in the United States is:*

A. enteric adenovirus.
B. a Norwalk-like virus.
C. rotavirus.
D. *Giardia lamblia.*

12–90 *For an uncomplicated* Salmonella *infection, the antibiotic of choice is:*

A. ampicillin (Polycillin).
B. amoxicillin (Amoxil).
C. trimethoprim-sulfamethoxazole (Bactrim).
D. No antibiotic is indicated

12–91 *An infant who is ruminating should be diagnosed and treated for:*

A. cystic fibrosis.
B. esophagitis.
C. Meckel's diverticulum.
D. intussusception.

12–92 *A palpable spleen 2 cm or less below the left costal margin in a 2-year-old child is:*

A. indicative of splenomegaly.
B. a sign of internal hemorrhaging.
C. normal.
D. a sign of infection.

12–93 *Mona is breast-feeding her 5-day-old daughter, who has just been found to have physiologic jaundice with a bilirubin level of more than 20 mg/dL. You should tell Mona that she:*

A. should stop breast-feeding altogether.
B. can continue breast-feeding.
C. should discontinue breast-feeding for 24 hours.
D. should alternate breast milk with formula for every other feeding.

12–94 *You are trying to differentiate between functional (acquired) constipation and Hirschsprung's disease in a neonate. Distinguishing features of Hirschsprung's disease include all of the following* ***except:***

A. small ribbonlike stools.
B. no abdominal pain.
C. female gender.
D. failure to thrive.

12–95 *Ellie, age 42, has a seizure disorder and has been taking phenytoin (Dilantin) for years. Which supplement should she also be taking if no other problems exist?*

A. Vitamin B_{12}
B. Iron
C. Folic acid
D. Calcium

12–96 *In counseling Maria, age 24, who is healthy, you advise her to limit her intake of sugar to prevent:*

A. dental caries.
B. obesity.
C. diabetes.
D. hyperactivity.

12–97 *The most common cause of mechanical bowel obstruction in all ages is:*

A. volvulus.
B. intussusception.
C. cancer.
D. a hernia.

12–98 *Nora, age 78, has terminal cancer and is wasting away. What should you order to stimulate her appetite?*

A. Megestrol (Megace)
B. Sertraline (Zoloft)
C. Vitamin C
D. Alprazolam (Xanax)

12–99 *More than 50% of older adults have all of the following conditions* ***except:***

A. hiatal hernia.
B. diverticulosis.
C. constipation.
D. colonic polyps.

12–100 *Zena just had a hemorrhoidectomy. You include all of the following points in your teaching* ***except:***

A. "Take a sitz bath after each bowel movement for 1–2 weeks after surgery."
B. "Drink at least 2000 mL of fluids per day."
C. "Decrease your dietary fiber for 1 month."
D. "Take stool softeners as prescribed."

12–101 *Sylvia, age 59, has acute hepatitis. You're told it's from a drug overdose. Which drug do you suspect?*

A. Flagyl
B. Acetaminophen
C. Sumatriptan
D. Hydrocortisone

12–102 *The majority of the population of the United States has antibodies against which type of hepatitis?*

A. Hepatitis A
B. Hepatitis B
C. Hepatitis C
D. Hepatitis D
E. Hepatitis E

12–103 *Sandy, age 52, presents with jaundice, dark urine, and light-colored stools, stating that she is slightly improved over last week's symptoms. Which stage of viral hepatitis do you suspect?*

A. Incubation
B. Prodromal
C. Icteric
D. Convalescent

12–104 *Which of the following statements about cirrhosis is true?*

A. Biliary cirrhosis is the most common type of cirrhosis in the United States.
B. Alcoholic cirrhosis only occurs in malnourished alcoholics.
C. Cirrhosis is reversible if diagnosed and treated at an early stage.
D. Women tend to develop cirrhosis more quickly with less alcohol intake than men.

12–105 *Marty, aged 52, notices a bulge in his midline every time he rises from bed in the morning. You tell him it's a ventral hernia, also known as:*

A. Inguinal hernia
B. Epigastric hernia
C. Umbilical hernia
D. Incisional hernia

12–106 *You suspect appendicitis in Andrew, who is 18. With his right hip and knee flexed, you slowly rotate his right leg internally to stretch a muscle. He states that it is painful over his right lower quadrant. Which sign did you elicit?*

A. Rovsing's sign
B. Psoas sign
C. Obturator sign
D. McBurney's sign

Answers

12–1 Answer C

Antidiarrheal agents are contraindicated in the presence of ulcerative colitis because they may precipitate colonic dilation. Sulfasalazine (Azulfidine) is often prescribed for its antibiotic and inflammatory effects; however, it interferes with folate metabolism, and therefore folate supplements may be required. A high-calorie, nonspicy, caffeine-free diet that is low in high-residue foods and milk products; corticosteroids in the acute phase; and a colectomy with permanent ileostomy in severe cases are all treatments for ulcerative colitis.

12–2 Answer A

In a 2-month-old infant with vomiting and diarrhea, the most effective way of determining a fluid deficit is to check for decreased peripheral perfusion. The body compensates for loss of fluid by shifting the interstitial fluid into the intravascular space, thereby maintaining perfusion of vital organs. If the fluid loss continues, circulating volume is diminished, and vasoconstriction occurs in the peripheral vessels, resulting in decreased perfusion.

12–3 Answer C

Although stress-related conditions such as anxiety and panic attacks and long-term use of nonsteroidal anti-inflammatory drugs may contribute to and aggravate peptic ulcer disease, about 90% of the cases of peptic ulcers have been found to be caused by infection with *Helicobacter pylori*.

12–4 Answer A

The American Cancer Society (ACS) recommends a sigmoidoscopy for colon cancer screening in persons at average risk every year, beginning at age 50 for 2 years, then every 3–5 years thereafter. The ACS also recommends an annual digital rectal exam beginning at age 40 and checking the stool for occult blood every year beginning at age 50.

12–5 Answer B

A false-positive result with the fecal occult blood test can result from a high dietary intake of rare-cooked beef or fruits and vegetables that contain peroxidases. Oral iron preparations have also been shown to produce a false-positive result in some, but not all, studies. False-negative results can occur in clients who ingest large amounts of vitamin C, have a colon neoplasm that is not bleeding, and from stool that has been stored before testing.

12–6 Answer A

Although the colon is the major site of gastrointestinal involvement in Crohn's disease (inflammatory bowel disease), it can affect all areas from the mouth to the anus.

12–7 Answer B

Escherichia coli is the pathogen most often responsible for traveler's diarrhea (infectious diarrhea). Other causes may include viruses, other bacteria, protozoa, or parasites.

12–8 Answer C

The most common causes of upper gastrointestinal hemorrhage, in descending order, are peptic ulcer disease, esophageal varices, esophagitis, erosive gastritis, carcinomas, and arteriovenous malformations.

12–9 Answer A

Bulking agents such as psyllium preparations or methylcellulose preparations are used for irritable bowel, chronic constipation, and diverticulitis. Stool softeners such as docusate sodium are frequently used for the prevention of constipation but most likely are not effective for chronic use. Saline laxatives such as magnesium hydroxide are indicated for intermittent use in chronic constipation and as a bowel preparation; stimulant irritant laxatives such as bisacodyl, senna, and cascara are used in acute constipation and should not be used for chronic constipation. Lubricants such as mineral oil are used in intermittent chronic constipation.

12–10 Answer A

Although drug metabolism by the liver is usually impaired in older adults, the metabolism of alcohol is unchanged.

12–11 Answer C

The proper order of assessing the abdomen is inspection, auscultation, percussion, and palpation. It is important to inspect the abdomen first before percussion or palpation to avoid causing any discomfort that might alter the client's position. Auscultation is important before percussion and palpation because these techniques can increase peristalsis, which would give a false interpretation of bowel sounds.

12–12 Answer A

Cullen's sign is a bluish periumbilical color that may indicate intra-abdominal bleeding.

12–13 Answer C

Striae are silvery-white linear, jagged marks (stretch marks) about 1–6 cm in length that result when elastic fibers in the reticular layer of the skin are broken as a result of rapid or prolonged stretching. This stretching may occur with pregnancy, excessive weight gain, or ascites.

12–14 Answer A

Hyperresonance is present when there is gaseous distention. Dullness occurs over a distended bladder or adipose tissue and when there is fluid or a mass present.

12–15 Answer B

Costovertebral angle tenderness occurs when one hand is "thumped" with the ulnar edge of the other fist over the 12th rib at the costovertebral angle on the back and tenderness or sharp pain occurs. It indicates inflammation of the kidney.

12–16 Answer C

A positive fluid wave test assesses for ascites, which is free fluid in the peritoneal cavity. Ascites may occur with congestive heart failure, portal hypertension, cirrhosis, hepatitis, pancreatitis, or cancer. It does not occur with inflammation of the spleen.

12–17 Answer A

Rebound tenderness is present when there is pain on release of pressure to the abdomen and is a reliable indicator of peritoneal inflammation.

12–18 Answer B

An infant's umbilical cord stump dries within 7 days, then hardens and falls off in 10–14 days. It then takes 3–4 weeks for skin to cover the area.

12–19 Answer C

Abdominal respirations cease by age 7 years. The absence of abdominal respirations under age 7 indicates peritoneal inflammation.

12–20 Answer A

Hyperactive bowel sounds (borborygmi) are present with laxative use, early mechanical bowel obstruction, gastroenteritis, and brisk diarrhea. They are not present with cirrhosis.

12–21 Answer D

A peritoneal friction rub, which sounds like a rough, grating sound, occurs over organs with a large surface area in contact with the peritoneum when there is peritoneal inflammation (peritonitis). When a peritoneal friction rub is heard over the lower right rib cage, it may be caused by an abscess or tumor of the liver. When heard over the lower left rib cage in the left anterior axillary line, it may indicate infection of the spleen or an abscess or tumor of the spleen.

12–22 Answer C

Lipids are broken down in the small intestine by the pancreatic lipases. Carbohydrates, proteins, and nucleic acids are also broken down in the small intestines by various enzymes.

12–23 Answer D

A distinct foul odor to the stool may indicate blood in the stool, ingestion of a high-fat diet, or colon cancer.

12–24 Answer D

There is no such thing as a "normal" pattern of defecation. Patterns of defecation vary widely and may in part be affected by dietary habits, fluid intake, bacteria in the stool, psychological stress, or voluntary postponement of defecation.

12–25 Answer D

Antacids may contain magnesium, which decreases bowel transit time and may contain poorly absorbed salts that result in an osmotic draw of fluid into the bowel. Fructose is present in apple juice, pear juice, grapes, honey, dates, nuts, figs, and fruit-flavored soft drinks. Sorbitol or mannitol is present in apple juice, pear juice, sugarless gums, and mints. Caffeine is present in coffee, tea, cola drinks, and over-the-counter analgesics.

12–26 Answer B

Diphenoxylate (Lomotil) and loperamide (Imodium), like all opiates and opium derivatives, help to relieve diarrhea by decreasing the motility of the ileum and colon, slowing the transit time, and promoting more water absorption. Anticholinergics such as atropine (Donnatal) and other belladonna alkaloids (Donnagel) reduce bowel spasticity and acid secretion in the stomach.

12–27 Answer C

Polyethylene glycol (GoLYTELY) should be taken in the early evening so as not to interfere with sleep because the first bowel movement begins within 1 hour and continues until the sigmoid colon is clear. The solution should be chilled to enhance palatability, taken on an empty stomach, and administered in 8-oz servings every 10 minutes until 1 gallon is consumed.

12–28 Answer C

Bulk-forming agents such as methylcellulose (Citrucel) are the only laxatives that are safe for long-term use. They contain natural vegetable fiber that is not absorbed. This creates bulk and draws water into the intestine, thus softening the stool. Mineral oil reduces the absorption of the fat-soluble vitamins A, D, E, and K, and may cause damage to the liver and spleen because of systemic absorption. Irritant or stimulant laxatives, such as bisacodyl (Dulcolax), work by stimulating the motility and secretion of the intestinal mucosa. Osmotic and saline laxatives and cathartics, such as magnesium hydroxide (milk of magnesia), when used over the long term, may suppress normal bowel reflexes.

12–29 Answer B

Food substances that reduce the lower esophageal sphincter pressure or irritate the gastric mucosa include alcohol; caffeinated beverages, chocolate, citrus fruits, decaffeinated coffee, fatty foods, onions, peppermint and spearmint, tomatoes, and tomato-based products. Nonfood substances that irritate GERD include anticholinergic drugs, beta-adrenergic blocking agents, calcium channel blockers, Diazepam, estrogens, nicotine, and theophylline.

12–30 Answer A

Rebound tenderness at McBurney's point, located midway between the umbilicus and the anterior iliac crest in the right lower quadrant, would alert you to appendicitis.

12–31 Answer C

Traveler's diarrhea caused by *Escherichia coli* is treated with a 3–5 day course of ciprofloxacin (Cipro), norfloxacin (Noroxin), or trimethoprim-sulfamethoxazole (Bactrim). Ampicillin (Polycillin) may be used to treat salmonellosis caused by *Salmonella* bacteria and shigellosis caused by *Shigella* bacteria. Ampicillin and tetracycline (Achromycin) are used to treat cholera, which is caused by *Vibrio cholerae*. Azithromycin (Zithromax) is a good choice for treating community-acquired pneumonia.

12–32 Answer B

Giardiasis, a protozoal infection of the upper small intestine, is caused by *Giardia lamblia*. It is the most common intestinal protozoal infection in the United States that also occurs worldwide. *Clostridium botulinum*, which causes botulism, is an enterotoxin, whereas *Salmonella*, causing salmonellosis, and *Shigella*, causing shigellosis, are both bacteria.

12–33 Answer C

Serum chloride level is increased with significant diarrhea when the diarrhea causes sodium loss that is greater than chloride loss. However, when there is severe diarrhea and vomiting, serum chloride levels may be decreased. Serum potassium and chloride levels are decreased as a result of loss through stool, and bicarbonate level is decreased in a metabolic acidotic state.

12–34 Answer C

Cryptosporidiosis, a common protozoal infection of the bowel, is common in immunocompromised clients. It causes villous atrophy and mild inflammatory changes and may secrete an enterotoxin. Giardiasis and amebiasis are also protozoal infections affecting the intestine, but because the question mentioned that Martina has AIDS, the answer must be cryptosporidiosis. *Escherichia coli* (*E. coli*) is a gram-positive bacterium.

12–35 Answer A

Ascariasis is the most common of the intestinal helminths (parasitic worms). It causes pulmonary manifestations such as low-grade fever, productive cough with blood-tinged sputum, wheezing, and dyspnea because the larvae are transmitted to the lungs from the vascular system. The larvae burrow through alveolar walls, migrating up the bronchial tree to the pharynx, and then down the esophagus back to the intestines. Nocturnal perianal and perineal pruritus occur with enterobiasis (pinworm infection). Diarrhea, cramps, and malaise are common with trichinosis. Ascites and facial and extremity edema are common with trichuriasis.

12–36 Answer A

Potato skins, potato chips, fried potatoes, brown rice, and whole-grain pasta products should be avoided if a client with ulcerative colitis is on a low-residue diet that was ordered to reduce intestinal motility and allow the bowel to rest.

12–37 Answer B

Self-care measures to teach a client with an ileostomy how to relieve food blockage include massaging the peristomal area, which may stimulate peristalsis and fecal elimination; assuming a knee-chest position to reduce intra-abdominal pressure; taking a warm shower or tub bath to relax the abdominal muscles; and drinking warm fluids or grape juice to produce a mild cathartic effect.

12–38 Answer C

Folic acid and serum levels of most vitamins, including A, B complex, C, and the fat-soluble vitamins, are decreased in Crohn's disease as a result of malabsorption. The sedimentation rate and liver enzymes and bilirubin levels are all increased.

12–39 Answer D

Celiac disease, also known as celiac sprue, may begin during early childhood or adulthood. Clients with sprue usually have steatorrhea, abdominal bloating and cramps, and diarrhea. Clients with celiac disease are often small in stature and have delayed maturity. The malabsorption that results may cause deficiencies such as anemia.

12–40 Answer C

Clients with celiac disease have an allergy to gliadin, a component of gluten; therefore they are placed on a gluten-free diet in which wheat and other grains containing analogues to wheat gluten, such as oats, barley, and rye, must be avoided.

12–41 Answer B

A classification of T1N2MX for colorectal cancer means that the tumor is invading the submucosa, there is metastasis in four or more lymph nodes, and the presence of distant metastasis cannot be assessed.

12–42 Answer A

Cheese, bread, pasta, rice, pretzels, and yogurt all help to thicken stools. Leafy green vegetables, raw fruits and vegetables, and dried beans may all loosen stools.

12–43 Answer D

An umbilical hernia may be congenital or acquired as the tissue around the umbilical ring weakens. Conditions resulting in umbilical hernias include pregnancy, including multiple pregnancies with prolonged labor; obesity; ascites; and large intra-abdominal tumors. An incisional or ventral hernia may develop at a previous surgical incision site.

12–44 Answer C

Clients with gastroesophageal reflux disease should be instructed to avoid coffee, alcohol, chocolate, peppermint, and spicy foods; eat smaller meals; stop smoking; remain upright for 2 hours after meals; elevate the head of the bed on 6–8 inch blocks; and refrain from eating for 3 hours before retiring. You should not suggest having a snack before retiring.

12–45 Answer B

The client with gastroesophageal reflux disease should avoid taking nonsteroidal anti-inflammatory drugs because they tend to aggravate the already irritated gastric mucosa.

12–46 Answer A

Achalasia is an absence of peristalsis of the esophagus and a high gastroesophageal sphincter pressure. After initial noninvasive treatments, clients may require a balloon dilation of the lower esophageal sphincter. Calcium channel blockers, not beta blockers, may be used to decrease symptoms of dysphagia. A fundoplication is done for a hiatal hernia. An esophagogastrectomy is performed for esophageal cancer.

12–47 Answer B

Clostridium botulinum is an anaerobic gram-positive bacillus that produces toxins. The primary source is canned foods. *Campylobacter jejuni* is found primarily in eggs and poultry but may be found in domestic animals. *Clostridium perfringens* is found in soil, feces, air, and water. Outbreaks are caused most often by contaminated meat. Staphylococcus is a common cause of food poisoning. It is caused by the ingestion of an enterotoxin found in improperly handled or stored foods.

12–48 Answer B

Vomiting is more common with gastric ulcers than duodenal ulcers. Stools are more often altered with duodenal ulcers. The possibility of perforation and obstruction of the gastrointestinal tract is present in both types of ulcers. Approximately half of the clients report relief of pain with food or antacids (especially with duodenal ulcers). Many clients deny the relationship of meals to the pain. Two-thirds of clients with duodenal ulcers and one-third with gastric ulcers have nocturnal pain that awakens them.

12–49 Answer B

Cushing's ulcers are stress ulcers that occur after a

head injury or intracranial disease. A Cushing's ulcer may also occur after a severe burn.

12–50 Answer C

A pyloroplasty surgically enlarges the opening between the stomach and duodenum to improve gastric emptying. A Billroth I is a gastroduodenostomy. A total gastrectomy is removal of the entire stomach and is rarely performed. It results in an anastomosis connecting the esophagus to the duodenum or jejunum. A vagotomy severs a portion or all of the vagus nerves to the stomach.

12–51 Answer B

An abrupt change in the defecation pattern of a middle-aged or older client must be evaluated for colorectal cancer.

12–52 Answer B

A urea breath test is the easiest, least expensive, and most reliable test for *Helicobacter pylori.* Its average sensitivity is 96% and specificity is 98%. An enzyme-linked immunosorbent assay titer, a rapid urease test (*Campylobacter*-like organism [CLO]) test, and an endoscopy may also be used. The CLO test and endoscopy require biopsy specimens and are therefore more invasive.

12–53 Answer C

A rapid onset of severe right upper quadrant (RUQ) abdominal cramping pain with nausea and vomiting is a classic presentation of acute cholecystitis; 90–95% of clients with acute cholecystitis also have gallstones. Other symptoms include low-grade fever, epigastric tenderness, guarding, and pain on inspiration during palpation of the RUQ (Murphy's sign).

12–54 Answer A

Ursodiol (Actigall) is an oral bile acid that dissolves gallstones. For dissolution, 8–10 mg/kg per day is given in two to three divided doses; for prevention, 300 mg bid is given. Nonsteroidal anti-inflammatory drugs such as ibuprofen (Advil) may be very irritating to the gastrointestinal mucosa. Steroids, such as prednisone (Deltasone), may mask an infection as well as be irritating to the gastric mucosa. Methyltertbutyl ether (MTBE) is a lipid solvent that is infused directly into the gallbladder via a T-tube.

12–55 Answer C

Hepatocellular damage from chronic alcohol abuse is the most frequent cause of elevated liver function tests (LFTs) in adults. Other causes include biliary tract obstruction, hepatitis, drug-induced injuries, vascular changes caused by anoxia, and congestive heart failure; however, chronic alcohol abuse remains the number one cause of abnormal LFTs.

12–56 Answer D

Increasing fluid intake has not been shown to decrease the risk of colorectal cancer. Current recommendations to aid in preventing colorectal cancer include decreased fat and increased fiber consumption and the daily use of aspirin. The daily use of aspirin has been shown to decrease the incidence of colorectal cancer as well as dramatically decreasing the incidence of metastasis.

12–57 Answer C

The pain associated with pelvic inflammatory disease can be palpated in both the right and left lower quadrants. Pain in the left upper quadrant may signify a gastric ulcer, gastritis, pancreatitis, splenic abscess, or pleurisy.

12–58 Answer B

Erythromycin (E-Mycin) is the antibiotic that causes the most cases of gastrointestinal upset such as nausea or vomiting. Other medications that commonly cause nausea and vomiting are opiates, estrogen, ipecac, digitalis, chemotherapy, and theophylline.

12–59 Answer C

Metoclopramide (Reglan) is used for diabetic gastroparesis and postoperative nausea and vomiting. It works by affecting the chemoreceptor trigger zone, thereby stimulating upper gastrointestinal motility and increasing lower esophageal sphincter pressure. Anticholinergics work at the site of the labyrinth receptors and the chemoreceptor trigger zones, that is, the vomiting center. Antidopaminergic agents work at the chemoreceptor trigger zone. The site and mechanism of tetrahydrocannabinols are unknown.

12–60 Answer A

Crohn's disease would show transmural inflammation, granulomas, focal involvement of the colon with some skipped areas, and sparing of the rectal mucosa. Ulcerative colitis would show acute inflammatory infiltrates, depleted goblet cells, negative cultures, and involvement of the rectum. Infectious colitis, because of the toxic products released, may induce periportal inflammation, mild hepatomegaly, and low-grade liver enzyme abnormalities, but usually without trophozoites in the liver. Ischemic colitis seen on colonoscopy reveals segmental inflammatory changes most often in the rectosigmoid and the splenic flexure, where there is more collateral circulation.

12–61 Answer A

Pruritus indicates that biliary obstruction is present with the liver disease. Increased abdominal girth indicates ascites is present from portal hypertension or hypoalbuminemia. Right upper quadrant pain may indicate hepatitis, cholecystitis, hepatocellular carcinoma, or abscess. Easy bruising may indicate splenomegaly secondary to portal hypertension with platelet sequestration, or coagulopathy secondary to decreased synthesis of clotting factors.

12–62 Answer D

Fecal output from an ileostomy is a malodorous, continuous, soft-to-watery effluent material that contains intestinal enzymes, which are very irritating to the skin around the stoma. Stomas further along the large colon will have more formed stools, and a sigmoid colostomy will result in stools that are almost normal in consistency.

12–63 Answer B

Grey Turner's sign is a bluish discoloration over the flanks. Cullen's sign is a bluish discoloration around the umbilicus. Other findings that can result from the pancreatic inflammatory process include left-sided pleural effusion, jaundice caused by impingement on the common bile duct, and an epigastric mass secondary to pseudocyst development.

12–64 Answer D

Gastrointestinal bleeding is uncommon with gastric cancer. Weight loss is usually the presenting symptom of gastric cancer, followed by dysphagia. Hematemesis occurs in 10–15% of all clients with gastric cancer.

12–65 Answer C

Once gastric cancer has been diagnosed, accurate staging can be determined by an endoscopic ultrasound. Ranson's criteria is a classification system to assess the severity of pancreatitis.

12–66 Answer B

About 95% of gastric ulcers are benign, even though some of these seem to look malignant on x-ray.

12–67 Answer B

The dumping syndrome may occur 1–3 weeks after gastric surgery when the client starts to consume larger meals. Food enters the intestine faster and in larger quantities than before the surgery, causing the client to experience epigastric fullness, distention, discomfort, abdominal cramping, nausea, and increased flatus.

12–68 Answer C

To help clients with dumping syndrome, suggest that they eat foods with a moderate fat and protein content. These foods tend to leave the stomach more slowly and do not draw fluid into the intestine. Also suggest that they reduce the amount of car-bohydrates consumed, eat six small meals per day, and take fluids between meals and not at mealtime.

12–69 Answer B

Because of Marvin's alcoholism and his resulting dietary insufficiencies, there is an inadequate amount of vitamin K in the liver for the thrombin to convert fibrinogen to fibrin; thus, the sequence of coagulation is disrupted.

12–70 Answer D

In 80% of the cases, gastroenteritis is viral in nature. This viral infection causes diarrhea by stimulating the secretion of electrolytes into the intestine. This is rapidly followed by water along the osmotic gradient, resulting in watery stools.

12–71 Answer C

Osteopenic bone disease may occur in celiac disease because there is decreased calcium absorption by the small intestine, decreased absorption of the fat-soluble vitamin D, and binding of calcium and magnesium in the intestinal lumen by unabsorbed dietary fatty acids. Clients should be identified as having celiac disease before menopause so that therapy to increase bone mass can be instituted before clients develop osteopenia.

12–72 Answer D

The diagnosis of celiac disease is classically established by a trial period of a gluten-free diet with an accompanying improvement in the mucosal histologic response. Laboratory tests may confirm malabsorption, but they are not diagnostic of celiac disease. A barium enema may show dilatation of the small intestine, but in mild celiac disease, the study may be normal. A peroral biopsy showing the gross absence of duodenal folds on endoscopy is a clue to the presence of celiac disease, but it is not diagnostic because this symptom may also occur in tropical sprue, intestinal lymphoma, Zollinger-Ellison syndrome, and other diseases.

12–73 Answer C

Infants with gastrointestinal reflux should be placed on their left side to prevent aspiration. They should be fed a formula thickened with rice cereal while being held in an upright position and kept in an elevated prone position for 1 hour after feeding so gravity helps prevent reflux.

12–74 Answer B

A history of irritable bowel syndrome has no association with diverticulitis. A client with diverticulitis would have left lower quadrant abdominal pain, a tender mass in the left lower quadrant, and an elevated temperature.

12–75 Answer A

Dehydration is the most common complication of viral gastroenteritis in children. Gastrointestinal bleeding is uncommon. Peritonitis and bacterial sepsis are other causes of diarrhea.

12–76 Answer D

Tenesmus is the spasmodic contraction of the anal or bladder sphincters, producing pain and the persistent desire to empty the bowel or bladder via involuntary ineffectual straining efforts. Rectal tenesmus is often experienced in ulcerative colitis.

12–77 Answer B

Advise clients who are lactose-intolerant to avoid foods containing whey. Whey is a lactose-rich ingredient found in some foods; therefore labels need to be read on all foods for clients who are lactose intolerant. To control symptoms, dietary lactose should be reduced or restricted by using lactose-reduced and lactose-free dairy products or by eating lactose-rich food in small amounts or in combination with low-lactose or lactose-free foods. Fermented dairy products such as aged or hard cheeses and cultured yogurt are easier to digest and contain less lactose than other dairy products. Most stores carry milk that has been pretreated with lactase, making it over 70% lactose-free. Lillian can eat oranges.

12–78 Answer A

Alcohol intake of one to two drinks per day has not been shown to contribute to a malignant neoplasm of the stomach. What has been shown to contribute to this type of cancer is a diet low in fruits and vegetables; a diet high in foods with additives such as smoked, pickled, or salted foods; and highly spiced foods such as some Asian foods.

12–79 Answer B

A portacaval shunt is the surgery often performed for bleeding esophageal varices. They are associated with alcoholic cirrhosis and portal hypertension, commonly the result of a history of alcohol abuse. Bleeding esophageal varices occur when the small esophageal veins become distended and rupture from increased pressure in the portal system.

12–80 Answer A

Diarrhea is a common problem after a gastroplasty because of the induced malabsorption. Clients usually do not end up losing too much weight because sometimes the only foods they can tolerate are high-caloric foods (simple sugars) such as ice cream.

12–81 Answer B

Performed for clients with ulcerative colitis, a Koch pouch (continent ileostomy) is the surgical removal of the rectum and colon and construction of an internal ileal reservoir, nipple valve, and stoma, allowing for intermittent drainage of ileal contents.

12–82 Answer C

The marker for permanent immunity, hepatitis B surface antibodies in the serum will be present 4–10 months after exposure and immunity to hepatitis B. Hepatitis B surface antigen is the earliest indicator of the presence of an acute infection and is present 4–12 weeks after exposure. This marker is also indicative of a chronic infection.

12–83 Answer B

A Schilling test is a timed urine test that evaluates the ability to absorb vitamin B_{12} from the gastrointestinal tract. It is used to diagnose pernicious anemia and malabsorption syndromes. The normal values range from 10 to 40%. A value less than 7% indicates pernicious anemia and some gastric lesions.

12–84 Answer D

Because the hepatitis C virus is transmitted in blood, including menstrual blood, clients should abstain from sex during menstruation. Clients should not donate blood, and there is a possibility of transmission through razors, toothbrushes, and tattoo instruments. No vaccine is available.

12–85 Answer A

All of the drugs listed are used in the eradication of *Helicobacter pylori*. Traditional 14-day "triple therapy" with bismuth subsalicylate (Pepto-Bismol), tetracycline (Achromycin) or amoxicillin (Amoxil), and metronidazole (Flagyl) has consistently produced eradication rates of approximately 90% and is the least-expensive therapy.

12–86 Answer B

To elicit information concerning nausea in a young child, ask the child about hunger because a young child cannot usually differentiate between hunger and mild nausea. Young children sometimes equate being "sick to their tummy" with vomiting and thus might answer "no" when questioned about nausea.

12–87 Answer C

There are many systemic causes of acute abdominal pain that also result in a rash. In the infectious category, these include Rocky Mountain spotted fever, measles, mumps, anaphylaxis, acute rheumatic fever, and infectious mononucleosis. A food allergy may also present itself as abdominal pain along with dermatitis. Appendicitis does not present with a rash.

12–88 Answer A

Constant periumbilical pain shifting to the right lower quadrant; vomiting following the pain; a small volume of diarrhea; no systemic symptoms such as a headache, malaise, or myalgia; a mild elevation of the white blood cell count with an early left shift; and white blood cells (WBCs) or red blood cells (RBCs) in the urine are indications of appendicitis. The WBC count becomes high only with gangrene or perforation of the appendix. The urine may have WBCs or RBCs if the bladder is irritated, and ketosis if there is prolonged vomiting.

12–89 Answer C

Rotavirus causes 15–35% of all the cases of diarrhea in the United States. It is followed by enteric adenovirus and Norwalk-like viruses. *Giardia lamblia* is a parasite that causes a high incidence of diarrhea in day care centers.

12–90 Answer D

Antibiotic therapy is not indicated for an uncomplicated salmonellosis because it is generally a self-limiting illness.

12–91 Answer B

In the process of rumination, food is regurgitated, mouthed or chewed, and then reswallowed. It may be psychogenic or self-stimulated. In some cases when there is an attempt to stimulate the gag reflex in infants, esophagitis has been shown to be present and the rumination is in response to the pain in the throat.

12–92 Answer C

A palpable spleen 2 cm or less below the left costal margin is a normal finding in a child under age 3 and may be a normal finding in an older child. Other symptoms would have to be present to warrant further evaluation.

12–93 Answer C

No treatment is necessary for physiologic jaundice unless the bilirubin level exceeds 20 mg/dL. In this case, the breast-feeding should be discontinued for 24 hours because this will result in a decreased bilirubin level.

12–94 Answer C

Hirschsprung's disease is common in male infants, results in small ribbonlike stools, usually has no accompanying abdominal pain unless there is obstruction, and may be accompanied by failure to thrive. The infant with functional (acquired) constipation is usually male and has very large stools and abdominal pain, but failure to thrive is uncommon.

12–95 Answer C

Clients taking phenytoin (Dilantin) should also be taking 0.4–1 mg/day of folic acid because this medication promotes a folate deficiency. Phenytoin may also contribute to demineralization of the bone, so the serum calcium levels should also be checked. If demineralization is detected, then vitamin D should be added.

12–96 Answer A

Reducing sugar intake is one of the preventive measures to take against dental caries. Other measures include regular brushing and flossing. Sugar has not been correlated with hyperactivity, and simple sugars do not cause diabetes. Dietary fat, rather than sugar, is the culprit in obesity.

12–97 Answer D

Hernias account for more cases of mechanical bowel obstruction in all ages than do volvulus, intussusception, or cancer.

12–98 Answer A

Although depression might be a contributing factor to Nora's wasting away, megestrol (Megace) can produce weight gain by stimulating appetite and food intake and by decreasing the nausea and vomiting that usually accompanies terminal cancer.

12–99 Answer D

More than 50% of the population age 65 and older have a hiatal hernia, diverticulosis, and constipation. Colonic polyps are fairly common, but do not approach 50%.

12–100 Answer C

For the client who has just had a hemorrhoidectomy, teaching would include advising the client to maintain an adequate intake of dietary fiber to maintain stool bulk, to take a sitz bath after each bowel movement for 1 to 2 weeks after surgery to promote relaxation and aid with discomfort, to drink at least 2000 mL of fluids per day, to take stool softeners as prescribed (for short-term relief only), and to exercise regularly to maintain stool bulk, softness, and regularity.

12–101 Answer B

The following drugs may cause acute hepatitis: acetaminophen, allopurinol, aspirin in high doses, captopril, carbamazepine, isoniazid, ketoconazole, methyldopa, NSAIDs, procainamide, and sulfonamides.

12–102 Answer A

The majority of the population in the United States has antibodies against Hepatitis A (HAV). Besides immunity, there is also a vaccine available.

12–103 Answer C

During the incubation period of viral hepatitis, there are no subjective or objective complaints. During the prodromal stage, there is anorexia, nausea, vomiting, malaise, upper respiratory infection (nasal discharge, pharyngitis), myalgia, arthralgia, easy fatigability, fever (HAV), and abdominal pain. In the icteric stage of viral hepatitis, there is jaundice, dark urine, and light-colored stools. There are continued prodromal complaints with gradual improvement. During the convalescent stage there is an increased sense of well-being; the appetite returns; and the jaundice, abdominal pain, and fatigability abate.

12–104 Answer D

Women tend to develop cirrhosis more quickly with less alcohol intake than men, which suggests that a smaller, leaner body mass and enhanced absorption are both factors in the development of alcoholic cirrhosis. Alcoholic cirrhosis, also known as Laënnec's, portal, fatty, or micronodular cirrhosis, is the most common type of cirrhosis in the U.S. Alcohol cirrhosis is often associated with nutritional and vitamin deficiencies but occurs in well-nourished individuals as well as alcoholics. Cirrhosis is the irreversible end stage of liver injury and may be caused by a variety of insults.

12–105 Answer B

A ventral hernia, also known as an epigastric hernia, occurs along the midline between the xiphoid process and the umbilicus. The fibers along the linea alba are brought together in a patchwork type closure; the defect exists within this decussation. As these fibers weaken, the contents can herniate through the abdomen. Epigastric hernias are three times more likely to occur in men than women. Umbilical hernias that develop in adulthood occur through a weakening in the abdominal wall around the umbilical ring. Incisional hernias can occur anywhere along a surgical incision into the abdomen. An inguinal hernia may be indirect or direct. Indirect inguinal hernias result when tissue herniates through the internal inguinal ring, which extends the length of the spermatic cord. A direct inguinal hernia occurs when the transversus abdominis and internal oblique muscles are attached, forming a high arch on the inferior border that results in a faulty shutter mechanism.

12–106 Answer C

The obturator sign is elicited when, with the patient's right hip and knee flexed, the examiner slowly rotates the right leg internally, which stretches the obturator muscle. Pain over the RLQ is considered a positive sign. Rovsing's sign is deep palpation over the LLQ with sudden, unexpected release of pressure. This causes tenderness over the RLQ and is considered a positive finding. Psoas sign is when the patient is instructed to try to lift the right leg against gentle pressure applied by the examiner or by placing the patient in the left lateral decubitus position and extending the patient's right leg at the hip. An increase in pain is considered positive and is an indication of the inflamed appendix irritating the psoas muscle. McBurney's sign is pressure applied to McBurney's point, which is located halfway between the umbilicus and the anterior spine of the ilium. Pain when pressure is applied to this area is considered a positive response.

References

Bradley, M, and Pupiales, M: Essential elements of ostomy care. Am J Nurs 97:7, 1997.

Damianos, AJ, and McGarrity, TJ: Treatment strategies for *Helicobacter pylori* infection. Am Fam Physician 55:8, 1997.

Dillon, PM: Nursing Health Assessment: A Critical Thinking, Case Studies Approach. FA Davis, Philadelphia, 2003.

Dunphy, LM, & Winland-Brown, JE: Primary Care: The Art and Science of Advanced Practice Nursing. FA Davis, Philadelphia, 2002.

Latif, A: Gastric cancer: Update on diagnosis, staging, and therapy. Postgrad Med 102:4, 1997.

Malnick, SDH, et al: Celiac disease: Diagnostic clues to unmask an impostor. Postgrad Med 101:6, 1997.

Martin, FL: Ulcerative colitis. Am J Nurs 97:8, 1997.

Picco, MF: Crohn's disease: Rational management. Consultant 42:2, 2002.

HOW WELL DID YOU DO?

85% AND ABOVE CONGRATULATIONS! THIS SCORE SHOWS APPLICATION OF TEST-TAKING PRINCIPLES AND ADEQUATE CONTENT KNOWLEDGE.

75–85% KEEP WORKING! REVIEW TEST-TAKING PRINCIPLES AND TRY AGAIN.

65–75% HANG IN THERE! SPEND SOME TIME REVIEWING CONCEPTS AND TEST-TAKING PRINCIPLES AND TRY THE TEST AGAIN.

Renal Problems 13

JILL E. WINLAND-BROWN
and
GRETCHEN HOPE MILLER HEERY

13–1 *The most common factor predisposing a woman to a urinary tract infection is:*

A. the use of an oral contraceptive.
B. the use of a diaphragm.
C. urinary stasis.
D. calculi.

13–2 *Sally, age 24, has frequent urinary tract infections. In teaching her about measures to prevent them, you instruct her about all of the following* ***except:***

A. voiding after intercourse.
B. avoiding bubble baths.
C. wearing underwear with pantyhose.
D. drinking 2–4 glasses of water per day.

13–3 *Which type of hematuria in an older adult is an ominous sign?*

A. Painless, gross hematuria
B. Flank pain with hematuria
C. Hematuria following trauma
D. Intermittent hematuria

13–4 *The most common cause of nephrotic syndrome is:*

A. systemic lupus erythematosus.
B. diabetes mellitus.
C. routine use of nonsteroidal anti-inflammatory drugs.
D. glomerulosclerosis.

13–5 *Sam, age 42, has had persistent proteinuria on the previous two office visits. Which action is warranted next?*

A. Schedule extensive blood work.
B. Order an intravenous pyelogram.
C. Admit Sam to the hospital.
D. Have Sam collect one urine specimen on first arising, then another 2 hours later.

13–6 *The urinary sediment finding indicative of pyelonephritis and interstitial nephritis is:*

A. hyaline casts.
B. granular casts.
C. red blood cell casts.
D. white blood cell casts.

13–7 *Which type of kidney stone is the most common?*

A. Calcium oxalate
B. Uric acid
C. Calcium phosphate
D. Cystine

13–8 *Transient urinary incontinence in women is caused by:*

A. atrophy of the vagina or urethra.
B. stool impaction.
C. use of anticholinergic agents.
D. all of the above.

13–9 *In clients receiving dialysis, which is the most common cause of end-stage renal disease in the United States?*

A. Diabetic nephropathy
B. Chronic renal failure secondary to vascular disorders
C. Acute tubular necrosis
D. Kidney trauma

13–10 *About 80% of all cases of dysuria are caused by ascending bacterial infection of the urinary tract by which organism?*

A. *Klebsiella*
B. *Proteus*
C. *Escherichia coli*
D. *Staphylococcus saprophyticus*

13–11 *Rita, age 16, appears with a 3-day history of red urine. In completing the history,you should inquire whether or not she has ingested any of the following* ***except:***

A. blackberries.
B. ibuprofen.
C. red food color.
D. watermelon.

13–12 *Which type of bloody urine is characteristic of bleeding from the upper urinary tract?*

A. Grossly bloody urine
B. Urine with blood clots
C. Brown, smoky, or tea-colored urine
D. Blood noted at the beginning or end of the stream

13–13 *The hormone(s) either activated or synthesized by the kidneys include all* ***except:***

A. the active form of vitamin D.
B. erythropoietin.
C. natriuretic hormone.
D. estrogen.

13–14 *Who is at risk of developing a prerenal type of acute renal failure?*

A. Joey, age 2, who is dehydrated from gastroenteritis
B. Tommy, age 3, who accidentally took an overdose of acetaminophen (Tylenol)
C. Justine, age 5, who nearly drowned in a swimming pool
D. Buddy, age 12, who was born with one kidney and just injured the other in a football game

13–15 *Why do middle-aged men not incur as many urinary tract infections as middle-aged women?*

A. Women are more prone to urinary stasis than men.
B. Men have the bacteriostatic effect of prostatic fluid and a longer urethra.
C. Women have a higher urine pH.
D. Men take more baths than women.

13–16 *Alice, age 29, is having an intravenous pyelogram (IVP). In teaching her about the procedure, you tell her that an IVP:*

A. takes about 30 minutes and uses x rays to show the structures of the kidney, ureters, and bladder after injection of a dye that is rapidly excreted in the urine.
B. involves first filling the bladder with a dye solution, then taking x rays of the filled bladder and of the bladder and urethra during urination.
C. involves the use of radioisotopes.
D. is the same as a renal arteriogram.

13–17 *Thiazide diuretics are used for the treatment of which type of renal calculi?*

A. Calcium phosphate and/or oxalate stones
B. Struvite stones
C. Uric acid stones
D. Cystine stones

13–18 *Jim has had several episodes of kidney stones. The last stone he passed was examined and found to be an oxalate stone. You tell him to avoid foods high in oxalate such as:*

A. beans and lentils, chocolate and cocoa, dried fruits, canned or smoked fish except tuna, flour, milk, and milk products.
B. cheese, cranberries, eggs, grapes, meat and poultry, plums and prunes, tomatoes, and whole grains.
C. asparagus, beer, beets, cabbage, celery, chocolate and cocoa, fruits, green beans, nuts, tea, colas, and tomatoes.
D. goose, organ meats, sardines, herring, and venison; and to have a moderate intake of beef, chicken, crab, pork, salmon, and veal.

13–19 *Jake is having a urinary diversion procedure performed because of a urinary tract tumor. He states that he heard about a Koch's pouch and asks you what it is. You respond:*

A. "It is a cutaneous ureterostomy in which one or both of the ureters create a stoma on the skin surface."
B. "It is an ileal conduit in which the ileum is formed into a pouch with an open stoma and the ureters are inserted into the pouch."
C. "It is a continent internal ileal reservoir in which nipple valves are formed on the skin. The filling pressure closes the valves, preventing leakage and reflux."
D. "It is a ureterosigmoidostomy in which the ureters are inserted into the sigmoid colon. Urine empties into the rectum and is expelled with defecation."

13–20 *Which medication is used primarily in the treatment of acute postoperative and postpartum urinary retention and for neurogenic bladder atony with urinary retention?*

A. Bethanechol chloride (Urecholine)
B. Neostigmine (Prostigmin)
C. Propantheline bromide (Pro-Banthine)
D. Oxybutynin (Ditropan)

13–21 *A factor contributing to stress incontinence is:*

A. a decreased estrogen level.
B. bladder irritation from a urinary tract infection.
C. prostatic hypertrophy.
D. a spinal cord lesion or trauma above S2.

13–22 *Postmenopausal women tend to have more recurrent urinary tract infections. This is not because of:*

A. postvoid residual urine.
B. estrogen depletion-related changes.
C. a decrease in lactobacilli.
D. a decrease in *Escherichia coli.*

13–23 *The clinical presentation of a client with urolithiasis would include:*

A. a gradual onset of nagging pain.
B. marked leukocytes in the urine.
C. a fever of 101°F or above.
D. pain starting in the flank and localizing in the costovertebral angle.

13–24 *Extracorporeal shock wave lithotripsy is not recommended for which type of kidney stones?*

A. Oxalate stones
B. Uric acid stones
C. Struvite stones
D. Cystine stones

13–25 *General recommendations for the prevention of kidney stones, regardless of the type of stone the client has, include:*

A. drinking 3–4 liters of mineral water per day.
B. reducing protein in the diet.
C. increasing vitamin C in the diet.
D. decreasing fiber in the diet.

13–26 *The inability to empty the bladder, resulting in overdistention and frequent loss of small amounts of urine, describes which type of urinary incontinence?*

A. Stress incontinence
B. Urge incontinence
C. Overflow incontinence
D. Reflex incontinence

13–27 *Decreased bladder capacity; bladder irritation from a urinary tract infection, tumor, stones, or irritants such as caffeine and alcohol; and central nervous system disorders or spinal cord lesions are all contributing factors to:*

A. stress urinary incontinence.
B. urge urinary incontinence.
C. overflow urinary incontinence.
D. reflex urinary incontinence.

13–28 *You explain to Yolanda that pelvic floor (Kegel) exercises help to restore and maintain continence by improving pelvic muscle strength, increasing urethral pressure, and decreasing abnormal detrusor muscle contractions. These exercises are used for her diagnosis of:*

A. stool incontinence.
B. full-bladder incontinence.
C. cystitis-related incontinence.
D. stress incontinence.

13–29 *Medications affected by a decreased glomerular filtration rate include all of the following* ***except:***

A. cardiac drugs, such as digoxin and procainamide.
B. antibiotics, such as aminoglycosides, tetracyclines, and cephalosporins.
C. histamine (H_2) antagonists, such as cimetidine.
D. hematinics, such as FER-IN-SOL, Slow Fe, and Niferex.

13–30 *Which of the following changes in laboratory values is associated with kidney disease?*

A. Serum creatinine greater than 4 mg/dL
B. Serum albumin greater than 5 g/dL
C. Serum sodium greater than 150 mEq/L
D. Serum calcium greater than 6.0 mEq/L

13–31 *Clinical manifestations including microscopic or gross hematuria, a palpable abdominal mass, fever, and flank pain may indicate a:*

A. pancreatic tumor.
B. liver tumor.
C. colon mass.
D. renal tumor.

13–32 *Cardiovascular failure is a major cause of which type of acute renal failure?*

A. Prerenal
B. Intrarenal
C. Postrenal
D. Perirenal

13–33 *If a client with acute renal failure excretes 400 mL of urine on Tuesday, how much fluid intake (both oral and intravenous) should the client have on Wednesday?*

A. 400 mL
B. 600 mL
C. 900 mL
D. 1200 mL

13–34 *Dietary management for the client in acute renal failure includes:*

A. decreasing carbohydrate intake.
B. increasing dietary sodium intake.
C. limiting protein intake.
D. increasing potassium.

13–35 *Goodpasture's syndrome is:*

A. characterized by glomerulonephritis and pulmonary hemorrhage resulting from immune complex damage to the glomerular and alveolar basement membranes.
B. characterized by massive proteinuria, hypoalbuminemia, hyperlipidemia, and edema.
C. an inflammatory autoimmune disorder affecting the connective tissue of the body with inflammatory lesions involving the supportive tissues of the glomerulus.
D. typically the end stage of other glomerular disorders, such as rapidly progressive glomerulonephritis, lupus nephritis, or diabetic nephropathy.

13–36 *The most common cause of chronic renal failure is:*

A. glomerulonephritis.
B. hypertension.
C. diabetic nephropathy.
D. other urologic disease.

13–37 *The most frequent complication during hemodialysis is:*

A. bleeding.
B. infection.
C. dialysis dementia.
D. hypotension.

13–38 *You should be concerned about the use of diuretics, chronic renal failure, a high-protein diet, gout, leukemia, or lymphoma when a serum uric acid level is:*

A. 4.0 mg/dL
B. 5.0 mg/dL
C. 6.0 mg/dL
D. greater than 7.0 mg/dL

13–39 *The most common cause of urinary tract obstruction is:*

A. edema resulting from trauma.
B. a tumor.
C. ureterolithiasis.
D. a vascular problem.

13–40 *The first step in the treatment of uric acid kidney stones is:*

A. encouraging hydration.
B. alkalinizing the urine.
C. prescribing allopurinol (Zyloprim).
D. reducing protein intake.

13–41 *Most calcium phosphate kidney stones are caused by:*

A. a high dietary calcium intake.
B. a high phosphorus dietary intake.
C. primary hyperparathyroidism.
D. hyperthyroidism.

13–42 *The most frequent sign of bladder cancer is:*

A. hematuria.
B. flank pain.
C. nocturia.
D. dysuria.

13–43 *Marie, age 16, fell off her bicycle and sustained a contusion of her left kidney. The treatment of choice is:*

A. surgery.
B. urethral catheterization.
C. conservative therapy.
D. to continue normal activity because it is only a contusion.

13–44 *Jill, who has had urinary incontinence for several months, wants to have an evaluation to determine if any therapy will be beneficial. After having an initial pelvic examination, she has a postvoid residual catheterization. A residual volume of more than how many mL is abnormal?*

A. 10 mL
B. 30 mL
C. 50 mL
D. 100 mL

13–45 *Urine tends to become colonized when indwelling urinary catheters are left in place for more than:*

A. 24 hours.
B. 36 hours.
C. 48 hours.
D. 72 hours.

13–46 *Samuel wants his son circumcised, but it is noted that the baby has hypospadias. What do you tell Samuel?*

A. "Your son should be circumcised as soon as possible."
B. "Wait until your son is 1 month old; then he can be circumcised."
C. "We first have to check to see where the opening is; then we can determine if your son can be circumcised or not."
D. "Your son should not be circumcised."

13–47 *Doug, age 6, appears with abdominal distention and pain, an abdominal mass on the right side, fever, and slight hematuria. There is no precipitating event. What do you suspect?*

A. A urinary tract infection
B. Appendicitis
C. Wilms's tumor
D. An intestinal obstruction

13–48 *Martha, age 42, states that she has intercourse only about once a month, but immediately afterward, she usually gets a urinary tract infection. She is frustrated with having to come to the office frequently to have an examination with a urine test. She says that she is ready to "kick her husband out of bed." How do you respond?*

A. "By taking a low-dose antibiotic every day, you can prevent a urinary tract infection."
B. "Take 200 mg of ofloxacin with a large glass of water after intercourse."
C. "I'll write you a prescription for a 3-day pack of antibiotics with several refills to take when you need it."
D. "Yes, not having sexual intercourse will resolve the problem."

13–49 *Because of infections related to long-term indwelling urinary catheterization, it should not be used routinely in clients who:*

A. have sacral ulcers.
B. have urinary retention that cannot be managed surgically or medically and for whom intermittent catheterization cannot be performed.
C. are terminally ill or severely impaired so that frequent changing of clothes or linen would be uncomfortable.
D. need assistance to get to the bathroom.

13–50 *The most common cause of sepsis in older adults is:*

A. urinary stasis.
B. a urinary tract infection.
C. a kidney stone.
D. a genitourinary problem.

13–51 *Tony is considering dialysis for his end-stage renal disease, but heard that he might not be a candidate. He asks you if there are any contraindications to dialysis. You tell him that the contraindication(s) to hemodialysis include all of the following* ***except:***

A. severe cardiac disease.
B. bleeding disorders.
C. inability to create or maintain arteriovenous access.
D. preexisting disease.

13–52 *The aging process begins to affect the kidneys with a progressive loss of nephron units by age:*

A. 40 years.
B. 50 years.
C. 60 years.
D. 70 years.

13–53 *In the older adult, which physiologic change does not affect pharmacokinetics?*

A. Decreased creatine clearance
B. Decreased lean muscle mass
C. Increased total body fat
D. Increased serum albumin level

13–54 *Which of the following groups is most prone to developing nephrolithiasis?*

A. White men
B. White women
C. Black men
D. Black women

13–55 *Who is at a higher risk for developing nephrolithiasis?*

A. Jean, who exercises every day and drinks copious amounts of water
B. Bill, who runs every day and takes excessive amounts of vitamin C
C. Mary Ann, who watches her weight and eats a low-sodium diet
D. Harvey, a "couch potato" who drinks a lot of no-sodium soda.

13–56 *Which diagnostic finding(s) may lead to a diagnosis of nephrolithiasis?*

A. Urinary uric acid output of less than 750 mg/24 hours
B. Urinary pH greater than 5.5
C. Urinary calcium output of greater than 300 mg/24 hours
D. Serum calcium of 8mg/dL

13–57 *For clients taking nonsteroidal anti-inflammatory drugs on a long-term basis, the following may not be found:*

A. Hemodynamically induced acute renal failure
B. Acute interstitial nephropathy
C. Salt and water retention
D. Hypokalemia

13–58 *Prevention of drug-induced nephrotoxicity is especially important in older adults and persons with kidney damage. Which of the following step(s) is/are helpful in preventing it?*

A. Select diagnostic procedures or therapeutic measures without nephrotoxic potential.
B. Avoid dehydration.
C. Limit total daily dosage and duration of treatment with certain drugs.
D. All of the above.

13–59 *Which of the following drugs is not associated with acute renal failure?*

A. Angiotensin-converting enzyme inhibitors
B. Cimetidine (Tagamet)

C. Nonsteroidal anti-inflammatory drugs
D. Erythromycin (E-Mycin)

13–60 *Janet has stress urinary incontinence and has been doing Kegel exercises with some success. What other simple action might help in relieving some of the problem?*

A. Stopping smoking.
B. Limiting fluids.
C. Taking a daily multivitamin.
D. Beginning lifting 2-lb weights.

13–61 *Mary Lou, who has stress urinary incontinence, is desperate for some relief and asks for your help. She already takes several pills a day and does not really want to take any more, but wants to do something about her problem. What do you suggest?*

A. Propantheine bromide (Pro-Banthine)
B. Dicyclomine hydrochloride (Bentyl)
C. Estrogen vaginal cream
D. Imipramine hydrochloride (Tofranil)

13–62 *Eric, age 5, has enuresis. The probable cause is:*

A. anatomic disease.
B. neurologic disease.
C. a psychological problem.
D. maturational delay.

13–63 *Which of the following does not cause urine to appear reddish in color?*

A. Cascara sagrada
B. Phenazopyridine (Pyridium)
C. Phenytoin (Dilantin)
D. Multivitamins

13–64 *Urine specific gravity is increased in clients with:*

A. dehydration.
B. diabetes insipidus.
C. chronic renal failure.
D. overhydration.

13–65 *An intravenous pyelogram is contraindicated in clients who:*

A. are allergic to shellfish or iodinated dyes.
B. are severely dehydrated.
C. have renal insufficiency.
D. all of the above.

13–66 *After a renal biopsy, the client should be instructed:*

A. that there may be some blood in the urine for the next several days.
B. to avoid strenuous activities for at least 2 weeks.
C. to drink 3–4 glasses of water per day.
D. about all of the above.

13–67 *A 24-hour urine test for vanillylmandelic acid and catecholamines is done to diagnose:*

A. a renal tumor.
B. hypertension secondary to pheochromocytoma.
C. renal artery stenosis.
D. hydronephrosis.

13–68 *A nuclear scan of the kidney is used:*

A. to detect renal infarctions.
B. to detect renal arterial atherosclerosis.
C. to monitor rejection of a transplanted kidney.
D. for all of the above.

13–69 *All of the following conditions usually cause flank pain* ***except:***

A. pyelonephritis.
B. ureterolithiasis.
C. vascular occlusion of the kidney (renal vein thrombosis).
D. renal cysts.

13–70 *Urine that appears red or reddish-orange may result from all of the following* ***except:***

A. beets.
B. bile.
C. rifampin (Rifadin).
D. phenazopyridine (Pyridium).

13–71 *What is the single best indicator of overall renal function?*

A. A urinalysis
B. Blood urea nitrogen
C. The glomerular filtration rate
D. Serum albumin

13–72 *Which of the following is defined as a pathophysiological process that occurs when there is a primary excess in the extracellular fluid of bicarbonate as a result of a loss of acid or the addition of excess bicarbonate?*

A. Metabolic acidosis
B. Metabolic alkalosis
C. Respiratory acidosis
D. Respiratory alkalosis

13–73 *Excessive alcohol ingestion can cause:*

A. metabolic acidosis.
B. metabolic alkalosis.
C. respiratory acidosis.
D. respiratory alkalosis.

13–74 *Clinical manifestations of metabolic alkalosis include:*

A. tetany.
B. nausea and vomiting.

C. weakness.
D. bradycardia.

13–75 *Sara, age 82, was unable to breathe for several minutes after choking on a piece of meat. A successful Heimlich maneuver was done and her arterial blood gases now are: pH 7.39, $PaCO_2$ 48, PaO_2 92, and HCO_3 24. What do you suspect?*

A. Respiratory alkalosis
B. Respiratory acidosis
C. Metabolic alkalosis
D. Metabolic acidosis

13–76 *Maury has renal failure and his arterial blood gas readings show a decreased pH, normal PCO_2, and decreased HCO_3. What do you suspect?*

A. Respiratory acidosis
B. Respiratory alkalosis
C. Metabolic acidosis
D. Metabolic alkalosis

13–77 *The kidneys excrete increased amounts of HCO_3 to lower the pH as a mode of compensation for which acid-base disturbance?*

A. Respiratory acidosis
B. Respiratory alkalosis
C. Metabolic acidosis
D. Metabolic alkalosis

13–78 *Before using the radial artery to draw blood for arterial blood gas (ABG) testing, which test should be performed?*

A. The ABG test
B. The Thomas test
C. The Weber test
D. The Allen test

13–79 *All of the following are implicated in the formation of urinary tract neoplasms* ***except:***

A. Cigarette smoke, both active and passive inhalation
B. Chemicals from plastic and rubber
C. Chronic use of phenacetin-containing analgesic agents
D. Working long hours and not voiding often

13–80 *Marvin, age 59, is going to have a total cystectomy to remove his bladder tumor. He states that when the surgeon was talking to him, he was not really listening, and he asks you about the incidence of impotence after such a surgery. How do you respond?*

A. "You'll have to talk to the surgeon; every case is unique."
B. "This surgery requires the removal of the prostate and seminal vessels, which does result in impotence. Let's talk about it."
C. "I'm not sure if this will be the case, but if it is, how would you feel about it?"
D. "How does your wife feel about the possibility?"

13–81 *Leslie, age 13, says that her mother has polycystic kidney disease and asks about her chances of developing it. How do you respond?*

A. "It is hereditary, but if you develop it, a cure is possible."
B. "It is hereditary and, unfortunately, incurable, but there are many measures we can use in dealing with it."
C. "It is not hereditary, but you may develop it anyway."
D. "It is hereditary, but skips generations."

13–82 *Which history is commonly found in a client with glomerulonephritis?*

A. Beta-hemolytic streptococcal infection
B. Frequent urinary tract infections
C. Kidney stones
D. Hypotension

13–83 *Which diuretic acts by inhibiting sodium chloride reabsorption in the thick ascending limb of the loop of Henle?*

A. Furosemide (Lasix)
B. Mannitol (Osmitrol)
C. Hydrochlorothiazide (Hydrodiuril)
D. Acetazolamide (Diamox)

13–84 *Which category of diuretic has the following side effects: hyperkalemia, headache, hyponatremia, nausea, diarrhea, urticaria, and menstrual disturbances?*

A. Osmotic diuretic
B. Loop diuretic
C. Potassium-sparing diuretic
D. Thiazide diuretic

13–85 *Which of the following diagnostic studies for the evaluation of renal function assesses for the lack of erythropoietin?*

A. Urine creatinine clearance
B. Blood urea nitrogen
C. Serum albumin
D. Serum hemoglobin and hematocrit

13–86 *Which of the following in the urinary sediment signifies an allergic reaction in the kidney?*

A. Leukocytes
B. Eosinophils
C. Crystals
D. Erythrocytes

13–87 *Which of the following radiologic studies provides direct imaging in several planes conducive to* *detecting renal cystic disease, inflammatory processes, and renal cell carcinoma?*

A. Cystoscopy
B. Ultrasonography
C. Computed tomography
D. Magnetic resonance imaging

13–88 *Which diagnostic procedure can visualize the renal outline and identify lower rib fractures?*

A. Intravenous pyelogram
B. Renal angiography
C. Computed tomography
D. A kidneys, ureters, and bladder film

13–89 *Why is the right kidney slightly lower than the left kidney?*

A. The spleen pushes the left kidney upward.
B. The liver pushes the right kidney downward.
C. The diaphragm displaces the left kidney.
D. The right kidney is structurally larger than the left kidney.

13–90 *What amount of urine in a 24-hour period represents oliguria?*

A. Less than 500 mL
B. 500–749 mL
C. 750–999 mL
D. 1000–1500 mL

13–91 *In an assessment of renal function, what is the maximum amount of urine in a 24-hour period that a client would produce for a diagnosis of anuria to be considered?*

A. No urine output at all
B. Less than 100 mL
C. 100–150 mL
D. 151–200 mL

13–92 *What is the most common cause of death in dialysis clients?*

A. Infection
B. Bleeding from the access site
C. Cardiovascular failure
D. Sepsis

13–93 *An acidic urine pH favors precipitation of which type of kidney stone?*

A. Cystine stones
B. Calcium phosphate stones
C. Struvite stones
D. Magnesium stones

13–94 *The most common metabolic condition that predisposes to the formation of kidney stones is:*

A. idiopathic hypercalciuria.
B. hyperuricosuria.
C. hyperoxaluria.
D. a low urinary citrate excretion.

13–95 *Which of the following is not a complication of a urinary tract obstruction?*

A. A decrease in glomerular filtration rate with a potential tubular abnormality
B. Infection
C. Renal stones
D. Hypotension

13–96 *Eosinophils are not present in the urine in:*

A. interstitial nephritis.
B. urinary tract infections.
C. acute tubular necrosis.
D. normal urine.

13–97 *Aging may affect the kidney by causing:*

A. a diminished glomerular filtration rate.
B. decreased creatine production.
C. urinary incontinence.
D. all of the above.

13–98 *The antihypertensive drugs contraindicated in clients with renal artery stenosis are:*

A. calcium channel blockers.
B. beta blockers.
C. angiotensin-converting enzyme inhibitors.
D. cardiac glycosides

13–99 *A urinary tract infection is best detected by performing:*

A. a nitrite dipstick test.
B. a urinalysis.
C. a urine culture.
D. urine sensitivity.

13–100 *The most frequent reason why a person would come to your office complaining of burning on urination is:*

A. prostatitis.
B. urethritis.
C. a urinary tract infection.
D. a sexually transmitted disease.

Answers

13–1 Answer C

Urinary stasis is the most common factor predisposing a woman to a urinary tract infection (UTI). It is followed by calculi and the presence of catheters, stents, and other foreign bodies. The use of an oral contraceptive (if the male partner is not using a condom) also predisposes a woman to a UTI because sexual intercourse increases the likelihood of developing a UTI. The use of a diaphragm increases the risk of a UTI because of the properties of the spermicidal agents used in conjunction with the diaphragm.

13–2 Answer D

Clients with frequent urinary tract infections (UTIs), and in fact all persons, should drink 8–10 glasses of water per day to help distribute the body's own antibodies. Other measures that should be taught to women prone to developing UTIs include voiding after intercourse, avoiding bubble baths, wearing underwear with pantyhose, and using methods of contraception other than diaphragms with spermicidal agents.

13–3 Answer A

Painless gross hematuria in an older adult is an ominous sign. It is usually the result of a malignancy (prostate cancer, transitional cell cancer, or renal cell carcinoma). Flank pain with hematuria is commonly caused by the presence of a kidney stone in the upper collecting system of the affected kidney. Hematuria after trauma is quite common.

13–4 Answer B

Diabetes mellitus is the most common cause of nephrotic syndrome. Systemic lupus erythematosus, the routine use of nonsteroidal anti-inflammatory drugs, glomerulosclerosis, and diabetes mellitus are all causes of proteinuria.

13–5 Answer D

Before beginning an extensive workup for proteinuria, the syndrome of postural proteinuria should be ruled out. In this benign condition, which occurs in healthy, otherwise asymptomatic clients, urine collected first thing in the morning does not show any protein. If protein is present in the urine after the client has been ambulating for several hours, the syndrome of postural proteinuria is confirmed. The prognosis is excellent because clients with postural proteinuria do not develop renal disease with any greater frequency than that seen in the general population.

13–6 Answer D

White blood cell casts are seen in pyelonephritis and interstitial nephritis. Hyaline casts may be present in normal urine; granular casts may be present in a wide variety of renal disorders; and red blood cell casts indicate glomerular bleeding that is strongly suggestive of glomerulonephritis.

13–7 Answer A

The most common type of kidney stones are calcium oxalate stones. They make up about 75% of all kidney stones and are usually less than 2 cm in diameter. Uric acid stones, which are radiolucent, make up about 5% of all stones. Calcium phosphate stones, which occur with renal tubular acidosis, make up about 5% of all stones. Cystine stones, which are hexagonal crystals, are the result of an autosomal recessive genetic trait and make up less than 1% of all kidney stones.

13–8 Answer D

Atrophy of the vagina or urethra, stool impaction, and the use of anticholinergic agents may all be responsible for transient urinary incontinence in women. Etiologies for transient urinary incontinence may be stated using a "DIAPERS" mnemonic: D for drugs, such as hypnotics, sedatives, anticholinergic agents, diuretics, and adrenergic agents, and delirium or altered mental status; I for infection; A for atrophy of the vagina or urethra; P for psychologic disorders such as functional depression; E for endocrine disorders, such as hyperglycemia or hypercalcemia; R for restricted mobility; and S for stool impaction.

13–9 Answer A

In clients receiving dialysis, diabetic nephropathy (Kimmelstiel-Wilson syndrome) is the most common cause of end-stage renal disease in the United States (about 25%). Both type I and type II diabetes are implicated, indicating the need for good diabetic control throughout clients' life spans. Most clients with acute tubular necrosis recover with conservative management (fluid monitoring, protein restriction, drug adjustments, and dietary and potassium control). Dialysis may become necessary; however, it is usually temporary. In clients with major renal vascular occlusive disease, vascular repair or percutaneous angioplasty has been shown to slow the progression of the disease.

13–10 Answer C

Escherichia coli causes about 80% of all infections of the urinary tract. *Klebsiella* is responsible for about 10% of urinary tract infections, *Proteus* for about 10%, and *Staphylococcus saprophyticus* for about 5%.

13–11 Answer D

Ingesting blackberries or beets; taking ibuprofen or phenazopyridine (Pyridium); and eating foods with red food color all may cause the urine to be pink, red, burgundy, or cola colored.

13–12 Answer C

Brown, smoky, or tea-colored urine indicates blood coming from the upper urinary tract. It is the result of the acidic urine changing the hemoglobin to hematin, which has a brown color. Grossly bloody urine and urine with blood clots come from the lower urinary tract. Blood noted at the beginning or end of the stream also indicates lower tract bleeding, whereas blood throughout the stream may suggest upper urinary tract bleeding.

13–13 Answer D

The active form of vitamin D, erythropoietin, and natriuretic hormone are all either activated or synthesized by the kidneys. Vitamin D is necessary for the absorption of calcium and phosphate by the small intestine. Erythropoietin stimulates the bone marrow to produce red blood cells in response to tissue hypoxia. Natriuretic hormone is released from the right atrium of the heart in response to increased volume and stretch, as occurs in increased extracellular volume.

13–14 Answer A

The prerenal classification of acute renal failure (ARF) may be caused by dehydration secondary to gastroenteritis, malnutrition, or diarrhea, as well as hemorrhage, hypovolemia, shock, and heart failure. Therefore, Joey is at risk for developing a prerenal type of ARF. The renal classification of ARF may be caused by nephrotoxins such as acetaminophen (Tylenol), nearly drowning (especially in fresh water), acute glomerulonephritis, severe infections, and diseases of the kidney and blood vessels. Postrenal causes of ARF include obstructions caused by tumor, hematoma, stones, renal vein thrombosis, or trauma to a solitary kidney or collecting system.

13–15 Answer B

Middle-aged men do not incur as many urinary tract infections as middle-aged women because men have the bacteriostatic effect of prostatic fluid and a longer urethra. However, prostatic hypertrophy commonly associated with aging increases the risk of cystitis for older men. Men and women are equally prone to urinary stasis and have the same urinary pH.

13–16 Answer A

The intravenous pyelogram is an examination that takes about 30 minutes and uses x rays to show the structures of the kidney, ureters, and bladder after injection of a dye that is rapidly excreted in the urine. A voiding cystourethrogram is when the bladder is filled with dye solution, then followed by x rays of the filled bladder and of the bladder and urethra during urination. Radioisotope studies provide information regarding renal anatomy; blood flow; and glomerular, tubular, and collecting system function. Renal arteriography or venography is indicated in children only when it is necessary to define vascular abnormalities such as renal artery stenosis before a surgical intervention. Usually other less invasive measures are used.

13–17 Answer A

Thiazide diuretics, along with phosphates and calcium-binding agents, are used for calcium phosphate and oxalate stones. Antibiotic therapy is used for the urinary tract infections that occur with struvite stones; allopurinol is used for uric acid stones; and penicillamine and sodium bicarbonate are used for cystine stones.

13–18 Answer C

Foods high in oxalate that a client with oxalate kidney stones should avoid include asparagus, beer, beets, cabbage, celery, chocolate and cocoa, fruits, green beans, nuts, tea, colas, and tomatoes. Foods high in calcium are beans and lentils, chocolate and cocoa, dried fruits, canned or smoked fish except tuna, flour, milk, and milk products. Acid ash foods to avoid with calcium phosphate or oxalate stones and struvite stones include cheese, cranberries, eggs, grapes, meat and poultry, plums and prunes, tomatoes, and whole grains. Purine-rich foods include goose, organ meats, sardines, herring, and venison. Purine levels are moderate in beef, chicken, crab, pork, salmon, and veal.

13–19 Answer C

A Koch's pouch is a continent internal ileal reservoir or continent ileal bladder conduit in which a pouch is created to be an ileal conduit. Nipple valves are formed on the skin by intussuscepting tissue backward into the reservoir to connect the pouch to the skin and the ureters to the pouch. The filling pressure closes valves, preventing leakage and reflux.

13–20 Answer A

Cholinergic drugs such as bethanechol chloride (Urecholine) are used primarily in the treatment of acute postoperative and postpartum urinary retention and for neurogenic bladder atony with urinary retention. Anticholinesterase agents such as neostigmine (Prostigmin) and pyridostigmine (Mestinon) are used primarily in the treatment of myasthenia gravis, but they are also useful in the treatment of urinary retention because they stimulate contraction of the detrusor muscle. Anticholinergic agents such as propantheline bromide (Pro-Banthine), dicyclomine (Bentyl), flavoxate hydrochloride (Urispas), and oxybutynin (Ditropan) act to relax the detrusor muscle and increase contraction of the internal sphincter. They serve to increase the bladder capacity of clients with spastic or hyperreflexive neurogenic bladder.

13–21 Answer A

A decreased estrogen level contributes to stress incontinence. Bladder irritation from a urinary tract infection contributes to urge incontinence; prostatic hypertrophy contributes to overflow incontinence; and spinal cord lesion or trauma contributes to reflex incontinence.

13–22 Answer D

Postmenopausal women tend to have more recurrent urinary tract infections because of postvoid residual urine secondary to anatomic changes such as a dropped bladder or uterus; estrogen depletion-related changes such as a dry, thin vaginal lining; a decrease in lactobacilli; and an increase in the colonization of the vagina by *Escherichia coli*.

13–23 Answer D

The clinical presentation of a client with urolithiasis includes pain that typically starts in the flank and may localize at the costovertebral angle. The pain may radiate to the lower abdomen, groin, or perineum and is often associated with nausea and vomiting. Fever is unlikely unless there is a coexisting urinary tract infection. Hematuria may be present, but the urine should not have any leukocytes unless an infection is also present. Because the question is asked only about a client with urolithiasis and did not mention any infection, an assumption of an infection being present should not be made.

13–24 Answer C

Extracorporeal shock-wave lithotripsy is not recommended for struvite stones because bacteria or endotoxins inside the stone may be systemically dispersed. Appropriate antibiotics are required.

13–25 Answer B

General recommendations for the prevention of kidney stones, regardless of the type of stone the client has, include reducing protein in the diet because protein enhances calcium, urate, and oxalate excretion; drinking 3–4 liters of water per day with the avoidance of nonsoftened and mineral water; avoiding vitamin C supplements because these stimulate oxalate excretion; increasing fiber to decrease calcium absorption; restricting sodium to 2.5 g/day to decrease excretion of urinary calcium; restricting the consumption of oxalate-containing foods; limiting calcium intake to 800–1000 mg/day; and restricting alcohol to no more than one to two drinks per day.

13–26 Answer C

Overflow incontinence is the inability to empty the bladder, resulting in overdistention and frequent loss of small amounts of urine. Stress incontinence is the loss of urine associated with increased intra-abdominal pressure such as occurs with sneezing, coughing, and lifting. The quantity of urine lost is usually small. Urge incontinence is the inability to inhibit urine flow long enough to reach the toilet after the urge sensation. Reflex incontinence is the involuntary loss of a moderate volume of urine without stimulus or warning. It may occur during the day or night.

13–27 Answer B

The contributing factors of urge urinary incontinence include decreased bladder capacity; bladder irritation from a urinary tract infection, tumor, stones, or irritants such as caffeine and alcohol; and central nervous system disorders or spinal cord lesions. Contributing factors of stress urinary incontinence include multiple pregnancies, decreased estrogen levels, a short urethra, weakness of the abdominal wall, prostate surgery, and increased intra-abdominal pressure as a result of tumor, ascites, or obesity. For overflow urinary incontinence, contributing factors include spinal cord injuries below S2, diabetic neuropathy, prostatic hypertrophy, fecal impaction, and drugs, especially those with an anticholinergic effect. For reflex urinary incontinence, contributing factors include a spinal cord lesion or trauma above S2, history of a cerebrovascular accident, neurologic disorders such as Parkinson's or Alzheimer's disease, and multiple sclerosis.

13–28 Answer D

Kegel exercises are essential for the APN to teach patients with stress incontinence to improve their quality of life. Pelvic floor (Kegel) exercises help to restore and maintain continence by improving pelvic muscle strength, increasing urethral pressure, decreasing abnormal detrusor muscle contraction, and decreasing pressure within the bladder.

13–29 Answer D

Medications affected by a decreased glomerular filtration rate (GFR) include cardiac drugs, antibiotics, histamine (H_2) antagonists, and antidiabetic agents such as chlorpropamide. A decreased GFR in the older adult reduces the clearance of drugs excreted through the kidneys. This reduced GFR prolongs the half-life of drugs and may necessitate lower drug dosages and longer dosing intervals. Hematinics are excreted through the liver, not the kidneys.

13–30 Answer A

A serum creatinine level greater than 4 mg/dL is associated with kidney disease and is indicative of severe impairment of renal function. A decreased serum albumin level occurs in nephrotic syndrome. Serum sodium is decreased in nephrotic syndrome and serum calcium is decreased in renal failure.

13–31 Answer D

Clinical manifestations of renal tumors include microscopic or gross hematuria, a palpable abdominal mass, fever, flank pain, fatigue, weight loss, and anemia or polycythemia.

13–32 Answer A

Cardiovascular failure and hypovolemia are the two major causes of prerenal acute renal failure. Vascular disease, glomerulonephritis, interstitial nephritis, and acute tubular necrosis are causes of intrarenal acute renal failure. Extrarenal obstruction, intrarenal obstruction, and bladder rupture are causes of postrenal acute renal failure.

13–33 Answer C

If a client with acute renal failure (ARF) excretes 400 mL of urine on Tuesday, the amount of fluid intake (both oral and intravenous) the client should have on Wednesday is 900 mL. A client with ARF is initially managed conservatively by fluid and dietary management. The permitted daily intake is calculated by allowing 500 mL for insensible losses (respiration, perspiration, bowel losses) and adding the amount excreted as urine in the previous 24 hours. The client excreted 400 mL as urine, so adding 500 mL for insensible loss equals 900 mL total intake for the next 24 hours.

13–34 Answer C

Dietary management for the client in acute renal failure (ARF) includes limiting protein intake to 0.7–1.0 g/kg of body weight per day to minimize the degree of azotemia. Carbohydrate intake is increased to maintain adequate calorie intake and provide a protein-sparing effect. Dietary sodium intake is decreased to assist in preventing fluid retention.

13–35 Answer A

Goodpasture's syndrome is characterized by glomerulonephritis and pulmonary hemorrhage resulting from immune complex damage to the glomerular and alveolar basement membranes. Nephrotic syndrome is characterized by massive proteinuria, hypoalbuminemia, hyperlipidemia, and edema. Lupus nephritis is an inflammatory autoimmune disorder affecting the connective tissue of the body with inflammatory lesions involving the supportive tissues of the glomerulus. Chronic glomerulonephritis is typically the end stage of other glomerular disorders such as rapidly progressive glomerulonephritis, lupus nephritis, or diabetic nephropathy.

13–36 Answer C

The most common cause of chronic renal failure (CRF) is diabetic nephropathy. Diabetic nephropathy makes up about 34% of all cases of CRF, followed by hypertension (29%), glomerulonephritis (11%), and other urologic diseases (6%).

13–37 Answer D

Hypotension is the most frequent complication seen during hemodialysis. It is related to many factors, such as changes in serum osmolality, rapid removal of fluid from the vascular compartment, and vasodilatation. Bleeding is the next most common complication because of both altered platelet function associated with uremia and the use of heparin during dialysis. Infection may either occur locally, at the site of the arteriovenous fistula, or be systemic. Dialysis dementia is a progressive, potentially fatal neurologic complication that affects clients on long-term hemodialysis.

13–38 Answer D

When a client has an elevated serum uric acid level (greater than 7.0 mg/dL), the following should be considered: the use of diuretics, chronic renal failure (CRF), a high-protein diet, gout, leukemia, and lymphoma. To specifically look for CRF, a serum creatinine level and a 24-hour urinary uric acid test need to be performed.

13–39 Answer C

Ureterolithiasis is the most common cause of urinary tract obstruction. Pain with ureteral obstruction is compounded by the stretching of the renal capsule by edema and swelling. Edema does not usually cause complete obstruction. Although a tumor may cause an obstruction, it is not as common as an obstruction caused by ureterolithiasis. Vascular problems may aggravate or potentiate a problem leading to an obstruction, but not be the actual cause.

13–40 Answer A

Encouraging hydration is the first step in the treatment of uric acid kidney stones. Additional steps include alkalinizing the urine with potassium citrate (Urocit-K) to keep the urine pH above 6.5. Reducing protein intake to 56 g/day will also help. As a last resort, allopurinol (Zyloprim) may be added. Usually clients with uric acid kidney stones will have a normal serum uric acid level but an elevated urine uric acid concentration.

13–41 Answer C

Most calcium phosphate stones are caused by primary hyperparathyroidism. Treatment involves surgical excision of the parathyroid adenoma. If the surgery is not successful or is impossible, treatment involves hydration and the administration of orthophosphate. The client is then observed for hypertension and sodium and water retention.

13–42 Answer A

The most frequent sign of bladder cancer is hematuria. With gross hematuria, an intravenous pyelogram should be performed to detect bladder cancer as early as possible. Flank pain is usually a sign of glomerulonephritis or kidney stones; nocturia is the number one symptom of benign prostatic hypertrophy; and dysuria is present with a urinary tract infection.

13–43 Answer C

The treatment of choice for a contusion of the kidney after trauma is conservative therapy, including bedrest and observation. With these injuries, bleeding is typically minor and self-limiting. Treatment of major renal injuries is usually surgical to stop hemorrhaging. A urethral catheterization will be done to assess the characteristics of the urine (quantity and color), but this is a procedure for the condition, not treatment, of the kidney contusion.

13–44 Answer B

A postvoid residual catheterization volume of more than 30 mL is abnormal.

13–45 Answer D

Urine tends to become colonized with bacteria when indwelling urinary catheters are left in place for more than 72 hours. If catheters are left in place only temporarily and removed quickly when the client can void, infection will usually not result. Antibacterial coverage is warranted if catheters are left in place for 5–10 days.

13–46 Answer D

A circumcision should never be done on a baby with hypospadias because the consulting surgeon may need the prepuce to repair the defect. Surgical correction should be undertaken by the time the child enters the first grade.

13–47 Answer C

A child with Wilms's tumor commonly has abdominal distention or an abdominal mass. There may also be fever, abdominal pain, or hematuria. This kidney tumor requires surgical removal, followed by chemotherapy. Radiation therapy is not necessary.

13–48 Answer B

Clients who recognize a similar association between a urinary tract infection and recent sexual intercourse, diaphragm and spermicide use, and/or pelvic exam, can be instructed to take a single small dose of an antibiotic, such as ofloxacin (Floxin), with a large glass of water after intercourse.

13–49 Answer D

Indwelling urinary catheters should never be used for convenience when patients are able to go to the bathroom. Assistance should be provided whenever necessary to avoid the use of catheters. Long-term indwelling urinary catheterizations have been shown to cause infections and should only be used for clients who have sacral ulcers, have urinary retention that cannot be managed surgically or medically and for whom intermittent catheterization cannot be performed, or are terminally ill or severely impaired so that frequent changing of clothes or linen would be uncomfortable.

13–50 Answer B

The most common cause of sepsis in the older adult is a urinary tract infection (UTI). An older adult who is ill with hypothermia or high fever, has a change in mental status and a documented UTI, or has a suspected UTI and sepsis should be treated vigorously with adequate hydration, immediate use of potent antibiotics, and support of blood pressure. Urinary stasis may precipitate a UTI, and kidney stones may accompany one, along with genitourinary problems, but a UTI alone is the most common cause of sepsis in the older adult.

13–51 Answer D

Contraindications to hemodialysis include severe cardiac disease, bleeding disorders, and the inability to create or maintain arteriovenous access.

13–52 Answer A

The aging process begins to affect the kidneys with a progressive loss of nephron units by age 40. The kidneys lose about 20% of their mass between ages 40 and 80.

13–53 Answer D

Pharmacokinetics refers to absorption, distribution, metabolism, and elimination of drugs and their metabolites. It is affected by the following physiologic changes in the older adult: decreased creatine clearance, decreased lean muscle mass, increased total body fat, decreased hepatic blood flow, decreased renal blood flow, decreased serum albumin level, and decreased total body water.

13–54 Answer A

White men are most prone to developing nephrolithiasis. The incidence of nephrolithiasis is four times higher in men than women, with white men having three times more attacks than black men, except for struvite stones, which occur more often in black men.

13–55 Answer B

Bill is at a higher risk for developing nephrolithiasis because of his intake of excessive amounts of vitamin C. Other risk factors for nephrolithiasis include use of certain medications, such as vitamin D supplements, calcium, corticosteroids, and acetazolamide (Diamox); a diet high in oxalate or sodium; a low fluid intake; and a history of chronic diarrhea, peptic ulcer disease, gout, recurrent urinary tract infection, skeletal fractures, jejunoileal bypass, or renal tubular acidosis.

13–56 Answer C

A urinary calcium output greater than 300 mg in 24 hours (hypercalcuria) may lead to a diagnosis of nephrolithiasis. The following disorders and diagnostic findings may also lead to a diagnosis of nephrolithiasis: hyperuricosuria (urinary uric acid output greater than 750 mg in 24 hours), hyperoxaluria (urinary oxalate output greater than 40 mg in 24 hours), hypocitraturia (urinary citrate output less than 320 mg/day), gouty diathesis (urinary pH less than 5.5 and gouty arthritis), and hypomagnesuria (urinary magnesium output less than 50 mg in 24 hours). Serum calcium of 8mg/dL is within normal range.

13–57 Answer D

For clients taking nonsteroidal anti-inflammatory drugs on a long-term basis, the following may be found: hemodynamically induced acute renal failure; acute interstitial nephropathy, with or without nephrotic syndrome; salt and water retention; papillary necrosis and chronic renal injury; hyperkalemia; and vasculitis and glomerulitis.

13–58 Answer D

The steps necessary to prevent drug-induced nephrotoxicity include selecting diagnostic procedures or therapeutic measures without nephrotoxic potential; avoiding dehydration; limiting total daily dosage and duration of treatment with certain drugs; being aware of the nephrotoxic potential of specific drugs; identifying clients at risk (those with renal insufficiency, dehydration, salt-retaining states, diabetes, and multiple myeloma); being aware of the increased risk in older adults; carefully assessing the benefits of radiologic procedures or prescribed drugs against potential risk; adjusting the daily dosage to reflect ongoing alterations in the glomerular filtration rate; and avoiding a combination of potentially nephrotoxic drugs.

13–59 Answer D

Erythromycin (E-Mycin) is not associated with acute renal failure (ARF). It is one of the safest antibiotics, even in pregnancy. Nonsteroidal anti-inflammatory drugs and angiotensin-converting enzyme inhibitors can cause the prerenal type of ARF by causing a decreased intrarenal arteriolar resistance. Cimetidine (Tagamet) can cause an elevation in serum creatinine levels without a change in glomerular filtration. Although this is not a problem in clients with normal renal function, there is a more profound effect on serum creatinine concentrations in clients with borderline renal dysfunction.

13–60 Answer A

If Janet stops smoking, her stress urinary incontinence may improve. Studies have shown that clients who smoke increase their risk of stress incontinence by 28% in spite of increased urethral sphincter tone. Limiting fluids, which may result in dehydration, may cause further problems. Although taking a multivitamin is good, it will not help with stress incontinence. In postmenopausal women not on hormone replacement therapy, using an estrogen vaginal cream has been shown to be effective. Lifting weights will not help with the urinary sphincter muscles. Kegel exercises have been proven effective.

13–61 Answer C

Propantheline bromide (Pro-Banthine), dicyclomine hydrochloride (Bentyl), and imipramine hydrochloride (Tofranil) all help urinary incontinence. If the client does not like taking pills, the best (and least invasive) agent to suggest is estrogen vaginal cream. One type of stress urinary incontinence is anatomic incontinence, which may be caused by hormone deprivation and atrophic vaginitis. Using estrogen replacement cream to correct the dryness will also improve bladder outlet function.

13–62 Answer D

Most children with voiding disturbances do not have an anatomic or neurologic disease or a psychological problem causing their enuresis. Although the cause of primary nocturnal enuresis has not been clearly established, it appears to be related to maturational delay of sleep and arousal mechanisms or to a delay in development of increased bladder capacity. Most children can be helped through parental involvement, such as restricting fluids after dinner, encouraging bladder training, awakening the child during the night to void, and using electronic devices that establish a conditioned reflex response to waken the child the moment urination starts. (Such devices are only mildly successful). Imipramine (Tofranil) is effective (50 mg po at bedtime) as well as desmopressin acetate (DDAVP) nasal spray (one spray in each nostril at bedtime).

13–63 Answer D

Cascara sagrada, a stimulant laxative, may cause urine color to be red in alkaline urine and yellow-brown in acid urine; phenazopyridine (Pyridium), a urinary tract analgesic, will cause urine to appear orange to red; and phenytoin (Dilantin), an anticonvulsant, may cause urine to appear pink, red, or red-brown.

13–64 Answer A

Urine specific gravity is increased in clients who are dehydrated, in those who have a pituitary tumor that causes the release of excessive amounts of antidiuretic hormone, and in those with decreased renal blood flow, glycosuria, or proteinuria. The specific gravity of urine is decreased in clients who are overhydrated and in those who have diabetes insipidus or chronic renal failure.

13–65 Answer D

An intravenous pyelogram is contraindicated in clients who are allergic to shellfish or iodinated dyes (if the clients are not properly prepared beforehand with prednisone and diphenhydramine); those who are severely dehydrated, unless the condition is corrected before the procedure; and those with renal insufficiency or multiple myeloma.

13–66 Answer B

After a renal biopsy, the client should be instructed to avoid strenuous activities for at least 2 weeks. These activities include heavy lifting, contact sports, or any other activity that will cause jolting of the kidney.

The client should also be warned that he or she may notice some blood in the urine for the first 24 hours following the procedure and be instructed to drink large amounts of fluid, such as 8–10 glasses of water per day, to prevent clot formation and urine retention. Caution should be used in an oliguric client in renal failure who might develop pulmonary edema with increased fluid intake.

13–67 Answer B

A 24 hour urine test for vanillylmandelic acid (VMA) and catecholamines is done to diagnose hypertension secondary to pheochromocytoma. A pheochromocytoma is an adrenal tumor that frequently secretes abnormally high levels of epinephrine and norepinephrine, resulting in episodic or persistent hypertension from arterial vasoconstriction.

13–68 Answer D

Renal scanning (kidney scan, radiorenography, radionuclide renal imagining, nuclear imaging of the kidney) is used to detect renal infarctions, renal arterial atherosclerosis or trauma, primary renal disease (such as glomerulonephritis or acute tubular necrosis), pathologic renal conditions in clients who cannot have an intravenous pyelogram because of dye allergies, and tumors, abscesses, or cysts; and to monitor rejection of a transplanted kidney and renovascular hypertension.

13–69 Answer D

Renal cysts are usually asymptomatic and usually do not cause flank pain. Pyelonephritis, ureterolithiasis, and vascular occlusion of the kidney (renal vein thrombosis) all usually cause flank pain.

13–70 Answer B

Bile produces urine that is brownish in color. Beets, rifampin (Rifadin), and phenazopyridine (Pyridium) can cause reddish or reddish-orange urine.

13–71 Answer C

The glomerular filtration rate (GFR) is the single best indicator of overall renal function. It increases from birth until age 4–6 years. The GFR is estimated by creatinine clearance, the normal rate of which is between 80 and 125 mL/minute, and decreases with age.

13–72 Answer B

Metabolic alkalosis is a pathophysiologic process that occurs when there is a primary excess in the extracellular fluid of bicarbonate because of loss of acid (hydrogen ions) or the addition of excess bicarbonate. Metabolic acidosis results from an accumulation in the blood of keto acids (derived from fat metabolism) at the expense of bicarbonate. Respiratory acidosis occurs with a reduction of alveolar ventilation, resulting in an accumulation of carbonic acid. Respiratory alkalosis occurs with an increase of alveolar ventilation, resulting in a decrease of carbonic acid.

13–73 Answer A

Excessive alcohol ingestion can cause metabolic acidosis, because alcohol results in excess acid levels in the blood.

13–74 Answer A

Clinical manifestations of metabolic alkalosis include tetany, hypotension, tachycardia, confusion, decreasing level of consciousness, hyperreflexia, dysrhythmias, seizures, and respiratory failure. Nausea and vomiting, weakness, and bradycardia are manifestations of metabolic acidosis.

13–75 Answer B

With arterial blood gas values of: pH 7.39, $PaCO_2$ 48, PaO_2 92, and HCO_3 24, all values are within normal range except for an elevated $PaCO_2$, which would indicate acute respiratory acidosis.

13–76 Answer C

A decreased pH, normal PCO_2, and decreased HCO_3 indicated metabolic acidosis. Renal failure, diabetes, shock, and intestinal fistulas all cause metabolic acidosis because of one of the following reasons: an increased production of metabolic acids from diabetic ketoacidosis, impaired excretion of metabolic acids from renal failure, an increased bicarbonate loss from loss of intestinal secretions and increased renal losses, or an increased chloride level from abnormal renal function.

13–77 Answer B

The kidneys excrete increased amounts of HCO_3 to lower the pH as a mode of compensation for respiratory alkalosis. In respiratory acidosis, renal compensatory mechanisms elevate the bicarbonate level, and eventually the pH approaches normal. Signs of compensation in metabolic acidosis are hyperventilation (causing increased intake of oxygen and increased blowing off of carbon dioxide), decreased $PaCO_2$ and increased amounts of ammonia in the urine. The compensatory response to metabolic alkalosis is retention of carbon dioxide.

13–78 Answer D

Before using the radial artery to draw blood for measurement of arterial blood gas values, the Allen test should be performed to evaluate the presence of the ulnar artery. To perform the Allen test, first cause the hand to blanch by obliterating both the radial and ulnar pulses. Then release the pressure over the ulnar artery only. If the flow is adequate, flushing will immediately be seen. The Allen test is then considered positive and the radial artery may be used to draw the blood.

13–79 Answer D

Cigarette smoke, from both active and passive inhalation, is a significant risk factor for urinary tract neoplasms and may account for half of the incidence of bladder tumors among men and a third among women. Other factors implicated in the formation of urinary tract neoplasms include chemicals and dyes used in the plastics, rubber, and cable industries; the chronic use of phenacetin-containing analgesic agents; and substances in the environment of textile workers, leather finishers, spray painters, hairdressers, and petroleum workers. The breakdown products of these chemicals and those from cigarette smoke are stored in the bladder and excreted in the urine, which causes a local influence on abnormal cell development. Working long hours with inability to void may often result in a bladder infection, not a neoplasm.

13–80 Answer B

With a total cystectomy in a man, the prostate and seminal vessels are also removed, resulting in impotence. With Marvin, it is important to state the facts, then explore his feelings. Referring to the surgeon when you know the answer is an evasive tactic. Asking Marvin how his wife feels negates his own feelings.

13–81 Answer B

Polycystic kidney disease is a hereditary, incurable renal disease in which multiple outpouchings (cysts) of the nephrons occur in both kidneys. The cysts may be filled with urine, serous fluid, blood, or a combination of these. As the cysts enlarge, they distort and compress surrounding renal tissue and blood vessels, causing ischemia and necrosis. Eventually, too few normal nephrons remain to support the client and end-stage renal disease slowly develops.

13–82 Answer A

Clients with glomerulonephritis commonly have a history of beta-hemolytic streptococcal infections as well as a history of systemic lupus erythematosus or other autoimmune diseases. Glomerulonephritis is usually caused by an immunologic response.

13–83 Answer A

Loop diuretics, such as furosemide (Lasix), bumetanide (Bumex), and ethacrynic acid (Edecrin), all act to inhibit sodium chloride reabsorption in the thick ascending limb of the loop of Henle. Mannitol (Osmitrol) is an osmotic diuretic, hydrochlorothiazide (Hydrodiuril) is a thiazide diuretic, and acetazolamide (Diamox) is a carbonic anhydrase inhibitor.

13–84 Answer C

Potassium-sparing diuretics have the following side effects: hyperkalemia, headache, hyponatremia, nausea, diarrhea, urticaria, and menstrual disturbances. Osmotic diuretics may precipitate congestive heart failure; high doses of loop diuretics may cause hearing loss; and thiazide diuretics may cause hypokalemia and hyperglycemia.

13–85 Answer D

Serum hemoglobin and hematocrit testing assesses bleeding or the lack of erythropoietin. A urine creatinine clearance rate measurement is a very specific indicator of renal function and is used to evaluate the glomerular filtration rate. Blood urea nitrogen level measures the nitrogen portion of urea, a product formed in the liver from protein metabolism. Serum albumin measurement is used to assist in the diagnosis of nephrotic syndrome.

13–86 Answer B

Eosinophils in the urinary sediment signify an allergic reaction in the kidney. Leukocytes are present in an infection and interstitial nephritis. Crystals are present in diseases of stone formation or following ethylene glycol intoxication. Erythrocytes are present in large amounts in active glomerulonephritis, interstitial nephritis, and infections.

13–87 Answer D

Magnetic resonance imaging provides direct imaging in several planes conducive to detecting renal cystic disease, inflammatory processes, and renal cell carcinoma. Cystoscopy detects bladder or urethral pathologic processes. Ultrasonography identifies hydronephrosis and fluid collections. Computed tomography identifies tumors and other pathologic conditions that create variations in body density.

13–88 Answer D

A kidneys, ureters, and bladder film can visualize the renal outline and identify lower rib fractures. An intravenous pyelogram compares the kidneys and shows distortion of the calyces and incomplete filling. Renal angiography provides information on the integrity of the renal vasculature. Computed tomography can determine the extent of injury in three dimensions.

13–89 Answer B

The liver on the right side displaces the right kidney slightly downward.

13–90 Answer A

Excretion of less than 500 mL of urine in a 24-hour period is considered oliguria.

13–91 Answer B

Anuria refers to a 24-hour urine volume of less than 100 mL. It indicates a severe reduction in urine volume commonly associated with obstruction, renal cortical necrosis, or severe acute tubular necrosis. It is important to make the distinction between oliguria and anuria so that the appropriate treatment may be initiated early.

13–92 Answer C

The most common cause of death in dialysis clients is cardiovascular failure, with hypotension and diabetes as predisposing factors. Sepsis is the next leading cause of death, followed by bleeding complications, cerebrovascular accidents, pericardial effusion with tamponade, and trauma. The mortality in dialysis clients remains significant, about 15% in the first year.

13–93 Answer A

An acidic urine pH favors precipitation of organic stones: uric acid and cystine. An alkaline urine pH favors the precipitation of inorganic stones: calcium phosphate and magnesium ammonium phosphate (struvite).

13–94 Answer A

The most common metabolic condition that predisposes clients to the formation of kidney stones is idiopathic hypercalciuria. Idiopathic hypercalciuria is present in approximately 50% of stone-forming clients, followed by a low urinary citrate excretion at a slightly lower percentage. Hyperuricosuria is present in approximately 30% of stone-forming clients and hyperoxaluria in approximately 15% of all stone-forming clients.

13–95 Answer D

Complications of urinary tract obstruction include a decrease in glomerular filtration rate with a potential tubular abnormality. Urinary stasis can predispose to infection, renal stones, and papillary necrosis. Sodium and water retention can lead to hypertension.

13–96 Answer D

Eosinophils are present in the urine in interstitial nephritis, urinary tract infections, and acute tubular necrosis (ATN). They are not present in normal urine, but are activated by antigens and antigen-induced hypersensitivity reactions.

13–97 Answer D

Aging affects the kidney by causing a diminished glomerular filtration rate, decreased creatinine production because of decreased muscle mass, urinary incontinence, and obstructive uropathy caused by benign prostatic hypertrophy.

13–98 Answer C

Angiotensin-converting enzyme (ACE) inhibitors are the antihypertensive drugs contraindicated in clients with renal artery stenosis. In bilateral renal artery stenosis or stenosis to a solitary kidney, the renal perfusion pressure and the glomerular filtration rate depend on the local renin-angiotensin system. When the system is blocked by an ACE inhibitor, a marked decrease in the efferent arterial pressure with subsequent decrease in renal perfusion pressure results, causing a diminished GFR.

13–99 Answer C

A urine culture is still the "gold standard" for detecting a urinary tract infection.

13–100 Answer C

Urinary tract infections (UTIs) are the most common cause of burning on urination. UTIs cause approximately 7 million episodes of acute cystitis per year.

References

Ahrens, T, and Prentice, D: Critical Care Certification, ed 4. Appleton & Lange, Norwalk, CT, 1998.

Brown, K: Management Guidelines For Women's Health Nurse Practitioners. FA Davis, Philadelphia, 2002.

Cantarovich, F, and Bodin, L: Functional acute renal failure. In:

Dunphy, LM, and Winland-Brown, J: Primary Care: The Art and Science of Advanced Practice Nursing. FA Davis, Philadelphia, 2004.

Dunphy, LM: Management Guidelines for Nurse Practitioners Working with Adults, ed 2. FA Davis, Philadelphia, 2004.

Fawzy, A, and Pool, J. Benign prostatic hypertrophy and the role of alpha-adrenergic blockade. Fam Med, September 2002.

Fuselier, HA, et al: Cystitis: Not always a simple problem. Patient Care 31(16):34, 1997.

Jaffe, MS, and McVan, BF (eds.): Laboratory and Diagnostic Test Handbook. FA Davis, Philadelphia, 2001.

Kennedy-Malone, L et al. (eds.): Management Guidelines for Gerontological Nurse Practitioners. FA Davis, Philadelphia, 2002.

Kliegman, RM (ed): Practical Strategies in Pediatric Diagnosis and Therapy. WB Saunders, Philadelphia, 2000.

Liano, F, et al: The spectrum of acute renal failure in the ICU compared to that seen in other settings: The Madrid acute renal failure study group. Kidney Int Suppl 53:16–24, 1998.

Nissenson, AR: Acute renal failure: definition and pathogenesis. Kidney Int. Suppl 66:7–10, 1998.

Nolan, CR, and Anderson, RJ: Hospital acquired acute renal failure. J Am Soc Nephrology 9:710–718, 1998.

Ronco, C, et al: Effects of different doses in continuous veno-venous hemofiltration on outcomes of acute renal failure: A prospective randomized trial. Lancet 356:26–30, 2000.

Schiffl, H, et al.: Daily hemodialysis and the outcome of acute renal failure. New Engl J Med 346:305–10, 2002.

Siroky, M, et al: Stress urinary incontinence: Expanding

treatment options. June 2003; available at *www.medscape.com/viewprogram/2484*

Sosa-Guerrero, S, and Gomez, NJ: Dealing with end-state renal disease. Am J Nurs 97(10):44, 1997.

Tierney, LM, et al: Current Medical Diagnosis and Treatment. Appleton & Lange, Stamford, CT, 1998.

Tran, D, et al: Short course versus conventional length antimicrobial therapy for uncomplicated lower UTI in children: A meta analysis of 1279 patients. J Pediatr 139:93-99, 2001.

HOW WELL DID YOU DO?

85% AND ABOVE CONGRATULATIONS! THIS SCORE SHOWS APPLICATION OF TEST-TAKING PRINCIPLES AND ADEQUATE CONTENT KNOWLEDGE.

75–85% KEEP WORKING! REVIEW TEST-TAKING PRINCIPLES AND TRY AGAIN.

65–75% HANG IN THERE! SPEND SOME TIME REVIEWING CONCEPTS AND TEST-TAKING PRINCIPLES AND TRY THE TEST AGAIN.

14 Male Genitourinary Problems

M. CHRISTOPHER SASLO,
JILL E. WINLAND-BROWN,
and
LYNNE M. DUNPHY

14–1 *Bill appears with a tender, ulcerated, exudative, papular lesion on his penis. It has an erythematous halo, surrounding edema, and a friable base. What do you suspect?*

A. A chancre
B. A chancroid
C. Condyloma acuminatum
D. Genital herpes

14–2 *Herb, who has diabetes, is complaining of a rash on his penis. Before examining him, you suspect that he may have:*

A. tinea cruris.
B. genital herpes.
C. *Candida*.
D. intraepithelial neoplasia.

14–3 *You are performing a school physical examination on Damon, age 5. You are unable to retract his foreskin over the glans penis while inspecting his penis. This is referred to as:*

A. phimosis.
B. paraphimosis.
C. microphallus.
D. priapism.

14–4 *When performing a newborn assessment of a male infant, you note that the urethral opening is on the dorsal side of the glans. This is referred to as:*

A. hypospadias.
B. Peyronie's disease.
C. priapism.
D. epispadias.

14–5 *Marty, age 16, states that he feels like he has a "bag of worms" on the left side of his scrotum. Even before examining him, what do you suspect?*

A. A varicocele
B. A hydrocele
C. Cystic nodules
D. A spermatocele

14–6 *Elliot's chief complaint is heaviness in the scrotum. You assess swelling of the testicle, along with warm scrotal skin. What do you suspect?*

A. Cryptorchidism
B. Orchitis
C. Testicular torsion
D. Epididymitis

14–7 *Joe comes in for an evaluation after a testicular self-examination. He states that it is probably nothing to worry about because his testicle is not tender, but he does have a tiny, hard nodule on the testicle. You confirm that there is a hard, fixed nodule on his testicle. Your next course of action would be to:*

A. order a urinalysis.
B. schedule Joe for a recheck next month.

C. refer Joe to a specialist.
D. tell Joe that it is a cyst and if it does not resolve by itself, he will have to have it excised.

14–8 *Max, age 70, is obese. He is complaining of a bulge in his groin that has been there for months. He states that it is not painful, but is annoying. You note that the origin of swelling is above the inguinal ligament directly behind and through the external ring. You diagnose this as a(n):*

A. indirect inguinal hernia.
B. direct inguinal hernia.
C. femoral hernia.
D. strangulated hernia.

14–9 *You are performing a rectal examination on James for follow-up of his melena. What do you expect his stool to look like if his condition has not resolved?*

A. Grayish tan
B. Bright red
C. Pale yellow, greasy, and fatty
D. Black and tarry

14–10 *When performing a prostate examination, you note a tender, warm prostate. What do you suspect?*

A. Benign prostatic hypertrophy
B. Prostatic abscess
C. Prostate cancer
D. Bacterial prostatitis

14–11 *The most common cause of urinary incontinence in men is:*

A. urethritis.
B. prostate cancer.
C. benign prostatic hypertrophy.
D. chronic bacteriuria.

14–12 *Which of the following medications causes retention of urine by inhibiting bladder contractibility and may cause overflow incontinence in certain individuals?*

A. Antispasmodics
B. Drugs that affect the sympathetic nervous system
C. Diuretics
D. Antihistamines

14–13 *Which type of urinary incontinence results from Parkinson's disease and multiple sclerosis?*

A. Overflow incontinence
B. Stress incontinence
C. Urge incontinence
D. Functional incontinence

14–14 *Which technique uses a learned method to target muscle contraction and relaxation to assist with urinary continence?*

A. Biofeedback
B. Kegel exercises
C. Bladder training
D. Prompted voiding

14–15 *In performing an assessment on an older man, you note that he is wearing an incontinence pad. He is very embarrassed. How do you respond?*

A. "It's okay. It's common in men your age."
B. "Let me suggest another method that won't show as much as this pad."
C. "My grandfather does the same thing."
D. "It must be embarrassing; how long have you been doing this?"

14–16 *Jake, age 62, has asymptomatic benign prostatic hypertrophy. You recommend:*

A. no treatment at this time.
B. surgery.
C. balloon dilation.
D. starting him on an alpha blocker.

14–17 *Which drug reduces the size of the prostate, leads to a small average increase in peak urinary flow rate, and reduces some of the symptoms of benign prostatic hypertrophy?*

A. Doxazosin (Cardura)
B. Prazosin (Minipress)
C. Finasteride (Proscar)
D. Terazosin (Hytrin)

14–18 *Which of the following optional tests is not recommended to initially evaluate the need for treatment in clients with benign prostatic hypertrophy?*

A. Postvoid residual urine measurement
B. Urethrocystoscopy
C. Urinary flow rate recording (uroflowmetry)
D. Pressure-flow studies

14–19 *If a client appears with symptoms of benign prostatic hypertrophy, a digital rectal exam is considered beneficial in order to:*

A. detect prostate or rectal malignancy.
B. evaluate for hypospadias.
C. rule out any neurologic problems that may cause the symptoms.
D. detect presence of prostatitis.

14–20 *Which test accurately identifies prostate cancer?*

A. Urinalysis
B. Creatinine measurement
C. Prostate-specific antigen
D. None of the above

14–21 *The most common type of genitourinary dysfunction after a transurethral resection of the prostate is:*

A. erectile dysfunction.
B. urinary incontinence.
C. retrograde ejaculation.
D. decreased libido.

14–22 *Samuel, who takes many different medications, is complaining of erectile dysfunction. You know that several medications could be the cause of Samuel's problem. Which of his medications is not the culprit?*

A. diuretic
B. antihypertensive
C. antipsychotic
D. anticholinergic

14–23 *Martin is complaining of erectile dysfunction. He also has a condition that has reduced arterial blood flow to his penis. This condition is:*

A. epilepsy.
B. multiple sclerosis.
C. diabetes mellitus.
D. Parkinson's disease.

14–24 *Morris is in a new relationship and is not sure whether his erectile dysfunction is caused by stress about his performance or is organic. What simple test do you suggest to determine if he has the ability to have an erection?*

A. Penile Doppler test
B. Penile duplex ultrasonography
C. Intracavernosal injection
D. Postage stamp test

14–25 *Sildenafil (Viagra) 50 mg taken 1 hour before sexual activity is ordered for Mitchell for his erectile dysfunction. What medication must you make sure he is not taking before writing the prescription?*

A. An antihistamine
B. Nitroglycerine
C. A stool softener
D. An anticoagulant

14–26 *Drew has an erectile dysfunction and says that a friend told him about a method that uses a constricting ring around the base of the penis. What is he referring to?*

A. Intracavernous injection therapy
B. External vacuum device
C. Urethral suppositories
D. Surgery

14–27 *Transillumination of fluid in the scrotum may be seen with:*

A. a varicocele.
B. a hydrocele.
C. testicular torsion.
D. testicular cancer.

14–28 *The following would suggest against a differential diagnosis of testicular cancer when examining a patient:*

A. Transillumination of the suspected mass.
B. White race.
C. Scandinavian background.
D. History of cryptorchidism.

14–29 *Which of the following men is more prone to prostatitis?*

A. Jim, age 52, who wears tight jeans and sits at a computer all day
B. Jerry, age 30, who is a cross-country runner
C. Marvin, age 46, who is a dog trainer
D. Justin, age 39, who is a boat salesman

14–30 *The most common gram-positive bacteria that causes both acute and chronic bacterial prostatitis is:*

A. *Staphylococcus aureus.*
B. *Klebsiella.*
C. *Escherichia coli.*
D. Enterobacteriaceae.

14–31 *Harry has benign prostatic hypertrophy and complains of some incontinence. Your first step in diagnosing overflow incontinence would be to order:*

A. urinalysis.
B. cystometrogram.
C. cystoscopy.
D. postvoid residual (PVR) urine measurement.

14–32 *Tim asks you about returning to his normal sex life after surgery for benign prostatic hypertrophy. You tell him:*

A. "You probably won't be able to have an erection after surgery, we need to discuss alternative ways of lovemaking."
B. "You need to wait several months after surgery to make sure the site has healed."
C. "You may resume sexual activity 4–6 weeks after surgery."
D. "You'll have to ask the surgeon."

14–33 *Milton, a 72-year-old unmarried, sexually active white man, presents to your clinic with complaints of hesitancy, urgency, and occasional dribbling. Although you suspect benign prostatic hypertrophy, your differential diagnoses should also include:*

A. Antihistamine use
B. Urethral stricture
C. Detrusson hyperreflexia
D. Renal calculi

14–34 *Jeff, age 19, is a bodybuilder who admits to "stacking" steroids (the practice of using combinations of injectable and oral steroids). You discuss all* *the potential hazards of this with him and stress that the most clearly demonstrated area of health risk with steroid use is to his:*

A. liver (hepatic system).
B. heart (cardiovascular system).
C. hormones (endocrine system).
D. behavior (psychological and neurological systems).

14–35 *George states that he heard that if he takes finasteride (Proscar), he may not need to have surgery for his benign prostatic hypertrophy or if he develops acute urinary retention. How do you respond?*

A. "When the symptoms of urinary obstruction appear, you will need to have surgery."
B. "Taking finasteride has been shown to be safe for only about 6 months."
C. "Proscar has been shown to reduce the probability of surgery and acute urinary retention."
D. "You should have surgery now because it is more effective before the prostate becomes too enlarged."

14–36 *John asks for a prescription for sildenafil (Viagra). He says that the only medication he takes is isosorbide mononitrate (Monoket) tablets and that he has diabetes, but it is controlled by diet alone. What do you tell him?*

A. "Let's try a sample and see how you do."
B. "It's contraindicated with isosorbide mononitrate; let's discuss other options."
C. "Because of your history of diabetes, we can't use it."
D. "I'd better refer you to a urologist."

14–37 *You have just treated Jay's condyloma acuminata with podophyllum in benzoin. What instructions do you give him?*

A. "Refrain from sexual relations for 48 hours."
B. "Don't take a shower until tomorrow morning."
C. "Wash the medication off within 1–2 hours."
D. "Go into the bathroom now and wash the medication off."

14–38 *Your client's chief complaint is blood in the urine. You know that the most common cause of gross hematuria is:*

A. a bladder infection.
B. benign prostatic hyperplasia.
C. bladder tumor.
D. prostatitis.

14–39 *The single most effective method of treating urinary calculi is:*

A. prescribing an antibiotic.
B. having the client increase his fluid intake.
C. performing lithotripsy.
D. performing cystoscopy.

14–40 *Bernard presents to the emergency room with a diagnosis of priapism. Despite application of cold compresses and pain medications, relief is unsuccessful. The treatment of choice is:*

A. Terbutaline 0.25 mg subcutaneously
B. Phenylephrine injection 0.3–0.5 mL into the corpora cavernosa
C. Doxasozin 5 mg sublingually
D. Lidocaine 1% via the glans

14–41 *The bladder tumor antigen test may also be positive with:*

A. testicular torsion.
B. the use of steroids for bodybuilding.
C. scrotal trauma.
D. symptomatic sexually transmitted disease.

14–42 *Michael complains of a urinary tract infection (UTI). Which of the following is a risk factor for a UTI in men?*

A. A history of circumcision
B. A history of testicular torsion
C. Homosexuality
D. Presence of a left inguinal hernia

14–43 *You percuss for pain at the costovertebral angle when examining Marlin. What condition are you assessing for?*

A. Urethritis
B. Pyelonephritis
C. Kidney stone
D. Bladder tumor

14–44 *Jordan appears with a rapid onset of unilateral scrotal pain radiating up to the groin and flank. You are trying to differentiate between epididymitis and testicular torsion. Which test to determine whether swelling is in the testis or the epididymis should be your first choice?*

A. X ray
B. Ultrasound
C. Technetium scan
D. Physical examination

14–45 *Barry, a 32-year-old gay man, has been diagnosed with acute bacterial prostatitis. In addition to providing education, you would encourage him to avoid the following:*

A. rest.
B. nonsteroidal anti-inflammatory drugs.
C. hydration and stool softeners.
D. engaging in any activity which would elicit prostatic massage.

14–46 *In deciding whether or not to treat Morrison, who has benign prostatic hypertrophy, you use the American Urological Association (AUA) scale. No treatment is indicated if the AUA score is:*

A. 36 or higher.
B. 20–35.
C. 8–19.
D. 7 or lower.

14–47 *Which statement is true about the use of alpha blockers in the treatment of symptomatic benign prostatic hypertrophy?*

A. They are safe and effective and should be given in the morning before breakfast.
B. They do not lower blood pressure in normotensive clients.
C. Pedal edema is the most common adverse effect.
D. Blood counts should be monitored periodically for reduction in the platelet count.

14–48 *Manny has been taking finasteride (Proscar) and states that he has had dramatic relief. He previously took terazosin (Hytrin), which also helped, and he asks you about taking that again. You tell him:*

A. "Yes, let's try the combination therapy because two are better than one."
B. "No, they are absolutely contraindicated together."
C. "There is no evidence to support combination therapy."
D. "When symptoms get so bad that you need two different medications, it's time for surgery."

14–49 *What differentiates prostate cancer symptoms from benign prostatic hypertrophy (BPH) symptoms?*

A. Urinary frequency, hesitancy, and intermittency are much worse with prostate cancer.
B. Nocturia is worse with BPH.
C. Dribbling and a weak stream are more indicative of BPH.
D. Symptoms of prostate cancer progress rapidly and develop over a few months, as compared to the long-term development of BPH.

14–50 *An accurate diagnostic tool for prostate cancer is:*

A. a digital rectal examination.
B. a prostate-specific antigen test.
C. a transrectal ultrasound examination.
D. a needle biopsy.

14–51 *Josh and Martha have five children and do not want any more. Josh said he heard about a no-scalpel vasectomy and asks how it works. You tell him:*

A. "For the vasectomy to be permanent, you must have the vas deferens excised."
B. "It's safer for Martha to be sterilized."
C. "A loop of vas deferens is occluded through the scrotal skin."
D. "The testes are twisted, which occludes the vas deferens."

14–52 *Josh has a no-scalpel vasectomy and asks if he can proceed immediately with sexual relations with his wife without worrying about getting her pregnant. You tell him:*

A. "Yes, you are now sterile."
B. "You must use protection for at least 2 weeks after the procedure."
C. "You must use protection for at least 6 weeks after the procedure."
D. "In 6 months, we'll do a sperm count to see if you can discontinue other precautions."

14–53 *Jack and Jane have been married for 6 months and are unable to conceive. They ask you to recommend an infertility specialist. What do you tell them?*

A. "Infertility is not an issue until you have had unprotected sex for at least 1 year."
B. "Let's run some routine tests first; then I'll recommend someone."
C. "Tell me about your sexual experiences."
D. "It's usually a problem with the woman, so let's have Jane examined first."

14–54 *The most common cause of male infertility is:*

A. azoospermia.
B. a problem with sperm motility.
C. a varicocele.
D. antisperm antibodies.

14–55 *Which client will never develop prostate cancer?*

A. Jacob, age 79, who had a transurethral resection of the prostate for benign prostatic hypertrophy
B. Jeffrey, age 11, who recently had an orchiectomy after a traumatic accident
C. Sid, age 70, who has a normal prostate-specific antigen level
D. Johnny, age 32, who is taking steroids for bodybuilding

14–56 *Clinical manifestations of prostate cancer may include symptoms from systems other than the genitourinary system. Which system is unlikely to be affected?*

A. Musculoskeletal
B. Neurologic
C. Systemic
D. Endocrine

14–57 *Nathan is trying to decide between undergoing a radical prostatectomy and radiation therapy for his prostate cancer. He asks you about them. You tell him:*

A. "A radical prostatectomy results in more erectile dysfunction after the surgery than radiation therapy."
B. "A urethral stricture is possible as a result of the radiation therapy as opposed to the surgery."
C. "Radiation therapy may result in diarrhea, proctitis, a rectal ulcer, bowel obstruction, and urinary incontinence."
D. "There is more potential for urinary incontinence after the surgery than after the radiation therapy."

14–58 *Which statement is true about prostatitis and prostatodynia?*

A. The terms are interchangeable.
B. Prostatodynia may be acute, chronic, or nonbacterial.
C. The symptoms of both are extremely irritating.
D. Prostatodynia results in the same symptoms as prostatitis, but there is no evidence of infection.

14–59 *Austin has been on finasteride (Proscar) for 6 months for benign prostatic hypertrophy. A decrease in his PSA from the original value of 5.4 has not occurred. Your initial expectation was:*

A. His PSA will remain stable, neither increasing nor decreasing.
B. Austin's dosage should be reduced only after he has been on the medication for approximately 12 months.
C. A significant reduction in the overall PSA is associated with true benign prostatic hypertrophy.
D. Elevation of the antigen will occur because of the effect of the alpha-andrenergic antagonist.

14–60 *Harvey is complaining of stress urinary incontinence. To assess the autonomic arch innervating the bladder, you test the:*

A. inguinal reflex.
B. neuronal reflex.
C. bulbocavernous reflex.
D. meatal resistance.

14–61 *Mikey had an undescended testicle at birth, and at age 2 it remains in the inguinal region. His mother is afraid of surgery and asks for your advice. How do you respond?*

A. "In many children, the testicle descends close to the sixth birthday."
B. "Even with only one normal testicle, he will have normal development."
C. "If it hasn't descended by now, it probably won't. He needs to have surgery by age 6."
D. "Don't worry, it can remain in that position forever with no problems."

14–62 *Sidney states that he was recently given a diagnosis of prostate cancer and that he has to return to the urologist for staging. He doesn't understand why because he says, "Cancer is still cancer. I just want to get rid of it." You tell him:*

A. "Staging determines the type of treatment required."
B. "You have time to decide on treatment until the cancer gets to the last stage."
C. "Staging will determine the extent of the spread of the cancer."
D. "You already know you have prostate cancer, you don't need another test unless you want to know how long you've had it."

14–63 *The most common sexually transmitted disease (STD) in men is:*

A. genital herpes.
B. genital warts.
C. urethritis.
D. syphilis.

14–64 *Tim, age 12, asks you how long it will take him to make the complete change from preadolescence to adulthood once he starts puberty. You tell him it will take approximately:*

A. 2 years.
B. 3 years.
C. 4 years.
D. all of his teen years.

14–65 *Jerry, age 13, notices a sparse growth of long, slightly pigmented, downy pubic hair at the base of his penis; slightly larger testes; and a larger, red scrotum with a different texture. What Tanner stage is he in?*

A. Stage 1
B. Stage 2
C. Stage 3
D. Stage 4

14–66 *Your friend, a nurse practitioner, states that there is a Tanner Stage 6. Which statement is true about this stage?*

A. Some men continue to develop past stage 5, and although it is slightly abnormal, it is labeled stage 6.
B. It is not a puberty change, but one that occurs in men in their mid-20s.
C. It is the stage that older men go through when their skin atrophies.
D. The testes decrease in size with protracted, debilitating illnesses.

14–67 *Precocious puberty is present if:*

A. a delay in any of the Tanner stages takes longer than 2 years from one stage to the next.
B. the adolescent has had sexual relations.
C. puberty starts before age 9.5 years.
D. an adolescent rushes through all Tanner stages in less than 2 years.

14–68 *Inflammation of the glans and prepuce is called:*

A. balanitis.
B. balanoposthitis.
C. phimosis.
D. paraphimosis.

14–69 *Gerard is complaining of a scrotal mass; however, it is so edematous that it is difficult to assess. How do you determine if it is a hernia or a hydrocele?*

A. You can always return a hernia's contents to the abdominal cavity.
B. Bowel sounds may be heard over a hernia.
C. You can transilluminate a hernia.
D. With a hydrocele, a bulge appears on straining.

14–70 *Harris is complaining of crooked, painful erections. He has palpable, nontender, hard plaques just beneath the skin of his penis. What do you suspect?*

A. Carcinoma of the penis
B. Genital herpes
C. Syphilitic chancre
D. Peyronie's disease

14–71 *Most lesions of the penis are nontender and painless. Which of the following conditions begins with a tender, painful lesion?*

A. Syphilitic chancre
B. Genital herpes
C. Carcinoma of the penis
D. Peyronie's disease

14–72 *Abnormalities of the scrotum are usually painless or nontender. Which of the following is an exception and is usually tender?*

A. Hydrocele
B. Tumor of the testis
C. Spermatocele
D. Tuberculous epididymitis

14–73 *Which of the following scrotal disorders is most common in adolescents?*

A. Acute epididymitis
B. Testicular torsion
C. Atrophic testes
D. Scrotal edema

14–74 *The most common type of hernia is a(n):*

A. indirect inguinal hernia.
B. direct inguinal hernia.
C. femoral hernia.
D. umbilical hernia.

14–75 *Bob just found out that he has syphilis. He asks how long it will be contagious; that is, how long he will be able to spread the disease sexually. You respond:*

A. "Only for the first year."
B. "For 4 years."
C. "For about 10 years."
D. "For life."

14–76 *When teaching Tom how to do a testicular self-examination, which of the following do you tell him?*

A. "Examine your testicles when you are cold because this makes them more sensitive."
B. "Make sure your hands are dry to create friction."
C. "If you feel firmness above and behind the testicle, make an appointment."
D. "Make an appointment if you note any hard lumps directly on the testicle."

14–77 *Balanitis may evolve into a chronic problem. If this occurs, the client is at risk for:*

A. cancer of the penis.
B. cancer of the bladder.
C. diabetes.
D. recurrent herpes simplex II infection.

14–78 *At what age does the foreskin become fully retractable?*

A. 3 months
B. 6 months
C. 9 months
D. 1 year

14–79 *Which of the following can cause phimosis?*

A. Paraphimosis
B. Smegma
C. Adhesions from infection
D. Priapism

14–80 *For inspecting the male genitalia, what is the ideal position for the client and examiner?*

A. The client should be in a modified lithotomy position with the examiner at the foot of the table.
B. The client should be in the dorsal recumbent position and the examiner should approach from the left side.
C. The client should stand and the examiner should assume a seated position in front of the client.
D. The client and examiner should both stand.

14–81 *You are rolling your fingers along the inguinal ligament and you encounter small, freely mobile lymph nodes in this area. What do you suspect?*

A. Nothing; this is not a cause for concern.
B. Something abnormal that warrants further evaluation and possible referral.
C. The lymph nodes should be biopsied.
D. The lymph nodes must be congenital in origin.

14–82 *Bloody penile discharge is unlikely to be associated with the following:*

A. Cancer
B. Ulcerations
C. Urethritis
D. Peyronie's disease

14–83 *When should a blood sample be drawn to measure serum acid phosphatase or prostate-specific antigen levels?*

A. Always before examination of the prostate
B. After examination of the prostate
C. Several days before seeing the client so that you have the results
D. Several days after the examination has shown evidence of an enlargement

14–84 *Urinary tract infections in the male patient are divided into upper- and lower-tract infections. A classic example of an upper-tract infection includes:*

A. cystitis
B. pyelonephritis
C. prostatitis
D. epididymitis

14–85 *The most common prostatitis syndrome found in males of any age is:*

A. bacterial prostatitis
B. prostodynia
C. nonbacterial prostatitis
D. epididymitis

14–86 *Benign prostatic hypertrophy is a common finding as men age. Classically, this condition may begin with difficulty initiating the urinary stream, hesitancy, urgency, postvoid dribbling, urinary frequency, nocturia, urinary retention, sensation of a full bladder immediately after voiding, and incontinence. Other differential diagnoses for these symptoms would most likely exclude:*

A. diabetes mellitus.
B. testicular cancer.
C. cancer of the prostate.
D. neurological disease.

14–87 *Cancer of the prostate often begins with subtle symptoms that develop very slowly over time and, if left untreated, will lead to metastatis. What prognostic finding is not a significant indicator of probable metastatic disease?*

A. Gleason score of 5
B. Sudden onset of weakness of the legs in an older African-American man with known prostate cancer
C. Crawford score of D-3
D. Bladder outlet obstruction

14–88 *Mycoses commonly affect the skin of the groin. Which fungus commonly affects the scrotum?*

A. Tinea cruris
B. *Candida albicans*
C. *Trichomonas*
D. *Trichophyton*

14–89 *At what point of fetal development does sexual differentiation occur?*

A. As soon as fertilization occurs
B. By 4 weeks' gestational age
C. By 8 weeks' gestational age
D. By 12 weeks' gestational age

14–90 *The testes in male infants descend from the retroperitoneal space through the inguinal canal and into the scrotal sacs. This most commonly occurs:*

A. during the second trimester.
B. during the third trimester.
C. during the neonatal period.
D. by age 6 months.

14–91 *Cryptorchidism is a risk factor for:*

A. cancer of the prostate.
B. testicular cancer.
C. bladder cancer.
D. a benign testicular tumor.

14–92 *Erectile dysfunction is a complex phenomenon with a variety of causes. The predominant cause is:*

A. psychological.
B. vascular.
C. neurogenic.
D. drug related.

14–93 *Erectile dysfunction (ED), which affects 18–30 million men in the United States, increases with age. In men over the age of 50, the most commonly found contibutors to ED are:*

A. Endocrine diseases
B. Vascular disorders
C. Neurogenic diseases
D. Psychiatric conditions

14–94 *When evaluating an adolescent boy using the Tanner sexual maturity rating scale, all the following statements are true* ***except:***

A. External genital changes precede pubic hair development.
B. Semen is contained in ejaculate from the time a boy first ejaculates.
C. The "growth spurt" or peak height velocity occurs before the genitalia change.
D. The scrotum enlarges and reddens before the penis.

14–95 *Tommy, age 15, comes to the clinic in acute distress with "belly pain." When obtaining his histo-*

ry, you find that he fell off his bike this morning and has vomited. Upon closer examination, you determine the "belly pain" to be left-sided groin pain or pain in his left testicle. He is afebrile and reports no dysuria. You suspect:

A. testicular torsion.
B. epididymitis.
C. a hydrocele.
D. a varicocele.

Answers

14–1 Answer B

A chancroid is a tender, ulcerated, exudative, papular lesion with an erythematous halo, surrounding edema, and a friable base. It is caused by inoculation of *Haemophilus ducreyi* through tiny breaks in epidermal tissue. A chancre is a small papular lesion that enlarges and undergoes superficial necrosis to produce a sharply marginated ulcer on a clean base and is the lesion of primary syphilis. Condyloma acuminatum (genital warts) range from pinhead-size papules to cauliflower-like groupings of skin-colored, pink, or red lesions. They are caused by human papillomavirus infection of the epithelial cells. Genital herpes simplex virus appears as erythematous plaques, developing into vesicular lesions that may become pustular.

14–2 Answer C

A *Candida* infection is fairly common in clients with diabetes. *Candida* on the penis appears as multiple, discrete, flat pustules with slight scaling and surrounding edema. It is a superficial mycotic infection that occurs in moist cutaneous sites. Other predisposing factors may include moisture, antibiotic therapy, and immunosuppression. Tinea cruris is a fungal infection of the groin that appears as erythematous plaques whose scaling, papular lesions have sharp margins and occasionally clear centers. Genital herpes is caused by skin-to-skin contact with the herpes simplex virus. It causes epidermal degeneration and erythematous plaques; the plaques develop into vesicular lesions that may become pustular. Intraepithelial neoplasia is a human papillomavirus infection with multicolored, multifocal maculopapular lesions.

14–3 Answer A

An unusually long foreskin or a foreskin that cannot be retracted over the glans penis during physical examination is referred to as phimosis. It occurs in uncircumcised males and is normal in infancy. At Damon's age, however, one should be able to retract the foreskin. He needs referral to a urologist. Paraphimosis occurs when the foreskin is retracted and is unable to be returned to the original position. The penis distal to the foreskin usually will become swollen and gangrenous. A microphallus is a normally formed penis that is smaller in size than expected. Priapism is a continuous and pathologic erection of the penis that does not occur as a result of sexual desire.

14–4 Answer D

Epispadias means that the urethral meatus opens on the dorsal side of the glans. Hypospadias means that the urethral meatus opens on the ventral side of the glans. Both must be reported to the physician because a circumcision should not be performed until these conditions are corrected. Peyronie's disease is a condition of penile curvature that occurs with erection. Priapism is a continuous and pathologic erection of the penis.

14–5 Answer A

A varicocele is enlargement of the veins of the spermatic cord that commonly occurs on the left side in adolescent males. It seldom requires treatment. A hydrocele is an accumulation of fluid between the two layers of the tunica vaginalis. It may occur on its own or in response to trauma, inguinal surgery, epididymitis, or testicular tumor. Cystic nodules are round, firm sebaceous cysts that are confined within the scrotal skin. A spermatocele results from blockage of the efferent ductules of the rete testis. It causes a sperm-filled cyst to be formed at the top of the testis or in the epididymis.

14–6 Answer B

Orchitis is an acute, painful onset of swelling of the testicle accompanied by warm scrotal skin. The client usually complains of a heavy feeling in the scrotum. It is typically unilateral, but after 1 week may progress to the other testicle. In cryptorchidism, one or both testicles are undescended. Testicular torsion is a twisting or torsion of the testis. The testicle is enlarged, retracted, and in a lateral position, and is extremely sensitive. The result is venous obstruction, secondary edema, and eventual arterial obstruction. It is a surgical emergency. Epididymitis is caused by a retrograde spreading of pathogenic organisms from the urethra to the epididymis. It results in an indurated, swollen, and tender epididymis. The testes are also usually enlarged and tender.

14–7 Answer C

Testicular cancer is suspected if a hard, fixed, nontender area or nodule is palpated on the testicle. The client should be referred for further evaluation and probably surgery. Testicular self-examination should be taught to all male clients beginning in adolescence. Testicular cancer is more common among men ages 16–35.

14–8 Answer B

A direct inguinal hernia usually occurs in middle-aged to older men and is the result of an acquired weakness caused by heavy lifting, obesity, or chronic obstructive pulmonary disease. The origin of swelling is above the inguinal ligament directly behind and through the external ring. An indirect inguinal hernia is congenital or acquired and is more common in infants younger than 1 year of age and in men age 16–25. The origin of swelling is above the inguinal ligament. The hernia sac enters the canal at the internal ring and exits at the external ring. A femoral hernia, which occurs more frequently in women, is acquired and results from an increase in abdominal pressure as well as muscle weakness. The origin of swelling is below the inguinal ligament. Because Max is not having any pain and the condition has been this way for months, you know that the hernia is not strangulated. A strangulated hernia, which requires immediate referral to a surgeon, results in no blood supply to the affected bowel and causes nausea, vomiting, and tenderness.

14–9 Answer A

Melena is black, tarry stool caused by upper gastrointestinal bleeding. Grayish-tan stool is caused by obstructive jaundice; bright-red stool results from rectal bleeding; and pale-yellow, greasy, fatty stool (steatorrhea) is caused by malabsorption syndromes such as cystic fibrosis or celiac disease.

14–10 Answer D

Bacterial prostatitis, in which the prostate feels very tender and warm, is usually caused by *Escherichia coli*. Clients with bacterial prostatitis usually also have a sudden onset of high fever, chills, malaise, myalgias, and arthralgias. In benign prostatic hypertrophy, the prostate gland would feel soft and nontender and would be enlarged. With prostatic abscess, the prostate feels like a firm, tender, or fluctuant mass. With prostate cancer, the prostate may have single or multiple nodules that are firm, hard, or indurated and are usually nontender.

14–11 Answer C

Benign prostatic hypertrophy is the most common cause of urologic incontinence in men. The enlarged prostate obstructs the bladder neck, resulting in a sensation of incomplete emptying. This results in hypertrophy of the pelvic muscle, which produces more forceful and uninhibited contractions, leading to urgency. Overflow incontinence is concomitant with this obstruction of the bladder neck. Urethritis, or inflammation of the ureter, can be a transient cause of incontinence, but is not that frequent. Although prostate cancer does not usually cause incontinence, the surgery for it might. If the nerves that supply the bladder or urethral sphincter are damaged during surgery, incontinence may persist after surgery. Chronic bacteriuria is common in older adults, but research has not shown a link between urinary incontinence and the presence of chronic asymptomatic bacteriuria.

14–12 Answer D

Antihistamines cause retention of urine by inhibiting bladder contractibility and may cause overflow incontinence in certain individuals. Other medications that may cause overflow incontinence include anticholinergics, antipsychotics, and antidepressants. Antispasmodics may cause excessive muscular relaxation and sphincter incompetency. Drugs that affect the sympathetic nervous system, such as alpha blockers, may relax the smooth muscle of the sphincter and decrease urethral pressure, which increases bladder emptying. Alpha stimulants may increase urethral closure pressure, which may lead to urinary retention. Diuretics may affect continence by causing frequent and large bladder volume that overwhelms the ability of the individual to reach the toilet in time.

14–13 Answer C

There are five types of urinary incontinence: overflow, stress, urge, functional, and transient. Urge incontinence results in the failure to store urine, which may be caused by conditions such as Parkinson's disease, multiple sclerosis, urinary tract infection, bladder stones, or tumors. Overflow incontinence is the failure to empty the bladder, such as occurs with prostatic hyperplasia. Stress incontinence is a failure to store urine. It may be caused by weak pelvic musculature or intrinsic sphincter deficiency. Functional incontinence is caused by the effects of medications, manual dexterity, or mobility. Transient incontinence is usually caused by delirium.

14–14 Answer B

Kegel exercises are a learned technique of pelvic muscle exercises that help with urinary incontinence after 4–5 weeks of consistent daily exercise. When used with biofeedback, they can improve pelvic floor tone and reduce uninhibited bladder contractions. Biofeedback consists of capturing information about a normally unconscious physiological process and subsequently using it in an educational process to accomplish specific therapeutic results, in this case, continence. Bladder training is a form of behavioral modification that helps to restore a normal pattern of voiding and normal bladder function. Clients void at fixed intervals whether the urge to void is present or not. Prompted voiding is also a form of behavioral modification that uses a toileting schedule, verbal feedback, and reinforcement.

14–15 Answer D

The response "It must be embarrassing" is one of empathy and caring. The other responses assume that incontinence is normal and that the client must just contain the urine. Practitioners should instead focus on restoring continence and finding out the cause. Asking, "How long have you been doing this?" helps to assess the problem so that further follow-up and corrective measures can be started.

14–16 Answer A

Asymptomatic clients with benign prostatic hypertrophy (BPH) rarely require treatment. Watchful waiting is an appropriate strategy for following the disease's progression and the development of any complications. Prostate surgery offers the best choice for symptom improvement. A transurethral resection of the prostate is the most commonly used surgical treatment for BPH. Balloon dilation of the prostatic urethra has fewer complications than surgery, but is not as effective in relieving the symptoms. Alpha blockers relax the bladder neck and prostate smooth muscle and offer relief for many clients, particularly in regard to nocturia.

14–17 Answer C

Finasteride (Proscar) is a 5-alpha-reductase inhibitor that blocks conversion of testosterone to dihydrotestosterone. It reduces the size of the prostate, leads to a small average increase in peak urinary flow rate, and results in a reduction of the symptoms of benign prostatic hypertrophy. Usually 6 months or more of treatment are required for maximal effects. Doxazosin (Cardura), prazosin (Minipress), and terazosin (Hytrin) are all alpha-adrenergic receptor blockers that relax the bladder neck and prostate smooth muscle. They also relieve some of the symptoms, but do not affect the size of the prostate.

14–18 Answer B

A urethrocystoscopy is not recommended to initially evaluate the need for treatment in clients with benign prostatic hypertrophy (BPH). A urethrocystoscopy is recommended for men with prostatism who have a history of microscopic or gross hematuria, urethral stricture disease, bladder cancer, or previous lower urinary tract surgery. The self-administered American Urological Association Symptom Index is recommended to evaluate the need for treatment in clients with BPH. Its seven questions relate to symptoms of prostatism and help determine their severity and how they affect the quality of life for the individual. Additional tests that are optional for men with prostatism include urinary flow rate recording (uroflowmetry), measurement of postvoid residual urine, and pressure-flow studies.

14–19 Answer D

Hypospadias is a disorder in which the meatus of the urethra is inferiorly located on the glans. If a client has symptoms of benign prostatic hypertrophy, a digital rectal exam (DRE), and a neurologic examination are performed to detect prostate or rectal malignancy, evaluate anal sphincter tone, and rule out any neurologic problems that may cause the symptoms. A DRE should be performed annually on men over age 40 regardless of symptoms. The American Urological Association Symptom Index is a good tool to use to assess how the symptoms are affecting the man's life.

14–20 Answer D

Although the prostate-specific antigen (PSA) is thought to be a tumor marker for prostate cancer and is used by most practitioners, it does not accurately identify prostate cancer. PSA is a glycoprotein produced by the epithelial cells that line the acini and ducts of the prostate gland. It is secreted into the prostatic ductal system. To be a valuable detector of early prostate cancer in clients with benign prostatic hypertrophy (BPH), a PSA test must be able to identify and distinguish curable cancer from purely benign conditions of the prostate. The PSA has mediocre sensitivity and specificity when the values are between 4 and 10 ng/mL. The normal range is 0.0–4.0 ng/mL. When a client appears with symptoms of BPH, a urinalysis is recommended to rule out a urinary tract infection and hematuria. A creatinine measurement is an assessment of renal function and is recommended in all clients with symptoms of prostatism.

14–21 Answer C

The most common type of genitourinary dysfunction occurring after a transurethral resection of the prostate is retrograde ejaculation (73.4%), followed by erectile dysfunction (13.6%), urinary incontinence (2.1%), and decreased libido (less than 2%).

14–22 Answer A

Many medications may cause erectile dysfunction (impotence); however, diuretics have not been shown to cause it. The following medications have been shown to cause erectile dysfunction: antiandrogens; antihypertensives; anticholinergics; antidepressants; antipsychotics; central nervous system depressants; and drugs of abuse such as alcohol, tobacco, and heroin.

14–23 Answer C

About 50% of men who have had diabetes for longer than 6 years develop erectile dysfunction to some extent as a result of pathological changes in the vascular wall, which lead to a reduction of arterial blood flow to the penis. Many other conditions can cause erectile dysfunction. They include cerebrovascular accidents, spinal cord injury, temporal lobe epilepsy, multiple sclerosis, chronic obstructive pulmonary disease, angina, chronic renal failure, and Parkinson's disease.

14–24 Answer D

The postage stamp test is a simple test the client may do at home by himself to determine if he has the ability to have a nocturnal erection, which would rule out an organic cause of erectile dysfunction. At night, have the client place a row of postage stamps around the penis and tape the ends together. (Self-stick stamps are not recommended.) If, in the morning, the row of stamps has been broken at the perforations, the client probably had an erection during the night.

The test may be done several nights in a row to make sure that the stamps did not come off in the client's sleep. In that case, the row of stamps usually rips randomly, not just at the perforations, as it does during an erection. Other tests that may be done to determine the cause of erectile dysfunction include the penile Doppler test (a noninvasive procedure comparing the penile pressure with the brachial artery pressure), a penile duplex ultrasonography (to assess the penile arteries and diagnose a vascular cause of erectile dysfunction), and an intracavernosal injection (to test for an erection, thus ruling out vascular disease).

14–25 Answer B

Sildenafil (Viagra) has shown promise in clients with erectile dysfunction. It is not effective in men with psychogenic impotence or those with neurological or arterial disease. It potentiates the hypotensive effect of nitrate and is contraindicated for clients receiving nitrates, such as nitroglycerine.

14–26 Answer B

An external vacuum device is a viable method for alleviating erectile dysfunction regardless of the cause of the disorder. A plastic cylinder is placed around the penis, a vacuum pump causes cavernosal engorgement, and a constrictor ring is applied around the base of the penis, allowing the client to hold an erection for 30 minutes. Intracavernous injection therapy consists of injecting the vasoactive drug alprostadil (Caverject) directly into the corpus cavernosom of the penis, causing an erection that lasts 40–60 minutes. Urethral suppositories such as alprostadil are also effective in causing an erection when inserted into the urethra after voiding. Surgery involves inserting a penile prosthesis, of which there are many different types.

14–27 Answer B

A hydrocele is a collection of fluid within the scrotum around the testes. It can be assessed by transillumination of the fluid, which should be performed in a darkened room using a penlight. The fluid will appear light pink, yellow, or red. The mass can be illuminated to show the full size and shape. Masses of the testicles, such as testicular cancer, do not transilluminate, nor do hematomas or testicular torsion. A varicocele is venous dilatation of the pampiniform plexus above the testes; it is typically painful and may not be transilluminated. In infancy, observation is the therapy of choice for a hydrocele. For adults, no treatment is required unless complications are present. If the hydrocele is painful, large, unsightly, or uncomfortable, then several options are available: surgery, sclerotherapy, or an endoscopic procedure.

14–28 Answer A

Transillumination is not clinically significant because a cancerous tumor cannot be succesfully transilluminated. The only undisputed risk factors that have been proven for testicular cancer are white race, especially Scandinavian background, and a history of undescended or partially descended testicles (cryptorchidism).

14–29 Answer B

Athletes who run long distances and those who perform vigorous exercises and workout regimens have a predisposition to prostatitis. Prostatitis, both bacterial and nonbacterial, occurs predominantly between ages 30 and 50 in sexually active men.

14–30 Answer A

The most common gram-positive bacterium that causes both acute and chronic bacterial prostatitis is *Staphylococcus aureus. Streptococcus faecalis* is also a cause. The most common aerobic gram-negative bacteria include *Klebsiella, Pseudomonas, Enterobacteriaceae, Escherichia coli, Proteus mirabilis,* and *Neisseria gonorrhoeae.*

14–31 Answer D

The first step in diagnosing overflow incontinence is to perform a postvoid residual (PVR) urine measurement. Clients with overflow incontinence cannot empty their bladders completely, so after voiding, residual urine remains and this measurement is elevated. A urinalysis, cystometrogram, and cystoscopy are also commonly performed to confirm the cause and diagnosis, but a PVR measurement is the most important component of the diagnosis.

14–32 Answer C

Many clients feel more comfortable talking to their primary care provider, with whom they have an established relationship, and the question of when to resume sex after prostate surgery for benign prostatic hypertrophy is no exception. They may not feel comfortable asking their surgeon; thus they may resume sexual activity too early or wait an exorbitant amount of time. Within 4–6 weeks after surgery, it is safe to resume a full sex life. Before this time, the spasmodic contractions that occur in the prostatic urethra at the time of ejaculation could trigger delayed bleeding. After 6 weeks, the risk of delayed bleeding is very slight. There may be slight discomfort because of the spasm if the area has not completely healed.

14–33 Answer B

Urethral strictures may develop as a result of sexually transmitted diseases and should be considered in a sexually active individual no matter what the age. Antihistamine use generally will result in hesitancy and urinary retention but not result in incontinence. Recent use of Viagra is not associated with urinary urgency. Detrusor hyperreflexia involves urge incontinence characterized by a strong, sudden urgency (not hesitancy), immediately followed by a bladder contraction, resulting in an involuntary loss of urine.

14–34 Answer A

The most clearly demonstrated area of health risk to men using steroids is to the liver (hepatic system). Peliosis hepatitis and hepatoma, cysts, and tumors of the liver are irreversible liver conditions associated with long-term steroid use. Hepatic cholestasis is another common condition, but it is reversible. Continued use of steroids also causes a reduced high-density liproprotein cholesterol level, which may predispose an individual to ischemic heart disease. Elevated blood pressure and fluid and water retention are other cardiovascular effects of steroid use. Steroid use suppresses the gonadotropin levels as well as the body's ability to produce its own testosterone. This may result in priapism, baldness, acne, gynecomastia, and suppressed sperm production. Behavioral problems associated with steroid use include increased aggression and an exaggerated sense of self and grandiosity.

14–35 Answer C

In a long-term (4-year) study in men with symptoms of urinary obstruction and prostatic enlargement, treatment with finasteride (Proscar) reduced symptoms and prostate volume, increased urinary flow rate, and reduced the probability of surgery and acute urinary retention. No other therapies have been shown to decrease the incidence of acute urinary retention in long-term studies. Reducing the risk of acute urinary retention has implications for reducing morbidity as well as reducing the number of men who need surgery. Previously, finasteride was used only for short intervals; this study shows that it is safe for long-term trials. Although alpha-adrenergic blockers also provide symptomatic relief, a reduced requirement for surgery has not been shown.

14–36 Answer B

Because sexual stimulation leads to the release of nitric oxide in the corpus cavernosum and sildenafil (Viagra) potentiates that release, there is a double hypotensive effect between sildenafil and the presence of an existing nitric oxide such as isosorbide mononitrate (Monoket, Imdur, Ismo). Sildenafil is not contraindicated with nitrates found in foods.

14–37 Answer C

The treatment of choice for the client with condyloma acuminata (warts) on the external genitalia is to "paint" them with podophyllum in benzoin. The client should wash the medication off in 1–2 hours because normal tissue may be destroyed along with the warts. Sometimes a repeat treatment is necessary. Carbon dioxide laser treatment might be more effective, but is done only by physicians.

14–38 Answer A

The most common cause of gross hematuria is bladder infection (22%), followed by bladder tumor (14.9%), benign prostatic hyperplasia (12.5%), and prostatitis (9%).

14–39 Answer B

The single most effective method of treating urinary calculi is having the client increase fluid intake to 3–4 L/day. If increased hydration is not effective, a cystoscopy, lithotripsy, or other surgery may need to be performed. Antibiotics are not indicated.

14–40 Answer B

Phenylephrine (Neo-Synephrine) is the drug of choice for first-line treatment of low-flow priapism because the drug has almost pure alpha-agonist effects and minimal beta activity. In short-term priapism (<6 h), especially for drug-induced priapism, intracavernosal injection of phenylephrine alone may result in detumescence. Terbutaline is considered for refractory priapism of greater than 6 hours in duration. Doxazosin is used to treat benign prostatic hypertrophy. Lidocaine is not considered to be efficacious for relief of priapism.

14–41 Answer D

Bladder tumor antigen in urine is a qualitative agglutination test for bladder cancer that detects basement membrane proteins. It tests positive for symptomatic sexually transmitted disease and is also positive within 14 days of prostate biopsy or resection, with renal or bladder calculi, and with genitourinary tract cancers.

14–42 Answer C

Young men can develop a urinary tract infection (UTI), similar to the type of uncomplicated UTI seen in women, which does not require any additional workup. Risk factors include homosexuality, lack of circumcision, a history of prostatitis, unprotected intercourse with a woman who harbors pathogens in her vagina, and sex with men with acquired immunodeficiency syndrome (AIDS) with a CD4 count less than 200/mL. Testicular torsion, a surgical emergency, is not a risk factor. Inguinal hernias have no documented impact on the development of urinary tract infections given anatomical proximity.

14–43 Answer B

Pyelonephritis typically begins with costovertebral angle pain, fever, low back pain, general malaise, and often dysuria, nausea and vomiting, or diarrhea. Physical examination may reveal flushing, tachycardia, hypotension, fever, and signs of dehydration. With urethritis, there is typically burning on urination and a urethral discharge. Kidney stones usually result in pain that "travels" as the stone moves from the kidney to the bladder to the urethra. A bladder tumor usually causes no pain and the initial sign is typically hematuria.

14–44 Answer B

If your client has a rapid onset of unilateral scrotal pain radiating up to the groin and flank and you are trying to differentiate between epididymitis and testicular torsion, an ultrasound test is useful to determine whether the swelling is in the testis or the epididymis and should be your first choice. Initially, before the swelling has reached its peak, a physical exam will probably differentiate, but within a few hours, when the testis also swells, it may not be possible to differentiate between epididymis and testis by palpation. A reactive hydrocele may also develop. A technetium scan will show an increased uptake in the case of epididymitis and decreased uptake in the case of torsion, but the least invasive and most inexpensive test is an ultrasound.

14–45 Answer D

The prostate should not be massaged in acute bacterial prostatitis because it may cause bacteremia and sepsis. In homosexual relationships among men, this is an important educational component. Antibiotics should be ordered as well as supportive therapy such as rest, analgesics, hydration, and stool softeners.

14–46 Answer D

If surgery for benign prostatic hypertrophy is not mandated by obstruction or severe symptoms, it is based on the results of the client's American Urological Association (AUA) scale and the client's choice. If the AUA score is 7 or lower, no treatment is indicated. If the score is 8–19 (moderate) or 20–35 (severe), then medical treatment or surgery can be presented to the client as an option.

14–47 Answer B

Alpha blockers are an effective treatment of symptomatic benign prostatic hypertrophy. They reduce symptoms in 60–70% of clients with nearly 50% improvement in urinary flow rates. They do not lower the blood pressure in normotensive clients. Dosing must begin with the lowest dose, preferably at bedtime, so the client will sleep through any mild adverse effects such as malaise, fatigue, dizziness, or orthostatic hypotension. Pedal edema is a rare adverse effect. Blood counts should be monitored occasionally for reduction in white or red blood cell counts.

14–48 Answer C

Combination therapy with an alpha blocker such as terazosin (Hytrin) or finasteride (Proscar) is not supported by the literature. One study showed no improvement when combination therapy was tried. Combination therapy involves extra expense and increased risk of adverse effects, and has unproven effectiveness; therefore, it should not be used until successful trials have ensued.

14–49 Answer D

Symptoms of prostate cancer can mimic the symptoms of benign prostatic hypertrophy (BPH); however, with prostate cancer the symptoms rapidly progress over a few months as compared to those of BPH, which may take several years to develop. Symptoms of both prostate cancer and BPH include urinary frequency, hesitancy, intermittency, nocturia, dribbling, and a weak urinary stream.

14–50 Answer D

A needle biopsy takes a histologic sampling of the prostate gland and is diagnostic for prostate cancer. A digital rectal exam accurately predicts prostate cancer in 24% of cases. An extremely elevated prostatic-specific antigen (PSA) level usually indicates prostate cancer; however, about 25% of men with prostate cancer will have a normal PSA level, and other conditions, such as benign prostatic hypertrophy, may raise the PSA level. Transrectal ultrasound is most commonly used to guide the needle biopsy; however, it is not a very accurate screening or diagnostic tool.

14–51 Answer C

A no-scalpel vasectomy (NSV) is a method of delivering a loop of vas deferens through the scrotal skin for occlusion. The skin is stretched to create an opening, which speeds the procedure and avoids the need for cutting through tissue Postoperative complications are minimized this way. It does result in permanent sterility. Because there is no excision, the NSV is safer than a tubal ligation would be for a woman. Minimal postoperative complications include swelling, bruising, and pain in the scrotal area.

14–52 Answer C

A man is still capable of fertilizing an egg for weeks after a no-scalpel vasectomy; therefore a sperm count should be obtained after 4 weeks. Sperm cannot survive in the ampulla of the vas for more than 3 weeks, and it takes about 15 ejaculations for most men to clear the ampulla of sperm. A repeat sperm count is done 2 weeks after the first, and if both show azoospermia, other precautions may be discontinued at that time.

14–53 Answer A

Infertility is defined as 1 year of unprotected intercourse in which conception has not occurred. Although routine tests, such as thyroid studies, may be performed, a specialist will usually not see a couple until they have been "trying" for 1 year. Although you may ask how often they have been having intercourse—because once a month is certainly different from 3 times a week—the definition of infertility remains the same. Although the cause of infertility is found in the man 26–30% of the time, most specialists perform a comprehensive diagnostic evaluation on both members of the couple.

14–54 Answer C

The most common cause of male infertility is a varicocele. Other causes include oligospermia or azoospermia, problems with sperm function or motility, abnormalities of sperm morphology, and, rarely, an antisperm antibody.

14–55 Answer B

In the early stages of prostate cancer, the tumor is androgen-dependent. Testosterone is the major androgen, and clients who have undergone an orchiectomy before puberty never develop adenocarcinoma of the prostate.

14–56 Answer D

Other systems besides the genitourinary system may be affected when prostate cancer is present. There may be musculoskeletal manifestations (bone or joint pain), neurological symptoms (bowel or bladder dysfunction, muscle spasms), and systemic symptoms (weight loss, fatigue).

14–57 Answer C

Radiation therapy may result in diarrhea, proctitis, rectal ulcer, bowel obstruction, and urinary incontinence. Urinary incontinence may also occur after a radical prostatectomy. Both therapies may cause erectile dysfunction and a urethral stricture.

14–58 Answer D

Prostatodynia is a condition in which the client experiences the symptoms of prostatitis but demonstrates no evidence of infection or inflammation. Prostatitis may be acute bacterial, chronic bacterial, or nonbacterial (the most common type).

14–59 Answer C

After 6 months of therapy with finasteride (Proscar) for benign prostatic hypertrophy, the prostate-specific antigen (PSA) level will decrease by about 50%. Testing can then be repeated annually. If the PSA level has not decreased, you should suspect prostate cancer and proceed to evaluate for such. Finasteride is a 5-alpha reductase inhibitor and will affect PSA levels, as opposed to other agents such as alpha-andrenergic antagonists, which do not affect PSA levels.

14–60 Answer C

After palpating the prostate gland, which is the first step in evaluating a male client complaining of stress urinary incontinence, you should evaluate the autonomic arch innervating the bladder by testing the bulbocavernous reflexes. By squeezing the glans penis, you should note contraction of the anal sphincter in an individual without incontinence. An absent reflex suggests that there has been an interruption of the normal neuronal arch. If the individual is able to contract the rectal sphincter voluntarily, neuronal competence is also positive.

14–61 Answer C

In boys with undescended testes, fewer than 1% have their testes descend after the first year. Orchiopexy needs to be performed before age 6 to promote normal spermatogenesis and hormone production, prevent tumor formation, and leave the testis in a location where it can be easily palpated. Testes that remain undescended by puberty should be removed.

14–62 Answer C

Staging will determine the extent of the spread of the cancer. The prostate cancer tissue is graded histologically. The most widely used system is the Gleason system, which rates cancer on a scale of 1–5 (1 is a well-differentiated cancer and 5 is anaplastic cancer). Another method is that of the American Urological Association, which uses a -D (localized disease) and D (metastatic disease) classification, with subcategories of 1 and 2 following the letters. Staging does not determine the type of treatment required, but helps the provider and the client discuss options available. Clients with localized prostate cancer should probably either have a surgical prostatectomy or radiotherapy. Watchful waiting has also been used at this stage. Advanced disease requires systemic chemotherapy or hormonal manipulation. Staging will not be able to establish how long a client has had prostate cancer.

14–63 Answer C

The most common sexually transmitted disease in men is urethritis. It may be gonococcal or nongonococcal. Gonococcal urethritis is caused by *Neisseria gonorrhoeae*. Nongonococcal urethritis is usually caused by *Chlamydia trachomatis*. The three most common genital ulcer diseases in order are genital herpes, syphilis, and chancroid.

14–64 Answer B

The complete sequence of anatomic changes that occur in the male genitalia from preadolescence to adulthood requires approximately 3 years. (In some individuals, it takes less than 2 years; in others, it spans almost 5 years). The first change, which usually begins between age 9.5–13.5, is an increase in the size of the testes. Next, pubic hair appears and the penis begins to grow.

14–65 Answer B

In Tanner stage 2, there is sparse growth of long, slightly pigmented, downy hair, straight or only slightly curled, chiefly at the base of the penis. There is slight or no enlargement of the penis, the testes are larger, and the scrotum is larger, somewhat reddened, and altered in texture. Stage 1 is the preadolescent stage. Stages 3 and 4 involve more evidence of maturity. Stage 5 is the adult phase.

14–66 Answer B

In most men (80%), after they are fully developed, pubic hair continues to spread further up the abdomen in a triangular pattern directed toward the umbilicus. This is not completed until they are in their mid-20s or later, if it is going to happen, and is Tanner stage 6. In older men, pubic hair decreases and becomes gray. The penis decreases in size and the testicles hang lower in the scrotum. Although the testes decrease in size with protracted, debilitating illnesses, they do not necessarily decrease with aging.

14–67 Answer C

Precocious puberty is present if puberty starts before age 9.5 years. Puberty is considered delayed if no testicular increase has occurred by age 13.5 and if pubic hair has not reached Tanner stage 2. Pubertal delay also occurs if the boy has not reached stage 3 within 4 years of reaching stage 2.

14–68 Answer B

Balanoposthitis is inflammation of the glans and prepuce. Balanitis is inflammation of the glans. Phimosis is a tight prepuce that cannot be retracted over the glans. Paraphimosis is a tight prepuce that, once retracted, gets caught behind the glans and cannot be returned, resulting in edema.

14–69 Answer B

Bowel sounds may be heard over a hernia, but not over a hydrocele. Some hernias are not able to be returned to the abdominal cavity. A hernia is incarcerated when its contents cannot be returned; it is strangulated when the blood supply to the entrapped contents is compromised. Scrotal swellings containing serous fluid transilluminate, whereas those containing blood or tissue do not. A bulge that appears on straining suggests a hernia.

14–70 Answer D

In Peyronie's disease, the client has palpable, nontender, hard plaques just beneath the dorsal skin of the penis and usually complains of crooked, painful erections. With carcinoma of the penis, there is usually an indurated, nontender nodule or ulcer, and usually the man is uncircumcised. Genital herpes appears as a cluster of small vesicles, followed by shallow, painful, nonindurated ulcers on red bases. They may appear anywhere on the penis, and the initial outbreak is usually the worst. A syphilitic chancre is an oval or round, dark red, painless erosion or ulcer with an indurated base. It feels like a button that is lying directly underneath the skin. It may also be associated with nontender, enlarged inguinal lymph nodes.

14–71 Answer B

Genital herpes begins with a tender, painful ulcer on the penis. Most other conditions begin with nontender, painless lesions such as those found with syphilitic chancre, carcinoma of the penis, Peyronie's disease, and venereal warts.

14–72 Answer D

Tuberculous epididymitis is a chronic inflammation of tuberculosis. It produces a firm enlargement of the epididymis, which is usually tender, and thickening or beading of the vas deferens. A hydrocele is a nontender, fluid-filled mass that is in the space within the tunica vaginalis. A spermatocele is a painless, movable cystic mass just above the testis. A tumor of the testis is usually a painless nodule.

14–73 Answer B

Testicular torsion or torsion of the testicle on its spermatic cord is the most common scrotal disorder in adolescents. It produces an acutely painful, tender, and swollen scrotum. Because of the potential of circulation being constricted, it is a surgical emergency. Acute epididymitis occurs chiefly in adults and is an acutely inflamed epididymis that is tender and swollen. Atrophic testes are small, soft testes associated with several conditions, such as cirrhosis, myotonia dystrophia, administration of estrogens, and hypopituitarism. Scrotal edema is usually associated with generalized edema in adults and is usually related to cardiac or nephrotic conditions.

14–74 Answer A

An indirect inguinal hernia is the most common type of hernia affecting all ages and both genders. The point of origin is above the inguinal ligament and often travels into the scrotum. A direct inguinal hernia is less common and usually occurs in men over age 40. The point of origin is above the inguinal ligament and rarely travels into the scrotum. The femoral hernia is the least common and occurs more often in women than in men. The point of origin is below the inguinal ligament and never travels into the scrotum in men. An umbilical hernia occurs more frequently in infants and is a protrusion of part of the intestine at the umbilicus.

14–75 Answer B

By the end of the fourth year, syphilis can no longer be spread sexually. Clients are most infectious (90% contagious) during the first year of infection and become less so with each following year (5% during the second year), until the end of the fourth year, when they no longer spread the disease sexually.

14–76 Answer D

Men should be advised to perform a monthly testicular self-examination and to call if they notice any hard lumps directly on the testicle, whether the lumps are tender or not. Testicles should be examined when taking a warm shower or bath with soapy hands to allow easy manipulation of the tissue. If parts of the testicle above and behind feel rather firm, this is the epididymis and is normal. The spermatic cord, a small, round, movable tube, extends up from the epididymis and feels firm and smooth.

14–77 Answer A

Balanitis is an inflammation of the glans penis and is a possible causative factor in the development of cancer of the penis. Balanitis may be a common problem in clients with diabetes; however, it does not cause diabetes. Although there may be some relationship between balanitis and recurrent herpes simplex II, herpes may occur anywhere. Balanitis refers specifically to inflammation, not necessarily of a vesicular variety, of the glans penis. Reiter's syndrome is frequently accompanied by circinate balanitis, a painless eruption on the glans that begins as small blebs that then coalesce into a large circular ring about the size of a dime.

14–78 Answer D

The foreskin of the penis is not fully retractable until age 1 year. Diaper rash can cause balanitis, an acute inflammation of the glans penis. Uncircumcised clients may develop phimosis after balanitis.

14–79 Answer C

Phimosis, defined as inability to retract the foreskin of the penis, may be caused by a congenital malformation or, secondarily, by adhesions resulting from infections. It normally takes until age 1 year for complete retraction of the foreskin. Paraphimosis is the term used to refer to the inability to replace the foreskin, once retracted, because of edema of the glans. (If examining an unconscious client, be sure to return the foreskin to its usual state; failure to do this may result in severe edema). Smegma refers to the cheesy, white material under the foreskin, which does not in and of itself cause phimosis. Priapism is a prolonged, generally painful erection, usually unaccompanied by sexual desire.

14–80 Answer C

To allow an effective visual inspection of the male genitalia, the client should stand in front of the examiner and the examiner should assume a seated position in front of the client. If the client is unable to stand or the examination continues with the client lying, a supine position is best.

14–81 Answer A

Lymph nodes in the inguinal area, if small and mobile, are not considered abnormal. The lymphatics from the perineum, legs, and feet drain into this area, and thus it is not surprising that small lymph nodes are frequently encountered.

14–82 Answer A

Bloody penile discharge does not occur with Peyronie's disease. Bloody penile discharge requires close investigation, including the length of time of the discharge. Ulcerations, neoplasms, and urethritis are all common causes of bloody penile discharge. A thick, yellow, purulent discharge is commonly associated with chronic prostatitis or gonococcal urethritis. With Peyronie's disease, also known as plastic induration of the penis, the client may complain of curvature of the penis during erection.

14–83 Answer B

The rectal and prostate examination does not cause false-positive elevations of levels of the serum acid phosphatase or prostatic-specific antigen (PSA) in clients with benign prostatic enlargements. Therefore, it is not necessary to draw blood to test these levels before the rectal and prostate examination. The exam can, however, cause a rise in the acid phosphatase level in clients with malignant prostatic enlargement or in those with malignancy that has become refractive to hormonal therapy. Thus, to improve the sensitivity of the serum acid phosphatase and the PSA tests for detecting prostatic malignancy, they should be drawn after the rectal and prostate exam.

14–84 Answer B

Pyelonephritis is a classic example of upper tract urinary infections in the male. Pyelonephritis results from hematogenous or asending infection. Bacteremia, particularly with virulent organisms such as *Staphylococcus aureus,* can result in pyelonephritis with focal renal abscesses. Prostatitis, epidiymitis, cystitis, and urethritis are some of the lower-tract diseases that affect males.

14–85 Answer A

Staphylococcus aureus is the pathogen least associated with prostatitis. All the others, *Escherichia coli, Klebsiella,* and *Proteus mirabilis,* including *Enterobacter,* do cause prostatitis.

14–86 Answer B

Testicular cancer appears as a hard, painless lump in the testes and usually affects men ages 20–34. Other differential diagnoses for symptoms classically seen in men with benign prostatic hypertrophy, such as difficulty initiating stream, hesitancy, urgency, postvoid dribbling, frequency, nocturia, retention, sensation of a full bladder immediately after voiding, and incontinence, include diabetes mellitus, cancer of the prostate, and some neurological diseases that can lead to voiding disorders.

14–87 Answer D

Bladder outlet obstruction (BOO) can have either a bacterial or physiological etiology, and does not necessarily indicate a metastatic process. Such disorders as bacterial urethritis can lead to BOO if left untreated. Gleason scores have been used to stage cancers and with a score of 4–5, metasastatic processes are considered likely. Likewise, a Crawford score of D2 indicates metastatis to bone and other organs. Sudden onset of weakness in the lower extremities can indicate metastisis to the spine with possible cord compression.

14–88 Answer B

Tinea cruris ("jock itch") tends to affect the groin, whereas *Candida albicans* commonly affects the scrotum. *Trichomonas* infection does not evidence itself as a skin rash. *Trichophyton* causes tinea of the feet.

14–89 Answer D

The external genitalia are identical for males and females at 8 weeks gestational age, but by 12 weeks sexual differentiation has occurred. Any fetal insult during weeks 8 and 9 of gestation may lead to major anomalies of the external genitalia.

14–90 Answer B

The testes most commonly descend from the retroperitoneal space through the inguinal canal and into the scrotal sacs during the third trimester. In some cases, one or both testes may still lie within the inguinal canal at birth, with the final descent into the scrotum occurring during the early neonatal period. Descent of the testicles may be arrested at any point or may follow an abnormal path.

14–91 Answer B

Cryptorchidism, failure of one or both of the testes to descend into the scrotum, is a risk factor for testicular cancer. Most testicular tumors are malignant. Testicular cancer is the most common solid tumor in young men age 17–34. It begins as an irregular, nontender mass fixed on the testes that does not transilluminate.

14–92 Answer B

Erectile dysfunction has an organic origin in approximately 70% of cases. Of those cases, approximately 80% are related to vascular problems. The most common problem is generalized atherosclerosis that interferes with normal arterial function. Other vascular etiologies include hypertension, peripheral vascular disease, arterial insufficiency, trauma, or congenital abnormalities. Neurogenic disorders of the somatic, parasympathetic (cholinergic), sympathetic, and central nervous systems can cause or contribute to erectile dysfunction. Other diseases associated with erectile dysfunction include Parkinson's disease, cerebrovascular accident, Alzheimer's disease, and diseases that create perfusion neuropathies such as diabetes and alcoholism. Erectile dysfunction is drug related in 25% of cases, with the common offenders being antihypertensive agents, nonsteroidal anti-inflammatory drugs, digoxin, antidepressants, sedatives, and antiandrogens.

14–93 Answer B

Vascular diseases account for nearly half of all cases of erectile dysfunction. These include atherosclerosis, peripheral vascular disease, myocardial infarction, and arterial hypertension. Less frequent but nonetheless important factors include systemic diseases such as diabetes, scleroderma, renal failure, and liver cirrhosis; and neurogenic diseases such as epilepsy, stroke, MS, and Alzheimer's disease. Other contributing factors include psychiatric conditions and penile, endocrine, nutritional, hematological, and medication-associated causes.

14–94 Answer B

Semen is not usually present in the first ejaculate. Ejaculation may occur by Tanner stage 3, but semen is usually not identified until later. In men, the growth of the penis, testes and scrotum, and pubic hair is used to assign sexual maturity ratings (or Tanner stages) from 1–5. The examiner should record two ratings, one for pubic hair and one for genitalia. If the development of the penis differs from that of the testes and scrotum, the two ratings should be averaged to determine the Tanner stage.

14–95 Answer A

Testicular torsion is a condition in which the testes twist on the spermatic cord, thereby compromising blood flow to the testes. This is a surgical emergency. Examination usually reveals a tender scrotal mass high in the hemiscrotum, and there is frequently a reactive hydrocele around the testes obscuring anatomic detail. The scrotum can become erythematous and edematous. The cremaster reflex is frequently blunted on the side of the torsion. Epididymitis usually is accompanied by fever, as well as urethral discharge, and usually occurs in boys older than Tommy. Although a hydrocele may develop secondary to the torsion, the intense discomfort and acute onset accompanied often by nausea distinguish the possibility of testicular torsion. A varicocele, which usually occurs in young men, may cause pain, but does not usually develop acutely.

References

Brosman, SA, and Leslie, SW: Erectile dysfunction. E-medicine Online Journal, November 2002.

Dunphy, LM, and Winland-Brown, JE: Primary Care: The Art & Science of Advanced Practice Nursing. FA Davis, Philadelphia, PA, 2001.

Estes, MEZ: Health Assessment and Physical Examination. Delmar, Albany, NY, 1998.

Gleich, P: Prostatitis: A state-of-the-art review of diagnosis and therapy. Consultant 38:2, 2001.

Kamel, HK, and Kaiser, FE: Erectile dysfunction: A guide to causes and current treatment options. Consultant 38:6, 2002.

Leveilee, RJ, et al: Prostate Hyperplasia, Benign. E-medicine Online Journal, February 2003.

Maloney, C: Urinary incontinence: A guide to the diagnosis of chronic and reversible causes in a primary care setting. Am J Nurse Pract 2:3, 1998.

McConnell, JD, et al: The effect of finasteride on the risk of acute urinary retention and the need for surgical treatment among men with benign prostatic hyperplasia. N Engl J Med 338:9, 1998.

Poole, RM: News from 98th Annual Meeting of the American Urological Association (AUA). Inpharma Weekly 1391:14–15, June 14, 2003.

Qureshi, S: Prostate Cancer: Metastatic and Advanced Disease. E-medicine Online Journal, March, 2002.

Rakel, RE: Textbook of Family Practice, ed 6. WB Saunders, Philadelphia, 2002.

Rous, SN: The Prostate Book: Sound Advice on Symptoms and Treatment.: WW Norton, New York, 1994.

Sabo, D, and Gordon, DF: Men's Health and Illness: Gender, Power, and the Body. Sage, Thousand Oaks, CA, 1995.

Sexually Transmitted Diseases Treatment Guidelines, 2002. Morbidity and Mortality Weekly Report 51:RR6, May 10, 2002.

Taylor, RB: Manual of Family Practice, ed 2. Lippincott Williams & Wilkins, Philadelphia, 2002.

Tubaro, A, et al: Early Treatment of Benign Prostatic Hyperplasia: Implications for Reducing the Risk of Permanent Bladder Damage. Drugs & Aging. 20(3):185–195, 2003

U.S. Department of Health and Human Services: Benign Prostatic Hyperplasia: Diagnosis and Treatment. AHCPR publication No. 94-0582. U.S. Department of Health and Human Services, Rockville, MD, 1994.

Wallach, J: Handbook of Interpretation of Diagnostic Tests. Lippincott-Raven, Philadelphia, 2000.

HOW WELL DID YOU DO?

85% AND ABOVE CONGRATULATIONS! THIS SCORE SHOWS APPLICATION OF TEST-TAKING PRINCIPLES AND ADEQUATE CONTENT KNOWLEDGE.

75–85% KEEP WORKING! REVIEW TEST-TAKING PRINCIPLES AND TRY AGAIN.

65–75% HANG IN THERE! SPEND SOME TIME REVIEWING CONCEPTS AND TEST-TAKING PRINCIPLES AND TRY THE TEST AGAIN.

Female Genitourinary Problems 15

JILL E. WINLAND-BROWN
GRETCHEN HOPE MILLER HEERY

15–1 *A sexually active woman should be aware that genital herpes simplex virus:*

A. may be transmitted to a partner or newborn even in the absence of lesions because of viral shedding.
B. is suppressed during menstruation, physical or emotional stress, immunosuppression, sexual intercourse, and pregnancy.
C. recurrences usually last the same length of time as the initial outbreak.
D. requires the use of condoms only during outbreaks.

15–2 *Jane is in her first trimester of pregnancy and is experiencing "morning sickness" because of:*

A. production of human chorionic gonadotropin.
B. suppression of estrogen.
C. suppression of linea alba.
D. suppression of progesterone.

15–3 *You have discussed the pros and cons of starting Mary, age 50, on hormone replacement therapy (HRT). She has a family history of osteoporosis and has begun having hot flashes, which she cannot tolerate. You have decided to initiate therapy for 1 year. She asks you if she also needs to take calcium or vitamin D for prevention of osteoporosis. How do you respond?*

A. "Research has shown that HRT alone is sufficient to protect against osteoporosis."
B. "Yes, calcium intake should be increased to 1200 mg/day along with 600 mg of vitamin D to decrease bone turnover and increase intestinal absorption."
C. "If you decide to take calcium and vitamin D, you can stop the HRT."
D. "If you are getting sufficient exercise, you don't need to take calcium and vitamin D."

15–4 *The* Mobiluncus *species causes which sexually transmitted disease?*

A. Condylomata acuminata
B. Bacterial vaginosis
C. Human papilloma virus
D. Lymphogranuloma venereum

15–5 *Reiter's syndrome is a complication of:*

A. bacterial vaginosis.
B. syphilis.
C. chlamydia.
D. gonorrhea.

15–6 *Why is ceftriaxone (Rocephin) the drug of choice for gonorrhea?*

A. It treats all strains of gonorrhea.
B. It is the least expensive.
C. It provides effective single-dose therapy.
D. All of the above.

15–7 *Genital herpes is:*

A. cured with acyclovir (Zovirax).
B. best managed with trichloroacetic acid 80–90% applied directly to the lesion.
C. expected to be completely resolved within 21 days (for the primary lesion).
D. not a factor in continuing with intercourse.

15–8 *Emotional support is best given to the client with a sexually transmitted disease by:*

A. offering many alternatives.
B. authentic active listening.
C. assuring the client that everything will be okay.
D. emphasizing the duration of the disease.

15–9 *Cynthia says that her healthcare provider wants to do a colposcopy. She asks you what this is. You tell her that a colposcopy:*

A. visualizes the cervical, vaginal, or vulvar epithelium under magnification to identify abnormal areas that may require a biopsy.
B. involves removal of one or more areas of the endometrium by means of a curette or small aspiration device without cervical dilation.
C. allows visual examination of the uterine cavity with a small fiberoptic endoscope passed through the cervix.
D. allows visualization of the abdominal and pelvic cavity through a small fiberoptic endoscope passed through a subumbilical incision.

15–10 *Human papilloma virus may lead to:*

A. pelvic inflammatory disease.
B. molluscum contagiosum.
C. cervical dysplasia.
D. genital herpes.

15–11 *Emergency contraception refers to:*

A. an induced abortion in an emergency room (ER).
B. quickly starting on birth control pills in anticipation of sexual intercourse.
C. having a medroxyprogesterone (Depo-Provera) injection in the ER every 12 weeks.
D. taking 2 doses of an estrogen-plus-progestin birth control pill 12 hours apart within 72 hours of unprotected coitus to induce abortion.

15–12 *Brianne, age 24, complains of urgency, frequency, and dysuria. Your dipstick test shows no hematuria and her urine culture shows no growth. What is your next action?*

A. You suspect a sexually transmitted disease, so you obtain a culture of the urethra, do a potassium hydroxide wet prep, and obtain another urine culture.
B. You suspect urethra irritation, so you tell her to take showers, not bubble baths, and wear white, dry underwear and loose-fitting clothing.
C. You suspect a urinary tract infection not visible yet on culture, so you start her on Bactrim DS.
D. You suspect that the vulva is irritated. You tell her to take a relaxing shower and dry the area well and come back in 1 week if there is no improvement.

15–13 *The most common type of vaginal infection is:*

A. candidiasis.
B. trichomoniasis.
C. gonorrhea.
D. bacterial vaginosis.

15–14 *Samantha has a diagnosis of a chlamydia vaginal infection. You think that it is questionable whether she will fill the prescription that you write or take it for 7 days as ordered. What would you do?*

A. Give azithromycin (Zithromax) 1 g po now.
B. Emphasize the importance of the drug and tell her the consequences of not taking it.
C. Send out the public health nurse to follow up on whether she takes the drug for 7 days.
D. Assume that Samantha is an adult and will follow your instructions.

15–15 *A dancer from an adult club down the street comes in for a renewal of her birth control pill prescription. She says that everything is fine. On examination, you find grayish-white vaginal discharge, greenish cervical discharge, and cervical motion tenderness. You might suspect all of the following* ***except:***

A. gonorrhea.
B. interstitial cystitis.
C. bacterial vaginosis.
D. chlamydia.

15–16 *Before performing a Pap smear, certain instructions should be given to the client. These include:*

A. "Insert nothing in the vagina for 24 hours before the exam."
B. "Douching enhances visualization of the cervix and should be done before the appointment."
C. "An infection or menstrual period is no reason to cancel the appointment."
D. "The procedure is completely painless."

15–17 *When a woman has extreme spasticity, which position should she assume for a Pap smear?*

A. "OB" stirrups position
B. Knee-chest position while prone
C. V-shaped position without stirrups
D. Side-lying position

15–18 *Signs and symptoms of a genital herpes infection include all of the following* ***except:***

A. painful or pruritic vesicles.
B. dysuria.
C. prodromal tingling or pruritus of the genital region.
D. white curdlike plaques on a red base in the vagina.

15–19 *Herpes simplex virus is potentially but least likely acquired by an infant:*

A. before labor.
B. during delivery.

C. postnatally.
D. during the neonatal period.

15–20 *Why does a woman with an intact uterus need to add progestin to her estrogen replacement therapy?*

A. Progestin assists in relieving the typical hot flashes of menopause.
B. Progestin reduces the incidence of endometrial hyperplasia and cancer.
C. Progestin decreases the risk of osteoporosis.
D. Progestin controls mood swings.

15–21 *Sandra says that her previous doctor never discussed why he took her off hormone replacement therapy (HRT). You share with her some of the results of the Women's Health Initiative (WHI). Which statement is true regarding the study?*

A. Estrogen plus progestin increases the risk of stroke in apparently healthy women.
B. Persons on HRT are at a higher risk of colorectal cancer.
C. Postmenopausal hormones do not actually prevent fractures of the hip.
D. Estrogen alone is associated with a greater risk of breast cancer than a combination of estrogen plus progestin.

15–22 *In a premenopausal woman, the biggest heart attack risk factor is:*

A. cigarette smoking.
B. family history.
C. sedentary lifestyle.
D. obesity.

15–23 *One of the leading causes of female infertility, Stein-Leventhal syndrome, is:*

A. pelvic inflammatory disease.
B. polycystic ovary disease.
C. multiple sex partners.
D. ectopic pregnancy syndrome.

15–24 *Characteristics of polycystic ovarian syndrome include:*

A. hirsutism, thinness, hypoinsulinemia.
B. menopausal onset, vitiligo.
C. alopecia, thinness, abdominal cramping.
D. premenarchial onset, obesity, hyperinsulinemia.

15–25 *First-line treatment for polycystic ovarian syndrome is:*

A. a bilateral oophorectomy.
B. beginning antiandrogen therapies.
C. a combination of diet modification, weight loss, and stress management.
D. a laparotomy with a bilateral wedge resection.

15–26 *Janice, age 26, who has genital herpes, asks if her partner has to use a condom during sexual intercourse even if she does not have a visible lesion. How do you respond?*

A. "Yes, we're not sure if it's still transmitted when the lesions are not visible, so it's better to be on the safe side."
B. "No, you're not 'contagious' when the lesions are not visible."
C. "No, use of a spermicidal agent is all that is required."
D. "Yes, shedding of the herpes simplex virus from mucocutaneous surfaces in the absence of visible lesions is a primary mode of transmission."

15–27 *A treatment used to improve the chance of pregnancy in an infertile woman who has minimal or mild endometriosis is:*

A. laparoscopic resection or ablation of the lesions.
B. dilation and curettage.
C. the use of gonadotropin-releasing hormone analogues.
D. the use of of birth control pills for 3 months, then abruptly stopping.

15–28 *Which of the following drugs given to nursing mothers may cause a reduction in the milk supply?*

A. Antihistamines
B. Antithyroid medication
C. Oral contraceptives
D. Laxatives

15–29 *Sarah, age 29, complains of premenstrual syndrome. She states she was told that changing her diet might help in managing some of the symptoms. What changes in her diet do you recommend?*

A. Increase intake of protein.
B. Increase intake of complex carbohydrates.
C. Increase intake of salt and salty foods.
D. Decrease intake of fatty foods.

15–30 *When premenstrual syndrome symptoms do not respond to other therapies, which of the following drugs might you try?*

A. Antidepressants
B. Diuretics
C. Gonadotropin-releasing hormone agonists
D. All of the above

15–31 *Julia is nursing her 8-week-old baby and states that he is very irritable and sleeps poorly. What medication or substance do you ask her if she is taking or using?*

A. Cimetidine (Tagamet)
B. Ergotamine (Ergostat)
C. Nicotine
D. Caffeine

15–32 *The simplest and safest method of suppressing lactation after it has started is to:*

A. wear a snug brassiere.
B. use ice packs.
C. gradually wean the baby to a bottle or a cup over a 3-week period.
D. begin oral hormones or long-acting hormonal injections.

15–33 *Which of the following conditions may result in dyspareunia?*

A. Vulvovaginitis
B. An incompletely stretched hymen
C. Vaginismus
D. All of the above

15–34 *Which of the following ovarian tumors or cysts has the potential for malignancy?*

A. Follicle cysts
B. Brenner's tumor
C. Fibroma
D. Secondary ovarian tumors

15–35 *Lynne, age 43, comes to your office in tears, stating that last night she had unprotected sex and forgot to take her birth control pill. She wants to know about the "morning-after pill." You tell her:*

A. "If your period does not start at the scheduled time, come back to see me."
B. "I'll go ahead and order the estrogen-only postcoital contraception pill."
C. "I'll go ahead and order the Yuzpe regimen."
D. "I'll refer you to a gynecologist."

15–36 *Lori, age 38, states that she has not had a pelvic exam in 5 years because she does not like having the digital rectal exam. How do you respond?*

A. "Let's schedule an exam now, because you don't need a rectal exam until you're 40."
B. "O.K., we'll do a pelvic, and I'll just put 'refused' on the chart to cover my liability."
C. "We really need to do one because the rectal exam has been shown to pick up many abnormalities such as rectal polyps."
D. "I'll try to be quick with the rectal exam and get it over with."

15–37 *The majority of breast carcinomas are found in which anatomic site in the breast?*

A. Around the areola
B. In the upper outer quadrant
C. In the lower half of the breast
D. Toward the sternum

15–38 *Which of the following conditions is a contraindication to using the copper intrauterine device?*

A. History of ectopic pregnancy
B. Nulliparity
C. Treated cervical dysplasia
D. Heart disease

15–39 *When a woman complains of dyspareunia in the lower back during orgasm, you should consider:*

A. endometriosis.
B. cystitis.
C. vaginitis.
D. pelvic inflammatory disease-related causes.

15–40 *The most likely cause of amenorrhea is:*

A. an anatomic deviation.
B. a genetic factor.
C. an endocrine abnormality.
D. pregnancy.

15–41 *Dysfunctional uterine bleeding is usually associated with:*

A. pregnancy.
B. anovulation.
C. genital tumor.
D. inflammation.

15–42 *The best method to diagnose uterine fibroids and polyps is:*

A. hysteroscopy.
B. dilation and curettage.
C. colposcopy.
D. laparoscopy.

15–43 *Toxic shock syndrome may be caused by all of the following* ***except:***

A. tampon contamination with *Staphylococcus aureus*.
B. damaged cervical and vaginal mucosa.
C. the use of superabsorbent tampons for an extended period of time.
D. a urinary tract infection involving the bladder and kidneys.

15–44 *Which of the following drugs may have their effects enhanced when used in combination with an oral contraceptive?*

A. Beta blockers
B. Oral anticoagulants
C. Antacids
D. Phenytoin (Dilantin)

15–45 *Which of the following drugs may have their effects diminished when used in combination with an oral contraceptive?*

A. Corticosteroids
B. Oral anticoagulants
C. Antibiotics
D. Anticonvulsants

15–46 *Which of the following drugs may diminish the effectiveness of oral contraceptives?*

A. Beta blockers
B. Oral anticoagulants
C. Antibiotics
D. Oral hypoglycemics

15–47 *Sydney, age 21, is taking an oral contraceptive (OC). She complains of acne. How should you adjust the estrogen in the OC?*

A. Increase it.
B. Decrease it.
C. Delete it.
D. No adjustment should be made.

15–48 *Marsha, age 40, has been given a diagnosis of rheumatoid arthritis. She asks you whether she should continue taking her birth control pills. You tell her:*

A. to check with her rheumatologist.
B. to stop.
C. to continue.
D. that the dose will have to be increased.

15–49 *Ursula, age 19, is going to begin taking birth control pills. She asks you if she is "safe" immediately. How do you respond?*

A. "Yes, you should not get pregnant once you start taking the pill. However, it doesn't protect you from STDs."
B. "For the first month, you need to be on a backup birth-control method. However, it doesn't protect you from STDs"
C. "A second birth control method needs to be used during intercourse for the first 7 days while taking the pill. However, it doesn't protect you from STDs"
D. "Until you have your second period (cycle) with the pill, you are not considered safe."

15–50 *Joanne wants to use some form of birth control, but, because she is getting married, she wants to be able to stop the birth control method and have her fertility restored almost immediately. Which method do you recommend for her?*

A. The birth control pill
B. Lunelle injections
C. Depo-medroxyprogesterone acetate (DMPA) injections
D. None of the above. Pregnancy will be delayed with all of these methods.

15–51 *For instructing women about their fertile period (when they are most likely to become pregnant), which of the following statements is false?*

A. Ovulation occurs on the 14th day, plus or minus 2 days, before the next menses.
B. Sperm are viable for 3 days.
C. The ovum is viable for 24 hours.
D. The ovaries always release one ovum per month.

15–52 *If a woman is using the basal body temperature (BBT) method of birth control and does not want to become pregnant, when would you tell her to avoid unprotected intercourse?*

A. From the beginning of the menstrual cycle until the BBT has been elevated for 3 days.
B. Whenever the BBT is elevated.
C. Whenever the BBT is lowered.
D. From the end of the menstrual cycle until the BBT has been low for 5 days

15–53 *Beth is breast-feeding her 3-month-old infant with no supplementation. She says she has heard that she cannot get pregnant during this time. What do you tell her?*

A. "It's highly likely that you may become pregnant, so you should use another method of birth control."
B. "Yes, you're safe for as long as you breast-feed."
C. "For the first 6 months, if you breast-feed and have very little supplementation, your chances are less than 2% that you'll get pregnant."
D. "You're more at risk for getting pregnant now because of your fluctuating hormone levels."

15–54 *Lynne states that she has heard that douching effectively washes out the sperm after intercourse and that she has been using this as a method of birth control. Which of the following statements about douching is true?*

A. Douching prevents sperm from entering the uterus.
B. Douching should be used at least once a month after menses if not used after intercourse
C. Douching is a reliable contraceptive.
D. Douching may increase the risk of ectopic pregnancy.

15–55 *The Joneses are thinking about going for infertility counseling because they have been married for 5 years and have been unable to conceive. They ask you whether the man or the woman is usually the cause of the infertility. What do you tell them about the etiology of infertility?*

A. "In most cases, infertility is related to a female factor."
B. "In most cases, infertility is related to a male factor"
C. "In the majority of cases, the etiology cannot be identified."
D. "Male and female infertility rates are almost the same in the majority of cases."

15–56 *Isabelle, age 50, asks how often she should do a breast self-examination. You tell her:*

A. "You don't need to continue; we'll just do a clinical breast exam every year along with your mammogram."
B. "You need to continue this every month."
C. "Every other month should be sufficient because you have no history of any breast disease."
D. "Because most problems begin at this age, you should try to do a breast exam every few weeks."

15–57 *Fibrocystic breast disease is exacerbated by many factors. Which of the following is not a factor?*

A. Caffeine intake.
B. Vitamin E.
C. Chocolate.
D. Wearing tight bras.

15–58 *The average age of menopause in the United States is:*

A. 45 years.
B. 48 years.
C. 50 years.
D. 53 years.

15–59 *Judi has a seizure disorder and wants to get pregnant. What is the drug of choice for her during pregnancy?*

A. Valproate (Depakene)
B. Trimethadione (Tridione)
C. Phenobarbital (Luminal)
D. Phenytoin (Dilantin)

15–60 *The most common virus known to be transmitted in utero is:*

A. cytomegalovirus.
B. rubella.
C. varicella.
D. toxoplasmosis.

15–61 *Menses at irregular intervals with excessive flow and duration are defined as:*

A. oligomenorrhea.
B. polymenorrhea.
C. menorrhagia.
D. metrorrhagia.

15–62 *Endometrial cancer, hirsutism, acne, breast cancer, increased risk of diabetes, infertility, menstrual bleeding problems, and an increased risk of cardiovascular disease are clinical consequences of:*

A. Mastalgia.
B. Menorrhagia.
C. Endometriosis.
D. Persistent anovulation.

15–63 *What is the definition of amenorrhea?*

A. No menses by age 14 in the absence of secondary sexual characteristics.
B. No menses by age 16 regardless of the appearance of secondary sexual characteristics.
C. Absence of three consecutive periods in a woman with established menstrual cycles.
D. All of the above.

15–64 *There are many causes of amenorrhea. In ballet dancers or marathon runners, where is the problem located?*

A. Outflow tract
B. Ovary
C. Anterior pituitary
D. Hypothalamus

15–65 *When performing a pelvic exam, you suspect an adnexal mass. Which of the following might be a differential diagnosis?*

A. Endometriosis
B. Diverticular disease
C. Distended bladder
D. All of the above

15–66 *Cervical neoplasia risk factors include all of the following* ***except:***

A. smoking.
B. human papillomavirus infection or having a sexual partner with the infection.
C. first sexual encounter before age 20.
D. monogamous relationship.

15–67 *Which of the following conditions is usually helped when women take an oral contraceptive?*

A. Human papillomavirus infection
B. Migraine headache
C. Iron-deficiency anemia
D. Herpes simplex virus

15–68 *In which Tanner stage is a girl when her pubic hair is adult in type, but over a smaller area, with no hair on the medial thigh?*

A. Stage 2
B. Stage 3
C. Stage 4
D. Stage 5

15–69 *For a diagnosis of premenstrual syndrome to be "assigned," all of the following criteria must be met* ***except:***

A. Symptoms must occur in the luteal phase and resolve within 1–2 days of onset of menses, followed by a symptom-free period during the follicular phase.
B. Symptoms must be documented through several menstrual cycles and be sufficient to disrupt a woman's life to some degree.

C. Other medical and psychological disorders must be ruled out.
D. The client's husband or significant other reports that the client has routine moodiness.

15–70 *Jennifer, age 27, is complaining of lower abdominal pain. After doing some lab studies, you find leukocytosis, an elevated erythrocyte sedimentation rate, and an elevated C-reactive protein level. What do you suspect?*

A. Ovarian cyst
B. Pelvic inflammatory disease
C. Tubal pregnancy
D. Diverticulitis

15–71 *Thelarche is the first sign of puberty in most girls. It usually occurs at about what age?*

A. 8 years
B. 10 years
C. 11 years
D. 13 years

15–72 *Which would not be an indication for a colposcopy?*

A. A pap smear showing dysplasia.
B. A history of diethylstilbestrol exposure.
C. Human immunodeficiency virus (HIV) infection.
D. All of the above.

15–73 *Of the symptoms listed below, the most commonly expressed symptom of women with premenstrual syndrome is:*

A. fatigue.
B. depression.
C. breast tenderness.
D. swelling of the extremities.

15–74 *Women with dysuria should have a thorough history taken. The most important question to ask to help you make a differential diagnosis is:*

A. "Do you have painful intercourse?"
B. "Do you have an associated vaginal discharge or irritation?"
C. "Do you also have a problem with defecation?"
D. "Do you have stress incontinence?"

15–75 *Candidiasis is more common in:*

A. teenage girls.
B. women on low-fat diets.
C. women with diabetes.
D. women with frequent urinary tract infections.

15–76 *If you diagnose a cervical gonococcal infection, which other infection is probably present?*

A. Candidiasis
B. Syphilis
C. Trichomoniasis
D. Chlamydia

15–77 *Which type of incontinence has an associated symptom of recurrent cystitis?*

A. Stress incontinence
B. Urge incontinence
C. Overflow incontinence
D. Functional incontinence

15–78 *Small-quantity incontinence with nearly continuous dribbling is symptomatic of which kind of incontinence?*

A. Stress incontinence
B. Urge incontinence
C. Overflow incontinence
D. Functional incontinence

15–79 *During a pelvic exam, if the client strains and a pouching is seen on the anterior wall of the vagina, what would you suspect?*

A. Cystocele
B. Rectocele
C. Enterocele
D. Uterine prolapse

15–80 *What is the position of the uterus when the cervix is on the anterior vaginal wall?*

A. Midposition
B. Retroverted
C. Retroflexed
D. Anteverted

15–81 *The most common type of invasive breast carcinoma is:*

A. infiltrating ductal.
B. medullary.
C. lobular.
D. infiltrating papillary.

15–82 *Elimination of the offensive agent and use of corticosteroids is the treatment of choice for which type of vulvovaginitis?*

A. Candidiasis
B. Reactive vaginitis
C. Atrophic vaginitis
D. Normal cervical or vaginal discharge vaginitis

15–83 *Which of the following is a sexually transmitted disease?*

A. Monilial vaginitis
B. Trichomonal vaginitis
C. Atrophic vaginitis
D. Bacterial vaginosis

15–84 *All of the following conditions have a vaginal pH of 5 or less* ***except:***

A. normal vaginal discharge.
B. candidiasis.
C. bacterial vaginosis.
D. reactive vaginitis.

15–85 *Which glands are posterior on each side of the vaginal orifice and open onto the sides of the vestibule in the groove between the labia minora and hymen?*

A. Bartholin's glands
B. Skene's glands
C. The paraurethral glands
D. Cystocele

15–86 *Which form of estrogen is the most potent and is secreted in the greatest amount by the ovaries during the reproductive years?*

A. Estrone (E1)
B. Estradiol (E2)
C. Estriol (E3)
D. The potency and secretion of all of the above are in equal amounts

15–87 *Unilateral galactorrhea is not present in:*

A. fibrocystic breast disease.
B. intraductal papilloma.
C. carcinoma.
D. pregnancy.

15–88 *The risk factor(s) that may predispose a woman to dysfunctional uterine bleeding is/are:*

A. stress
B. extreme weight change
C. use of oral contraceptive agents
D. all of the above

15–89 *Procidentia is a:*

A. cystocele.
B. rectocele.
C. vaginal fistula.
D. third-degree uterine prolapse.

15–90 *Which type of cyst or polyp of the female reproductive system results in pain, redness, a perineal mass, and dyspareunia?*

A. Ovarian cyst
B. Bartholin's cyst
C. Endometrial polyp
D. Cervical polyp

15–91 *Which tumor marker is highly specific to epithelial ovarian cancer?*

A. PSA
B. CA 125
C. CA 15-3
D. CA 19-9

15–92 *Psychogenic causes of dyspareunia include all of the following* ***except:***

A. fear of vaginal penetration.
B. sexual dysfunction as a result of vaginismus.
C. pain from vaginal penetration.
D. lack of lubrication.

15–93 *Which of the following lifestyle factors is associated with an increased risk for breast cancer?*

A. Being underweight
B. Having one to two drinks of alcohol per day
C. Smoking
D. Eating a low-fat diet

15–94 *Which type of breast cancer involves infiltration of the nipple epithelium and has an initial symptom of itching or burning of the nipple?*

A. Ductal cancer
B. Paget's disease
C. Mammary duct ectasia
D. Fibroadenoma

15–95 *Minnie, age 52, states that she is going to have a TRAM procedure after her breast surgery. However, she was in shock from the diagnosis when the surgeon explained the procedure. She asks you to explain it. How do you respond?*

A. "It's when a breast implant is inserted under the pectoris muscle."
B. "It's an autogenous procedure that uses skin from the latissimus dorsi muscle to fashion a breast."
C. "It's an autogenous procedure that uses skin from the rectus abdominis muscle to fashion a breast."
D. "It's a breast implant that is done after the mastectomy scar heals."

Answers

15–1 Answer A

A sexually active woman should be aware that genital herpes simplex virus may be transmitted to a partner or newborn even in the absence of lesions because of viral shedding. Genital herpes may be transmitted to a partner at any time; therefore, condoms should always be used. Menstruation, physical or emotional stress, immunosuppression, sexual intercourse, and pregnancy may actually trigger herpes recurrences. Herpes recurrences usually do not last as long as the initial occurrence.

15–2 Answer A

Nausea and vomiting occurring during the first trimester are probably a result of hormonal changes such as the production of human chorionic gonadotropin. Women also experience pyrosis because of esophageal reflux caused by a decrease in gastrointestinal motility, leading to prolonged gastric emptying time.

15–3 Answer B

Hormone replacement therapy (HRT) may be used for short-term effectiveness in treating hot flashes in the absence of a personal or family history of breast cancer or a previous problem with venous thrombosis.

It is no longer considered cardioprotective. It continues to be effective in preventing bone loss. Prevention of osteoporosis includes HRT, exercise to help decrease bone turnover, and 1200 mg of calcium and 600 mg of vitamin D per day. For women not on HRT, calcium should be increased to 1500 mg/day.

15–4 Answer B

The *Mobiluncus* species causes bacterial vaginosis. The human papilloma virus is responsible for condylomata acuminata (genital warts). Lymphogranuloma venereum is a sexually transmitted disease characterized by localized lymphatic infection with a chlamydia origin.

15–5 Answer D

Gonorrhea may precipitate Reiter's syndrome (reactive arthritis). Bacterial vaginosis seldom results in complications. Syphilis may result in disseminated disease, but not Reiter's syndrome. Left untreated in women, *Chlamydia* infections may cause scarring in the uterine tubes, leading to infertility and ectopic (tubal) pregnancies.

15–6 Answer C

Ceftriaxone (Rocephin) is the drug of choice for treating gonorrhea because it provides effective single-dose therapy. It does not treat all strains of gonorrhea, and treatment failure may result with one of the resistant strains. Because it is a cephalosporin, ceftriaxone is relatively expensive.

15–7 Answer C

Although the primary lesion of genital herpes normally resolves within 21 days, the client usually has recurrent episodes. Acyclovir (Zovirax) is a palliative management option, but the drug does not cure herpes simplex. Topical trichloroacetic acid is the treatment for genital warts. Intercourse should be avoided when a lesion is present.

15–8 Answer B

Emotional support is best given to the client with a sexually transmitted disease (STD) by authentic active listening. During times of increased psychological stress, minimizing choices is better than offering too many choices. The client with an STD needs support from others, and emphasis should focus on the prevention of recurrences rather than the specifics of the duration of the disease.

15–9 Answer A

A colposcopy visualizes the cervical, vaginal, or vulvar epithelium under magnification to identify abnormal areas that may require a biopsy. It is performed in the office. An endometrial biopsy removes one or more areas of the endometrium by means of a curette or small aspiration device without cervical dilation. A hysteroscopy allows visual examination of the uterine cavity with a small fiberoptic endoscope passed through the cervix. A laparoscopy allows visualization of the abdominal and pelvic cavity through a small fiberoptic endoscope passed through a subumbilical incision.

15–10 Answer C

When human papilloma virus (condylomata acuminata) causes genital warts, it may lead to cervical dysplasia and cervical cancer. Pelvic inflammatory disease is usually secondary to gonorrhea or *Chlamydia* infection. Molluscum contagiosum is a sexually transmitted disease that causes a benign viral skin infection. Genital herpes is caused by herpes simplex virus.

15–11 Answer D

Emergency (postcoital)contraception refers to taking 2 doses of an estrogen-plus-progestin birth control pill 12 hours apart within 48 hours after unprotected coitus to induce abortion.

15–12 Answer A

Your next action for Brianne is to obtain a culture of the urethra, do a potassium hydroxide wet prep, and obtain another urine culture. Doing so is the most efficient way of treating Brianne now. Discussing her social history might help you determine which course of action is most appropriate. However, if you do only one test now and it is negative, you might have to perform another diagnostic test, thereby delaying treatment again. A wet mount is done for bacterial vaginosis. A diagnosis of *Chlamydia* infection is accomplished by culture or smears for gram staining, but this is expensive and takes 2–6 days for results to be available. Other techniques include direct immunofluorescence assay and enzyme immunoassay. Diagnosis of gonorrhea is accomplished through cultures of the discharge (urethral, endocervical, rectal, pharyngeal, or conjunctive) using a modified Thayer-Martin medium or by gram staining to look for typical gram-negative intracellular diplococci. Diagnosis of herpes simplex viruses is accomplished by the enzyme-linked immunosorbent assay technique or viral cultures. Another, less reliable method of diagnosis consists of serologic antibody testing. The diagnosis of human papilloma virus infection is made by colposcopy. Trichomoniasis is diagnosed by pH, which, as in bacterial vaginosis, is greater than 4.5, and by a microscopic finding of flagellated motile organisms resembling whips that are larger than white blood cells. By just treating the symptoms as a urinary trract infection or irritation, you could be ignoring the true problem giving it time to spread. Medicating with antibiotics without identifying a definitive organism leads to antibiotic resistance.

15–13 Answer D

Bacterial vaginosis (BV) is the most common vaginal infection (about 40% of all cases). The infecting organisms are identified as *Gardnerella vaginalis*, *Mobiluncus* species, and other anaerobes. Bacterial vaginosis results in an overgrowth condition within the vagina for as yet unknown reasons. The incubation period is 5–10 days. About half of all clients with BV are asymptomatic. Those with symptoms typically describe a gray-white, malodorous or fishy smelling, pruritic discharge that is accompanied by burning. It may be scant to profuse and adheres to the vaginal walls. The differential diagnoses include any other known cause for vaginitis (such as trichomoniasis or candidiasis) and cervicitis (such as gonorrhea or *Chlamydia* infection). Diagnosis is made through microscopic examination of the specimen by wet mount. The practitioner should look for clue cells, which look like pepper, appear on the surface of cells, and are diagnostic of BV.

15–14 Answer A

An appropriate first-line drug for a *Chlamydia* vaginal infection is azithromycin (Zithromax) 1 g po. Although doxycycline (Vibramycin) 100 mg po bid for 7 days is the most tried and true and least expensive treatment, azithromycin is the most convenient option for single-dose administration. Azithromycin is contraindicated in pregnant women. For this population, erythromycin 500 mg po qid for 7 days should be ordered.

15–15 Answer B

A client who presents with grayish-white vaginal discharge, greenish cervical discharge, and cervical motion tenderness may have gonorrhea, bacterial vaginosis, or *Chlamydia* infection. Interstitial cystitis is a chronic disease with none of the symptoms listed. Gonorrhea may be asymptomatic or the client may present with yellowish urethral or vaginal discharge. The discharge of bacterial vaginosis is typically gray-white, malodorous or fishy smelling, and pruritic. *Chlamydia* infection may present with or without a vaginal or urethral discharge.

15–16 Answer A

Nothing should be inserted in the vagina for 24 hours before performing a Pap smear. Douching should be discouraged in all women because it changes the normal flora, increasing the likelihood of an infection. An acute infection or heavy menses preclude Pap testing because they alter the ability of the practitioner to obtain an adequate sample. Some women find the Pap test physically or emotionally very uncomfortable; therefore reassurance about its necessity should be provided.

15–17 Answer B

The woman who has extreme spasticity should assume a knee-chest position while prone for a Pap smear. Assistance may be required to keep the legs away from the perineal area. The "OB" stirrups position allows a woman who has difficulty using foot stirrups to assume the standard pelvic examination position. The client may need assistance in putting her legs into the stirrups up to the knees, which can be padded for comfort. The V-shaped position may be used without stirrups or with one foot in a stirrup. One or two assistants may be required to help the woman maintain this position by supporting each straightened leg at the knee and ankle. The client's comfort may be increased by elevating her legs slightly or by using a pillow under the small of her back or coccyx. The speculum must be inserted with the handle up. The side-lying position does not require stirrups and is most appropriate for the client who feels most comfortable and balanced lying on her side. An assistant may help elevate one leg if the client cannot spread her legs. The speculum can be inserted with the handle pointing either toward the woman's back or front, but the clinician should be sure to angle the speculum toward the small of the client's back and not straight up toward her head.

15–18 Answer D

Signs and symptoms of a genital herpes infection include tender inguinal lymph nodes, as well as painful or pruritic vesicles, dysuria, prodromal tingling or pruritus of the genital region, and cervical ulcerations. White curdlike plaques on a red base in the vagina are seen with monilial vaginitis.

15–19 Answer D

Herpes simplex virus may be acquired before labor, during delivery, or postnatally. About 5% of infants with neonatal herpes acquire the virus before labor. Direct contact with the maternal genitalia or secretions during delivery accounts for about 85% of neonatal herpes infections. Intrauterine infection occurs in about 5% of cases. Postnatal acquisition occurs by direct contact with an infected caretaker and accounts for the other 10% of neonatal herpes infections.

15–20 Answer B

A woman with an intact uterus needs to add progestin to her estrogen replacement therapy (ERT) because it reduces the incidence of endometrial hyperplasia and cancer, both of which are associated with long-term estrogen use. Decreased estrogen levels account for hot flashes as well as increasing the risk of fractures from osteoporosis. Discussion about discontinuing hormone replacement therapy should begin.

15–21 Answer A

The Women's Health Initiative found that estrogen plus progestin increases the risk of stroke in apparently healthy women. Users of postmenopausal hormones are actually at a lower risk of colorectal cancer. The mechanisms by which hormone use might reduce risk are unclear. The WHI is the first trial with definitive data supporting the ability of postmenopausal hormones to prevent fractures of the hip, vertebrae, and other sites. Estrogen plus progestin appears to be associated with greater risk of breast cancer than estrogen alone.

15–22 Answer A

In a premenopausal woman, the biggest heart attack risk factor is cigarette smoking. If a woman is premenopausal, her own estrogen is most likely to protect her from heart disease, but there are still risk factors associated with heart disease. The more risk factors that apply, the greater the danger. Smoking is the biggest risk factor. Others include a family history of premature heart disease (paternal side before age 55, maternal side before age 65), being over age 54, going through premature menopause, not using hormone replacement therapy (HRT), sedentary lifestyle, and a history of diabetes or high blood pressure.

15–23 Answer B

One of the leading causes of female infertility, Stein-Leventhal syndrome is polycystic ovary syndrome (PCOS). It is a condition that afflicts many women during their childbearing years. Symptoms of PCOS, which are related to androgen excess and not associated with estrogen deficiency, include amenorrhea, hirsutism, acne, and obesity.

15–24 Answer D

Characteristics of polycystic ovary syndrome (PCOS) include premenarchal onset, obesity, hyperinsulinemia, hyperandrogenism (hirsutism, seborrhea, acne, alopecia), menstrual disturbances, and infertility. Visible signs of the syndrome are obesity, acne, and hirsutism. Clients with PCOS typically present with complaints of amenorrhea or irregular menstrual cycles, whereas some have the initial complaint of infertility. About 10–20% of clients with PCOS are symptomatic. PCOS should be considered in all clients presenting with amenorrhea, infertility, or hirsutism.

15–25 Answer C

First-line treatment for polycystic ovary syndrome (PCOS) is a combination of diet modification, weight loss, and stress management, because obesity and stress alone can contribute to androgen excess. Oral estrogens are considered the first-line treatment for hyperandrogenism, with combination (estrogen and progesterone) oral contraceptives being the medication of choice. Treatment of uncomplicated amenorrhea in PCOS requires, at a minimum, monthly or bimonthly administration of medroxyprogesterone acetate (Depo-Provera). A laparotomy with a bilateral wedge resection is a treatment for anovulation. Because of the possibility of adhesions and ovarian atrophy, surgical interventions are used only in women who have tried and failed clomiphene citrate ovulation induction and when all other noninvasive options have been considered.

15–26 Answer D

A condom should be worn during sexual intercourse when one partner has genital herpes, even though there may not be a visible lesion. Shedding of the herpes simplex virus from mucocutaneous surfaces in the absence of visible lesions is a primary mode of transmission both horizontally (to sexual partners) and vertically (to the fetus).

15–27 Answer A

A treatment used to improve the chance of pregnancy in an infertile woman who has minimal or mild endometriosis is laparoscopic resection or ablation of the lesions. Although dilation and curettage removes tissue, it may not be the specific endometrial tissue involved. Gonadotropin-releasing hormone analogues suppress endometriosis by creating a pseudomenopause.

15–28 Answer C

Oral contraceptives, even in low doses, may cause a reduction in the milk supply to an infant. The progestin-only minipill can be used. Antihistamines are contraindicated because of the increased sensitivity of newborns and infants to antihistamines. Antithyroid medications such as methimazole (Tapazole) are contraindicated because they may cause goiter or agranulocytosis. The antithyroid drug propylthiouracil is considered safe. Laxatives may cause diarrhea in an infant.

15–29 Answer B

In the client complaining of premenstrual syndrome, advise her to increase her intake of complex carbohydrates. A diet high in complex carbohydrates, such as whole grains and cereals, fruits, and vegetables, helps prevent low blood sugar levels and reduce fatigue, jitteriness, and irritability. It may also raise serotonin levels, thus improving mood. Eating several small meals at frequent intervals rather than three large ones also keeps blood sugar on an even level and reduces the feeling of bloating. Women should also restrict their intake of salt, caffeine, and alcohol during the week before their cycle.

15–30 Answer D

When premenstrual syndrome symptoms do not respond to other treatments, you may prescribe any of the following drugs to aid in alleviating the symptoms: antidepressants to raise the levels of serotonin, such as paroxetine (Paxil), fluoxetine (Prozac), or sertraline (Zoloft); diuretics to help relieve bloating; gonadotropin-releasing hormone agonists to suppress the menstrual cycle; antianxiety agents such as alprazolam (Xanax); and an oral progesterone to help relieve bloating and moodiness.

15–31 Answer D

Caffeine in large amounts will make the infant who is being nursed irritable and give him or her a poor sleep pattern. Cimetidine (Tagamet) and ranitidine (Zantac) are concentrated in breast milk and may suppress the infant's gastric acidity and cause central nervous system stimulation. Ergotamine (Ergostat) in doses sufficient to treat a migraine may cause vomiting, diarrhea, and convulsions as well as suppressing lactation. Nicotine increases the incidence of respiratory disease in infants exposed to smoke.

15–32 Answer C

The simplest and safest method of suppressing lactation after it has started is to gradually wean the baby to a bottle or a cup over a 3-week period. If nursing must be stopped abruptly, avoiding nipple stimulation, refraining from expressing milk, and wearing a snug brassiere will help. Ice packs and analgesics are also helpful. The practice of using oral and long-acting injections of hormonal preparations has been abandoned because of their questionable efficacy and their associated adverse effects, such as thromboembolic episodes and hair growth.

15–33 Answer D

Dyspareunia (painful intercourse) may be caused by vulvovaginitis, an incompletely (or inadequately) stretched hymen during the initial intercourse, vaginismus, endometriosis, tumors or other pathologic conditions, or psychosexual conflicts.

15–34 Answer D

Secondary ovarian tumors account for about 10% of the fatal malignant diseases in women. They are usually the result of bowel or breast metastases to the ovary, and all of the tumors are malignant. Follicle cysts are frequent in the menstrual years, never occur in the postmenopausal years, and do not have a potential for malignancy. Follicle cysts often disappear after a 2-month regimen of oral contraceptives. Fibromas account for fewer than 5% of the ovarian tumors and very rarely have the potential for malignancy. Brenner's tumor accounts for about 1% of ovarian tumors, occurs more than 50% of the time in postmenopausal women, and very rarely has the potential for malignancy.

15–35 Answer C

Emergency contraception, referred to as postcoital contraception, prevents pregnancy after unprotected sexual intercourse. It should ideally be taken within 72 hours after unprotected intercourse. Waiting for menses to start or referring the client to a gynecologist is too late. In the United States three methods are available. The Yuzpe regimen consists of taking 2 birth control pills within 72 hours and 2 more 12 hours later. This is 75% effective. A medication for nausea should be taken before the birth control pills. An alternative plan is to take progestin-only postcoital contraceptives, which reduce the risk of pregnancy by 89%. One pill (levonorgestrel 75 mg) is taken within 72 hours of unprotected sex and another 12 hours later. The third method of postcoital contraception involves inserting a copper IUD up to 7 days after unprotected sex. This method reduces the risk of pregnancy by 99%.

15–36 Answer A

A large retrospective study showed that the digital rectal exam (DRE) is not warranted in women under 40 years of age. No significant findings were recorded in the DRE in women younger than age 40. In addition to the lack of diagnostic yield, the time, discomfort, and embarrassment associated with the DRE should discourage its use as part of a routine pelvic examination. One physician recorded results of DREs over 50 years of practice, and discovered only three cases of rectal polyps during that span of time.

15–37 Answer B

Of all breast carcinomas, 60% are found in the upper outer quadrant of the breast, 5% around the areola and nipple, 15% in the upper inner quadrant (toward the sternum), 15% in the lower outer quadrant, and 5% in the lower inner quadrant.

15–38 Answer D

The following conditions were previously believed to preclude the use of intrauterine devices (IUDs), including the copper IUD, but are no longer contraindications: history of ectopic pregnancy (remains a contraindication to use with the progesterone-containing IUDs), nulliparity, treated cervical dysplasia, diabetes mellitus, valvular heart disease, irregular menses as a result of anovulation, breast-feeding, corticosteroid use, and age under 25 years. The conditions that preclude systemic hormonal methods (breast cancer, venous thromboembolism or phlebitis, arterial vascular disease, active liver disease, and age over 35 combined with smoking) do not preclude intrauterine contraception. Heart disease is considered a contraindication because the patient may be susceptible to bacterial endocarditis.

15–39 Answer A

When a client complains of dyspareunia in the lower back during orgasm, you should consider a diagnosis of endometriosis. Cystitis and vaginitis should be considered when pain occurs at the vaginal canal and adjacent structures with the penis in midvagina. Pelvic inflammatory disease should be considered if pain occurs in the deep pelvis when there is deep penile penetration with thrusting. Causes of dyspareunia are many and diverse and depend on when and where the pain occurs.

15–40 Answer D

Although pregnancy seems like an obvious choice as the most likely cause of amenorrhea, it is sometimes overlooked, especially if the client denies the possibility of pregnancy and is seeking a pathological reason for the amenorrhea. The most likely physiological causes of amenorrhea that should be considered are pregnancy, lactation, and menopause, if appropriate. Among women who are in the childbearing years, amenorrhea unrelated to pregnancy may signal stress or a life-threatening disease. These conditions may include anatomic deviations, genetic factors, endocrine abnormalities or imbalances, defective enzyme systems, autoimmune diseases, tumors, eating disorders, excessive exercise, and medications. With amenorrhea, a pregnancy test should always be done first to rule out pregnancy or its related complications: ectopic pregnancies, complete or incomplete abortions, and trophoblastic neoplasms. The most accurate test is the serum beta human chorionic gonadotropin test.

15–41 Answer B

Dysfunctional uterine bleeding (DUB) is excessive, prolonged, and unpatterned bleeding from the endometrium in the absence of any structural pelvic pathology. It is usually associated with anovulation. Dysfunctional uterine bleeding is not related to pregnancy, inflammation, genital tumor, or other anatomic uterine lesion. Although no organic problems are associated with DUB, a history and physical examination and pelvic and rectal examinations are done to rule out neoplasia. These are followed by diagnostic tests and blood work.

15–42 Answer A

The best method to diagnose uterine fibroids and polyps is hysteroscopy. A hysteroscopy is visualization of the endometrium through a scope to assess for uterine fibroids, polyps, or structural abnormalities. Tissue sampling and removal of the polyps can be done through the hysteroscope. A dilation and curettage consists of scraping the walls of the uterus. A colposcopy is used to examine the vulva, vagina, and cervix. A laparoscopy examines the peritoneal cavity.

15–43 Answer D

A urinary tract infection involving the bladder and kidneys does not cause toxic shock syndrome (TSS). TSS is a potentially lethal disorder that is caused in almost all cases by absorption of one or more toxins produced by colonized *Staphylococcus aureus*. Several mechanisms are implicated as causative, although not proven. They include tampon contamination with *S. aureus,* damaged cervical and vaginal mucosa, the use of superabsorbent tampons (or the synthetic materials they are made of) for an extended period of time, absorption of bacteriostatic cervical secretions, alterations in the normal vaginal flora, mechanical blockage of menstrual fluids, and the enhanced multiplication of the organism in the menstrual efflux. The incidence of TSS has decreased steadily as a result of education, altered patterns of tampon use, and the removal of extremely high-absorbency tampons from the market.

15–44 Answer A

The effects of beta blockers as well as alcohol, corticosteroids, theophylline, and diazepam (Valium), may be enhanced when they are used in combination with oral contraceptives. Other drugs whose effects may be enhanced when used in combination with an oral contraceptive include tricyclic antidepressants and some benzodiazepines.

15–45 Answer B

The effects of oral anticoagulants, acetaminophen, some benzodiazepines, oral hypoglycemic agents, and methyldopa may be diminished when used in combination with oral contraceptives.

15–46 Answer C

Antibiotics, antacids, anticonvulsants, and barbiturates may diminish the effectiveness of oral contraceptives. Clients should be urged to use other methods of birth control when taking antibiotics.

15–47 Answer A

If a client taking an oral contraceptive (OC) complains of acne, the estrogen in the OC should be increased or the progestin decreased. In addition, you should also discuss hygiene, diet, and topical antibiotic drug therapy.

15–48 Answer C

If your client with rheumatoid arthritis (RA) is taking birth control pills, she should continue taking them as well as any medications for her RA.

15–49 Answer C

When a client is first starting to take birth control pills, she should be instructed to use a second birth control method during intercourse, such as condoms or a diaphragm used with spermicide, for the first 7 days. Another contraceptive method should always be kept on hand to use in case of missed pills, when taking another medication that might interfere with pill effectiveness, such as an antibiotic, or when vomiting or diarrhea occurs.

15–50 Answer B

There may be a temporary delay in conception after discontinuing oral contraceptives, although the exact time is unclear. Return to fertility with depo-medroxyprogesterone acetate (DMPA) may be delayed regardless of the duration of its use. However, return to fertility occurs rapidly after discontinuation of Lunelle injections. DMPA injections are given every 3 months, Lunelle injections are given monthly.

15–51 Answer D

When instructing women about their fertile period (when they are most likely to become pregnant), tell them that ovulation occurs on the 14th day, plus or minus 2 days, before the next menses; sperm are viable for 3 days; and the ovum is viable for 24 hours. It is essential for women to know these facts if they are using the calendar or rhythm method for preventing a pregnancy. The ovaries may release more than one ovum per month or none at all, depending on the fertility status of the woman.

15–52 Answer A

If a woman is using the basal body temperature (BBT) method of birth control and does not want to become pregnant, tell her to avoid unprotected intercourse from the beginning of the menstrual cycle (or at least from day 4) until the BBT has been elevated for 3 days. When using the BBT method, the temperature is taken daily after a minimum of 3 hours of sleep, before rising, eating, or drinking, and is recorded. The preovulatory temperatures are suppressed by estrogen, whereas postovulatory temperatures are increased under the influence of heat-inducing progesterone. Temperatures typically rise within a day or two after ovulation has occurred and remain elevated for 2 weeks until menstruation begins.

15–53 Answer C

Women have less than a 2% chance of getting pregnant as long as they are amenorrheic for 2 months postpartum; are fully breastfeeding, with a supplementation not exceeding 15%; and are less than 6 months postpartum. If any of these conditions is not present, the woman needs to begin to use another form of contraceptive.

15–54 Answer D

Douching will not prevent sperm from entering the uterus because sperm may enter the cervical canal as soon as 15 seconds after ejaculation. Douching may even enhance the movement of sperm up the canal because it washes fluids deeper into the vagina and washes away the protective mucus. Douching has been associated with an increased risk of pelvic infection and ectopic pregnancy and most gynecologists do not recommend it at any time.

15–55 Answer D

The etiology of infertility can be identified in 90% of couples. Male and female factor infertility are almost the same (males 30%, females 35%), and in 20% of cases there is a combination of male and female factors. It should also be stressed that infertility is no one's "fault," and that many things may be tried to assist the couple to conceive.

15–56 Answer B

Breast self-exams should be performed on a monthly basis from age 20 throughout the life span. From ages 20–39, a clinical breast exam should be done every 3 years. From ages 40–49, an annual clinical breast exam should be performed as well as a mammogram every 1–2 years. From age 50 on, an annual clinical breast exam should be done as well as an annual mammogram.

15–57 Answer D

There are many interventions that will alleviate the pain of fibrocystic breast disease as well as help decrease the proliferation of breast tissue. Caffeine intake should be reduced because this may alleviate breast tenderness and reduce nodularity. Clients should also reduce the intake of chocolate, tea, colas, and drugs containing caffeine. Vitamin E has been shown to decrease the pain and tenderness associated with fibrocystic change as well as the proliferation of breast tissue. Wearing a tight-fitting bra does not exacerbate the condition, but may increase tenderness.

15–58 Answer C

The average age of menopause in the United States is 50 years. Menopause is defined by the World Health Organization as the permanent cessation of menstruation resulting from loss of ovarian follicular activity and 12 months of amenorrhea at the time of midlife.

15–59 Answer C

Phenobarbital (Luminal) is the drug of choice in a pregnant woman with a seizure disorder. Ideally, if the woman has not had a seizure for 5 years before the pregnancy, a prepregnancy trial of withdrawal from seizure medication should be tried. Valproate (Depakene) and trimethadione (Tridione) are contraindicated during pregnancy and phenytoin (Dilantin) is teratogenic during the first trimester. If phenobarbital is used, serum levels should be measured in each trimester and the dosage should be such that it maintains the serum levels in the low-normal therapeutic range.

15–60 Answer A

The most common virus known to be transmitted in utero is cytomegalovirus (CMV). Transmission of CMV can take place as a consequence of either primary or reactivated infection in the mother. Children in day-care settings can also transmit the virus to their mothers or day-care workers. If the woman is infected in pregnancy, there is a 40% chance of transmission to the fetus, and 15% of infants born with CMV have symptoms such as hepatosplenomegaly, petechiae, small size for gestational age, direct hyperbilirubinemia, or thrombocytopenia. The risk is even higher for the infant if the mother acquires the disease early in the pregnancy. If a mother is infected with rubella in the first trimester, the rate of infection in utero is as high as 80%, but after the first trimester, the rate drops drastically. Congenital varicella is very rare. Toxoplasmosis is caused by a parasite, not a virus. When infection of the mother with toxoplasmosis occurs during pregnancy, almost 40% of their infants become infected in utero, and about 15% of those children have severe clinical damage.

15–61 Answer D

Metrorrhagia is menses with irregular intervals and excessive flow and duration. Oligomenorrhea is menses with an interval of more than 35 days. Polymenorrhea is menses with intervals of less than 21 days. Menorrhagia is menses of regular normal intervals, but with excessive flow and duration.

15–62 Answer D

The clinical consequences of persistent anovulation include infertility; menstrual bleeding problems, ranging from amenorrhea to dysfunctional uterine bleeding; an increased risk of cardiovascular disease; hirsutism and acne; an increased risk of endometrial cancer and breast cancer; and an increased risk of diabetes mellitus in clients with hyperinsulinemia. Therapy depends on the client. If the client wants to get pregnant, she is a candidate for the medical induction of ovulation. For the client who does not wish to become pregnant and does not complain of hirsutism, but is anovulatory and has irregular bleeding, therapy is directed toward interruption of the steady-state effect on the endometrium and breast. Cyclic mastalgia is the most common breast-related complaint seen in women's health practice. The breast is a complex organ that is sensitive to hormones. Estradiol and progesterone stimulate breast tissue. Breast pain that positively correlates with menses is cyclic mastalgia. Menorrhagia is a term used to describe irregular bleeding. Endometriosis is extrauterine growth of the endometrial glands or stroma. It is believed to occur through retrograde menstruation, or differentiation of totipotential cells, or both.

15–63 Answer D

Primary amenorrhea is defined as no menses by age 14 in the absence of secondary sexual characteristics, or no menses by age 16 regardless of the appearance of secondary sexual characteristics. Secondary amenorrhea is the absence of three consecutive periods in a woman with established menstrual cycles.

15–64 Answer D

In exercise-induced amenorrhea, such as occurs in ballet dancers and marathon runners, the location of the problem is the hypothalamus. The outflow tract is the location of the problem, with developmental absence of the vagina or uterus, obstruction of the outflow tract, scarred uterine lining, and cervical obstruction. The location of the problem is the ovary in primary amenorrhea if the etiology is a congenital chromosomal abnormality, such as Turner's syndrome. The location of the problem is the anterior pituitary, with amenorrhea resulting from prolactin-secreting tumors or nonfunctioning adenomas.

15–65 Answer D

The differential diagnosis for an adnexal mass may involve five different sites with many different masses, such as the ovary for endometriosis, functional cyst, or benign neoplasm; the gastrointestinal tract for diverticular disease, appendicitis, inflammatory bowel disease, or colon cancer; the urinary tract for a distended bladder; the fallopian tube for an ectopic pregnancy or a malignant neoplasm; the uterus for a fibroid; or the retroperitoneum for a benign neoplasm, sarcoma, or abdominal wall hematoma or abscess.

15–66 Answer D

Risk factors for cervical neoplasia include smoking, human papillomavirus infection or having a sexual partner with the infection, first sexual encounter before age 20, a previous abnormal Pap smear, more than two lifetime sexual partners or having a sexual partner who has had more than two partners, and human immunodeficiency virus infection or other immunosuppressed states.

15–67 Answer C

Iron-deficiency anemia is usually helped when women take an oral contraceptive (OC) because women on an OC tend to lose less blood each month. Other noncontraceptive benefits or conditions for which OC use offers protection include ovarian and endometrial carcinoma, ectopic pregnancy, pelvic inflammatory disease, functional ovarian cysts, menstrual irregularities, dysmenorrhea, benign breast disease, and premenstrual syndrome.

15–68 Answer C

Tanner's sexual maturity rating stage 4 in a girl is when pubic hair is adult in type, but over a smaller area, with none on the medial thigh. In girls, stage 1 is preadolescent with no pubic hair. In stage 2, pubic hair growth is sparse and mostly on the labia. The hair is long and downy, slightly pigmented, and straight or only slightly curly. In stage 3, the pubic hair is sparse and spreads over the mons pubis. The hair is darker, coarser, and curlier. In stage 5, pubic hair is adult in type and patterned as an inverse triangle. Hair also appears on the medial thigh surface.

15–69 Answer D

For a diagnosis of premenstrual syndrome (PMS) to be "assigned," the following criteria must be met: symptoms occur in the luteal phase and resolve within 1–2 days of onset of menses, followed by a symptom-free period during the follicular phase; symptoms must be documented through several menstrual cycles and are sufficient to disrupt a woman's life to some degree; and other medical and psychological disorders have been ruled out. PMS occurs only in the presence of cyclic hormonal changes.

15–70 Answer B

In clients with pelvic inflammatory disease, leukocytosis is present in about 50% of the cases, the erythrocyte sedimentation rate is classically elevated, and the C-reactive protein level is usually elevated (exceeding 20 mg/L) in about 74% the cases.

15–71 Answer C

Thelarche (breast bud development) is the first sign of puberty in most girls. It occurs at an average age of 11 years. It is considered premature if it occurs before age 8. Premature thelarche without other signs of pubertal development or accelerated growth is usually benign and requires no treatment. It should be diagnosed after a medical evaluation is performed to exclude true precocious puberty, estrogen-producing tumors, ovarian cysts, and exogenous estrogen exposure.

15–72 Answer D

Indications for a colposcopy include a Pap smear showing dysplasia or cancer; history of diethylstilbestrol exposure; human immunodeficiency virus infection; persistent unexplained atypia of a Pap with evidence of human papillomavirus; suspicious visible lesion of the cervix, vagina, or vulva; and as a follow-up for previously treated clients. It is also highly recommended for clients with visible condylomata, unexplained vaginal discharge, or a sexual partner with condylomata.

15–73 Answer A

Of the symptoms listed in the question, the most commonly expressed symptom of women with premenstrual syndrome is fatigue (90%). Depression occurs about 80% of the time; breast tenderness about 85%; and swelling of the extremities about 67%. Other common symptoms include irritability (91%) and abdominal bloating (90%).

15–74 Answer B

Women with dysuria should be questioned about an associated vaginal discharge or irritation. Dysuria often represents a vaginal infection rather than a urinary tract infection. Women with dysuria from cystitis usually describe an internal discomfort, whereas women with dysuria from vaginitis usually describe a more external discomfort with the burning sensation in the vagina or labia, a result of urine flow over an inflamed vaginal mucosa.

15–75 Answer C

Candida albicans infection is more common in women with diabetes, as well as those who are pregnant, immunosuppressed, or using antibiotics or oral contraceptives.

15–76 Answer D

Simultaneous chlamydial infections are present in 30–50% of clients who have cervical gonococcal infections. Treatment should automatically be done for both when one has been diagnosed. The most common therapies are azithromycin (Zithromax) 1 g po for 1 dose for *Chlamydia* infection and ceftriaxone (Rocephin) 125 mg IM for 1 dose for gonorrhea.

15–77 Answer A

Recurrent cystitis is an associated symptom of stress incontinence. An associated symptom of urge incontinence (unstable detrusor contractions) is the inability to delay voiding long enough to reach the toilet. Recurrent cystitis occurs more frequently in clients who have persistent residual urine resulting from an atonic bladder, cystocele, or diabetes mellitus. Neurogenic disorders are frequently associated with urge incontinence. Overflow incontinence is usually associated with benign prostatic hyperplasia and neurogenic conditions. Functional incontinence is incontinence caused by functional disabilities such as those associated with Alzheimer's disease or a cerebrovascular accident, rather than any problem with structure.

15–78 Answer C

Small-quantity incontinence, which produces nearly continuous dribbling, is symptomatic of overflow incontinence. Stress incontinence is symptomized by small-quantity incontinence on coughing, sneezing, laughing, and running. Urge incontinence involves an uncontrolled urge to void and is symptomized by large-quantity incontinence. Functional incontinence involves voiding normally with assistance.

15–79 Answer A

A cystocele is the prolapse into the vagina of the anterior vaginal wall and the bladder. Clinically, a pouching is seen on the anterior wall as the client strains. A rectocele is a prolapse into the vagina of the posterior vaginal wall and the rectum and is seen on the posterior wall as the client strains. An enterocele is a hernia of the pouch of Douglas into the vagina and would be seen as a bulge emerging from the posterior fornix. In first-degree uterine prolapse, the cervix appears at the introitus when the client strains.

15–80 Answer D

When the uterus is anteverted, the position of the cervix is on the anterior vaginal wall. When the position of the uterus is midposition, the cervix is at the apex of the vagina. When it is retroverted, the cervix is on the posterior vaginal wall. When the uterus is retroflexed, the position of the cervix may be on the anterior or posterior vaginal wall or the apex.

15–81 Answer A

The most common type of invasive breast carcinoma is infiltrating ductal carcinoma (70–80%). This is followed by lobular (5–10%); medullary (5–7%); and Paget's, inflammatory, infiltrating papillary, tubular, and mucinous breast carcinomas (less than 5%).

15–82 Answer B

Elimination of the offensive agent and use of corticosteroids is the treatment of choice for reactive vaginitis. An antifungal agent needs to be administered for candidiasis, and topical estrogen is used for atrophic vaginitis. No treatment or povidone-iodine is used for normal cervical or vaginal-discharge vaginitis.

15–83 Answer B

Trichomonal vaginitis is a sexually transmitted disease. Monilial vaginitis, atrophic vaginitis, and bacterial vaginosis are all nonsexually transmitted types of vaginitis. Vulvovaginal candidiasis (formerly *Monilia* species), although not an STD, may be transmitted between partners and between mother and newborn. Atrophic vaginitis is present in postmenopausal women who are not on hormone replacement therapy. Bacterial vaginosis is the most common vaginitis in women of reproductive age and is caused by *Gardnerella vaginalis*.

15–84 Answer C

The gray, mucoid, pasty vaginal discharge of bacterial vaginosis has a pH of 5 or higher (usually 5–6). The normal vaginal discharge has a pH of 3.8–4.2. The vaginal pH in candidiasis and reactive vaginitis is 5 or less. This might have significance in the office if the pH on a gray, mucoid, pasty vaginal discharge is above 5. Treatment for bacterial vaginosis can then be initiated immediately.

15–85 Answer A

Bartholin's (greater vestibular) glands are posterior on each side of the vaginal orifice and open onto the sides of the vestibule in the groove between the labia minor and hymen. Skene's (lesser vestibular, paraurethral) glands open onto the vestibule on each side of the urethra. Cystocele is a herniation of posterior bladder into the anterior vagina with a primary symptom of incontinence.

15–86 Answer B

Estradiol (E2) is the most potent form of estrogen and is secreted in the greatest amount by the ovaries during the reproductive years. Estrogens are secreted throughout the menstrual cycle, although at varying levels. They are essential for the development and maintenance of secondary sex characteristics and, along with progesterone and androgen, stimulate the female reproductive organs to prepare for the growth of a fetus. As ovarian function decreases, the production of estradiol decreases and is ultimately replaced by estrone (E1) as the major ovarian estrogen. Estrone has only a fraction of the potency of estradiol. During this time, the second ovarian hormone, progesterone, also is markedly reduced.

15–87 Answer D

Galactorrhea (lactation not associated with pregnancy or nursing) is sometimes associated with a pituitary tumor. Unilateral discharge from one or two ducts can be seen in fibrocystic breast disease, intraductal papilloma, and carcinoma.

15–88 Answer D

Risk factors that may predispose a woman to dysfunctional uterine bleeding (DUB) include stress, extreme weight change, use of oral contraceptive agents or intrauterine devices, and postmenopausal status. DUB is the most frequently reported health-care problem in women and the leading cause of hysterectomy. DUB is usually related to hormonal imbalances or benign or malignant pelvic neoplasms.

15–89 Answer D

Procidentia is a third-degree uterine prolapse. Prolapse of the uterus can vary from mild to complete. In procidentia, also referred to as hysteroptosia, the uterus prolapses completely outside the body, with inversion of the vagina. It is generally attributable to the relation of the tissues that provide support for the pelvic organs. A cystocele is a herniation of the urinary bladder into the vagina. A rectocele is a hernial protrusion of part of the rectum into the vagina. A vesicovaginal fistula is an abnormal opening between the urinary bladder and the vagina, leading to incontinent leakage of urine through the vagina. A rectovaginal fistula is an abnormal opening between the rectum and vagina, causing incontinent leakage of stool or flatus through the vagina. This type is less common than the vesicovaginal fistula.

15–90 Answer B

Bartholin's cyst is an obstruction or infection of the Bartholin's gland. It results in pain, redness, a perineal mass, and dyspareunia. An ovarian cyst may be functional or inflammatory. A functional cyst occurs during ovulation and may be asymptomatic and resolve spontaneously, or it can cause pain, menstrual irregularity, or amenorrhea. An inflammatory cyst is an infection of the ovary or uterine tube and results in an elevated white blood cell count, a low-grade fever, pain, and excessive menstrual flow. An endometrial polyp results in bleeding between periods. A cervical polyp can cause bleeding after intercourse or between periods.

15–91 Answer B

CA 125 is a tumor marker that is highly specific to epithelial ovarian cancer. Increased levels (above 35 U/mL) may indicate peritoneal diseases such as endometriosis, although significant elevations are usually found with ovarian cancer. The PSA is the tumor marker for prostate cancer, although high levels have also been shown with benign prostatic hypertrophy, prostate massage, prostate surgery, and prostatitis. CA 15-3 level is elevated in metastatic breast disease and may be elevated in benign breast or ovarian disease. CA 19-9 level is elevated in pancreatic and hepatobiliary cancer.

15–92 Answer D

Dyspareunia (pain during intercourse) may be caused by organic or psychogenic factors. Psychogenic causes include fear of vaginal penetration, which may be helped by desensitization therapy and gradual, progressive dilation; sexual dysfunction caused by vaginismus (painful spasm of the vagina from the contraction of the muscles surrounding it), which may be a result of real, imagined, or anticipated attempts at vaginal penetration; and pain caused by vaginal penetration. Desensitization therapy may be helpful in all these cases as well as sexual education regarding "normal" functioning and psychotherapy to resolve underlying conflicts that may be present and that inhibit the sexual act.

15–93 Answer C

Smoking is one of the lifestyle factors associated with an increased risk for breast cancer. Others include a high-fat diet, two or more drinks of alcohol per day, overweight, a high socioeconomic status, and breast trauma.

15–94 Answer B

Paget's disease (Paget's carcinoma) is a rare type of breast cancer involving infiltration of the nipple epithelium. It begins with itching or burning of the nipple combined with superficial erosion, crusting, or ulceration. It is usually misdiagnosed as an infection. It has an excellent prognosis if the cancerous changes are confined to the nipple. Mammary duct ectasia, also known as plasma cell mastitis, is a palpable lumpiness found beneath the areola. Duct ectasia involves periductal inflammation, dilation of the ductal system, and an accumulation of fluid and dead cells that block the involved ducts. It is sometimes difficult to differentiate from cancer because it also occurs in perimenopausal or late premenopausal women. Fibroadenomas are overgrowths of periductal stromal connective tissue that compress ducts into well-defined lumps with circumscribed edges and smooth boundaries. They are mobile, firm, and nontender lumps, and usually occur in women younger than age 25.

15–95 Answer C

A trans-rectus abdominis muscle flap procedure (TRAM) is a type of breast reconstruction surgery. It is an autogenous procedure in which skin is transferred from the rectus abdominis muscle to fashion a breast. It is performed immediately after the removal of the breast cancer. The abdominal muscle is fashioned into a new breast and a new nipple is created or the client's own one is used. Women seem to prefer this type of breast reconstructive surgery because a "tummy tuck" is done at the same time.

Bibliography

Agras, WS, et al: Outcome predictors for the cognitive behavior treatment of bulimia nervosa: Data from a multisite study. Am J Psychiatry 157:1307, 2000.

Baker, D, et al: Role of primary care physician in evaluating and managing genital herpes. Fam Med, January, 2003.

Barclay, L. Advance provision of emergency contraceptives safe, appropriate postpartum. Fam Med, July, 2003.

Brown, KMP (ed): Management Guidelines for Nurse Practitioners Working with Women (2nd ed). FA Davis, Philadelphia, 2004.

Campbell, KA, and Shaughnessy, AF: Diagnostic utility of the digital rectal examination as part of the routine pelvic examination. J Fam Pract 46:2, 1998.

Caufield, KA: Controlling fertility. In Youngkin, EQ, and Davis, MS (eds): Women's Health: A Primary Care Clinical Guide. Appleton & Lange, Norwalk, CT, 1998.

Fairburn, C, et al: The natural course of bulimia nervosa and binge eating disorder in young women. Arch Gen Psychiatry 57:659, 2000.

Fogel, CI: Women and sexuality. In Youngkin, EQ, and Davis, MS (eds): Women's Health: A Primary Care Clinical Guide. Norwalk, CT: Appleton & Lange, 1998.

Fredman, S, and Rosenbaum, JF: Mood disorders and their treatment in women across the reproductive life cycle. Fam Med, June, 2003.

Keel, PK, et al: Long term impact of treatment in women diagnosed with bulimia nervosa. Int J Eat Disord 31:151, 2002.

Marantides, D: Management of polycystic ovary syndrome. Nurse Pract 22:12, 1997.

Millikan, L: The proposed inflammatory pathophysiology of rosacea: Implications for treatment. Fam Med, March 17, 2003.

Ninia, JG: New approaches to varicose and telangiectatic leg veins. Female Client 23:1, 1998.

Reas, DL, et al: Prognostic value of duration of illness and early intervention in bulimia nervosa: A systematic review of outcome literature. Int J Eat Disord 30:1, 2001.

Scharbo-DeHaan, M, et al: The CDC 2002 guidelines for the treatment of STDs: Implications for women's healthcare. J Midwifery Women's Health, May, 2003.

Speroff, L, et al: Preventing cardiovascular disease in women: A work in progress. Fam Med, October, 2002.

Strober, M, et al: Controlled family study of anorexia nervosa and bulimia nervosa: Evidence of shared liability and transmission of partial syndromes. Am J Psychiatry 157:393, 2000.

Wade, TD, et al: Anorexia nervosa and major depression: Shared genetic and environmental risk factors. Am J Psychiatry 157:469, 2000.

Wolf, J: Acne and Rosacea: Differential diagnosis and treatment in the primary care setting. Fam Med, September, 2002.

Writing Group for the Women's Health Initiative Investigators: Risks and benefits of estrogen plus progestin in healthy postmenopausal women—Principal results from the Women's Health Initiative Randomized Control Trial. JAMA 288:321–333, 2002.

HOW WELL DID YOU DO?

85% AND ABOVE CONGRATULATIONS! THIS SCORE SHOWS APPLICATION OF TEST-TAKING PRINCIPLES AND ADEQUATE CONTENT KNOWLEDGE.

75–85% KEEP WORKING! REVIEW TEST-TAKING PRINCIPLES AND TRY AGAIN.

65–75% HANG IN THERE! SPEND SOME TIME REVIEWING CONCEPTS AND TEST-TAKING PRINCIPLES AND TRY THE TEST AGAIN.

Musculoskeletal Problems 16

JILL E. WINLAND-BROWN

16–1 *Mrs. Matthews has rheumatoid arthritis. On reviewing an x ray of her hip, you notice that there is a marked absence of articular cartilage. What mechanism is responsible for this?*

A. Antigen-antibody formation
B. Lymphocyte response
C. Immune complex formation
D. Lysosomal degradation

16–2 *Mrs. Kelly, age 80, has a curvature of the spine. This is likely to indicate which age-related change?*

A. Lordosis
B. Dorsal kyphosis
C. Scoliosis
D. Kyphoscoliosis

16–3 *Mr. McKinsey was recently given a diagnosis of degenerative joint disease. Which assessment test would you use to check for effusion on his knee?*

A. Thomas test
B. Tinel's test
C. Bulge test
D. Phalen's tool

16–4 *During a sports preparticipation physical examination, when you ask the client to rise up on his toes and raise his heels, you are observing for:*

A. calf symmetry and leg strength.
B. symmetry and knee and ankle effusion.
C. hip, knee, and ankle motion.
D. scoliosis, hip motion, and hamstring tightness.

16–5 *A clinical manifestation of symmetric neurogenic pain may indicate:*

A. radiculopathy
B. reflex sympathetic dystrophy
C. entrapment neuropathy
D. peripheral neuropathy

16–6 *Which test is used to diagnose an Achilles tendon rupture?*

A. Boutonnière test
B. Lachman test
C. Thompson test
D. Drawer test

16–7 *James, age 17, has been complaining of a painful knob below his right knee that has prevented him from actively participating in sports. He has recently been given a diagnosis of Osgood-Schlatter disease and asks you about his treatment options. You tell him that the initial treatment is:*

A. relative rest; he could benefit from hamstring stretching, heel cord stretching, and quadriceps stretching exercises.
B. immobilization; a long-leg knee immobilizer is recommended.
C. surgical intervention; removal of the bony fragments is necessary.
D. bedrest for 1 week.

16–8 *Dennis, age 4, has an apparent hypertrophy of the calf muscles, which seem doughy on palpation. His mother is concerned because Dennis is unable to* *raise himself from the floor without bracing his knees with his hands. You suspect:*

A. Duchenne's muscular dystrophy.
B. cerebral palsy.
C. Legg-Calvé-Perthes disease.
D. multiple sclerosis.

16–9 *C5 innervates:*

A. wrist extension.
B. elbow extension.
C. abduction and lateral rotation of the shoulders.
D. ulnar deviation at the wrist.

16–10 *Janine, age 69, has a class III case of rheumatoid arthritis. According to the American Rheumatism Association, her function would be:*

A. adequate for normal activities despite a handicap of discomfort or limited motion at one or more joints.
B. incapacitated, largely or wholly bedridden, or confined to a wheelchair with little or no self-care.
C. completely able to carry on all usual duties without handicaps.
D. limited only to few or none of the duties of usual occupation or self-care.

16–11 *Risk factors for congenital hip dislocation include all of the following* ***except:***

A. being the firstborn female child.
B. orthopedic malformation in utero.
C. family history of congenital dislocation of the hip.
D. breech presentation.

16–12 *Modifiable risk factors for osteoporosis include all of the following* ***except:***

A. calcium deficiency.
B. estrogen deficiency.
C. smoking.
D. excessive exercise.

16–13 *Sam, age 50, presents with Paget's disease that has been stable for several years. Recently, his serum alkaline phosphatase level has been steadily rising. You determine that it is time to start him on:*

A. ibuprofen (Motrin).
B. indomethacin (Indocin).
C. calcitonin.
D. plicamycin (Mithracin).

16–14 *John, age 17, works as a stock boy at the local supermarket. He is in the office for a routine visit. You notice that he had an episode of low back pain 6 months ago from improperly lifting heavy boxes. In discussing proper body mechanics with him to prevent future injuries, you tell him all of the following* ***except:***

A. "Bend your knees and face the object straight on."
B. "Hold boxes close to your body, not at arm's length."
C. "Your back brace should be worn only when you plan on lifting very heavy objects."
D. "Spread your feet about shoulder width apart."

16–15 *Dan, age 49, developed osteomyelitis of the femur after a motorcycle accident. Which of the following statements about the clinical manifestations of osteomyelitis is correct?*

A. Integumentary effects include swelling, erythema, and warmth at the involved site.
B. There is a low-grade fever with intermittent chills.
C. Musculoskeletal effects include tenderness of the entire leg.
D. Cardiovascular effects include bradycardia.

16–16 *You are assessing Laura, a 69-year-old Asian woman, for the first time. You are trying to differentiate between scoliosis and kyphosis. Kyphosis involves:*

A. asymmetry of the shoulders, scapulae, and waist creases.
B. a lateral curvature and vertebral rotation on posteroanterior x rays.
C. severe back pain.
D. a posterior rounding at the thoracic level.

16–17 *Mr. Miller is a 72-year-old African-American with insulin-dependent diabetes mellitus. He has been a chronic smoker for 50 years. He has been told recently that he must have an above-the-knee amputation because of a gangrenous foot. He has lost the will to live and states, "They shoot horses, don't they?" How do you respond?*

A. "You should be thankful they can save your life, if not your leg."
B. "Your wife needs you; you must think of her at this time."
C. "How do you feel this surgery will affect you?"
D. "I will stay with you before, during, and after the surgery because I know that this is a difficult time for you."

16–18 *Mary, age 21, presents today with another muscle strain from one of her many sports activities. You think that she was probably never taught about health promotion and maintenance regarding physical activity. What information do you include in your teaching?*

A. "After an activity, if any part hurts, apply ice for 20 minutes."
B. "You must first get in shape with a rigorous schedule of weight training and then you can participate in any activity once you are physically fit."

C. "After any strenuous activity, you must completely rest your muscles before beginning your next activity."
D. "Stretching and warmup exercises are an important part of any exercise routine."

16–19 *Jim, age 18, sprained his ankle playing ice hockey. He is confused as to whether to apply heat or cold. What do you tell him?*

A. "Use continuous heat for the first 12 hours, then use heat or cold to your own preference."
B. "Use continuous cold for the first 12 hours, then use heat or cold to your own preference."
C. "Apply cold for 20 minutes, then take it off for 15 minutes; repeat for the first 24 hours, then repeat the same procedure using heat."
D. "Alternate between cold and heat for 20 minutes each for the first 24 hours."

16–20 *Joyce, age 87, broke her wrist after falling off a curb. She just had a plaster cast applied to her wrist. In instructing her family on allowing the cast to dry properly, tell them to:*

A. continuously elevate Joyce's arm on a pillow.
B. change the position of Joyce's arm every hour.
C. position a fan near Joyce during the night to ensure even drying of the cast.
D. put a blanket over the cast to absorb the dampness.

16–21 *John, age 26, has a cast on his right arm because of a rollerblading accident. Twelve hours after the cast was applied, he complains of severe pain even though he recently took his pain medication. His fingers are pink, yet he states that they are tingling and feel slightly numb. What do you suspect?*

A. Compartment syndrome
B. Phlebitis
C. Osteomyelitis
D. Muscle contraction

16–22 *Mike, a golf pro, has had chronic back pain for many years. His workup reveals that it is not the result of a degenerative disc problem. His back "goes out" about twice per year and he is out of work for about a week each time. Which of the following is not indicated?*

A. Surgery
B. A planned exercise program to strengthen back muscles
C. Reinforcement of teaching regarding appropriate body mechanics in lifting and reaching
D. Modifying the workplace or environment to minimize stress to the lower back

16–23 *Your client has just been told that he has a primary bone tumor. He was so upset when the physician told him that he focused only on the word "malignant" and not on the prognosis or type of tumor. Which of the following tumors is malignant?*

A. Osteochondroma
B. Chondroma
C. Osteosarcoma
D. Giant-cell tumor

16–24 *Paul has a malignant fibrosarcoma of the femur. He recently had surgery and is now on radiation therapy. You want to order a test to determine the extent of the tumor invasion of the surrounding tissues and the response of the bone tumor to the radiation. Which of the following tests should you order?*

A. An x ray
B. A magnetic resonance imaging scan
C. A computed tomography scan
D. A needle biopsy

16–25 *Mickey is on a chemotherapeutic antibiotic for a musculoskeletal neoplasm. Which drug do you think he is taking?*

A. Cyclophosphamide (Cytoxan)
B. Bleomycin (Blenoxane)
C. Methotrexate (Rheumatrex)
D. Cisplatin (Platinol)

16–26 *Jane, age 64, comes in for a visit. She has a cast on her right arm and tells you that she has a comminuted fracture of her radius. When she asks what that means, you tell her that a comminuted fracture is when the:*

A. bony fragments are in many pieces.
B. broken ends of the bone protrude through the soft tissues and skin.
C. bone breaks cleanly but does not penetrate the skin.
D. bone is crushed.

16–27 *Grating of the bones or entrance of air into an open fracture is manifested as:*

A. swelling.
B. ecchymosis.
C. crepitus.
D. pain and tenderness.

16–28 *There are many precursors of deep venous thrombosis, such as decreased blood flow, injury to the blood vessel wall, and altered blood coagulation. Which one is the result of blood loss whereby the body attempts to maintain homeostasis by increasing the production of platelets and clotting factors?*

A. Altered blood coagulation
B. Decreased blood flow
C. Injury to the blood vessel wall
D. None of the above

16–29 *When Johnny, age 12, slid into home plate while playing softball, he injured his ankle. You are trying to differentiate between a sprain and a strain. You know that a strain includes all the following* ***except:***

A. the presence of sharp or dull pain.
B. pain that is often increased with isometric contraction of the muscle.
C. the presence of swelling and local tenderness.
D. the possibility of joint instability.

16–30 *Jill, age 49, has recently begun a rigorous weight-lifting regimen. She presents in your office with an anterior shoulder dislocation. All of the following are clinical manifestations of an anterior shoulder dislocation* ***except:***

A. inability to shrug the shoulder.
B. pain.
C. inability to rotate the shoulder externally.
D. lengthening of the arm.

16–31 *Colchicine may be used to terminate an acute attack of gouty arthritis as well as to prevent recurrent episodes. The mechanism of action is to:*

A. interrupt the cycle of urate crystal deposition and inflammatory response.
B. increase serum uric acid levels.
C. potentiate the excretion of uric acid.
D. inhibit the tubular reabsorption of urate, promoting the excretion of uric acid.

16–32 *Jim, age 64, has rheumatoid arthritis. Which of the following drugs would you not order?*

A. Acetylsalicylic acid
B. Acetaminophen (Tylenol)
C. Valdecoxib (Bextra)
D. Nabumetone (Relafen)

16–33 *For your client with a knee injury, you order a nonsteroidal anti-inflammatory drug (NSAID) to be taken on a routine basis for the next 2 weeks. Your teaching would include all the following* ***except:***

A. "Do not take these drugs on an empty stomach, take with food or milk."
B. "Do not drive or operate machinery if you notice drowsiness while taking an NSAID."
C. "Call immediately if you notice any bloody urine, coffee-ground emesis, or blood in the stool."
D. "If you have additional pain, an occasional aspirin is permitted in between the usual doses of the NSAID."

16–34 *Jessie, age 49, states that she thinks she has rheumatoid arthritis. Before any diagnostic tests are ordered, you complete a physical exam and make a tentative diagnosis of osteoarthritis rather than rheumatoid arthritis. Which clinical manifestation ruled out rheumatoid arthritis?*

A. Fatigue.
B. Affected joints are swollen, cool, and bony-hard on palpation.
C. Decreased range of motion.
D. Stiffness.

16–35 *Marsha, age 34, presents with symptoms resembling both fibromyalgia and chronic fatigue syndrome, which have many similarities. Which of the following is not characteristic of chronic fatigue syndrome?*

A. Musculoskeletal pain
B. Difficulty sleeping
C. Depression
D. Fatigue

16–36 *Steve, age 32, fell off a roof while shingling it. He is complaining of pain in his left hip and leg area. Other than an x-ray, what would make you suspect a fractured pelvis?*

A. A clicking sensation when moving the hips
B. A positive pelvic tilt test
C. Hematuria
D. Absence of distal reflexes

16–37 *Stan, age 34, fractured his femur when his horse tripped over a jump. With this type of injury, you know that Stan is at risk for fat emboli. Early assessment findings for this complication include:*

A. fever, tachycardia, rapid respiration, and mental confusion.
B. mental confusion, temperature elevation, bradycardia, and pallor.
C. hostility; combativeness; substernal pain; and weak, thready pulse.
D. lethargy, hypothermia, paresthesia, and absent peripheral pulses.

16–38 *Manny, age 52, is a postal worker who drives a truck every day. He presents with lower back pain and has decreased sensation to a pinprick in the lateral leg and web of the great toe. This indicates discogenic disease in which area?*

A. L3/L4 (L4 root involvement)
B. L4/L5 (L5 root involvement)
C. L5/S1 (S1 root involvement)
D. None of the above

16–39 *You are driving home from work and stop at the scene of a motorcycle accident that must have just occurred because there are no rescue vehicles at the scene. The driver is lying at the side of the road unconscious with an obvious open fracture of his femur. Which of the following actions should take priority?*

A. Stop the bleeding from the wound.
B. Determine if there has been a cervical fracture.
C. Establish an airway.
D. Feel the peripheral pulses.

16–40 *You are assessing Mike, age 16, after a football injury to his right knee. You elicit a positive anterior/posterior drawer sign. This test indicates an injury to the:*

A. lateral meniscus.
B. cruciate ligament.
C. medial meniscus.
D. posterior meniscus.

16–41 *A positive McBurney's point, a positive psoas sign, and a positive obturator test are all indicative of which condition?*

A. pancreatitis
B. cholecystitis
C. bursitis
D. appendicitis

16–42 *To plan for a community education program, the nurse practitioner needs to know that persons at highest risk for developing thoracic outlet syndrome are:*

A. bicycle riders.
B. dancers.
C. computer programmers.
D. swimming instructors.

16–43 *Which muscle enzyme is elevated in polymyositis?*

A. Aldolase A
B. Aspartate aminotransferase
C. Creatine kinase
D. Lactate dehydrogenase

16–44 *Management of fibromyalgia includes all of the following* ***except:***

A. Giving psychotropic drugs, such as amitriptyline (Elavil), in a low dose at bedtime.
B. Injecting trigger points with local anesthetics and steroids.
C. Using acetaminophen (Tylenol) or a nonsteroidal anti-inflammatory drug.
D. Avoiding exercise.

16–45 *When should a bone mass measurement be taken to assess whether a female client is at high risk for osteoporosis?*

A. At the beginning of menopause
B. When she is in her 30s
C. During perimenopause
D. When the client is estrogen deficient

16–46 *In assessing the head and neck, you palpate for lymphadenopathy. Which of the following sites for lymph node enlargement indicates the most serious problem?*

A. Epitrochlear
B. Deep cervical chain
C. Posterior auricular
D. Supraclavicular

16–47 *In assessing the skeletal muscles, you turn the forearm so that the palm is up. This is called:*

A. supination.
B. pronation.
C. abduction.
D. eversion.

16–48 *The largest joint in the body is the:*

A. hip.
B. shoulder.
C. knee.
D. elbow.

16–49 *Sarah, age 70, was told that she has osteoporosis. When she asks you what this is, you respond that osteoporosis:*

A. develops when loss of bone matrix (resorption) occurs more rapidly than new bone growth (deposition).
B. is a degenerative joint disease characterized by degeneration and loss of articular cartilage in synovial joints.
C. is a chronic, systemic inflammatory disorder characterized by persistent synovitis of multiple joints.
D. is a metabolic bone disorder characterized by inadequate mineralization of bone matrix.

16–50 *Black men have a relatively low incidence of osteoporosis because they have:*

A. increased bone resorption.
B. long, narrow, and dense long bones.
C. wide and thick long bones.
D. decreased bone deposition.

16–51 *When grading muscle strength, a grade of 4 indicates:*

A. full range of motion (ROM) against gravity with full resistance.
B. full ROM against gravity with some resistance.
C. full ROM with gravity.
D. full ROM with gravity eliminated (passive motion).

16–52 *In assessing your client, you place the tips of your first two fingers in front of each ear and ask him to open and close his mouth. Then you drop your fingers into the depressed area over the joint and note for smooth motion of the mandible. With this action, you are assessing for:*

A. maxillomandibular integrity.
B. well-positioned permanent teeth or well-fitting dentures.
C. temporomandibular joint syndrome.
D. a calcium imbalance.

16–53 *If any limitation or any increase in range of motion occurs when assessing the musculoskeletal system, the angles of the bones should be measured by using:*

A. Phalen's tool.
B. skeletometry.
C. the Thomas joint measure.
D. a goniometer.

16–54 *During your assessment of your client's foot, you note that the foot is in alignment with the long axis of the lower leg and that weight bearing falls on the middle of the foot, from the heel, along the mid-foot, to between the second and third toes. You diagnose:*

A. a normal foot.
B. hallux valgus.
C. talipes equinovarus.
D. hammer toes.

16–55 *In assessing an infant for congenital hip dislocation, the practitioner places the infant supine; flexes the knees by holding the thumbs on the inner midthighs, with fingers outside on the hips touching the greater trochanters; then adducts the legs until the practitioner's thumbs touch. The legs are then abducted, moving the knees apart and down so that their lateral aspects touch the table. If this external rotation feels smooth with no sound present, there is no hip dislocation. This is the:*

A. Allis test.
B. Laseque's test.
C. McMurray test.
D. Ortolani maneuver.

16–56 *When teaching Amanda, age 67, to use a cane because of osteoarthritis of her left knee, an important point to stress is to tell her to:*

A. carry the cane in the ipsilateral hand.
B. advance the cane with the ipsilateral leg.
C. make sure that the cane length equals the height of the iliac crest.
D. use the cane to aid in joint protection and safety.

16–57 *To diagnose fibromyalgia, there must be tenderness on digital palpation in at least 11 of 18 (9 pairs) tender-point sites in all of the following* ***except:***

A. the occiput.
B. the second rib.
C. the gluteal.
D. the ankle.

16–58 *Gerry, age 46, presents with a tender, red, swollen knee. A presumptive diagnosis of acute gout may be made by all of the following* ***except:***

A. a negative joint culture.
B. hyperuricemia.
C. a significant response to colchicine or a nonsteroidal anti-inflammatory drug.
D. a positive antinuclear antibody test.

16–59 *First-line drug therapy for acute low back pain includes the use of:*

A. nonsteroidal anti-inflammatory drugs.
B. muscle relaxants.
C. opioids.
D. a combination of the above.

16–60 *Jim, age 22, a stockboy, has an acute episode of low back pain. You order a nonsteroidal anti-inflammatory drug and tell him to do all of the following* ***except:***

A. stay in bed for 3–4 days.
B. resume normal activity within the limits imposed by the pain.
C. begin lower back strengthening exercises depending on pain tolerance.
D. use cold packs, heat, or a combination of both.

16–61 *A Baker's cyst is:*

A. an inflammation of the bursa.
B. a form of tendinitis.
C. the buildup of synovial fluid in the knee.
D. the result of a "twisted" ligament.

16–62 *The straight-leg-raising maneuver can be used to diagnose:*

A. nerve root compression.
B. a fractured hip.
C. an anterior cruciate ligament tear.
D. tendinitis.

16–63 *Ginny, age 38, has rheumatoid arthritis and gets achy and stiff after sitting through a long movie. This is referred to as:*

A. longevity stiffness.
B. gelling.
C. intermittent arthritis.
D. molding.

16–64 *Marie states that she has a maternal history of rheumatoid disease but that she has never been affected. Today she presents with complaints of dryness of the eyes and mouth. What do you suspect?*

A. Rheumatoid arthritis
B. Systemic lupus erythematosus
C. Sjögren's syndrome
D. Rosacea

16–65 *Sandra, a computer programmer, has just been given a diagnosis of carpal tunnel syndrome. Your next step is to:*

A. suggest surgery.
B. take a more complete history.

C. try neutral position wrist splinting and order an oral nonsteroidal anti-inflammatory drug.
D. do electrophysiologic testing.

16–66 *All of the following serum levels are low in osteomalacia **except:***

A. serum calcium.
B. alkaline phosphatase.
C. creatinine excretion.
D. serum phosphorus.

16–67 *Lois, age 42, is pregnant and was just given a diagnosis of carpal tunnel syndrome. She is worried that this will affect her in caring for the baby. What do you tell her?*

A. "Don't worry, we'll find a brace that is very malleable."
B. "After childbirth, your carpal tunnel syndrome may clear up."
C. "If we do surgery now, you'll be recovered by the time the baby arrives."
D. "Let's wait and see how bad it gets before you jump to conclusions."

16–68 *You suspect adolescent idiopathic scoliosis in Maura, age 15, who is in her growth spurt. You perform the Adams forward-bending test and note a right-sided rib hump. This is indicative of:*

A. right lumbar shifting.
B. right thoracic curvature.
C. right truncal shift.
D. spondylolysis.

16–69 *Mindy, age 52, who has just been given a diagnosis of sarcoidosis, has joint symptoms including arthralgias and arthritis. Your next plan of action would be to:*

A. order a bone scan.
B. obtain a tissue biopsy.
C. begin a course of glucocorticoids.
D. obtain an electrocardiogram.

16–70 *Jeffrey, age 16, was involved in a motor vehicle accident. He walks into the office with an obvious facial fracture, then collapses. Your first action would be to:*

A. call his parents for permission to treat.
B. assess for an adequate airway.
C. obtain facial x-rays.
D. assess for a septal hematoma.

16–71 *The type of joint that is freely movable, such as the shoulder joint, is called:*

A. a synarthrosis joint.
B. an amphiarthrosis joint.
C. a diarthrosis joint.
D. none of the above.

16–72 *Julie says that she has heard that caffeine can cause osteoporosis and asks you why. How do you respond?*

A. "Caffeine has no effect on osteoporosis."
B. "A high caffeine intake has a diuretic effect that causes calcium to be excreted more rapidly."
C. "Caffeine affects bone metabolism by altering intestinal absorption of calcium and assimilation of calcium into the bone matrix."
D. "Caffeine increases bone resorption."

16–73 *Sally, who is postmenopausal, is taking 1500 mg of calcium, but does not understand why she also needs to take vitamin D. You tell her that:*

A. a deficiency of vitamin D results in an inadequate mineralization of bone matrix.
B. all vitamins need to be supplemented.
C. vitamin D increases intestinal absorption of dietary calcium and mobilizes calcium from the bone.
D. vitamin D binds with calcium to allow active transport into the cells.

16–74 *The American College of Obstetricians and Gynecologists' guidelines for exercise during pregnancy and after delivery include which of the following?*

A. Women can continue to perform moderate exercise routines three times per week.
B. Exercise in the supine position is the position of choice.
C. Anaerobic exercise during pregnancy is preferred over aerobic exercise
D. Exercise should be discontinued upon discovery of pregnancy and be resumed after delivery.

16–75 *What pathophysiology associated with transient pain after exercising usually lasts a few hours with soreness and may last up to a week?*

A. Increased lactic acid production, muscle breakdown, and minor inflammation.
B. Mild musculotendinous inflammation.
C. Major musculotendinous inflammation, periostitis, and bone microtrauma.
D. Breakdown in soft tissue and stress fracture.

16–76 *Greg, age 26, runs marathons and frequently complains of painful contractions of his calf muscles after running. You attribute this to:*

A. hypokalemia.
B. hyponatremia.
C. heat exhaustion.
D. dehydration.

16–77 *Jake, age 16, comes into the office with a human bite on his fist. What is the first course of action?*

A. Débride and irrigate the wound thoroughly.
B. Initiate broad-spectrum antibiotics.

C. Leave the wound open for drainage.
D. Administer a tetanus injection.

16–78 *When you elicit a painful Finkelstein's sign, you are testing for:*

A. carpal tunnel syndrome.
B. bursitis of the shoulder.
C. de Quervain's disease.
D. tennis elbow.

16–79 *A coccygeal fracture is treated:*

A. with traction.
B. by surgical repair.
C. conservatively with analgesia and by use of a "donut" cushion when sitting.
D. by bedrest.

16–80 *Martin, aged 58, presents with urethritis, conjunctivitis, and shallow, painful oral ulcers. You suspect the following condition:*

A. syphilis
B. gonorrhea.
C. HIV.
D. Reiter's syndome.

16–81 *Deborah, age 62, has swollen, bony proximal interphalangeal joints. You describe these as:*

A. Heberden's nodes.
B. Bouchard's nodes.
C. Osler's nodes.
D. Murphy's nodes.

16–82 *In analyzing the synovial fluid, a greenish-yellow color may indicate which of the following:*

A. trauma
B. gout
C. a bacterial infection
D. rheumatoid arthritis

16–83 *Which test assesses for thoracic outlet syndrome by having the client abduct his or her arms 90 degrees externally rotated with the elbows flexed 90 degrees, and then having the client open and close his or her hands for 3 minutes?*

A. Neer test.
B. Speed test.
C. Hawkins test.
D. Roos test.

16–84 *How can you differentiate between a ganglion cyst and a neoplasm?*

A. A neoplasm is more painful.
B. Ganglia transilluminate.
C. Ganglia cause more swelling.
D. A neoplasm may fluctuate in size.

16–85 *When wrist and finger extension causes pain over the extensor carpi radialis brevis tendon, the extensor carpi radialis longus tendon, and the extensor digitorum communis, you would suspect:*

A. tennis elbow.
B. golfer's elbow.
C. de Quervain's disease.
D. trigger finger intersection syndrome.

16–86 *Sandy, age 49, presents with loss of anal sphincter tone, impaired micturition, incontinence, and progressive loss of strength in the legs. You suspect cauda equina syndrome. What is your next action?*

A. Order physical therapy.
B. Teach bowel and bladder training.
C. Order extensive lab work.
D. Refer to a neurologist.

16–87 *Linda, age 29, is a nurse who has an acute episode of back pain. You have determined that it is a simple "mechanical" backache and order:*

A. bedrest for 2 days.
B. muscle relaxants.
C. "let pain be your guide" and continue activities.
D. back-strengthening exercises.

16–88 *Mary has a 15-year-old son who wants to play sports; however, she is very leery because she has heard of so many accidents. Which one of the following sports does the American Academy of Pediatrics list as a limited contact/impact sport?*

A. Field hockey
B. Soccer
C. Basketball
D. Lacrosse

16–89 *Steve, age 15, has only one testicle. When he asks you if he can play on the soccer team at school, how do you respond?*

A. "No, you'd be taking too much of a chance of injuring your remaining testicle."
B. "You can play any noncontact sport; however, soccer is too strenuous."
C. "As long as you can protect the remaining testicle, go for it."
D. "It should have no bearing on any activity."

16–90 *Which test is routinely recommended for a preparticipation sports physical?*

A. A complete blood count.
B. A chest x ray.
C. An electrocardiogram.
D. A Snellen eye test.

16–91 *The top three common causes of sudden death in athletes younger than age 30 include all of the following* ***except:***

A. bronchospasm from exercise-induced asthma.
B. hypertrophic cardiomyopathy.
C. idiopathic left ventricular hypertrophy.
D. coronary artery anomalies.

16–92 *Morris, age 52, is a chef who just cut off two of his fingers with a meat cutter. You would recommend all the following* ***except:***

A. transporting the fingers to the emergency room along with Morris.
B. sealing the fingers in a plastic bag.
C. maintaining the fingers at body temperature.
D. packing the fingers in a saline-soaked dressing.

16–93 *What part of the body is affected by Dupuytren's contracture?*

A. The fourth and fifth fingers
B. The great toe
C. The tibia
D. The penis

16–94 *You have just completed a workup on Michael, age 13, and confirmed Osgood-Schlatter disease. You should do all of the following* ***except:***

A. refer for early surgical correction.
B. recommend quadriceps-strengthening exercises.
C. teach heel-cord–stretching exercises.
D. discuss how Michael can modify his activities.

16–95 *Juliette, age 72, has severe osteoarthritis of her right knee. She obtains much relief from corticosteroid injections. When she asks you how often she can have them, how do you respond?*

A. Only once a year
B. No more than twice a year
C. No more than three times a year
D. No more than four times a year

16–96 *Nathan, age 48, has asymptomatic hyperuricemia. What is your initial therapy?*

A. Nonsteroidal anti-inflammatory drugs
B. Dietary counseling
C. Colchicine
D. Allopurinol (Zyloprim)

16–97 *To aid in the diagnosis of meniscus damage, you should:*

A. perform the bulge test.
B. perform the Lachman test.
C. perform the drawer test.
D. elicit Apley's sign.

16–98 *Which of the following can assist in the diagnosis of myasthenia gravis?*

A. The Tensilon test
B. The presence of cogwheel rigidity
C. Chvostek's sign.
D. Trousseau's sign

16–99 *Common causes of in-toeing in childhood include all the following* ***except:***

A. medial femoral torsion.
B. metatarsus adductus.
C. calcaneovalgus feet.
D. talipes equinovarus.

16–100 *Elaine, the mother of a 2-year-old, is concerned because her daughter walks on her toes all the time. What do you tell her?*

A. "Toe-walking is considered normal until age 3."
B. "Don't worry, she'll outgrow it."
C. "Toe-walking is normal until she starts preschool."
D. "We should do further testing now."

16–101 *Which of the following tests and signs assesses for de Quervain's disease?*

A. Allen's test
B. Finkelstein's test
C. Phalen's test
D. Tinel's sign

16–102 *Sammy is 45, of Northern European ancestry, and has a dysfunctional and disfiguring condition affecting the palmar tissue between the skin and the distal palm and fourth and fifth fingers. What do you suspect?*

A. Carpal tunnel syndrome
B. De Quervain's tenosynovitis
C. Dupuyten's contracture
D. Trigger finger

16–103 *June, a 59 year old cashier, presents with back pain with no precipitating event. Pain is over her lower back and muscles without sciatica, and it is aggravated by sitting, standing, and certain movements. It is alleviated with rest. Palpation localizes the pain, and muscle spasms are felt. There is an insidious onset with no progressive improvement. What is your initial diagnosis?*

A. Ankylosing spondylitis
B. Musculoskeletal strain
C. Spondylolisthesis
D. Herniated disk

16–104 *You suspect a herniated disk on Sarah, aged 72. You elevate her affected leg when she is in the supine position and it elicits pain, which indicates a positive test. This is known as which test or sign?*

A. Sciatic stretch test
B. Cross straight-leg-raising test
C. Doorbell sign
D. Lasegue's sign

16–105 *Margaret, age 72, states that her DEXA (dual-energy x-ray absorptiometry) or bone mass density (BMD) test revealed a BMD of > 1 standard deviation with a T score of −1. She asks you what this indicates. How do you respond?*

A. "This is a normal test."
B. "This means you have osteopenia."
C. "You have osteoporosis."
D. "You have severe osteoporosis."

16–106 *Beth, aged 49, comes in with low back pain. You do an x ray and it is negative. Which of the following diagnoses do you explore further?*

A. Scoliosis
B. Osteoarthritis
C. Spinal stenosis
D. Herniated nucleus pulposus

Answers

16–1 Answer D

Lysosomal degradation results when leukocytes produce lysosomal enzymes that destroy articular cartilage in rheumatoid arthritis. The collagen fibers and the protein polysaccharides of articular cartilage are broken down by the enzymes. Immune complexes initiate the inflammatory process that brings leukocytes to the cartilage. Immune complexes are formed by the combination of immunoglobulin G with rheumatoid factors that are the result of antigen-antibody formation.

16–2 Answer B

Dorsal kyphosis, an exaggerated convexity of the thoracic curvature, typically accompanies the aging process. Lordosis occurs when the normal lumbar concavity is further accentuated, such as with pregnancy or obesity. Scoliosis, which is more prevalent in adolescent girls, is a lateral S-shaped curvature of the thoracic and lumbar spine and is usually involved with vertebral rotation.

16–3 Answer C

The bulge test assesses for effusion on the knee. If effusion is present, a bulge will appear to the sides of or below the patella when the practitioner compresses the area above the patella. Thomas's test is used to assess for hip problems. Both the Tinel and Phalen tests assess for carpal tunnel syndrome.

16–4 Answer A

To observe for calf symmetry and leg strength, the practitioner asks the client to rise up on the toes and raise the heels. The athletic activity required to assess for symmetry and knee and ankle effusion would be to tighten and then relax the quadriceps. The "duck walk" of four steps away from the examiner with buttocks on heels would be used to observe for hip, knee, and ankle motion. Standing with the knees straight and then touching the toes is to check for scoliosis, hip motion, and hamstring tightness.

16–5 Answer D

Symmetric neurogenic pain (burning, numbness, paresthesia) will include peripheral neuropathy and myelopathy. Asymmetric neurogenic pain will include radiculopathy, reflex sympathetic dystrophy, and entrapment neuropathy. A claudication pain pattern will be present in peripheral vascular disease, giant-cell arteritis (with jaw pain), and lumbar spinal stenosis. These conditions all include the clinical manifestations of neurogenic pain.

16–6 Answer C

The Thompson test is used to diagnose an Achilles tendon rupture. With an Achilles tendon rupture, there is local swelling and bruising and a weak push-off. The Thompson test is positive when the gastrocnemius muscle belly is firmly squeezed and the foot does not plantarflex. Boutonnière deformity, not test, results from a direct laceration over the proximal interphalangeal joint, involving the extensor slip that attaches to the middle phalanx. The Lachman test assesses for an anterior cruciate ligament (ACL) tear. The knee is flexed 30 degrees, the femur is stabilized, and a forward force is applied to the proximal calf of the leg. Any perceived side-to side difference is usually significant. The drawer test (or sign) is also used to assess for an ACL tear, but it is much less reliable than the Lachman test.

16–7 Answer A

Osgood-Schlatter disease results from repetitive hyperextension strain caused by the pull of the patellar tendon on the tibial tuberosity. Treating the client as an adolescent will avoid many of the recurring problems in the active individual. Initially, relative rest should be used with hamstring stretching, heel cord stretching, and quadriceps stretching exercises. If the problem persists, a long-leg knee immobilizer may be used. Surgical intervention is rarely needed, but if so, only in an adult.

16–8 Answer A

Duchenne's muscular dystrophy, inherited in a sex-linked recessive pattern, afflicts boys, with the onset usually occurring around age 3–5. The inability of the child to raise himself without supporting his knees because of weakness beginning primarily in the quadriceps and hip extensor muscles is characteristic. Cerebral palsy affects motor function along with occasionally affecting intellect, emotional behavior, speech, sight, hearing, and touch. Damage occurs to the upper motor neurons during the prenatal or neonatal period. Legg-Calvé-Perthes disease is avascular necrosis of the capital femoral epiphysis. A limp would be present. Multiple sclerosis usually appears in the client around age 25–30. The most common symptoms involve visual, sensory, and gait disturbances.

16–9 Answer C

C5 innervates abduction and lateral rotation of the shoulders. Wrist extension results from the nerves at C6, elbow extension from the nerves at C7, and ulnar deviation from the nerves at the wrist at C8.

16–10 Answer D

The American Rheumatism Association has identified functional classes from I–IV depending on the client's ability to accomplish activities of daily living. Because Janine is a class III, her function would be limited to few or none of the duties of usual occupation or self-care. Class I refers to the client who can carry on all usual duties without handicaps. Class II refers to the client whose function is adequate for normal activities despite a handicap of discomfort or limited motion at one or more joints. Class IV refers to the client who is incapacitated, largely or wholly bedridden, or confined to a wheelchair with little or no self-care.

16–11 Answer B

Congenital hip dislocation occurs in approximately 1% of live births. Risk factors include being the firstborn female child, a family history of congenital dislocation of the hip, and breech presentation. Orthopedic malformation in utero is not a risk factor.

16–12 Answer D

Modifiable risk factors for osteoporosis include calcium deficiency, estrogen deficiency, and smoking. Excessive exercise is not a modifiable risk factor. Instead, a sedentary lifestyle is a risk factor. Other risk factors are a high caffeine intake and a high alcohol intake. Over the course of their lives, women tend to lose up to one-third of their original bone mass, ultimately affecting 80% of their skeletal system. It is essential that modifiable risk factors be modified because there are many that cannot be modified, including increasing age, status as a white woman, postmenopausal status, pale complexion, and long-term glucocorticoid therapy.

16–13 Answer C

Ibuprofen (Motrin), indomethacin (Indocin), and other nonsteroidal anti-inflammatory drugs are helpful for clients with Paget's disease who have mild symptoms and pain. However, once the serum alkaline phosphatase level rises, which indicates that the disease has progressed, calcitonin is the preferred treatment. Salmon calcitonin (Calcimar) and human calcitonin (Cibacalcin) are the two choices. Plicamycin (Mithracin) is a toxic cancer medication that is occasionally used with clients who fail to respond to other medications. It is extremely toxic to the liver, kidneys, and bone marrow, and thus it is a last resort.

16–14 Answer C

In discussing proper body mechanics with John to prevent future injuries, you tell him that a back brace should be worn at all times at work, not so much to prevent an injury but as a constant reminder to use proper mechanics. Even lifting a medium-weight box can cause a lumbosacral injury if poor body mechanics are used. You would also tell him to bend his knees and face the object straight on, to hold boxes close to his body and not at arm's length, and to spread his feet about shoulder-width apart. Using legs as well as arms, facing objects straight on, and keeping a wide stance, thereby giving oneself a broad base of support, use supporting muscles instead of isolating strictly back muscles.

16–15 Answer A

The clinical manifestations of osteomyelitis include the integumentary effects of swelling, erythema, and warmth at the involved site as well as drainage and ulceration and lymph node involvement, especially in the involved extremity. The client with osteomyelitis may also have tachycardia, localized tenderness, and a high fever with chills.

16–16 Answer D

Kyphosis involves a posterior rounding at the thoracic level and a kyphotic curve of over 45 degrees on x-ray. There may be moderate pain with kyphosis. Scoliosis involves asymmetry of the shoulders, scapulae, and waist creases, a lateral curvature and vertebral rotation on the posteroanterior x-rays, and severe back pain.

16–17 Answer C

Exploring Mr. Miller's feelings and getting more clarification of how the surgery will affect him will allow you to know him better and be better able to assist him in dealing with the situation.

16–18 Answer D

Health promotion and maintenance information regarding physical activity that should be included in client teaching includes reminding the client that stretching and warm-up exercises are an important part of any exercise routine. After proper stretching and warm-up exercises, muscles should not hurt after most sports activities if engaged in on a regular basis. If the activity is new, an extremity may be slightly sore, in which case ice applied to the area may help relieve the discomfort. Any rigorous exercise should be avoided until one is in proper physical condition.

This is usually obtained after a conservative, lengthy program of physical fitness activities. After any strenuous activity, a cool-down period should be employed.

16–19 Answer C

Tell a client who has sprained his ankle to apply cold for 20 minutes, then take it off for 15 minutes and repeat for the first 24 hours, then repeat the same procedure using heat. Cold for the first 24 hours will cause vasoconstriction, preventing any further bleeding into the tissues. After that length of time, heat may reduce muscle spasm and pain. Neither heat nor cold should be applied continuously because both would hinder proper circulation. After any sprain, use the principles of RICE: R for rest, I for ice, C for compression, and E for elevation.

16–20 Answer B

Instructions to the client and family on how to allow a cast to dry properly should include advising them to change the position of the part with the cast every hour. In this case, Joyce's arm should be repositioned frequently to prevent indentations in the cast itself (caused by continuous placement on a pillow) and to ensure drying on all the surfaces of the cast. Elevating her arm will prevent edema, but is not needed continuously. A fan will dry only the outside of the cast, not the inside, and may cause Joyce further problems, such as an upper respiratory infection. A blanket will prevent drying of the cast.

16–21 Answer A

Compartment syndrome occurs when external pressure constricts the structures within a compartment, compromising tissue perfusion. The pressure causes compressed nerves, muscles, and blood vessels. Cellular acidosis results, followed by edema, further increasing compartment pressures. This develops within the first 48 hours of injury. Phlebitis usually involves the lower extremities. Osteomyelitis might be considered if the fracture were an open one and bacteria entered through the open wound, but it would not develop this soon after the injury. Osteomyelitis can occur at any age, but children under age 12 and adults over age 50 are the usual victims. When assessing circulation, think of the five Ps: pain, pulselessness, pallor, paresthesias, and poikilothermia. A muscle contraction is a normal physiologic function and would not result in these symptoms.

16–22 Answer A

Surgery is recommended only for clients with low back pain caused by degenerative disk disorders, and then only when severe neurologic involvement has occurred. Surgery benefits only 1% of persons with low back problems. In this case, Mike may benefit from the following during nonpain intervals: a planned exercise program to strengthen back muscles, reinforcement of teaching regarding appropriate body mechanics in lifting and reaching, and modifying the workplace or environment to minimize stress to the lower back.

16–23 Answer C

An osteosarcoma is the most common malignant tumor that occurs in the long bones and the knee. An osteochondroma is the most common benign tumor and usually occurs in the pelvis, scapula, and ribs. A chondroma occurs in the hands, feet, ribs, spine, sternum, or long bones. A giant-cell tumor is a tumor of the bone marrow cells in the shaft of the long bones, such as the femur, tibia, radius, and humerus.

16–24 Answer B

For Paul, who has a malignant fibrosarcoma of the femur, a magnetic resonance imaging scan will determine the extent of the tumor invasion on the surrounding tissues and the response of the bone tumor to the radiation. It will also determine response to chemotherapy and will detect recurrent disease. A conventional x ray will show the location of the tumor and the extent of bone involvement. Metastatic bone destruction has a characteristic "moth-eaten" pattern in which the growth has a poorly defined margin that cannot be separated from normal bone. A computed tomography scan will evaluate the extent of the tumor invasion into bone, soft tissues, and neurovascular structures. A needle biopsy, usually performed at the time of surgery, will determine the type of tumor.

16–25 Answer B

The only antibiotic listed is bleomycin (Blenoxane). All of the other medications are chemotherapeutic agents frequently used for musculoskeletal neoplasms. Cyclophosphamide (Cytoxan) is an alkylating agent, methotrexate (Rheumatrex) is an antimetabolite, and cisplatin (Platinol) is a synthetic agent.

16–26 Answer A

A comminuted fracture occurs when the bony fragments are in many pieces. An open fracture occurs when the broken ends of the bone protrude through soft tissues and skin. A closed fracture occurs when the bone breaks cleanly but does not penetrate the skin. A compression fracture occurs when the bone is crushed.

16–27 Answer C

Grating of the bones or entrance of air into an open fracture is manifested as crepitus. The extremity should not be manipulated to elicit crepitus because it may cause additional damage. Swelling is manifested by edema from localization of serous fluid and bleeding. Ecchymosis results from extravasation of blood into the subcutaneous tissue. Pain and tenderness result from muscle spasm, direct tissue trauma, nerve pressure, or movement of the fractured bone.

16–28 Answer A

One of the precursors of deep vein thrombosis is altered blood coagulation, which may result from active blood loss. The body then attempts to compensate by increasing the production of platelets and clotting factors. Decreased blood flow is common in clients with a fracture and those who are immobilized and not as active. Venous flow can be decreased by 50% in bedridden persons. Injury to the blood vessel wall may occur as a direct result of force, such as from a fracture, or may occur during surgery.

16–29 Answer D

A strain is defined as a microscopic tear in a muscle. It includes the presence of sharp or dull pain, pain that is often increased with isometric contraction of the muscle, and the presence of swelling and localized tenderness. A sprain is defined as an injury to a ligament that results from a twisting motion and may cause joint instability.

16–30 Answer C

Clinical manifestations of an anterior shoulder dislocation include the inability to shrug the shoulder, pain, and lengthening of the arm. The inability to rotate the shoulder externally is a clinical manifestation of a posterior shoulder dislocation, along with the inability to elevate the arm.

16–31 Answer A

The mechanism of action of colchicine is to interrupt the cycle of urate crystal deposition and inflammatory response. Used to treat an acute attack of gout, colchicine does not alter serum uric acid levels. After the acute attack is over, uricosuric drugs may be ordered to prevent recurrent attacks of acute gouty arthritis and treat chronic gout. Probenecid (Benemid) inhibits the tubular reabsorption of urate, which promotes the excretion of uric acid, thus decreasing the levels. Sulfinpyrazone (Anturane) is also a uricosuric drug that potentiates the renal excretion of uric acid and reduces serum uric acid levels. Allopurinol (Zyloprim) acts on purine metabolism, which reduces the production of uric acid and decreases serum and urinary concentrations of uric acid. It is useful for primary or secondary gout.

16–32 Answer B

The client with rheumatoid arthritis (RA) benefits from the anti-inflammatory effects of nonsteroidal anti-inflammatory drugs (NSAIDs). Acetaminophen (Tylenol) is not an NSAID and therefore does not have anti-inflammatory effects. Acetylsalicylic acid, valdecoxib (Bextra), and nabumetone (Relafen) are all NSAIDs and would benefit the client with RA.

16–33 Answer D

When teaching clients about nonsteroidal anti-inflammatory drugs (NSAIDs), tell them not to take these drugs on an empty stomach but to take them with food or milk, not to drive or operate machinery if they notice drowsiness while taking the NSAID, and to call immediately if they notice any bloody urine, coffee-ground emesis, or blood in the stool. If the client is having additional pain, acetaminophen (Tylenol) may be taken as needed for pain relief, but not aspirin, which is also an NSAID and might potentiate gastric bleeding.

16–34 Answer B

In osteoarthritis, the affected joints are swollen, cool, and bony hard on palpation. With rheumatoid arthritis, the affected joints appear red, hot, and swollen and are boggy and tender on palpation. Fatigue, decreased range of motion, and joint stiffness are common to both.

16–35 Answer A

Musculoskeletal pain is not characteristic of chronic fatigue syndrome; rather, it is characteristic of fibromyalgia. The musculoskeletal pain, usually an achy muscle pain that may be localized or involve the entire body, is usually gradual in onset, although the onset may be sudden, occasionally after a viral illness. Fatigue is a more significant feature of chronic fatigue syndrome. With both disorders, difficulty sleeping and depression occur.

16–36 Answer C

To determine if a client has a fractured pelvis, a test for hematuria will usually prove positive. A fracture of the pelvis usually results in hypovolemia caused by a generally significant associated blood loss. Surrounding blood vessels rupture and result in a large retroperitoneal hematoma with shock. Pelvic fractures also commonly injure the urinary bladder or urethra. A client with a fracture in several locations of the pelvis may need a pneumatic antishock garment to control the blood loss and stabilize the pelvis. Only x-ray studies will confirm the diagnosis.

16–37 Answer A

Fat emboli are a common complication after a long-bone fracture. They usually occur within 72 hours after the injury. Fat emboli commonly lodge in the lung and produce sudden-onset respiratory problems resulting in hypoxemia. Symptoms include fever, tachycardia, rapid respirations, and mental confusion.

16–38 Answer B

If a client presents with lower back pain and has decreased sensation to a pinprick in the lateral leg and web of the great toe, this indicates discogenic disease in the L4/L5 area (L5 root involvement). L3/4 innervates the motor function of knee extension, and L5/S1 innervates the motor function of knee flexion.

16–39 Answer C

Follow the ABCs of first aid: airway, breathing, circulation. Establishing the airway is the first priority, followed by breathing, then circulation. Stopping the bleeding from the wound, assessing if there has been a cervical fracture, and feeling the peripheral pulses are all important actions, but if the client is not breathing, the other actions will not be needed.

16–40 Answer B

A positive anterior/posterior drawer sign indicates an injury to the cruciate ligament. A medial meniscus tear is the most common cause of knee joint pain or strain. The most consistent physical finding of a meniscal tear is tenderness to palpation along the joint line anterior and posterior to the collateral ligament. To examine for a lateral meniscal tear, flex the knee and internally rotate the leg slowly. Then extend the leg slowly while you try to elicit a painful click. There is no posterior meniscus.

16–41 Answer D

A positive McBurney's point, a positive psoas sign, and a positive obturator sign are all indicative of appendicitis. A positive McBurney's point is rebound tenderness in the right lower quadrant. The psoas sign (iliopsoas test) is when extension and elevation of the right leg against resistance produces pain and it is positive with appendicitis. A positive obturator sign is pain on inward rotation of the hip.

16–42 Answer C

Predisposing factors for thoracic outlet syndrome include faulty posture, chronic illness, and occupations that result in compression of the neurovascular structures supplying the upper extremity, such as computer programming and piano playing. Clients with thoracic outlet syndrome often have a history of trauma to the head and neck area, so soccer players may also be at slight risk.

16–43 Answer C

Increased levels of creatine kinase are found in polymyositis, traumatic injuries, and progressive muscular dystrophy. Aldolase A level is elevated in muscular dystrophy and dermatomyositis. Aspartate aminotransferase is found in skeletal muscle, but mainly in heart and renal cells. Lactate dehydrogenase level is elevated in skeletal muscle necrosis, extensive cancer, and progressive muscular dystrophy.

16–44 Answer D

Although clients with fibromyalgia are fatigued and have stiff joints and muscle pain, physical therapy, including exercise, is an important aspect of care. Management also includes giving psychotropic drugs, such as amitriptyline (Elavil), in a low dose at bedtime; injecting trigger points with local anesthetics and steroids; and using acetaminophen (Tylenol) or a nonsteroidal anti-inflammatory drug.

16–45 Answer D

The Scientific Advisory Board of the National Osteoporosis Foundation states that bone mass measurements should be performed in estrogen-deficient women. This would allow decisions to be made about hormone replacement therapy. Because women start to lose bone mass at least several years before their last menses, the perimenopausal years might be the ideal time to do this, but mass screening is not cost-effective.

16–46 Answer D

An enlarged supraclavicular node may indicate a neoplasm in the abdomen or thorax.

16–47 Answer A

Turning the forearm so that the palm is up is supination. Turning the forearm so that the palm is down is pronation. Abduction is moving a limb away from the midline of the body. Eversion is moving the sole of the foot outward at the ankle.

16–48 Answer C

The knee is the largest joint in the body, with the articulation of three bones, the femur, tibia, and patella, in one common articular cavity. It is a hinge joint, permitting flexion and extension of the lower leg. The knee also has the body's largest synovial membrane.

16–49 Answer A

Osteoporosis develops when bone resorption occurs more rapidly than bone deposition. Osteoarthritis is a degenerative joint disease characterized by degeneration and loss of articular cartilage in synovial joints. Rheumatoid arthritis is a chronic, systemic inflammatory disorder characterized by persistent synovitis of multiple joints. Osteomalacia is a metabolic bone disorder characterized by inadequate mineralization of bone matrix.

16–50 Answer B

Black men have a relatively low incidence of osteoporosis because they have the densest bones. Osteoporosis has the highest incidence in white women.

16–51 Answer B

In grading muscle strength, a grade of 4 indicates full range of motion (ROM) against gravity with some resistance. A grade of 5 is full ROM against gravity with full resistance. A grade of 3 is full ROM with gravity. A grade of 2 is full ROM with gravity eliminated (passive motion). A grade of 1 indicates slight muscle contraction. A grade of 0 indicates no muscle contraction.

16–52 Answer C

In assessing your client, place the tips of your first two fingers in front of each ear and ask him to open and close his mouth. Then drop your fingers into the depressed area over the temporomandibular joint (TMJ) and note for smooth motion of the mandible. With this action, you are assessing for TMJ syndrome. Clicking or popping noises, decreased range of motion, pain, or swelling may indicate TMJ syndrome. However, an audible and palpable snap or click does occur in many normal people as they open their mouths. In rare cases, this may indicate osteoarthritis.

16–53 Answer D

If any limitation or increase in range of motion (ROM) occurs when assessing the musculoskeletal system, the angles of the bones should be measured by using a goniometer, which gives precise measurements of joint ROM. Phalen's test is used to diagnose carpal tunnel syndrome; it is not a tool.

16–54 Answer A

If, during your assessment of your client's foot, you note that the foot is in alignment with the long axis of the lower leg, and weight bearing falls on the middle of the foot, from the heel, along the midfoot, to between the second and third toes, you would diagnose a normal foot. Hallux valgus is a common deformity in which a lateral or outward deviation of the toe with medial prominence of the head of the first metatarsal is present. A hammer-toe deformity is common in hallus valgus and is a deformity in the second, third, fourth, or fifth toes that includes hyperextension of the metatarsophalangeal joint and flexion of the proximal interphalangeal joint. Talipes equinovarus (clubfoot) is a congenital, rigid, and fixed malposition of the foot including inversion, forefoot adduction, and the foot pointing downward.

16–55 Answer D

In performing the Ortolani maneuver to assess for congenital hip dislocation, the practitioner places the infant supine, flexes the knees by holding the thumbs on the inner midthighs, with fingers outside on the hips touching the greater trochanters, then adducts the legs until the practitioner's thumbs touch. The legs are then abducted, moving the knees apart and down so that their lateral aspects touch the table. If this external rotation feels smooth with no sound present, there is no hip dislocation. The Allis test is also used to check for hip dislocation by comparing leg lengths. LaSeque's test is straight-leg raising, which helps to confirm the presence of a herniated nucleus pulposus. McMurray's test is performed to confirm a torn meniscus.

16–56 Answer B

When teaching clients about using a cane, tell them to advance the cane with the ipsilateral (affected) leg. The cane should be carried in the contralateral hand and the cane length should equal the height of the greater trochanter. The use of assistive devices is an important strategy to protect the joints as well as provide safety, but clients must be taught the proper use of all devices.

16–57 Answer D

To diagnose fibromyalgia, there must be tenderness on digital palpation in at least 11 of 18 (9 pairs) tender-point sites, including the occiput, low cervical, trapezius, supraspinatus, second rib, lateral epicondyle, gluteal, greater trochanter, and knee. The ankle is not one of the tender point sites.

16–58 Answer D

A positive antinuclear antibody test may indicate systemic lupus erythematosus or scleroderma. To diagnose gout, there should be a negative joint culture, hyperuricemia, and a significant response to colchicine or a nonsteroidal anti-inflammatory drug.

16–59 Answer A

First-line drug therapy for acute low back pain includes the use of nonsteroidal anti-inflammatory drugs (NSAIDs). NSAIDs, as well as aspirin and acetaminophen (Tylenol), have been shown to be as effective as muscle relaxants and opioids for the control of acute low-back pain but without the potential for dependence and abuse. Muscle relaxants have not been shown to be any more effective than NSAIDs and combination therapy has no more effect than NSAIDs used alone.

16–60 Answer A

Years ago, muscle relaxants and bedrest were the treatments of choice for low back pain. Studies have now shown that resuming normal activity within the limits imposed by the pain has as good an effect as, if not better than, 2 days of bedrest. Exercise should begin as soon as possible after the acute injury and is directed at building endurance and stamina with consideration given to one's pain tolerance. The client's preference, cold or hot packs or both, is the desired treatment.

16–61 Answer C

A Baker's cyst, also called popliteal bursitis, is the buildup of synovial fluid in the knee. It usually occurs in men between the ages of 15 and 30 and consists of local pain, inability to extend the knee, and symptoms related to compression of surrounding structures. The latter symptoms may mimic venous thrombophlebitis.

16–62 Answer A

The straight-leg-raising maneuver can be used to diagnose nerve root compression by eliciting back pain. The leg is straight and lifted by the heel. The leg may also be brought across the body to increase the sensitivity of this maneuver. Leg shortening and external rotation may be present with a fractured hip. Extending the knee would elicit pain if an anterior cruciate ligament tear were present. Pressure over an affected tendon would elicit pain if tendinitis were present.

16–63 Answer B

Gelling refers to the achiness and stiffness that occur in clients with rheumatoid arthritis after a period of inactivity.

16–64 Answer C

Sjögren's syndrome, which affects the salivary and lacrimal glands, causes clients to have dry eyes and mouths. It is an inflammatory disease of the exocrine glands and may be an isolated entity or may be associated with another rheumatic disease, such as rheumatoid arthritis (RA) or systemic lupus erythematosus (SLE). Because Marie has no other symptoms of RA or SLE, Sjögren's syndrome should be considered first. Rosacea is a chronic facial disorder with a vascular component.

16–65 Answer C

For the client who has just been given a diagnosis of carpal tunnel syndrome, your next step is to try neutral position wrist splinting and order an oral nonsteroidal anti-inflammatory drug. For symptoms of less than 10 months' duration, conservative treatment should be tried first. Electrophysiological testing confirms focal median nerve conduction delay within the carpal canal and also provides information about disease severity. Taking a more complete history is not essential at this point because a diagnosis has already been made. For refractory cases, median nerve decompression may be accomplished by surgery, but complete recovery is not possible if atrophy is pronounced.

16–66 Answer B

The alkaline phosphatase level is moderately elevated in osteomalacia. Serum calcium and phosphorus, urinary calcium, and creatinine excretion levels are all low in osteomalacia.

16–67 Answer B

Clients with medical conditions that are reversible or temporary, such as pregnancy, often have their carpal tunnel syndrome resolve when the condition is corrected. In this case, it may resolve when Lois delivers.

16–68 Answer B

When you have a client bend forward to assess the spine (the Adams forward-bending test) and you note a right-sided rib hump, this is indicative of a right thoracic curve. Adolescent idiopathic scoliosis is a lateral spinal curvature of greater than 10 degrees when no pathological cause has been determined. Management consists of the three Os: observation, orthosis, and operation. Spondylolysis is a bony defect of the pars interarticularis.

16–69 Answer C

Sarcoidosis is the result of an exaggerated immune system response to a class of antigens or self-antigens. Glucocorticoids are prescribed to suppress the immune process, thus relieving symptoms; 50% of clients experience joint symptoms, including arthralgia and arthritis. About 5% show some form of cardiac dysfunction.

16–70 Answer B

The primary concern in the management of facial fractures is to ensure an adequate and stable airway. Displaced soft tissues, blood, secretions, or other foreign material may obstruct the airway and cause asphyxia. Septal hematomas are more commonly seen in children than in adults, but the first priority is to maintain an adequate airway. Once his airway is established and he is stabilized, permission to treat Jeffrey can be obtained from his parents. Facial x rays would then be obtained.

16–71 Answer C

The type of joint that is freely movable, such as the shoulder joint, is called a diarthrosis joint. Diarthrosis joints are freely movable joints, such as the joints of the limbs, shoulders, and hips. Synarthrosis joints are immovable, and include skull sutures, epiphyseal plates, ribs, and the manubrium of the sternum. Amphiarthrosis joints are slightly movable joints, such as the vertebral joints and the joint of the pubic symphysis.

16–72 Answer B

The effect of caffeine in causing osteoporosis is a diuretic effect that causes calcium to be excreted more rapidly. A high alcohol intake also alters intestinal absorption of calcium and the assimilation of calcium into the bone matrix.

16–73 Answer C

Advise clients taking calcium supplements that they also need to take vitamin D because vitamin D raises serum calcium levels by increasing the intestinal absorption of dietary calcium and mobilizing calcium from the bone. Vitamin D deficiency does result in an inadequate mineralization of bone matrix, more commonly seen in children.

16–74 Answer A

The American College of Obstetricians and Gynecologists guidelines for exercise during pregnancy and after delivery include the following: Women can continue to perform mild to moderate exercise routines three times per week (this is preferable to intermittent activity); exercise in the supine position should be avoided after the first trimester because this position is associated with a decreased cardiac output; and because of decreased oxygen available for aerobic exercise during pregnancy, the intensity of the workout should be based on maternal symptoms.

16–75 Answer A

The pathophysiology associated with transient pain after exercising that usually lasts a few hours with soreness and may last up to a week is increased lactic acid level, muscle breakdown, and minor inflammation. When there is longer-lasting pain late in an activity or immediately after, it is caused by mild musculotendinous inflammation. When there is pain in the beginning or middle of the activity, there is major musculotendinous inflammation, periostitis, and bone microtrauma. When the pain begins before or early in the exercise, preventing or affecting the performance, it is the result of breakdown in soft tissue, stress fracture, or compartment syndrome.

16–76 Answer B

Painful contractions of muscles after exertion, such as heat cramps, may be related to hyponatremia or other electrolyte imbalances. Usually the gastrocnemius and hamstring muscles are involved. Treatment of heat cramps includes passive muscle stretching, cessation of activities, transfer to a cooler environment, and drinking cool liquids. Sports drinks such as Gatorade that contain electrolytes may be beneficial. Heat exhaustion is a more serious condition, with symptoms ranging from nausea, vomiting, headache, loss of appetite, and dizziness to irritability, tachycardia, and hyperventilation. Hypokalemia may cause muscular weakness, fatigue, and muscle cramps. This would be a good second-choice answer. Greg's dehydration is attributed to his hyponatremia.

16–77 Answer A

When a client has a human bite, the first immediate course of action must be to débride and irrigate the wound thoroughly after it has been cultured for both anaerobic and aerobic bacteria. Then, an x ray should be taken to rule out osteomyelitis, fractures, and retained teeth from the offender. Broad-spectrum antibiotics such as gentamicin sulfate (Garamycin) should be started and the wound left open for drainage. Rabies is not a concern with human bites. Clients should then be evaluated for the need for a tetanus injection.

16–78 Answer C

When you elicit a painful Finkelstein's sign, you are testing for de Quervain's disease (stenosing tenosynovitis at the base of the thumb). The diagnosis is made by testing the thumb for pain in resisted extension and abduction of the thumb. Gliding the inflamed tendons will produce pain. A radial deviation with a sudden flexion of the thumb causes pain, called Finkelstein's sign. Tinel's sign and Phalen's maneuver are used to diagnose carpal tunnel syndrome. The tennis elbow test evaluates for lateral epicondylitis. The examiner holds the client's elbow with the thumb on the lateral epicondyle. The client's forearm is pronated, the wrist flexed fully, and the elbow extended. Tennis elbow is present if pain is elicited over the lateral epicondyle of the humerus. There is no specific test for shoulder bursitis.

16–79 Answer C

A coccygeal fracture, usually incurred by a direct blow such as a fall from a bicycle, is treated conservatively with analgesia and by using a "donut" cushion when sitting.

16–80 Answer D

Reiter's syndrome is arthritis of the lower extremities and is more common in white men. Associated symptoms include urethritis; mild conjunctivitis; shallow, painless oral ulcers; plantar fasciitis; diffuse swelling of the toes; and onychodystrophy.

16–81 Answer B

Swollen, bony proximal interphalangeal joints are Bouchard's nodes. Bony enlargements of the distal interphalangeal joints are Heberden's nodes. Both suggest osteoarthritis. Osler's nodes are painful, raised lesions of the fingers, toes, or feet that occur with infective endocarditis. There are no Murphy's nodes.

16–82 Answer D

Synovial fluid that is turbid or greenish yellow on analysis indicates an inflammation such as rheumatoid arthritis. Normal synovial fluid is clear or straw colored. With trauma, the color would be clear, turbid red, or zanthrochromic. With osteoarthritis, it is clear or straw colored. With gout, synovial fluid is turbid or white in color. With a septic infection such as a bacterial infection or TB the color is turbid, gray, or yellow.

16–83 Answer D

The Roos test suggests thoracic outlet syndrome if ischemic pain or paresthesias are present when the client abducts the arms 90 degrees externally rotated with the elbows flexed 90 degrees and then opens and closes his or her hands for 3 minutes. The Neer test suggests inflammation or injury to the structures in the subacromial space when pain is experienced when the client is seated and maximal forced flexion of the shoulder is imposed with the forearm pronated. The Speed test suggests tendinitis of the long head of the biceps when there is pain at the bicipital groove with forward elevation of the shoulders plus resistance. The Hawkins test assesses for inflammation or injury to the structures in the subacromial space when pain is elicited with forced internal rotation of the shoulder.

16–84 Answer B

Ganglia can be distinguished from neoplasms by their ability to transilluminate. Large ganglia and neoplasms may restrict joint motion, but usually pain and swelling are the main features of ganglia. Ganglia may fluctuate in size depending on the individual's activity level, and occasionally will spontaneously resolve.

16–85 Answer A

With tennis elbow, wrist and finger extension causes pain over the extensor carpi radialis brevis tendon, the extensor carpi radialis longus tendon, and the extensor digitorum communis. With golfer's elbow, pain is experienced on wrist flexion over the flexor carpi radialis, the flexor carpi ulnaris, and the pronator teres tendons. With de Quervain's disease, pain is experienced on thumb extension over the abductor pollicis longus and the extensor pollicis brevis tendons. With trigger finger intersection syndrome, pain is experienced with a grip and wrist extension over the extensor carpi radialis brevis and the extensor carpi radialis longus tendons.

16–86 Answer D

A prompt referral to a neurologist is required when a diagnosis of cauda equina syndrome is made. Cauda equina syndrome is a widespread neurologic disorder in which there is loss of anal sphincter tone; impaired micturition; and incontinence; saddle anesthesia at the anus, perineum, or genitals; progressive loss of strength in the legs; and maybe even gait disturbances.

16–87 Answer C

Faster symptomatic recovery has been seen in clients with a simple "mechanical" backache who continue normal activities as much as they can with "pain being their guide" than in clients who use traditional medical treatments, such as bedrest and use of nonsteroidal anti-inflammatory drugs (NSAIDs). Muscle relaxants should be ordered only if muscle spasms are actually present, although acetaminophen (Tylenol) and NSAIDs have also been shown to help the muscle spasms adequately. Back-strengthening exercises should be started within 6 weeks of the onset of pain.

16–88 Answer C

Basketball is listed as a limited contact/impact sport by the American Academy of Pediatrics Committee on Sports Medicine. Field hockey, soccer, and lacrosse all involve high-speed running and have the potential for collision and serious injury.

16–89 Answer C

For the client with only one testicle, as long as the remaining testicle can be protected, the client can participate in any sport.

16–90 Answer D

Other than a gross eye exam, no tests are routinely recommended for a preparticipation sports physical.

16–91 Answer A

Although exercise-induced asthma is common among athletes, it is not a common cause of sudden death. The three most common causes of sudden death in athletes younger than age 30 include hypertrophic cardiomyopathy, idiopathic left ventricular hypertrophy, and coronary artery anomalies.

16–92 Answer C

If a client has severed his fingers, the fingers should be wrapped in a saline-soaked dressing, placed in a plastic bag, and transported to the emergency room along with the client. The fingers should be cooled on ice, not frozen or kept at body temperature.

16–93 Answer A

Dupuytren's contracture manifests itself by nodular thickening of one or both hands, usually affecting the fourth and fifth fingers. There is tenderness with the inability to extend the fingers. Peyronie's disease results in painful curvature of the erect penis.

16–94 Answer A

Surgical correction for Osgood-Schlatter disease is not recommended until all other options have been tried and have failed. Conservative techniques such as quadriceps strengthening exercises, hamstring and heel cord stretching exercises, and modifying the client's activities should initially be tried.

16–95 Answer C

Intra-articular corticosteroid injections provide much needed pain relief in weight-bearing joints of clients with osteoarthritis; however, they should be limited to no more than three per year because of potential damage to the cartilage if given more frequently.

16–96 Answer B

Asymptomatic hyperuricemia does not require any therapy. Dietary counseling to avoid foods high in purine and alcoholic beverages may be helpful. An acute attack of gout may be treated with colchicine or a nonsteroidal anti-inflammatory drug. Allopurinol (Zyloprim) decreases uric acid production but should not be given during an acute gouty attack.

16–97 Answer D

To aid in the diagnosis of meniscus damage such as a torn meniscus, you should elicit Apley's sign. Apley's sign is elicited with the client in the prone position. The suspected knee is flexed to 90 degrees, then downward pressure is exerted on the foot so that the tibia is firmly opposed to the femur. On rotating the leg externally and internally, if the knee locks and there is pain with this maneuver or the sound of clicks, it is indicative of a loose body, such as a torn cartilage, trapped in the articulation. The bulge test assesses for effusions in the knee joint. The Lachman test is an indicator of injury to the anterior cruciate ligament. The drawer test assesses for stability of the anterior and posterior cruciate ligaments.

16–98 Answer A

The Tensilon test aids in the diagnosis of myasthenia gravis. Edrophonium chloride (Tensilon) 2 mg is administered while the examiner watches the client's eyelids. If there is no change after 1 minute, another 8 mg is administered. In clients with myasthenia gravis, the ptosis is markedly improved after the Tensilon is injected because of improved muscle strength. Cogwheel rigidity is present in Parkinson's disease. Chvostek's and Trousseau's signs are indications of tetanic cramps.

16–99 Answer C

Calcaneovalgus feet are a cause of out-toeing. Medial femoral torsion, metatarsus adduction, and talipes equinovarus (clubfoot) are all causes of in-toeing.

16–100 Answer A

Toe walking is considered normal until age 3 years. Constant toe walking after that age is considered abnormal and requires further investigation for neuromuscular disorders.

16–101 Answer B

Finkelstein's test assesses for de Quervain's disease. Have the client touch his thumb into the palm and make a fist. The test is positive if moving the wrist into ulnar deviation causes pain. Allen's test assesses the patency of the radial and ulnar arteries and the arterial arch. Phalen's test and Tinel's sign are tests done for carpal tunnel syndrome.

16–102 Answer C

Dupuytren's contracture affects the palmar tissue between the skin and the distal palm and fingers, most often in the fourth and fifth fingers but also in the thumb-index finger web space. It is progressive and results in flexor contracture while not affecting the flexor tendons. Most frequently occuring in males between the ages of 40–60, it is common among persons of Northern European ancestry. It is dysfunctional and disfiguring. While not actually painful, it may be tender. Surgery is the only cure.

16–103 Answer B

Musculoskeletal strain is pain over the lower back and spine as well as the muscles without sciatica. Often there is no precipitating event. It is aggravated by sitting, standing, and certain movements, and is alleviated with rest. Palpation localizes the pain, and muscle spasms may be felt. There is an insidious onset with progressive improvement. Ankylosing spondylitis is back pain and stiffness over several months. There is relief with exercise and reduced mobility of the spine. There are painful or ankylosed sacroiliac joints and reduced chest wall expansion. A herniated disk is often preceded by years of recurrent episodes of localized back pain and there is usually leg pain which overshadows the back pain. With spondylolisthesis, there is a systemic inflammatory condition of the vertebral column and sacroiliac joints,and it most frequently affects males between the ages of 20–30 with chronic low back pain that is worse in the morning, and excessive thoracic kyphosis is present.

16–104 Answer A

All the following tests are done for the purpose of assessing for a herniated disk. The sciatic stretch test is when you elevate the affected leg when the client is in the supine position and pain is elicited. The cross straight-leg-raising test is when elevation of the normal leg produces sciatica down the other leg. The doorbell sign is when deep palpation of the spinous process over the protruded disk reproduces sciatica. Lasègue's sign is done with the client supine and the hip flexed. Dorsiflexion of the ankle accentuates sciatic pain or a muscle spasm in the posterior thigh.

16–105 Answer B

The World Health Organization diagnostic criteria for osteoporosis consider a normal reading of bone mineral density (BMD) to be within 1 standard deviation of a young-adult reference mean. Osteopenia is considered a BMD of >1 standard deviation below the young adult reference mean with a T score of –1. Osteoporosis is a BMD >2.5 with a T score of –2.5. Severe osteoporosis is a BMD >2.5 with a T score of –2.5 and the presence of osteoporotic fractures.

16–106 Answer D

A plain x-ray film will not show a herniated nucleus pulposus nor a muscle strain. It will show spondylolisthesis, scoliosis, osteoarthritis, and spinal stenosis.

Bibliography

Carithers, JS, and Koch, BB: Evaluation and management of facial fractures. Am Fam Physician 55:8, 1997.

Dillon, PM. Nursing Health Assessment: A Critical Thinking, Case Studies Approach. FA Davis, Philadelphia, 2003.

Haasbeek, JF: Adolescent idiopathic scoliosis. Postgrad Med 101:6, 1997.

Jones, AK: Primary care management of acute low back pain. Nurse Pract 22:7, 1997.

Plank, LM, and Dunphy, LM, in Dunphy, LM, and Winland-Brown, JE (eds): Primary Care: The Art and Science of Advanced Practice Nursing, chap 17. FA Davis, Philadelphia, 2002.

Zitkus, BS: Sarcoidosis. Am J Nurs 97:10, 1997.

Zollo, AJ: Medical Secrets, ed 2. Hanley & Belfus, Philadelphia, 1997.

HOW WELL DID YOU DO?

85% AND ABOVE CONGRATULATIONS! THIS SCORE SHOWS APPLICATION OF TEST-TAKING PRINCIPLES AND ADEQUATE CONTENT KNOWLEDGE.

75–85% KEEP WORKING! REVIEW TEST-TAKING PRINCIPLES AND TRY AGAIN.

65–75% HANG IN THERE! SPEND SOME TIME REVIEWING CONCEPTS AND TEST-TAKING PRINCIPLES AND TRY THE TEST AGAIN.

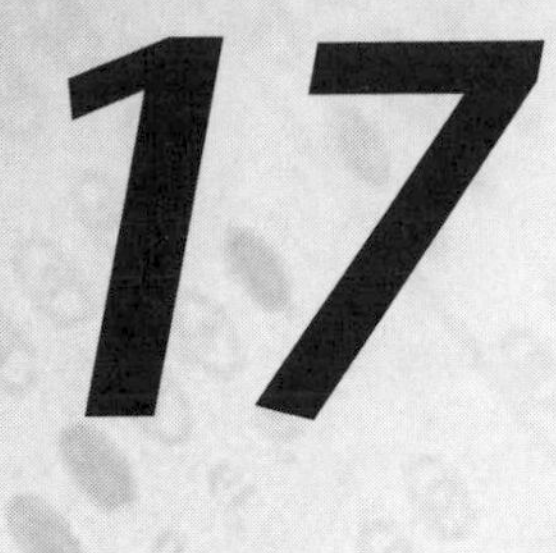

17 Endocrine and Metabolic Problems

JILL E. WINLAND-BROWN
and
GRETCHEN HOPE MILLER HEERY

17–1 *The American Diabetes Association recommends which of the following quarterly blood tests to be performed on all clients with diabetes?*

A. Urine
B. Liver function
C. Glycohemoglobin
D. Serum glucose

17–2 *What percentage of cases of type 2 diabetes is associated with excess body weight?*

A. 20%
B. 40%
C. 60%
D. 80%

17–3 *Nancy, age 52, has been on a sulfonylurea medication for type 2 diabetes, but it is still not under good control. Your next step would be to:*

A. stop the sulfonylurea and start metformin (Glucophage).
B. add insulin to the sulfonylurea regimen.
C. add metformin (Glucophage) to the sulfonylurea.
D. increase the dosage of the sulfonylurea.

17–4 *The three "Ps" of diabetes include all of the following* ***except:***

A. polyuria.
B. polydipsia.
C. paresthesias.
D. polyphagia.

17–5 *You are counseling your client with diabetes about diet. You would tell the client all of the following statements* ***except:***

A. "You can substitute two Oreo cookies for a fresh pear."
B. "You can have an occasional glass of chardonnay."
C. "You should monitor the amount of carbohydrates you eat at each meal."
D. "As long as you monitor your blood sugar and it's normal, you can eat anything."

17–6 *Peter, age 62, has diabetes and wants to start an exercise program. Which type of exercise would you not recommend?*

A. Swimming
B. Jogging
C. Tennis
D. Dancing

17–7 *Which class of antihypertensive agents is contraindicated for clients with diabetes?*

A. Angiotensin-converting enzyme inhibitors
B. Calcium channel blockers
C. Beta blockers
D. Alpha blockers

17–8 *Your diabetic patient asks you about Lantus. You tell her that:*

A. it may be administered SC at home, or IV in the hospital if need be.
B. the onset of action is 15 minutes.

C. Lantus stays in your system for 24 hours.
D. that it can be mixed with any other insulin.

17–9 *Jenny, age 46, has hypertension that has been controlled with hydrochlorothiazide (Hydrodiuril) 50 mg every day for the past 3 years. She is 5 feet 8 inches tall and weighs 220 lb. Her fasting blood sugar (FBS) level is 300 mg/dL, serum cholesterol level is 250 mg/dL, serum potassium level is 3.4 mEq, and she has 4+ glycosuria. Your next course of action would be to:*

A. discontinue her hydrochlorothiazide.
B. order a glucose tolerance test (GTT).
C. repeat her FBS test.
D. start insulin therapy.

17–10 *Harriet, age 62, has type 1 diabetes that is well controlled by insulin. Recently, she has been having marital difficulties that have left her emotionally upset. As a result of this stress, it is possible that she will:*

A. have an insulin reaction more readily than usual.
B. have an increased blood sugar level.
C. need less daily insulin.
D. need more carbohydrates.

17–11 *Clients with diabetes are more prone to cardiovascular disease than those without diabetes. This is probably because:*

A. of their difficulty in metabolizing fats and proteins, the end products of which accumulate in the blood vessels.
B. they are usually overweight, which increases the workload on the heart and blood vessels.
C. most are older adults, who are more likely to have degenerative cardiovascular disease.
D. the high levels of glucose and fat that occur with poor control result in atherosclerotic changes in the blood vessels.

17–12 *Betty, age 40, has had insulin-dependent diabetes for 20 years and takes a combination of neutral protamine Hagedorn (NPH) and regular insulin every day. She comes to the office because she has developed a severe upper respiratory infection with chills, fever, and production of yellow sputum. Because of her acute infection, you know that Betty is likely to require:*

A. a decrease in her daily insulin dosage.
B. an increase in her daily insulin dosage.
C. a high-caloric dietary intake and with no insulin change.
D. a change in her insulin from NPH to Lente insulin.

17–13 *Ben, a client with insulin-dependent diabetes, is hospitalized with an admitting diagnosis of diabetic ketoacidosis. Which of the following signs and symptoms would not be consistent with this condition?*

A. Hyperglycemia and glycosuria
B. Ketonuria and polyuria
C. Polydipsia and decreased blood pH
D. Decreased respiratory rate with shallow respirations

17–14 *Marie, age 50, has insulin-dependent diabetes mellitus and checks her blood glucose level several times every day. Her blood glucose level ranges from 250–280 mg/dL in the morning and is usually about 140 at lunch, about 120 at dinner, and about 100 at bedtime. In the morning she takes 30 units of neutral protamine Hagedorn (NPH) insulin and 4 units of regular insulin, and before dinner she takes 18 units of NPH insulin and 4 units of regular insulin. Although she has had her insulin dosage adjusted several times in the past month, it has had no effect on her high morning blood glucose level. What is your next course of action?*

A. Increase the evening NPH insulin dosage by 2 more units.
B. Have her check her blood glucose level between 2 and 4 AM for the next several days.
C. Increase the morning regular insulin dosage by 2 units.
D. Order a fasting blood sugar test.

17–15 *Angiotensin-converting enzyme inhibitors are given to clients with diabetes who have:*

A. an elevated glycohemoglobin level.
B. insulin sensitivity.
C. persistent proteinuria.
D. an elevated serum creatinine level.

17–16 *When inspecting the integumentary system of clients with endocrine disorders, coarse hair may be an indicator of:*

A. Addison's disease.
B. diabetes mellitus.
C. Cushing's syndrome.
D. hypothyroidism.

17–17 *Trousseau's sign assesses for:*

A. hypocalcemia.
B. hyponatremia.
C. hypercalcemia.
D. hypermagnesemia.

17–18 *Martin, age 62, has acute nontransient abdominal pain that grows steadily worse in the epigastric area and radiates straight through to the back. The pain has lasted for days. He is also complaining of nausea, vomiting, sweating, weakness, and pallor. Physical examination reveals abdominal tenderness and distention and a low-grade fever. What do you suspect?*

A. Cholecystitis
B. Acute pancreatitis

C. Cirrhosis
D. Cushing's syndrome

17–19 *Scott has type 2 diabetes and asks if he needs to do self-monitoring of his blood glucose (SMBG) level. You tell him:*

A. "No, it is only indicated in type 1 diabetes."
B. "Yes, definitely; you should be performing SMBG at least on a daily basis."
C. "You should be doing SMBG at least three times a week."
D. "We'll just test your serum glucose each month and you'll be OK."

17–20 *Which of the following contributes to macrovascular disease in type 2 diabetes?*

A. Hypertriglyceridemia
B. Hypertension
C. Altered coagulation
D. All of the above

17–21 *Morton has type 2 diabetes. His treatment, which includes diet, exercise, and oral antidiabetic agents, is insufficient to achieve acceptable glycemic control. Your next course of action is to:*

A. increase the dosage of the oral antidiabetic agents.
B. add a dosage of insulin at bedtime to the regimen.
C. discontinue the oral antidiabetic agents and start insulin therapy.
D. suggest treatment using an insulin pump.

17–22 *Sigrid, age 48, appears with a 3-month history of heat intolerance, increased sweating, palpitations, tachycardia, nervousness, irritability, fatigue, and muscle weakness. Which test would you order first?*

A. A blood chemistry panel
B. Thyroid-stimulating hormone level
C. Liver function studies
D. Electrocardiogram

17–23 *To lower the serum concentration of thyroid hormones and re-establish a eumetabolic state in the client with Graves' disease, all of the following therapies may be used* ***except:***

A. radioactive iodine (^{131}I).
B. antithyroid drugs.
C. chemotherapy.
D. thyroid surgery.

17–24 *Which blood test should be obtained before initiating antithyroid drugs for Graves' disease?*

A. Serum electrolytes
B. Liver function studies
C. White blood cell count
D. Complete chemistry profile

17–25 *Marsha, age 24, is preparing for radioactive iodine therapy for her Graves' disease. Which test must she undergo first?*

A. Beta human chorionic gonadotropin
B. Basal metabolism rate
C. Lithium level
D. Serum calcium

17–26 *After establishing clinical and biochemical euthyroidism after a thyroidectomy, you should perform a measurement of the serum thyroid-stimulating hormone level every:*

A. 3 months.
B. 6 months.
C. 1 year.
D. 2 years.

17–27 *Minnie is pregnant. She has hypothyroidism and has been on the same levothyroxine medication for years. What might you expect to do with her levothyroxine medication?*

A. Increase the dosage.
B. Maintain her established dose.
C. Decrease her dosage.
D. Increase the dose during the first trimester, then decrease it during the second and third trimesters.

17–28 *Alice, age 48, has a benign thyroid nodule. The most common treatment involves:*

A. surgery.
B. administration of levothyroxine therapy.
C. watchful waiting with an annual follow-up.
D. radioactive iodine therapy.

17–29 *Henry, age 72, has a fasting blood sugar (FBS) level of 176 mg/dL. He has never been given a diagnosis of diabetes before. Your next step would be to:*

A. repeat the FBS.
B. order an oral glucose tolerance test.
C. start him on an oral hypoglycemic agent.
D. order a glycohemoglobin measurement.

17–30 *Sidney has been taking a sulfonylurea for 5 years for his type 2 diabetes. He asks how long he needs to be taking the medication before he tries another medication. You tell him:*

A. "Sulfonylureas are usually effective for 7 to 10 years in most clients."
B. "You'll probably be on this medication for the rest of your life."
C. "After about 5 years, you will need to start on insulin therapy."
D. "After a few years, you can stop altogether and just regulate your diabetes with your diet."

17–31 *The thyroid-stimulating hormone (TSH) test measures the:*

A. total serum level of thyroxine.
B. serum level of T_3 and T_4.
C. pituitary's response to peripheral levels of thyroid hormone.
D. combined serum levels of T_3 and T_4.

17–32 *Which of the following is a sign of hypothyroidism?*

A. A thyroid bruit
B. Brittle hair
C. Gynecomastia
D. Warm, smooth, moist skin

17–33 *A low level of thyroid-stimulating hormone indicates:*

A. hypothyroidism.
B. myxedema.
C. hyperthyroidism.
D. thyroid nodule.

17–34 *When teaching Marcy how to use her new insulin pump, you tell her that she needs to monitor her blood glucose level:*

A. at least once a day.
B. only occasionally, because glycemic levels are maintained very steadily.
C. at least four times a day.
D. on an as-needed basis when she feels she needs to give herself an extra dose of insulin.

17–35 *Jim, a type 2 diabetic, overheard the nurse practitioner talking to the physician about putting him on "BIDS." He asks what this means. You respond:*

A. "BID (twice a day) sulfonylurea."
B. "Bedtime insulin, daytime sulfonylurea."
C. "Blood indicator daily sulfonylurea."
D. "Baby insulin dose several times daily."

17–36 *Diabetes and coronary artery disease have a close interrelationship. The following lists relationships between the two. Which is true?*

A. Hyperinsulinemia increases sympathetic tone and cardiac contractility by increasing plasma catecholamines, epinephrine, and norepinephrine.
B. An increase of glucose causes the distal nephrons of the kidneys to absorb more sodium, resulting in more fluid, expanding the intravascular volume and increasing the blood pressure.
C. Hyperinsulinemia causes a large number of vascular smooth muscle cells to be formed and deposited on the walls of vessels, eventually decreasing flow space.
D. All of the above.

17–37 *Morris has had type 1 diabetes for 10 years. Several recent urinalysis reports have shown microalbuminuria. Your next step would be to:*

A. order a 24-hour urinalysis.
B. start him on an angiotensin-converting enzyme inhibitor.
C. stress the importance of strict blood sugar control.
D. send him to a dietitian because he obviously has not been following his diet.

17–38 *As a result of the Diabetes Control and Complications Trial, elements of the intensive management of diabetes now include all of the following* ***except:***

A. testing blood sugar levels at least two times a day.
B. four daily insulin injections or use of an insulin pump.
C. adjustment of insulin doses according to food intake and exercise.
D. a diet and exercise plan.

17–39 *The Diabetes Control and Complications Trial recommends intensive management of diabetes for:*

A. children under age 13.
B. older adults.
C. persons who already have a diagnosis of beginning nephropathy, neuropathy, or retinopathy.
D. individuals with a history of frequent severe hypoglycemia.

17–40 *Sasha, who has diabetes and is postmenopausal, asks you about starting hormone replacement therapy (HRT). How do you respond?*

A. "Because HRT preparations tend to adversely affect glucose homeostasis, HRT is not recommended."
B. "It is not recommended because all major HRT preparations include a package insert warning about glucose intolerance."
C. "We should start you on hormone replacement therapy today because it will probably decrease the morbidity and mortality associated with heart disease and osteoporosis."
D. "Hormone replacement therapy tends to raise your lipid levels; therefore, I don't want to start you on it."

17–41 *Mary, age 72, has been taking insulin for several years. She just called you because she realized that yesterday she put her short-acting insulin in the long-acting insulin box and vice versa. She just took 22 units of regular insulin when she was supposed to take only 5 units. She says that she tried to do a fingerstick to test her glucose level, but was unable to obtain any blood. She states that she feels fine. What do you tell her to do first?*

A. "Keep trying to get a fingerstick and call me back with the results."
B. "Call 911 before you collapse."
C. "Drive immediately to the ER."
D. "Drink four ounces of fruit juice."

17–42 *Pancreatic juice carries all of the following digestive enzymes* ***except:***

A. pancreatic amylase.
B. pancreatic lipase.
C. pancreatic protease.
D. pancreatic trypsin.

17–43 *The process of aging results in:*

A. an increase in liver weight and mass.
B. a decreased absorption of fat-soluble vitamins.
C. an increase in enzyme activity.
D. constricted pancreatic ducts.

17–44 *After an oral cholecystogram, Sam complains of burning on urination. This is because of:*

A. a mild reaction to the contrast medium.
B. biliary obstruction.
C. contraction of the gallbladder.
D. the presence of dye in the urine.

17–45 *How long after the acute illness of hepatitis A do immunoglobulin M anti–hepatitis A virus titers disappear?*

A. 1 week
B. 3–6 months
C. 1 year
D. 2 years

17–46 *If a client has hepatitis, abdominal pain in the right upper quadrant is a result of what pathophysiologic basis?*

A. Reduced prothrombin synthesis by injured hepatic cells
B. Bile salt accumulation
C. Release of pyrogens
D. Stretching of Glisson's capsule

17–47 *You suspect myxedema in your client because she exhibits:*

A. smooth, moist skin.
B. pitting edema.
C. abnormal deposits of mucin in the skin.
D. abdominal bloating.

17–48 *Which of the following antithyroid drugs blocks thyroid hormone production and release?*

A. Propylthiouracil
B. Methimazole (Tapazole)
C. Saturated solution of potassium iodide
D. Radioactive iodine (^{131}I)

17–49 *You suspect that Sharon has hypoparathyroidism because, in addition to her other signs and symptoms, she has:*

A. elevated serum phosphate levels.
B. elevated serum calcium levels.
C. decreased neuromuscular irritability.
D. increased bone resorption, as implied by her bone density test.

17–50 *Risk factors for primary adrenal insufficiency include:*

A. taking glucocorticoids for longer than 3 weeks with sudden cessation.
B. adrenalectomy.
C. tuberculosis.
D. all of the above.

17–51 *Marty has pheochromocytoma. You instruct him to:*

A. void in small amounts.
B. not exercise for more than 30 minutes at a time.
C. avoid sleeping in the prone position.
D. take steroids.

17–52 *The most common cause of chronic hypocalcemia is:*

A. alkalosis.
B. burn trauma.
C. hypoalbuminemia.
D. renal failure.

17–53 *Sandy is being treated for chronic hypocalcemia. When her serum calcium level returns to normal, you assess her urinary calcium level and note that it is greater than 250 mg in a 24-hour sample. This indicates that:*

A. her vitamin D dosage should be increased.
B. her vitamin D dosage should be decreased.
C. she needs to restrict foods high in calcium.
D. she needs to eat more foods high in calcium.

17–54 *Jeffrey, age 17, has gynecomastia. You should also assess him for:*

A. obesity.
B. endocrine abnormalities.
C. testicular cancer.
D. tuberculosis.

17–55 *All of the following medications can produce gynecomastia* ***except:***

A. cimetidine (Tagamet).
B. cholesterol-lowering medications.
C. marijuana.
D. digoxin (Lanoxin).

17–56 *Kelley has a score of 8 on the Ferriman-Gallivey scale. This is diagnostic for:*

A. gynecomastia.
B. hirsutism.
C. adrenal hyperplasia.
D. an ovarian cyst.

17–57 *Polydipsia occurs in diabetes as a result of a high serum glucose level, which:*

A. interferes with the release of antidiuretic hormone.
B. has an osmotic effect on fluids and eventually triggers the thirst mechanism for compensation.
C. causes a dry mouth, increasing the client's thirst to the point of drinking compulsively.
D. disrupts fluid and electrolyte imbalance, increasing the thirst mechanism to compensate for fluid loss or gain.

17–58 *The most common cause of hyperthyroidism is:*

A. Graves' disease.
B. a toxic uninodular goiter.
C. subacute thyroiditis.
D. a pituitary tumor.

17–59 *All of the following statements are true about the ophthalmopathy in Graves' disease* ***except:***

A. Propranolol (Inderal) initially helps to control symptoms related to ophthalmopathy.
B. Treatment often includes diuretics and ophthalmic prednisone.
C. Severe cases may require radiation or surgical decompression.
D. Radioactive iodine may worsen it.

17–60 *The most common worldwide cause of hypothyroidism is:*

A. an autoimmune process.
B. Hashimoto's thyroiditis.
C. iodine deficiency.
D. iatrogenic hypothyroidism.

17–61 *The major risk factor for development of thyroid cancer is:*

A. inadequate iodine intake.
B. presence of a goiter.
C. exposure to radiation.
D. smoking.

17–62 *Lynne has Cushing's syndrome. You would expect her to have or develop:*

A. onychomycosis.
B. tinea versicolor.
C. a skin wound that heals very slowly.
D. any of the above.

17–63 *Dena said that she read on her husband's hospital chart that he has podagra. She asks what this is. You tell her it is:*

A. rheumatoid arthritis.
B. a fungal nail infection.
C. an ingrown toenail.
D. gout.

17–64 *The medication of choice for an initial acute attack of gout is:*

A. a nonsteroidal anti-inflammatory drug.
B. colchicine.
C. a corticosteroid.
D. allopurinol (Zyloprim).

17–65 *Joy has gout. In teaching her about her disease, you tell her to avoid all of the following foods* ***except:***

A. asparagus.
B. beans.
C. broccoli.
D. mushrooms.

17–66 *Mandy has type 2 diabetes. She says she heard that if she becomes pregnant, she must go on insulin therapy. How do you respond?*

A. "You're under good glycemic control now with your oral agents. As long as you stay in good control, you'll stay on the medication you are on now."
B. "Don't worry about it now; wait until you get pregnant."
C. "Yes, you should use insulin during your pregnancy. Then, after delivery, we'll try to get you back to your old routine of oral agents."
D. "You need to start on insulin therapy now before you get pregnant. You'll also need it throughout your pregnancy."

17–67 *Eunice, age 32, has type 2 diabetes. She said that she heard that she should take an aspirin a day after she reaches menopause for its cardioprotective action. She does not have coronary artery disease, but her father does. How do you respond?*

A. "You're right. Your hormones protect you against coronary artery diseases until menopause; then you should start on aspirin therapy."
B. "The American Diabetes Association recommends that you start on aspirin therapy now."
C. "Aspirin therapy is recommended only if you have a family history of coronary artery disease."
D. "If you maintain good glycemic control, you don't need aspirin therapy."

17–68 *Sari is having a glucose tolerance test (GTT) done to confirm the diagnosis of diabetes. Which of the following may cause an abnormal GTT?*

A. Oral contraceptives
B. A urinary tract infection (UTI)
C. Diuretics
D. Any of the above

17–69 *An infant with intrauterine growth retardation is prone to hypoglycemia because of:*

A. an imbalance in insulin-glucagon secretion resulting from hyperinsulinemia from islet cell hyperplasia.
B. few carbon stores in the form of glycogen and body fat.
C. an inborn error of metabolism: glycogen storage disease.
D. a complication of birth asphyxia.

17–70 *Susie has insulin-dependent diabetes mellitus. To forestall hypoglycemia, how much carbohydrate must she eat if she misses a regular meal?*

A. 5–15 g
B. 15–30 g
C. 30–35 g
D. more than 35 g

17–71 *Mark is insulin dependent and has mild hyperglycemia. What effect does physical activity (exercise) have on his blood glucose level?*

A. It may vary a little.
B. It may drop.
C. It may rise.
D. It may fluctuate greatly either way.

17–72 *Which of the following statements is true about the insulin lispro?*

A. It works faster than regular insulin because its amino acid composition has been slightly modified.
B. When taken 30 minutes before a meal, it reduces after-meal hyperglycemia.
C. Its duration of action is about 4–5 hours.
D. It is taken with the first bite of food.

17–73 *Jane has insulin-dependent diabetes mellitus and has been experiencing hyperglycemia before dinner. A possible solution to this problem is to:*

A. adjust her morning dose of rapid-acting insulin.
B. increase her midafternoon snack.
C. add physical activity between lunch and dinner.
D. reduce the amount of carbohydrate at dinner.

17–74 *Jane, who has insulin-dependent diabetes mellitus, has been hypoglycemic at bedtime. To correct this, she could try all of the following strategies* ***except:***

A. adjusting her insulin dose before dinner.
B. adding carbohydrate at dinner.
C. adding an afternoon snack.
D. changing the time of dinner.

17–75 *Mason, age 52, has diabetes and is overweight. You now find that he is hypertensive. How should you treat his hypertension?*

A. The same as a client without diabetes.
B. Because insulin affects most of the antihypertensive drugs, you should try diet and exercise first before any antihypertensives are ordered.
C. Very aggressively.
D. Initiate therapy when the blood pressure is 5–10 mm Hg more than the conventional therapeutic guidelines.

17–76 *All of the following steps can be taken to avoid or slow the progression of diabetic nephropathy* ***except:***

A. control of blood pressure.
B. use of angiotensin-converting enzyme inhibitors.
C. restriction of protein intake.
D. use of calcium channel blockers.

17–77 *Older clients with diabetes are predisposed to which of the following types of ear infections?*

A. Simple otitis externa
B. Malignant otitis externa
C. Otitis media
D. Serous otitis media

17–78 *Virilization in a woman is characterized by all the following* ***except:***

A. increased androgen response.
B. increased muscle mass.
C. clitoral enlargement.
D. excessive hair distribution.

17–79 *Which of the following statements regarding osteoporosis and gender is true?*

A. Men and women are equally prone to osteoporosis.
B. Because of menopause, women are more prone to osteoporosis.
C. Men who develop osteoporosis usually have fractures of the wrist and ankle.
D. Women who have had hysterectomies are more prone to developing osteoporosis

17–80 *Margie has hypoparathyroidism. Which of the following would you assess during your exam?*

A. Skin turgor
B. Heart tones
C. Chvostek's sign
D. Homan's sign

17–81 *Jason, age 14, appears with tender discoid breast tissue enlargement (2–3 cm in diameter) beneath the areola. Your next action would be to:*

A. perform watchful waiting for 1 year.
B. order an ultrasound.
C. obtain laboratory tests.
D. refer Jason to an endocrinologist.

17–82 *June stopped breastfeeding 2 years ago. Yesterday, when doing a breast self-exam, she noticed a small amount of yellowish liquid when she squeezed her nipples. She is concerned that this is one of the signs of breast cancer. You tell her:*

A. "Let's get a mammogram to be on the safe side."
B. "Let's wait for a month and reassess."
C. "A small amount of breast milk can be expressed from the nipple in many parous women and is not a cause for concern."
D. "We should do an ultrasound."

17–83 *Steve, age 42, has never been hypertensive, but appears today in the office with a blood pressure of 162/100 mm Hg. He also complains of "attacks" of headache, perspiration, and palpitations with frequent attacks of nausea, pain, weakness, dyspnea, and visual disturbances. He has lost 10 lb over the past 2 months and seems very anxious today. Your next action would be to:*

A. start him on an antianxiety agent.
B. obtain a 24-hour urine test.
C. start him on a diuretic or beta blocker.
D. recheck his blood pressure in 1 week.

17–84 *Leah has had diabetes for many years. When teaching her about foot care, you want to stress:*

A. that her calluses will protect her from infection.
B. the need to assess the bottom of her feet carefully after walking barefoot.
C. that painless ulceration might occur and feet should be examined with a mirror.
D. that mild pain is to be expected because of neuropathies.

17–85 *Early-morning increases in blood glucose concentration that occur with no corresponding hypoglycemia during the night are referred to as:*

A. the Somogyi phenomenon.
B. insulin shock.
C. diabetic ketoacidosis.
D. the dawn phenomenon.

17–86 *After a subtotal thyroidectomy, it is crucial to assess:*

A. heart tones.
B. for peripheral edema.
C. speaking ability.
D. skin turgor.

17–87 *Which of the following serum laboratory findings are found in the client with Cushing's syndrome?*

A. Increased cortisol, decreased sodium, and decreased potassium levels
B. Decreased cortisol, decreased potassium, and decreased glucose levels
C. Increased cortisol, increased sodium, and decreased potassium levels
D. Normal blood urea nitrogen, increased sodium, and decreased potassium levels

17–88 *Joan has severe asthma and has been on high doses of oral corticosteroids for 2 years. She has been reading some home remedy books and stops all of her medications. What condition may she develop?*

A. Myxedema crisis
B. Diabetes insipidus
C. Hypoparathyroidism
D. Addisonian crisis

17–89 *Sara has diabetes and is now experiencing anhidrosis on the hands and feet, increased sweating on the face and trunk, dysphagia, anorexia, and heartburn. Which complication of diabetes do you suspect?*

A. Macrocirculation changes
B. Microcirculation changes
C. Somatic neuropathies
D. Visceral neuropathies

17–90 *Pathologic changes that occur with diabetic neuropathies include:*

A. a thinning of the walls of the blood vessels that supply nerves.
B. the formation and accumulation of amino glycosol within the Schwann cells, which impairs nerve conduction.
C. demyelinization of the Schwann cells, which results in slowed nerve conduction.
D. increase of nutrients clogging the vessels that supply nerve endings.

17–91 *Mindy is scheduled to have an oral glucose tolerance test. For 3 days before the test, she should discontinue all of the following medications that she takes* ***except:***

A. vitamin C.
B. aspirin.
C. calcium.
D. her oral contraceptive.

17–92 *Sandra, who has diabetes, states that she heard that fiber is especially good to include in her diet. How do you respond?*

A. "Fiber is important in all diets."
B. "Too much fiber interferes with insulin, so only include a moderate amount in your diet."
C. "Fiber, especially soluble fiber, helps improve carbohydrate metabolism, so it is more important in the diet of persons with diabetes."
D. "You get just the amount of fiber you need with a normal diet."

17–93 *Sandra has diabetes and frequently develops vaginitis. You instruct her to:*

A. wipe from back to front after voiding.
B. wear white nylon underwear.
C. wear pantyhose if wearing tight jeans.
D. avoid douching.

17–94 *Sadie, age 40, has just been given a diagnosis of Graves' disease. She has recently lost 25 lb, has* *palpitations, is very irritable, feels very warm, and has a noticeable bulge on her neck. The most likely cause of her increased thyroid function is:*

A. hyperplasia of the thyroid.
B. an anterior pituitary tumor.
C. a thyroid carcinoma.
D. an autoimmune response.

17–95 *Marisa, age 16, is an active cheerleader who just became insulin dependent. She is worried that she will not fit in with her friends any more because she does not think she can have all the same snacks they have. How do you respond?*

A. "As long as your snacks are low in fats and carbohydrates, you'll be fine."
B. "Any snacks that are sufficient in calories to maintain your normal weight are okay."
C. "Just be sure that your snacks are high in fats and proteins."
D. "Be sure to stick to snacks that are high in simple carbohydrates."

17–96 *Jay has had insulin-dependent diabetes for 10 years. He recently had a physical and was told he has some evidence of renal nephropathy. What is the first manifestation of this renal dysfunction?*

A. Proteinuria
B. Development of Kimmelstiel-Wilson nodules
C. Decreased blood urea nitrogen levels
D. Increased serum creatine levels

17–97 *Diane has had Cushing's disease for 20 years and has been taking hydrocortisone since then. Today, she appears with a thick trunk and thin extremities. She has a "moon face," a "buffalo hump," thin skin with visible capillaries, and a number of bruises that appear to be slow in healing. To what do you attribute these symptoms?*

A. Decreased adrenal androgen levels
B. Malfunctioning of the adrenal cortex
C. Excessive levels of circulating cortisol
D. Ectopic secretion of adrenocorticotropic hormone

17–98 *How do you explain the fact that someone with Cushing's disease bruises easily?*

A. Decreased skin turgor
B. A loss of neurologic sensation
C. Decreased prothrombin levels
D. Protein wasting and collagen loss

17–99 *The major causes of death in clients with Cushing's disease are related to:*

A. untreated infections.
B. hypertensive disease.
C. arteriosclerosis.
D. All of the above.

17–100 *The anterior pituitary gland secretes all of the following major hormones* ***except:***

A. thyroid-stimulating hormone.
B. growth hormone.
C. follicle-stimulating hormone.
D. aldosterone.

Answers

17–1 Answer C

Although a serum glucose test is an excellent test for clients with diabetes, it reports only the serum glucose of that day. The American Diabetes Association (ADA) therefore recommends that the glycohemoglobin test be performed quarterly because it reports the serum glucose concentration of the previous 3 months. The ADA also recommends an annual urine test to assess for urine protein that might indicate an early sign of kidney damage. Liver function studies should be done on an annual basis as part of a routine exam.

17–2 Answer D

Eighty percent of cases of type 2 diabetes are associated with excess body weight. Although heredity is an important consideration, a normal-weight client with two parents who have diabetes has a better chance of avoiding the disease than an overweight client with healthy parents.

17–3 Answer C

The first line of therapy for a client with type 2 diabetes is usually a sulfonylurea medication, which lowers blood sugar levels by prompting the pancreas to pump out more insulin. If the sulfonylurea fails to control the blood sugar, metformin (Glucophage) is added to the regimen to reduce the amount of glucose the liver releases into the blood. If the combination therapy does not work, insulin is the final treatment choice and may be added to the combination therapy.

17–4 Answer C

Although paresthesias (tingling or numbness in the hands or feet) may be one of the warning signs of diabetes, the classic symptoms remain the three polys—polyuria, polydipsia, and polyphagia.

17–5 Answer D

While the diabetic diet has "relaxed" over the years, it is still not possible to eat everything. It is now acceptable to substitute two Oreo cookies for a fresh pear. Until recently, sugar was forbidden to clients with diabetes. The belief was that simple carbohydrates, like candy, were quickly digested, allowing blood sugar to soar, whereas the body took more time to process complex carbohydrates such as bread. Research now shows that both types of carbohydrates—simple and complex—affect glucose levels at comparable speeds. It is still important to monitor the amount of total carbohydrates per meal because they have the greatest impact on blood sugar. Drinking may increase the risk of low blood sugar, so if your client has an occasional glass of wine, stress the idea that alcohol should not be consumed on an empty stomach.

17–6 Answer B

Jogging is not a wise choice for clients with diabetes because of the potential underlying nerve damage to their feet or eyes. Although tennis is physically taxing, it does not require a constant bouncing up and down on the feet, and even if played at night, courts are well lit. Swimming and dancing are excellent forms of exercise.

17–7 Answer C

Beta blockers should not be used for clients with diabetes because of their blockade of hypoglycemic responses. Angiotensin-converting enzyme inhibitors are the first choice for clients with diabetes who have hypertension because they slow the progression of diabetic nephropathy. Calcium channel blockers provide pressure reduction without adverse effects on lipids and glucose control. Alpha-blocking agents provide a smooth control and an improved lipid profile.

17–8 Answer C

Lantus (insulin glargine) has an onset of action in just over 1 hour and stays in your system for 24 hours. Regular insulin is the only insulin that may be administered by the IV route. Lantus may not be mixed with any other insulin.

17–9 Answer C

Jenny's fasting blood sugar (FBS) test should be repeated before you order a glucose tolerance test (GTT) to confirm a diagnosis of diabetes. Diabetes is not diagnosed with a single high glucose reading. Hyperglycemia is an adverse reaction to hydrocholorothiazide, but the first action would be to repeat the FBS. If it is high for a second reading, the diuretic should be changed. A GTT may be ordered to diagnose diabetes mellitus if the second FBS is high. Certainly insulin therapy would not be started until Jenny was given a positive diagnosis, and even then oral hypoglycemic agents would be tried first.

17–10 Answer B

Stress causes the adrenal glands to secrete more cortisol, which leads to gluconeogenesis and insulin antagonism, raising the blood sugar. It is possible then that Harriet will have an increased blood sugar level. She will not need less daily insulin or more carbohydrates and will not have an insulin reaction, such as hypoglycemia, more readily than usual. Harriet may, in fact, need to increase her insulin use.

17–11 Answer D

Clients with diabetes are more prone to cardiovascular disease than those without diabetes. The most likely reason for this is that the high levels of glucose and fat that occur with poor control result in atherosclerotic changes in the blood vessels. The client with diabetes may also be overweight, but that is not the primary contributing factor to the development of cardiovascular disease. Diabetes is associated with a greater incidence of high blood lipid levels, high blood pressure, and obesity, all of which are risk factors for cardiovascular disease. Diabetes affects both small and large blood vessels, which contributes to the process of atherosclerosis. In women, diabetes negates the protective effects of estrogen. The amount of protein in the diet of a client with diabetes is restricted to help prevent or delay renal complications, not cardiovascular ones. The reason why clients with diabetes, especially older adults, are more prone to cardiovascular disease than those without diabetes is the high levels of glucose and fat, which result in atherosclerotic changes in the blood vessels.

17–12 Answer B

For insulin-dependent clients with diabetes, an increase in their daily insulin dosage is usually required in the presence of an acute infection. Betty should begin by increasing her regular insulin dosage by just 2 units, then monitoring her blood sugar level.

17–13 Answer D

A decreased respiratory rate with shallow respirations is not a sign or symptom of diabetic ketoacidosis. Signs and symptoms of diabetic ketoacidosis include Kussmaul breathing (very deep respiratory movements), hyperglycemia, glycosuria, polyuria, polydipsia, anorexia, and headache, as well as ketonuria and a decreased blood pH.

17–14 Answer B

Marie is experiencing the Somogyi phenomenon (nocturnal rebound hyperglycemia). If her 2–4 AM blood glucose level is greater than 70 mg/dL, the evening dosage of neutral protamine Hagedorn insulin should be increased and changed from before dinner to before bedtime. These actions should prevent most cases of nocturnal rebound hypoglycemia, which results in morning hyperglycemia. A fasting blood sugar test will not confirm the Somogyi phenomenon. The blood sugar level needs to be checked during the night to "catch" the Somogyi phenomenon.

17–15 Answer C

Angiotensin-converting enzyme (ACE) inhibitors are given to clients with diabetes who have persistent proteinuria. Proteinuria is one of the early signs of diabetic nephropathy, with or without the presence of hypertension. Urine protein must be measured to monitor the effectiveness of the ACE inhibitor. ACE inhibitors may be effective in decreasing urinary excretion of albumin even in clients without hypertension; therefore, a urinalysis should be performed and a serum creatinine level determined at least yearly. Detection of microalbuminuria alerts one that nephropathy is developing. When serum creatinine level reaches about 3 mg/dL, a referral to a diabetologist and nephrologist should be done. Intensive treatment can delay or improve diabetic nephropathy in its early stages. There is evidence that, with good control of hypertension, proteinuria can be reduced and the expected decline in the glomerular filtration rate can be slowed.

17–16 Answer D

During inspection of the integumentary system of clients with endocrine disorders, coarse hair may be an indicator of hypothyroidism. Fine hair is seen in clients with hyperthyroidism; hirsutism with Cushing's syndrome; hyperpigmentation with Addison's disease or Cushing's syndrome; hypopigmentation with diabetes mellitus, hyperthyroidism, or hypothyroidism; and purple striae over the abdomen and bruising with Cushing's syndrome.

17–17 Answer A

Trousseau's sign assesses for hypocalcemia. It is assessed by inflating a blood pressure cuff above the client's antecubital space to occlude the blood supply to the arm, then deflating it. Decreased calcium levels (hypocalcemia/tetany) cause the client's hand and fingers to contract in a carpal spasm. Hypocalcemia may also be assessed by checking for Chvostek's sign, which is performed by tapping fingers in front of the client's ear at the angle of the jaw. If hypocalcemia is present, the client's lateral facial muscle will contract.

17–18 Answer B

Acute pancreatitis is an inflammation of the pancreas caused by the release of activated pancreatic enzymes into the surrounding parenchyma with the subsequent destruction of tissue, blood vessels, and supporting structures. Although pancreatitis may be acute or chronic, acute symptoms include continuous abdominal pain for several days duration that increases in the epigastric area and radiates to the back, nausea, vomiting, sweating, weakness, pallor, abdominal tenderness, distention, and a low-grade fever. Pancreatitis occurs primarily in middle-aged adults and slightly more often in women than in men. The pain is in the upper right quadrant with cholecystitis and is intermittent, usually after a fatty meal. The gastrointestinal (GI) manifestations of cirrhosis include parotid enlargement, esophageal or rectal varices, peptic ulcers, and gastritis. The clinical manifestation of Cushing's syndrome related to the GI system is a peptic ulcer, which would result in intermittent pain related to meals.

17–19 Answer C

Although it is generally accepted that self-monitoring of blood glucose (SMBG) is a necessary component of the management of type 1 diabetes, its use in type 2 diabetes is controversial. Although individuals with type 2 diabetes may be treated with diet, oral agents, insulin, or combination therapy, the frequency of SMBG depends on the particular therapeutic interventions. The minimum recommended frequency is three times a week at selected intervals. The frequency obviously depends on the client's success in achieving treatment goals.

17–20 Answer D

Many factors contribute to macrovascular disease in type 2 diabetes. Some of the factors are related to insulin resistance and the hyperinsulinemia that may be seen developing in clients for years before pancreatic cells have been exhausted. These include hypertriglyceridemia, hypertension, obesity, and the potentially adverse effects of hyperinsulinemia on the vessel walls. Altered coagulation, platelet function, fibrinolysis, and modest hypercholesterolemia are also associated with type 2 diabetes and may contribute to macrovascular disease.

17–21 Answer B

If treatment with diet, exercise, and oral antidiabetic agents is insufficient to achieve acceptable glycemic control in clients with type 2 diabetes, adding a dose of insulin at bedtime to the regimen may be needed. As a first step, the addition of a bedtime injection of an intermediate-acting insulin such as neutral protamine Hagedorn (NPH) is recommended. Initially, the dosage is 10–15 units at bedtime; then the dose is adjusted to reduce overnight hepatic glucose production and achieve a normal or near-normal fasting blood glucose concentration. If this regimen does not achieve the desired effect, the oral antidiabetic agents should be discontinued and insulin therapy (two or more times a day) should be started. Finally, more intensified insulin regimens may be required in some clients, using multiple daily injections or insulin pump therapy.

17–22 Answer B

For a client with the symptoms experienced by Sigrid, a thyroid-stimulating hormone (TSH) level measurement should be ordered first because the symptoms suggest hyperthyroidism. The TSH level is the single best screening test for hyperthyroidism. Other laboratory and isotope tests for hyperthyroidism include a free T_4 or T_4 level, T_3 resin uptake, and thyroid autoantibodies including TSH receptor antibody (TSH or TRab). Tests that are not routinely performed, but may be helpful in selected cases such as hyperthyroidism during pregnancy, include radioactive iodine uptake and a thyroid scan (with iodine-123 or technetium-99m), which help to determine the etiology of the hyperthyroidism and assess the functional status of any palpable thyroid irregularities or nodules associated with the toxic goiter. Liver function studies and a chemistry panel will probably not show any abnormalities. An electrocardiogram may be ordered because of the palpitations, but once the thyroid is stabilized, the cardiac rhythm usually returns to normal.

17–23 Answer C

The treatment of Graves' disease (hyperthyroidism) is directed toward lowering the serum concentrations of thyroid hormones to re-establish a eumetabolic state. Chemotherapy is not used. Therapies that may be used include radioactive iodine (^{131}I), antithyroid drugs (ATDs), and thyroid surgery. For clients with hyperthyroidism and a low radioactive iodine uptake, none of these therapies are indicated because low-uptake hyperthyroidism usually implies thyroiditis, which generally resolves spontaneously. Therapy with beta-blocking agents is usually sufficient to control the symptoms of hyperthyroidism in these individuals. In addition, lithium carbonate and stable iodine have been used to block release of thyroid hormone from the thyroid gland in clients who are intolerant to ATDs.

17–24 Answer C

Clients should be cautioned about the adverse effects of antithyroid drugs (ATDs) before the initiation of therapy. Some providers obtain a white blood cell (WBC) count before initiating ATDs, because mild leukopenia is common in Graves' disease. A baseline WBC count may be useful for comparison if any problems arise. Serum electrolyte measurements and liver function studies will probably not be affected by ATD therapy.

17–25 Answer A

Radioactive iodine therapy is the most commonly used treatment in the United States for Graves' disease (hyperthyroidism); however, it is contraindicated during pregnancy. Therefore, for women, a pregnancy test (beta human chorionic gonadotropin) needs to be performed before initiating therapy. Women of child-bearing age should also be told to delay conception for a few months after radioactive iodine therapy. It is also contraindicated in women who are breast-feeding. Older adults or clients at risk for developing cardiac complications may be pretreated with antithyroid drugs (ATDs) before therapy to deplete the thyroid gland of stored hormone, thereby minimizing the risk of exacerbation of hyperthyroidism because of radioactive iodine (^{131}I)–induced thyroiditis. Marsha's basal metabolism rate will be affected by her Graves' disease, but has no bearing on her preparation for radioactive iodine therapy. Lithium levels are usually not performed before radioactive iodine therapy. They may be done if lithium is being used to block the release of thyroid hormone from the thyroid gland in clients who are intolerant of ATDs. Although parathyroid hormone secretion is dependent on the serum calcium level, it is usually not necessary to obtain a serum calcium level measurement before radioactive iodine therapy.

17–26 Answer C

After establishing clinical and biochemical euthyroidism after a thyroidectomy, you should perform a serum thyroid-stimulating hormone (TSH) level every year. Should it be necessary to adjust a client's dosage of levothyroxine, a repeat TSH level measurement should be done in 2–3 months to assess the therapeutic response. Once clinical and biochemical euthyroidism is reestablished, you may return to obtaining an annual serum TSH level.

17–27 Answer A

During pregnancy, many clients with hypothyroidism require an increase in levothyroxine, which would require an increase in the dosage of levothyroxine medication. This need would be detected by performing a thyroid-stimulating hormone (TSH) level test. The woman's TSH level should be checked every trimester to make sure the TSH level is normal. Adjustments to the medication dosage should be made as indicated. Usually, the levothyroxine medication dosage is returned to the prepregnancy dosage immediately after delivery. A serum TSH level reading should be obtained at the 6-week postpartum visit.

17–28 Answer C

Thyroid specialists agree that most benign thyroid nodules require no management beyond watchful waiting and an annual follow-up to evaluate their size. In rare cases, surgery may be indicated if a nodule enlarges to the point of interfering with breathing. Surgery may also be a cosmetic choice. There are conflicting studies regarding the use of levothyroxine to shrink thyroid nodules; because of this, the practice remains unclear. The choice of treatment for malignant thyroid nodules usually calls for subtotal or total thyroidectomy followed by radioactive iodine therapy to destroy residual thyroid tissue.

17–29 Answer A

If a client has a fasting blood sugar (FBS) level greater than 126 mg/dL, experts now prefer that the FBS test be repeated 8 hours after caloric intake. An oral glucose tolerance test, which is inconvenient and distasteful, is usually used for pregnant clients and those participating in research. Medication should not be started until the diagnosis of diabetes has been confirmed by two consecutive tests. Measurements of glycohemoglobin or other glycosylated proteins is not recommended for diagnosing diabetes. It is, however, the gold standard measure of long-term glycemic control in persons with diagnosed diabetes.

17–30 Answer A

For sulfonylurea medications to be effective, reasonable pancreatic insulin reserve is necessary. This reserve tends to dwindle over time; therefore, sulfonylureas tend to be effective for only 7–10 years in most clients. After they lose their effectiveness as a sole agent, another antidiabetic agent may be added to the regimen, insulin may be started, or both. It is unlikely that after being on an oral hypoglycemic agent for 7–10 years, the client will no longer require it and that diet alone would be effective.

17–31 Answer C

The thyroid-stimulating hormone (TSH) test measures the pituitary's response to peripheral levels of thyroid hormone. If the circulating level of T_4 is low, the pituitary will increase the production of TSH to try to increase the thyroid gland to produce more thyroid hormone.

17–32 Answer B

Brittle hair is a sign of hypothyroidism. A thyroid bruit, gynecomastia, and warm, smooth, moist skin are all signs of hyperthyroidism.

17–33 Answer C

A low level of thyroid-stimulating hormone (TSH) indicates hyperthyroidism. Hyperthyroidism results in an excess of circulating thyroid hormones, which will suppress the level of TSH produced by the pituitary. The TSH would be increased in primary hypothyroidism. In myxedema, there would be a deficiency of thyroxine. Most thyroid nodules secrete thyroid hormone, so those levels would be elevated.

17–34 Answer C

Clients using an insulin pump need to monitor their blood glucose levels at least four times a day. The client can develop diabetic ketoacidosis in as little as 4 hours if there is mechanical failure of the pump, because the only insulin used in the pump is rapid acting.

17–35 Answer B

BIDS refers to bedtime insulin, daytime sulfonylurea. It is a form of therapy in which a sulfonylurea medication is taken in the morning and insulin is taken at bedtime. The bedtime insulin suppresses hepatic glucose output and controls the blood glucose levels overnight, allowing the beta cells to recuperate so that they will function more effectively in the morning. The sulfonylurea stimulates the pancreas's insulin secretion in response to eating, thus giving an extra jolt to diabetes control. This combination therapy has been shown to reduce hyperglycemia and the dosage of insulin required.

17–36 Answer D

There is a major link between diabetes mellitus and coronary artery disease (CAD). There are many theories about the pathophysiology of diabetes mellitus and how it leads to CAD. Some of these mechanisms include the following: Hyperinsulinemia increases sympathetic tone and cardiac contractility by increasing plasma catecholamine, epinephrine, and norepinephrine levels; an increase of glucose level causes the distal nephrons of the kidneys to absorb more sodium, resulting in more fluid, expanding the intravascular volume and increasing blood pressure; and hyperinsulinemia causes a large number of vascular smooth muscle cells to be formed and deposited on the walls of vessels, causing buildup and eventual blockage.

17–37 Answer B

Morris should be started on an angiotensin-converting enzyme (ACE) inhibitor, such as captopril (Capoten) or enalapril (Vasotec). ACE inhibitors have renoprotective effects by reducing the intraglomerular pressure. They do this by inhibiting the renin-angiotensin system, which causes efferent dilation, and improving glomerular permeability, which causes a reduction of glomerulosclerosis. ACE inhibitors have this beneficial effect on clients with diabetes who are normotensive and hypotensive. Diabetic nephropathy is the leading cause of end-stage renal disease in the United States. Monitoring for microalbuminuria is a method for identifying early nephropathy. Ordering a 24-hour urinalysis will not give you any additional information. You do want to stress tight glycemic control and possibly send Morris to a dietitian, but he needs to be started on an ACE inhibitor now because he is already exhibiting microalbuminuria.

17–38 Answer A

A major element of the Diabetes Control and Complications Trial (DCCT) is testing blood sugar levels four or more times a day. The DCCT was a clinical study conducted from 1983–1993 by the National Institute of Diabetes and Digestive and Kidney Diseases. The study showed that by maintaining good glycemic control (as close to normal as possible), the onset and progression of retinopathy, nephropathy, neuropathy, and cardiovascular disease will be slowed. The other elements of intensive management in the DCCT include four daily insulin injections or use of an insulin pump; adjustment of insulin doses according to food intake and exercise; a diet and exercise plan; and monthly visits to a healthcare team composed of a physician, nurse educator, dietitian, and behavioral therapist.

17–39 Answer C

The Diabetes Control and Complications Trial recommends intensive management of diabetes for persons who already have a diagnosis of beginning nephropathy, neuropathy, or retinopathy. Intensive management of diabetes is recommended for clients with diabetes to prevent or reduce the risk for developing retinopathy, nephropathy, or neuropathy. Having one of these conditions does not preclude therapy. Intensive therapy may slow the progression of the disease if already present. However, because the most significant adverse effect of intensive treatment is an increase in the risk of severe hypoglycemic episodes, intensive therapy is not recommended for children under age 13; older adults; or people with heart disease, advanced complications, or a history of frequent severe hypoglycemia.

17–40 Answer C

Postmenopausal women with diabetes often fall into the category of high-risk clients who are most likely to benefit from long-term hormone replacement therapy (HRT) because of its ability to decrease morbidity and mortality associated with heart disease and osteoporosis. HRT preparations do not affect glucose homeostasis adversely in any significant manner, although it is wise to monitor blood glucose levels closely when women with diabetes begin HRT and throughout therapy. Although the package inserts of HRT preparations include a warning about glucose intolerance, this caution is not a reflection of their effect on glucose homeostasis, but rather a reminder that glycemic control has been observed to deteriorate in women who take high-dose oral contraceptive pills. Estrogen replacement therapy in women who do not have diabetes has been shown to increase high-density lipoprotein cholesterol levels and decrease low-density lipo-protein cholesterol levels by about 15% each; however, there is not much research on this effect in women with diabetes on HRT. One study did show significant improvements in cholesterol levels in this population. Because of the higher incidence of cardiovascular disease in women with diabetes and the lack of data that confirm an adverse effect of HRT in this group of women, the benefits of HRT seem to be greater for women with diabetes than for the general population.

17–41 Answer D

The first action a client should take for treating hypoglycemia (which is assumed because Mary took more than 4 times the usual dose of her short-acting insulin) is to ingest 10–15 g of a rapidly absorbable carbohydrate, such as 3–5 pieces of hard candy, 2–3 packets of sugar, or 4 ounces of fruit juice, to abort the episode. This should be repeated in 15 minutes, as necessary. Mary should continue to try to obtain her blood glucose level and should certainly not drive. You should ask Mary to call you back in about $^1/_2$ to 1 hour after ingesting the carbohydrate and after checking her glucose level (or sooner if she feels any different).

17–42 Answer C

Pancreatic protease is not carried in pancreatic juice. Pancreatic juice carries pancreatic amylase, pancreatic lipase, and pancreatic trypsin. Proteolytic enzymes are activated by trypsin, which is activated in the intestine. Pancreatic amylase splits carbohydrates into dextrins and maltose. Pancreatic lipase hydrolyzes fat to yield glycerol and fatty acids. Pancreatic trypsin is one of a group of enzymes, including chymotrypsin and carboxypolypeptidase, that split proteins.

17–43 Answer B

The process of aging results in a decreased absorption of fat-soluble vitamins. There is a decrease in the number and size of hepatic cells, leading to a decrease in liver weight and mass. There is also a decrease in enzyme activity, which diminishes the liver's ability to detoxify drugs. This increases the risk of toxic levels of many medications in older adults. There is calcification of the pancreatic vessels and the ducts distend and dilate. These changes lead to a decrease in the production of lipase.

17–44 Answer D

After an oral cholecystogram, some persons experience burning on urination because of the presence of dye in the urine. This is helped by forcing fluids. An oral cholecystogram is done to assess for biliary obstruction. Contraction of the gallbladder may be desirable during a cholecystogram to obtain a better reading and may be accomplished by having the client consume a high-fat meal during the procedure. A reaction to the contrast medium would produce symptoms such as urticaria, nausea, vomiting, or dyspnea.

17–45 Answer B

Immunoglobulin M (IgM) anti–hepatitis A virus (HAV) titers peak during the first week of the infection with acute hepatitis A and usually disappear within 3–6 months. Detection of IgM anti-HAV is a valid test for demonstrating acute hepatitis A. IgG anti-HAV titers peak after 1 month of the disease, but may stay elevated for years; therefore, it is an indicator of past infection.

17–46 Answer D

For the client with hepatitis, abdominal pain in the right upper quadrant is caused by stretching of Glisson's capsule surrounding the liver, which occurs because of inflammation; bleeding tendencies are a result of reduced prothrombin synthesis by injured hepatic cells; pruritus is caused by bile salt accumulation in the skin; and fever is the result of the release of pyrogens in the inflammatory process.

17–47 Answer C

Myxedema is characterized by abnormal deposits of mucin in the skin and other tissues; a dry, waxy type of swelling in the skin; and nonpitting edema in the pretibial and facial areas. Myxedema is most common in hypothyroid women in their 60s. Untreated myxedema has been associated with severe atherosclerosis and has been attributed to the increase in serum cholesterol concentrations, particularity low-density lipoprotein. Thyroid hormone replacement improves these changes.

17–48 Answer C

Saturated solution of potassium iodide is an antithyroid drug that blocks thyroid hormone production and release. It is used to treat hyperthyroidism before thyroidectomy. Propylthiouracil and methimazole (Tapazole) treat hyperthyroidism by inhibiting thyroid hormone synthesis. Radioactive iodine (^{131}I) treats hyperthyroidism and may be used to treat thryoid cancer by destroying thyroid tissue.

17–49 Answer A

Signs of hypoparathyroidism include elevated serum phosphate levels; decreased serum calcium levels; increased neuromuscular activity, which may progress to tetany; decreased bone resorption; hypocalciuria; and hypophosphaturia.

17–50 Answer D

Risk factors for primary adrenal insufficiency include taking glucocorticoids for longer than 3 weeks with sudden cessation and a history of tuberculosis, other endocrine disorders, or adrenalectomy.

17–51 Answer A

Clients with pheochromocytoma should be told to void in small amounts and to avoid a full bladder. In addition, to prevent stimulating a paroxysm in pheochromocytoma, also advise the client to avoid smoking; drugs that may influence catecholamine release, such as histamines, some anesthetics, atropine, opiates, steroids, and glucagon; and activities that might displace abdominal organs, such as bending, exercising, straining, and vigorous palpation of the abdomen. For women, pregnancy should be discouraged.

17–52 Answer C

The most common cause of chronic hypocalcemia is hypoalbuminemia. Other causes of hypocalcemia include vitamin D deficiency, alkalosis, hypoparathyroidism, malabsorption syndromes, pancreatitis, laxative abuse, peritonitis, pregnancy, renal failure, phosphate excess, burn trauma, osteomalacia, and overwhelming infections.

17–53 Answer B

When serum calcium levels return to normal, urinary calcium should be assessed. Hypercalciuria (greater than 250 mg in a 24-hour sample) indicates that the client's vitamin D dosage should be decreased. Once the dosages of calcium and vitamin D are regulated to achieve normal serum calcium levels, urinary calcium levels should be assessed every 3 months.

17–54 Answer C

Gynecomastia may be the first sign of testicular cancer. It is also associated with breast, adrenal, pituitary, lung, and hepatic malignancies. Hypogonadism produces low testosterone levels in men with normal estrogen levels. Alteration in breast tissue responsiveness to hormonal activity can result in gynecomastia. Gynecomastia can occur secondary to cirrhosis, chronic obstructive lung disease, malnutrition, hyperthyroidism and other endocrine imbalances, tuberculosis, and chronic renal disease.

17–55 Answer B

Cholesterol-lowering medications do not produce gynecomastia. Medications such as cimetidine (Tagamet), digoxin (Lanoxin), spironolactone (Aldactone), phenothiazines, antituberculosis agents, as well as marijuana, heroin, and alcohol can produce gynecomastia. In addition, men receiving estrogen therapy for the treatment of prostate cancer are likely to experience gynecomastia.

17–56 Answer B

The Ferriman-Gallivey scale has been used to define and grade hirsutism. The clinician evaluates hair growth in nine androgen-sensitive hair-growth areas. No hair growth is indicated by 0, and 4 is designated for frank virile hair growth. A score of 8 is diagnostic for hirsutism.

17–57 Answer B

Polydipsia occurs in diabetes as a result of high serum glucose levels that have an osmotic effect on fluids, which eventually triggers the thirst mechanism for compensation. The osmotic effect draws fluid from the cells into the intravascular space, creating a dehydrated state triggering the thirst mechanism for compensation. With a deficiency of antidiuretic hormone, as in diabetes insipidus, copious amounts of urine are excreted by the client, stimulating the thirst mechanism to replace fluid losses. Certain drugs such as phenothiazines and anticholinergics can cause dry mouth, increasing the client's thirst to the point of drinking compulsively. Excessive ingestion of salt, glucose, and other hyperosmolar substances can disrupt fluid and electrolyte imbalance, increasing the thirst mechanism to compensate for fluid loss or gain.

17–58 Answer A

The most common cause of hyperthyroidism is an autoimmune condition known as Graves's disease. It accounts for 90% of hyperthyroid conditions in young adults. Graves's disease is a result of a diffuse toxic goiter. A toxic uninodular goiter is the second most common cause of hyperthyroidism. Other causes include toxic hyperfunctioning multinodular goiter, subacute thyroiditis, metastatic follicular thyroid carcinoma, ingestion of iodide-containing drugs and contrast media, a pituitary tumor, a human chorionic gonadotropin-secreting tumor, and a testicular embryonal carcinoma.

17–59 Answer A

Propranolol (Inderal) is usually given initially to control symptoms of tachycardia, palpitations, or tremors during the initiation of radioactive iodine therapy. It is not used to help control symptoms related to ophthalmopathy in Graves' disease. Treatment for ophthalmopathy in Graves' disease often includes diuretics and ophthalmic prednisone drops, and severe cases may require radiation or surgical decompression. Radioactive iodine may worsen the ophthalmopathy in Graves' disease. Clients with ophthalmopathy require a referral to an ophthalmologist.

17–60 Answer C

Iodine deficiency is the most common worldwide cause of hypothyroidism. In the United States, where iodine ingestion is adequate, autoimmune processes are the primary cause of hypothyroidism. Hashimoto's thyroiditis, a type of primary hypothyroidism, is the most common form of autoimmune thyroid disease. Iatrogenic hypothyroidism, which occurs after treatment with radioactive iodine for hyperthyroidism or surgery for hyperthyroidism, thyroid nodules, or carcinoma, is the next most common cause of hypothyroidism.

17–61 Answer C

The major risk factor for development of thyroid cancer is exposure to radiation, usually from treatment to the head and neck. Until 1950, radiation treatments were given to children for an enlarged thymus, enlarged tonsils, and acne. Several million children were exposed in this manner. It may also occur in individuals who have had radiation therapy to the face or upper chest. There is also an increased incidence of thyroid cancer in areas where iodine deficiency and goiter are more common. Cigarette smoking is a risk factor for bladder and lung cancer, but not thyroid cancer.

17–62 Answer D

Cushing's syndrome results in an excessive amount of adrenocorticotropic hormone, which stimulates the secretion of glucocorticoids, mineralocorticoids, and androgenic steroids from the adrenal cortex. In the presence of excessive cortisol, fungal infections of the skin, nails, and oral mucosa, such as onychomycosis and tinea versicolor, are common and, in addition, skin wounds heal very slowly.

17–63 Answer D

Podagra is gout of the first metatarsophalangeal joint, the joint most frequently affected in the initial attack. Podagra is experienced by 90% of clients with gout. An acute attack of gout is usually monoarticular (affecting only one joint). Subsequent attacks may progress to include several joints (polyarticular).

17–64 Answer A

The medication of choice for an initial acute attack of gout is a nonsteroidal anti-inflammatory drug (NSAID). Indomethacin (Indocin) is the most commonly prescribed NSAID for this use. An initial dose of 50–75 mg is given, followed by 25–50 mg every 8 hours for 5–10 days. An alternative to indomethacin is naproxen (Naprosyn). The first dose of naproxen is 750 mg, followed by 250 mg every 8 hours for 5–10 days. Colchicine is an effective medication to terminate an acute attack only if administered within 48 hours of the initial onset of symptoms. Unfortunately, the attack is usually not diagnosed within this time frame. Corticosteroids can provide dramatic systematic relief, but are contraindicated in septic conditions; therefore, they should not be administered before analysis of the synovial aspirate. Allopurinol (Zyloprim) is used to decrease uric acid production. Although it is effective, it may take weeks to decrease the uric acid level, and therefore is not the initial choice in an acute attack.

17–65 Answer C

Foods high in purine should be avoided by clients with gout. Broccoli is not high in purine. Foods high in purine include all meats and seafood, meat extracts and gravies, yeast and yeast extracts, beans, peas, lentils, oatmeal, spinach, asparagus, cauliflower, and mushrooms. Wine and alcohol in excessive amounts impair the kidney's ability to excrete uric acid and should be used in moderation.

17–66 Answer C

Women with type 2 diabetes need to use insulin during their pregnancy to maintain good glycemic control. It would be ideal, although unrealistic, to put all women with type 2 diabetes who are thinking of conceiving on insulin. There is a risk of having a malformed infant if conception occurs when the blood sugar is not well controlled. Insulin is used, rather than oral antidiabetic medications, to achieve good glycemic control because the effects of most of the oral preparations on the human embryo and fetus are not well known. Many clients do not require antidiabetic therapy for the first several weeks after delivery and most women can return to their preconception regimen within 6–12 weeks. Sulfonylureas and angiotensin-converting enzyme inhibitors may be transferred to the fetus via breast milk, so they should not be resumed until breastfeeding is discontinued.

17–67 Answer B

The American Diabetes Association position statement on aspirin therapy in diabetes recommends aspirin use as a secondary prevention strategy in men and women with diabetes who have evidence of large-vessel disease, such as a history of myocardial infarction, vascular bypass procedures, and stroke. They also recommend aspirin therapy as a primary prevention strategy in high-risk men and women with type 1 or type 2 diabetes who have a family history of coronary heart disease and for individuals who smoke, are hypertensive or obese, or who have albuminuria, cholesterol levels greater than 200 mg/dL, low-density lipoprotein cholesterol levels greater than 130 mg/dL, high-density lipoprotein cholesterol levels less than 40 mg/dL, and triglyceride levels greater than 250 mg/dL.

17–68 Answer D

Many factors can cause an abnormal glucose tolerance test. They include medications such as oral contraceptives, diuretics, and cortisone; an infection, such as a urinary tract infection; trauma; bedrest; and stress. Because so many factors can render the test invalid, the current trend is to rely more on fasting blood sugar levels and postprandial blood sugar levels for the diagnosis of diabetes, unless the purpose is to assess for transitional gestational glucose intolerance.

17–69 Answer B

The infant with intrauterine growth retardation has very scant carbon stores in the form of glycogen and body fat and is prone to hypoglycemia even with appropriate endocrine adjustments at birth. The infant whose mother has diabetes has abundant glucose stores in the form of glycogen and fat and also develops hypoglycemia because of an imbalance in insulin-glucagon secretion resulting from hyperinsulinemia caused by islet cell hyperplasia. Other causes of hypoglycemia are associated with islet cell hyperplasia, inborn errors of metabolism such as glycogen storage disease and galactosemia, and as a complication of birth, asphyxia, hypoxia secondary to cardiorespiratory disease, or other stresses such as bacterial and viral sepsis.

17–70 Answer B

A client with insulin-dependent diabetes mellitus who misses a meal needs to eat about 15–30 g of complex carbohydrate to forestall hypoglycemia. If the client's appetite is poor, this may be accomplished through juice, flavored gelatin, soft drinks, or frozen juice bars.

17–71 Answer B

Clients with insulin-dependent diabetes mellitus (type 1) who have mild hyperglycemia may experience a drop in their blood glucose level during physical activity, whereas those with marked hyperglycemia may experience a rise in their blood glucose level. Clients with IDDM should check their blood glucose level before exercising and refrain from exercising if their blood glucose levels are too high (greater than 300 mg). For individuals without diabetes, the blood glucose level generally varies little during physical activity unless the activity is intense and of very long duration, such as marathon running.

17–72 Answer A

Insulin lispro is a rapid-acting human insulin whose amino acid composition has been slightly modified to make it work faster. It is administered 5–10 minutes before meals and reduces after-meal hyperglycemia to a greater extent than regular insulin. Its duration of action is about 3 hours rather than the 5–6 hours of regular insulin. Because of this, lispro reduces the risk of hypoglycemia between meals and during the night.

17–73 Answer C

If Jane has insulin-dependent diabetes mellitus and has been experiencing hyperglycemia before dinner, a possible solution to this problem is to add physical activity between lunch and dinner. In addition, she may try the following strategies: adjust her afternoon dose of rapid-acting insulin, reduce her carbohydrate consumption at lunch, reduce or omit her mid-afternoon snack, or change the time of her lunch or mid-afternoon snack. Adjusting her morning dose of rapid-acting insulin may be necessary if she is hyperglycemic before lunch. Reducing the amount of carbohydrate at dinner may be needed if she is hyperglycemic at bedtime.

17–74 Answer C

Jane, who has insulin-dependent diabetes mellitus, has been hypoglycemic at bedtime. To correct this, she could try all of the following strategies except adding an afternoon snack. This would be a strategy to try if the client is hypoglycemic before dinner. Strategies to try to correct hypoglycemia at bedtime include adjusting her insulin dose before dinner, adding carbohydrates at dinner, changing the time of dinner or evening snack, or adding an evening snack.

17–75 Answer C

Because hypertension is implicated in accelerating the microangiopathy of diabetes (especially retinopathy and nephropathy), therapy for hypertension in a client with diabetes should be more aggressive and initiated at a blood pressure 5–10 mm Hg less than the conventional therapeutic guidelines indicate (either systolic or diastolic pressure consistently over 140/90 mm Hg).

17–76 Answer D

Calcium channel blockers do not slow the progression of diabetic nephropathy in clients with diabetes. The steps that can be taken to avoid or slow the progression of diabetic nephropathy include maintaining excellent blood pressure control, using angiotensin-converting enzyme inhibitors, restricting protein, and maintaining excellent glucose control.

17–77 Answer B

Older clients with diabetes are predisposed to malignant otitis externa, caused by *Pseudomonas aeruginosa*. It is an invasive and necrotizing infection with a high mortality, mainly because of meningitis. The client complains of pain in the ear with or without a purulent drainage, swelling of the parotid gland, trismus (tonic contraction of the muscles of mastication), and paralysis of the sixth through twelfth cranial nerves.

17–78 Answer D

Hirsutism is excessive hair distribution. Virilization involves an increased androgen response, including increased muscle mass, clitoral enlargement, lowered voice, and behavioral changes.

17–79 Answer A

Men and women are equally prone to osteoporosis, but it usually occurs later in life in men. Men develop the classic fractures of osteoporosis: Colles's, vertebral, and hip. In women, the loss of sex steroids at menopause or after a hysterectomy leads to an increase in bone turnover through activation of bone remodeling. This results in an overall bone loss and loss of cancellous (trabecular) bone. In addition, with loss of estrogen, the amount of bone resorbed is greater than that replaced, leading to a continuing decline in overall bone mass and worsening microarchitecture. Hormone replacement for older men is not an option as it is in women because of the detrimental effects of testosterone on blood pressure and serum lipids. Prevention of osteoporosis in men is limited to maintenance of exercise, calcium supplementation, and cessation of smoking.

17–80 Answer C

Chvostek's sign is seen in tetany and is a spasm of the facial muscles after a tap on one side of the face over the facial nerve. To diagnose hypoparathyroidism, the following are usually present: a positive Chvostek's sign and Trousseau's sign, tetany, carpopedal spasms, tingling of the lips and hands, muscular and abdominal cramps, low serum calcium level, high serum phosphate level, and reduced urine calcium excretion.

17–81 Answer A

Pubertal gynecomastia is common and is characterized by tender discoid breast tissue enlargement of about 2–3 cm in diameter beneath the areola. The swelling usually subsides spontaneously within a year, and watchful waiting along with reassurance is recommended for that time period.

17–82 Answer C

Galactorrhea is lactation that occurs in the absence of nursing. A small amount of breast milk can be expressed from the nipple in many parous women and is not of concern. Normal breast milk may vary in color and not always be white. If there are significant amounts, or if galactorrhea occurs in nulliparous women or in conjunction with amenorrhea, headache, or visual field abnormalities, it might imply a systemic illness.

17–83 Answer B

Starting Steve on an antianxiety agent, starting him on a diuretic and/or beta blocker, or rechecking his blood pressure in 1 week will only delay the correct diagnosis. Steve's signs and symptoms are diagnostic of a pheochromocytoma, which can be detected with an assay of urinary catecholamine levels (total and fractionated), metanephrine, vanillylmandelic acid, and creatinine levels. A 24-hour urine specimen is usually obtained, but an overnight or shorter collection may also be obtained. Pheochromocytoma typically causes attacks of severe headache (85%), palpitations (65%), and profuse sweating (65%). The absence of all three of these symptoms can exclude the diagnosis of pheochromocytoma to a 99% certainty.

17–84 Answer C

Painless ulcerations are very common in clients with diabetes, and the only way to assess for them in the feet is for clients to use a mirror to examine the bottoms of their feet. Leah should not be walking barefoot because her sensations are probably decreased because of neuropathy, and she should try to avoid the development of calluses because preparations used to remove them are very caustic.

17–85 Answer D

The dawn phenomenon is an early-morning increase in blood glucose concentration occurring with no corresponding hypoglycemia during the night. It is secondary to the nocturnal elevations of growth hormone. The Somogyi phenomenon is a rebound effect caused by too much insulin at night, resulting in hypoglycemia during the night. This results in the secretion of certain anti-insulin hormones, including epinephrine, glucagon, glucocorticoids, and growth hormones, which result in hyperglycemia. Insulin shock is a hypoglycemic reaction. Diabetic ketoacidosis implies that there is hyperglycemia at all times during the day, not only in the early morning.

17–86 Answer C

Laryngeal nerve damage is a potential danger after a subtotal thyroidectomy. You should assess the client's speaking ability, including the ability to speak aloud, along with the quality and tone of the voice. The location of the laryngeal nerve increases the risk of damage during thyroid surgery. Hoarseness may be present because of edema or the endotracheal tube during surgery and will subside, but permanent hoarseness or loss of vocal volume is a sign of laryngeal nerve damage.

17–87 Answer C

Serum laboratory findings in the client with Cushing's syndrome usually include increased cortisol, increased sodium, decreased potassium, decreased glucose, and normal blood urea nitrogen levels.

17–88 Answer D

Addisonian crisis is a serious, life-threatening response to acute adrenal insufficiency and may be precipitated by abruptly stopping glucocorticoid medications. Other causes include major stressors, especially if the person has poorly controlled Addison's disease, and hemorrhage into the adrenal glands from either septicemia or anticoagulant therapy. The primary problems in Addisonian crisis are severe hypotension, circulatory collapse, shock, and coma. Treatment involves rapid intravenous replacement of fluids and glucocorticoids.

17–89 Answer D

Visceral neuropathies include anhidrosis (absence of sweating) on the hands and feet, increased sweating on the face or trunk, dysphagia, anorexia, heartburn, constricted pupils, nausea and vomiting, constipation, and diabetic diarrhea. Macrocirculation changes include an early onset of atherosclerosis, and peripheral vascular insufficiency with claudication, ulcerations, and gangrene of the legs. Microcirculation changes include diabetic retinopathy with retinal ischemia and loss of vision and diabetic nephropathy with hypertension, albuminuria, edema, and progressive renal failure. Somatic neuropathies include changes in sensation in the feet and hands; palsy of cranial nerve III with headache, eye pain, and inability to move the eye up, down, or to the middle; pain or loss of cutaneous sensation over the chest; and motor and sensory deficits in the anterior thigh and medial calf.

17–90 Answer C

Diabetic neuropathies involve three pathologic changes: a thickening of the walls of the blood vessels that supply nerves, which causes a decrease in nutrients; the formation and accumulation of sorbitol within the Schwann cells, which impairs nerve conduction; and demyelinization of the Schwann cells that surround and insulate nerves, which results in slowed nerve conduction. The locations of the lesions determine where the neuropathies occur.

17–91 Answer C

Calcium does not affect an oral glucose tolerance test (OGTT). The following medications may interfere with the results of an OGTT and should be discontinued for 3 days before the test: vitamin C, aspirin, oral contraceptives, corticosteroids, synthetic estrogens, phenytoin (Dilantin), thiazide diuretics, and nicotinic acid.

17–92 Answer C

Fiber is important in the dietary management of diabetes. A diet high in fiber, especially soluble fiber, helps improve carbohydrate metabolism, lowers total cholesterol level, and lowers low-density lipoprotein cholesterol. Soluble fiber is found in dried beans, oats, barley, and in some vegetables and fruits (peas, corn, zucchini, cauliflower, broccoli, prunes, pears, apples, bananas, and oranges). It should not be assumed that individuals will get enough fiber in their diet, because most dietary habits are not perfect. An intake of 20–30 g of fiber per day is recommended.

17–93 Answer D

Women who have diabetes and frequently develop vaginitis should avoid douching. They should also maintain good personal hygiene, wipe from front to back after voiding, wear cotton underwear, avoid wearing tight jeans with nylon pantyhose, and void after intercourse.

17–94 Answer D

The cause of Graves' disease is an autoimmune response wherein the body produces antibodies that act against its own organs and tissues. Thyroid-stimulating immunoglobulins are found in 95% of persons with Graves' disease and are evidence of this autoimmune process. Although thyroid carcinoma and pituitary tumors can cause hyperthyroidism, they do not cause Graves' disease. Hyperplasia of the thyroid results from hyperthyroidism; it does not cause it.

17–95 Answer B

Marisa can have snacks that are sufficient in calories to maintain her normal weight. She should consume adequate amounts of carbohydrates, fats, and proteins in a well-balanced diet. The majority of the fats should be unsaturated to decrease the incidence of vascular changes. The carbohydrates should be complex rather than simple to provide a more constant blood glucose level. She can still go out with her friends and consume most of the same snacks. Pizza, hamburgers, and many other "fast foods" are on the American Diabetes Association diet.

17–96 Answer A

Proteinuria is the first symptom indicative of renal nephropathy in clients who have had diabetes for about 10 years (although some studies suggest 5 years). There is increased permeability of the capillaries, with resultant leakage of albumin into the glomerular filtrate, causing albuminuria. The development of Kimmelstiel-Wilson nodules occurs in persons with type 1 diabetes, but does not necessarily precede the proteinuria. As renal function deteriorates, both the serum creatine and the blood urea nitrogen levels increase.

17–97 Answer C

Diane's symptoms today are the result of excessive levels of circulating cortisol. Ordinarily, there is a feedback loop that controls the circulating adrenocorticotropic hormone (ACTH) and cortisol levels. In Cushing's disease, the anterior pituitary is constantly producing excessive ACTH, which increases the levels of both cortisol and adrenal androgens. Her symptoms were precipitated by the administration of pharmaceutical cortisone preparations given in large doses over a long period of time.

17–98 Answer D

When clients have been on long-term cortisol therapy, increased protein breakdown or catabolism leads to loss of adipose and lymphatic tissue. The collagen loss is a result of protein wasting, which causes individuals to bruise easily. The skin is susceptible to rupture because the loss of collagenous support around the vessels makes them vulnerable. The skin becomes thin and atrophic.

17–99 Answer D

The major causes of death in clients with Cushing's disease are related to untreated infections, hypertensive disease, arteriosclerosis, and depression. Clients need to be taught to monitor their blood pressure closely, get an annual flu shot, avoid infections, and avoid stress-provoking confrontations. Because depression is one of the major causes of death, they should be encouraged to seek counseling.

17–100 Answer D

Aldosterone is a mineralocorticoid hormone secreted by the adrenal cortex. Follicle-stimulating hormone, thyroid-stimulating hormone, and growth hormones are all secreted by the anterior pituitary gland.

Bibliography

Aiello, JH: Preventing diabetic nephropathy: The role of primary care. Nurse Pract 23:2, 1998.

Amanti, M, and Schumann, L: Coronary artery disease: A link between hypertension, diabetes mellitus, hyperlipidemia, and obesity. J Am Acad Nurse Pract 10:2, 1998.

Barclay, L. Starting therapy with high dose levothyroxine is safe in asymptomatic cardiac clients. Medscape Medical News, June 2003. available at *www.medscape.com/viewarticle/457629*

Bengel, FM, et al: Cardiac oxidative metabolism, function and metabolic performance in mild hyperthyroidism: A noninvasive study using positron emission tomography and magnetic resonance imaging. Thyroid, July 2003.

Canaris GJ, Manowitz NR, Mayor G, et al. The Colorado thyroid disease prevalence study. Arch Int Med 2000 160:526, 2000.

DCCT/Epidemiology of Diabetes Interventions and Complications Research Group. Retinopathy and nephropathy in clients with type 1 diabetes 4 years after a trial of intensive therapy. New Engl J Med 342:381, 2000.

Deglin, JH, and Vallerand, AH: Davis's Drug Guide for Nurses (8th ed). FA Davis, Philadelphia, 2003.

Dunphy, LM, and Winland-Brown, JE (eds): Primary Care: The Art and Science of Advanced Practice Nursing. FA Davis, Philadelphia, 2001.

Dunphy LM: Management Guidelines for Nurse Practitioners Working with Adults (2nd ed). FA Davis, Philadelphia, 2004.

Genuth, S, et al: Effect of intensive therapy on the microvascular complications of type 1 diabetes mellitus. JAMA 287:2563, 2002.

Grey, M, et al: Coping skills training for youth with diabetes mellitus has long lasting effects on metabolic control and quality of life. J Pediatr 137:107, 2000.

Hak, AE, et al: Subclinical hypothyroidism is an independent risk factor for artherosclerosis and myocardial infarction in elderly women: The Rotterdam study. Ann Intern Med 132:270, 2000.

Heinig, R. Evidence-based primary care of clients with diabetes and cardiovascular disease. Fam Med, December 2002.

Holman, R, et al: The role of protein kinase C in diabetic microvascular damage. Fam Med, February 2003.

Hu, FB, et al: Physical activity and risk for cardiovascular events in diabetic women. Ann Int Med 134:96, 2001.

Krieger, DR, et al: Insulin: Recent developments and common quandaries. Client Care 32:3, 1998.

Kulkarni, K. Managing type 2 diabetes: The struggle to maintain control. Clinican Reviews, September 2002.

Lawrence, J, and Robinson, A: Screening for diabetes in general practice. Prev Cardiol, May 2003.

McKay JM. Diabetes mellitus and the elderly: A review of the 2003 California Health Care Foundation/American Geriatrics Society guidelines. Fam Med, 2003.

Meigs, J, et al: The natural history of progression from normal glucose tolerance to type 2 diabetes in the Baltimore longitudinal study of aging. Diabetes, July 2003.

Mukamai, KJ, et al: Impact of diabetes on long term survival after acute myocardial infarction. Diabetes Care 24: 1422, 2001.

HOW WELL DID YOU DO?

85% AND ABOVE CONGRATULATIONS! THIS SCORE SHOWS APPLICATION OF TEST-TAKING PRINCIPLES AND ADEQUATE CONTENT KNOWLEDGE.

75–85% KEEP WORKING! REVIEW TEST-TAKING PRINCIPLES AND TRY AGAIN.

65–75% HANG IN THERE! SPEND SOME TIME REVIEWING CONCEPTS AND TEST-TAKING PRINCIPLES AND TRY THE TEST AGAIN.

18 Hematologic and Immune Problems

LYNNE M. DUNPHY
and
JILL E. WINLAND-BROWN

18–1 *Which of the following multidrug-resistant community-acquired bacterial pathogens is (are) causing community healthcare concerns?*

A. *Mycobacterium tuberculosis*
B. *Neisseria gonorrhoeae*
C. *Streptococcus pneumoniae*
D. All of the above

18–2 *Clients with acquired immunodeficiency syndrome (AIDS) typically experience the neurological symptomatic triad consisting of:*

A. cognitive, motor, and behavioral changes.
B. seizures, paresthesias, and dysesthesias.
C. Kaposi's sarcoma, cryptococcal meningitis, and depression.
D. seizures, depression, and paresthesias.

18–3 *Barbie, age 27, had her spleen removed after an automobile accident. You are seeing her in the office for the first time after her discharge from the hospital. She asks you how her surgery will affect her in the future. How do you respond?*

A. "Your red blood cell production will be slowed."
B. "Your lymphatic system may have difficulty transporting lymph fluid to the blood vessels."
C. "You'll have difficulty storing the nutritional agents needed to make red blood cells."
D. "You may have difficulty salvaging iron from old red blood cells for reuse."

18–4 *Sara comes today with numerous petechiae on her arms. You know that she is not taking warfarin (Coumadin). What other drugs do you ask her about?*

A. Aspirin or aspirin compounds
B. Antihypertensive agents
C. Oral contraceptives
D. Anticonvulsants

18–5 *Screening infants for anemia should occur at what age?*

A. 6 months.
B. No screening is recommended.
C. 9 months.
D. 12 months.

18–6 *Despite successful primary prophylaxis, which infection remains a common acquired immunodeficiency syndrome-defining diagnosis?*

A. Pneumocystis carinii pneumonia (PCP)
B. Cryptococcosis
C. Cryptosporidiosis
D. Candidiasis

18–7 *Which of the following indicates that Jim, a 32-year-old client with acquired immunodeficiency syndrome, has oropharyngeal candidiasis?*

A. Small vesicles
B. Fissured white thickened patches
C. Removable white plaques
D. Flat-topped papules with thin, bluish-white spider-web lines

18–8 *Stu, age 49, has slightly reduced hemoglobin and hematocrit readings. What is your next action after you ask him about his diet?*

A. Repeat the laboratory tests.
B. Perform a fecal occult blood test.
C. Start Stu on an iron preparation.
D. Start Stu on folic acid.

18–9 *Sue has sickle cell anemia. In regulating her and monitoring her hemoglobin and hematocrit levels, you want to maintain them:*

A. slightly below normal.
B. strictly at normal.
C. slightly above normal.
D. around normal with only minor fluctuations.

18–10 *A metastatic tumor from below the diaphragm is suspected when you palpate which of the following nodes in the left supraclavicular space?*

A. Wringer's node
B. Sims's node
C. Wiscott-Aldrich's node
D. Virchow's node

18–11 *Which of the following is an X-linked recessive disorder commonly seen in African-American men?*

A. Sickle cell anemia
B. Glucose-6-phosphate dehydrogenase deficiency
C. Pyruvate kinase deficiency
D. Bernard-Soulier syndrome

18–12 *When Judy tells you that she has hemophilia, you know that:*

A. both of her parents also have the disease.
B. her maternal grandfather probably had the disease and it skipped a generation.
C. her father had the disease and her mother was a carrier.
D. her mother had the disease.

18–13 *Which of the following laboratory tests measures the amount of actively replicating human immunodeficiency virus and correlates with the disease progression and response to antiretroviral drugs?*

A. Western blot
B. HIV viral load tests
C. Absolute CD4 lymphocyte count
D. CD4 lymphocyte percentage

18–14 *Which is the most abundant immunoglobulin (Ig) found in the blood, lymph, and intestines?*

A. IgG
B. IgA
C. IgM
D. IgD

18–15 *Which of the following white blood cell types is elevated in parasitic infections, hypersensitivity reactions, and autoimmune disorders?*

A. Neutrophils
B. Eosinophils
C. Basophils
D. Monocytes

18–16 *Lorie, age 29, appears with the following signs: pale conjunctiva and nailbeds, tachycardia, heart murmur, cheilosis, stomatitis, splenomegaly, koilonychia, and glossitis. What do you suspect?*

A. Vitamin B_{12} deficiency
B. Folate deficiency
C. Iron-deficiency anemia
D. Chronic fatigue syndrome

18–17 *Antibodies (inhibitors) directed against factor VIII can arise spontaneously in a number of situations. These include:*

A. clients who have mitral regurgitation.
B. as sequelae to a strep infection.
C. clients on antibiotics.
D. women who are several weeks postpartum after a normal labor and delivery.

18–18 *Skip, age 4, is brought in to the office by his mother. His symptoms are pallor, fatigue, bleeding, fever, bone pain, adenopathy, arthralgias, and hepatosplenomegaly. You refer him to a specialist. Which of the following tests do you expect the specialist to perform to confirm a diagnosis?*

A. An enzyme-linked immunosorbent assay
B. A monospot test
C. A prothrombin time, partial thromboplastin time, bleeding time, complete blood count, and peripheral smear
D. A bone marrow smear

18–19 *When a neonate is initially protected against measles, mumps, and rubella because the mother is immune, this is an example of which type of immunity?*

A. Natural active
B. Artificial active
C. Natural passive
D. Artificial passive

18–20 *Systemic lupus erythematosus is diagnosed on the basis of the following:*

A. positive antinuclear antibody (ANA), malar rash, and photosensitivity.
B. positive ANA, weight loss, and night sweats.
C. negative ANA, photosensitivity, and renal disease.
D. leukopenia, negative ANA, and photosensitivity.

18–21 *When the donor and recipient of a transplant are identical twins, this is referred to as a(n):*

A. isograft.
B. autograft.
C. allograft.
D. xenograft.

18–22 *Your client, Mr. Jones, has Sjögren's syndrome. You suggest the following treatment:*

A. Artificial tears and chewing sugarless gum
B. Frequent rinsing out of the mouth with mouthwash
C. Drinking at least one glass of milk per day
D. Removing wax from the ears at regular intervals

18–23 *The first choice of therapy for a client who is positive for human immunodeficiency virus and has oral candidiasis is:*

A. fluconazole (Diflucan) 100 mg PO qd.
B. ketoconazole (Nizoral) 200 mg PO qd.
C. clotrimazole troches (10 mg) 5 times daily or nystatin (Mycostatin) suspension 500,000–1,000,000 units 3–5 times daily.
D. griseofulvin (Grisactin) 500 mg bid.

18–24 *A client with human immunodeficiency virus (HIV) infection has a CD4 count of 305 and an HIV RNA level of 13,549. The client is asymptomatic. What is your course of action?*

A. Negotiate with your client a time to start therapy.
B. Recheck the laboratory results in 1 month. If the counts remain like this, start treatment.
C. Start therapy now because the client's CD4 count is less than 500 and their HIV RNA level is greater than 10,000.
D. Wait to start therapy until the client becomes symptomatic.

18–25 *The three most common signs and symptoms of primary human immunodeficiency virus infection are:*

A. weight loss, pharyngitis, and fatigue.
B. fever, fatigue, and pharyngitis.
C. night sweats, rash, and headache.
D. myalgias, fatigue, and fever.

18–26 *Mrs. Jameson complains of unilateral blurry vision and partial blindness in the left eye. On physical examination, you find decreased peripheral vision on her left side. Fundoscopic exam reveals cotton-wool spots. Your most likely diagnosis is:*

A. cryptococcosis.
B. toxoplasmosis.
C. cytomegalovirus infection.
D. herpes simplex virus infection.

18–27 *The "gold standard" for definitive diagnosis of sickle cell anemia is:*

A. a reticulocyte count.
B. the sickle cell test.
C. a hemoglobin electrophoresis.
D. a peripheral blood smear.

18–28 *Jimmy is a 6-month-old with newly diagnosed sickle cell disease. His mother brings him to the clinic for a well-baby visit. Which of the following should you do on this visit?*

A. Tell the parents that Jimmy will not be immunized because of his diagnosis.
B. Tell the parents that Jimmy should not go to day care.
C. Immunize Jimmy with diphtheria, tetanus, and pertussis; *Haemophilus influenzae* type B (HIB); hepatitis B (HBV); and poliomyelitis vaccines.
D. Immunize Jimmy with measles, mumps, and rubella; HIB; and HBV vaccines only.

18–29 *Health maintenance in adults with sickle cell anemia includes which of the following?*

A. Early sterilization should be performed to prevent transmission of the disease.
B. Administer hepatitis A vaccine.
C. Avoid use of oral contraceptives because of increased risk of clotting.
D. Give folic acid 1 mg PO daily.

18–30 *Which of the following situations might precipitate a sickle cell crisis in an infant?*

A. Taking the infant to visit a relative.
B. Hepatitis B immunization.
C. Taking the infant to a home Miami Dolphins football game.
E. Having the infant sleep on its back.

18–31 *Tina, age 2, had a complete blood count (CBC) drawn at her last visit. It indicates that she has a microcytic hypochromic anemia. What should you do now at this visit?*

A. Obtain a lead level.
B. Instruct Tina's parents to increase the amount of milk in her diet.
C. Start Tina on ferrous sulfate (Feosol) and check the CBC in 6 weeks.
D. All of the above.

18–32 *You have just started Susie, age 4, on iron supplements. Counseling for her parents should include telling them that:*

A. iron is better absorbed if taken with vitamin C.
B. tea, coffee, and milk inhibit iron absorption.
C. iron is a common cause of accidental poisoning.
D. all of the above.

18–33 *Mindy, age 6, recently was discharged from the hospital after a sickle cell crisis. You are teaching her parents to be alert to the manifestations of splenic sequestration and tell them to be alert to:*

A. vomiting and diarrhea.
B. decreased mental acuity.

C. abdominal pain, pallor, and tachycardia.
D. abdominal pain and vomiting.

18–34 *The Centers for Disease Control and Prevention's definition of acquired immunodeficiency syndrome includes the presence of which of the following disorders, with or without laboratory evidence of human immunodeficiency virus infection?*

A. Pneumonia in clients under age 60
B. Dementia in clients under age 60
C. Kaposi's sarcoma in clients under age 60
D. Primary brain lymphoma in clients over age 60

18–35 *The most significant increase in cancer death rates have been that seen with:*

A. brain cancer.
B. prostate cancer.
C. lung cancer in women.
D. cancer of the cervix.

18–36 *A loss of DNA control over differentiation that occurs in response to adverse conditions is referred to as:*

A. hyperplasia.
B. metaplasia.
C. anaplasia.
D. dysplasia.

18–37 *Which of the following cancers is associated with Epstein-Barr virus?*

A. Burkitt's lymphoma
B. Kaposi's sarcoma
C. Lymphoma
D. Adult T-cell leukemia

18–38 *Prostate cancer is associated with which of the following viruses?*

A. Herpes simplex virus types I and II
B. Human herpesvirus 6
C. Human cytomegalovirus
D. Human T-lymphotropic viruses

18–39 *Which of the following is a genotoxic carcinogen?*

A. Vinyl chloride polymers
B. Chemotherapy drugs
C. Asbestos
D. Wood and leather dust

18–40 *Tobacco is responsible for all the following types of cancer* ***except:***

A. pancreatic cancer.
B. bladder cancer.
C. laryngeal cancer.
D. cervical cancer.

18–41 *Shelley has esophageal cancer and asks you if alcohol played a part in its development. How do you respond?*

A. "Your cancer was caused by your cigarette smoking, nothing else."
B. "Alcohol is also a carcinogen."
C. "Alcohol directly alters the DNA and causes mutations."
D. "Alcohol modifies the metabolism of carcinogens in the esophagus and increases their effectiveness."

18–42 *Maria asks if being overweight predisposes her to cancer. How do you respond?*

A. "No, you have the same risk as a normal-weight individual."
B. "You have less of a risk of cancer than normal-weight individuals because you have protein stores to combat mutant cells."
C. "Yes, you have an increased risk for hormone-dependent cancers because of your obesity."
D. "Yes, you have an increased risk because you have many more cells in all the organs of your body."

18–43 *Kathy, age 64, is a sun worshiper. She tells you that because she did not get skin cancer in her youth, she certainly will not get it now. How do you respond?*

A. "You're probably right; if you haven't had it by now, you're probably safe."
B. "As you age, you have decreased pigment in your skin, which puts you at more risk."
C. "Your skin elasticity is decreased, so you have more of a chance of contracting skin cancer as you age."
D. "Skin cancer is not dependent on age, anyone can get it."

18–44 *Which of the following is a benign neoplasm?*

A. Leiomyoma
B. Osteosarcoma
C. Glioma
D. Seminoma

18–45 *Marsha states that a relative is having a carcinoembryonic antigen (CEA) test done to detect some type of cancer. She wants to know what kind. You tell her a CEA is performed to detect:*

A. adenocarcinoma of the prostate.
B. medullary cancer of the thyroid.
C. adenocarcinomas of the colon, lung, breast, ovary, stomach, and pancreas.
D. multiple myeloma.

18–46 *The placement of a high dose of radioactive material directly into a malignant tumor and giving a lower dose to the normal tissues is referred to as:*

A. radiotherapy.
B. teletherapy.
C. brachytherapy.
D. ionization therapy.

18–47 *In teaching your client about the American Cancer Society's CAUTION model, which identifies signs of many cancers, you teach her that the "N" stands for:*

A. night sweats.
B. nagging cough.
C. nausea and vomiting.
D. noxious odor.

18–48 *Nancy recently had a mastectomy and refuses to look at the site. Her husband does all the dressing changes. When she comes into the office for a postoperative checkup, what would you say to her?*

A. "You'll look at it when you're ready."
B. "You must look at it today."
C. "Everything's going to be OK. It looks fine."
D. "You have to accept this eventually, just glance at it today."

18–49 *Trisha is going to undergo chemotherapy and is very worried about losing her hair. When she asks if there is anything that she can do to prevent it, how do you respond?*

A. "You need to accept the eventual loss. Buy a wig now and start wearing it so that it will seem natural when the time comes."
B. "If you wear a hot pack on your head during chemotherapy, it might help."
C. "Tell people you wanted to look like Demi Moore in the movie 'G.I. Jane'."
D. "Use an ice cap or a tight headband during the chemotherapy."

18–50 *What is the most significant reason why alcohol use is discouraged in persons with human immunodeficiency virus infection or acquired immunodeficiency syndrome (AIDS)?*

A. Alcohol interferes with the pharmacokinetics of most AIDS drugs.
B. Filling up on the empty calories of alcohol replaces the desire for food.
C. Alcohol decreases the ability of persons to adhere to a prescribed medical regimen.
D. If clients become addicted to alcohol, when AIDS advances, they will become addicted to painkillers.

18–51 *Sam is being worked up for pancreatic cancer. He states that the doctor wants to put a "scope" in and inject dye into his ducts. He wants to know more about this. What procedure is he referring to?*

A. Percutaneous transhepatic cholangiography
B. An endoscopic retrograde cholangiopancreatography
C. An angiography
D. An upper gastrointestinal (GI) series

18–52 *Jan is having biological therapy for her pancreatic cancer. What kind of treatment is this?*

A. Surgery
B. Radiation therapy
C. Immunotherapy
D. Chemotherapy

18–53 *Which of the following increases the risk of pancreatic cancer?*

A. A high-carbohydrate diet.
B. Cigarette smoking, diabetes, and a high-fat diet.
C. Diabetes and lack of activity.
D. Yo-yo dieting.

18–54 *One major approach to cancer prevention is:*

A. colonoscopy.
B. new drug trials.
C. Pap smears for women of all ages.
D. host modification.

18–55 *Which ethnic group has the highest overall cancer incidence rate?*

A. Native Americans
B. Asian and Pacific Islanders
C. Hispanics
D. African Americans

18–56 *Joan had a modified mastectomy with radiation therapy 10 years ago. She asks when she can have her blood pressure or needlesticks taken in the affected arm. How do you respond?*

A. "If it's been 10 years and you've had no problems, you can discontinue those precautions."
B. "Because you didn't have a radical mastectomy, you can do those things now."
C. "You must observe these precautions forever."
D. "As long as you do limb exercises and have established collateral drainage, you can discontinue these precautions."

18–57 *Which of the following is not an effective strategy to prevent the nausea and vomiting associated with the effects of radiation and chemotherapy?*

A. Decreasing the amount of liquids
B. Eating a soft, bland diet low in fat and sugar
C. Relaxation
D. Distraction

18–58 *Which of the following cancers does not have an effect on fertility?*

A. Uterine cancer
B. Cervical cancer after a cone biopsy
C. Hodgkin's lymphoma
D. Prostate cancer

18–59 *What is the earliest visual sign of oral and pharyngeal squamous cell carcinomas?*

A. Leukoplakia
B. Mucosal erythroplasia
C. Loss of sensation in the tongue
D. Difficulty chewing or swallowing

18–60 *Fecal occult blood testing is most effective in identifying:*

A. cancers in the right colon.
B. polyps.
C. cancers in the sigmoid colon.
D. cancers in the transverse colon.

18–61 *The "T" in the TNM staging system refers to:*

A. tolerance.
B. primary tumor.
C. tumor marker.
D. turgor.

18–62 *Bladder cancer can be detected early by:*

A. an annual urine culture.
B. a bladder tumor marker blood test.
C. an annual cystoscopy.
D. none of the above; there is no early detection.

18–63 *Which bone tumor arises from cartilage and is usually located in the pelvis, femur, proximal humerus, or ribs?*

A. Osteosarcoma
B. Chondrosarcoma
C. Ewing's sarcoma
D. Fibrosarcoma

18–64 *Which tumor marker may detect a tumor of the ovary or testis?*

A. Alpha fetoprotein
B. Carcinoembryonic antigen
C. Human chorionic gonadotropin
D. Cancer antigen 125

18–65 *Select a statement that is true about the erythrocyte sedimentation rate (ESR):*

A. It is a very specific indicator of inflammation.
B. A rise in the ESR is a normal part of aging.
C. It is useful in detecting pancreatic cancer.
D. It is diagnostic for rheumatoid arthritis.

18–66 *Julie's brother has chronic lymphatic leukemia. She overheard that he was in stage IV and asks what this means. According to the Rai classification system, stage IV is a stage:*

A. at which the lymphocytes are greater than 10,000 cu mm.
B. with an absolute lymphocytosis, in which the client may live 7–10 years or more.
C. of thrombocytopenia, in which the life expectancy may be only 2 years.
D. of anemia.

18–67 *Before initiating cancer therapy, the first crucial step is to:*

A. stage the disease.
B. define the goals of therapy.
C. confirm the diagnosis using tissue biopsy.
D. choose a treatment plan from the many therapeutic options.

18–68 *Which cancer can be cured with chemotherapy alone?*

A. Breast cancer
B. Malignant melanoma
C. Bladder cancer
D. Testicular cancer

18–69 *Clients with cancer have multiple sources and sites of pain. Guidelines for opioid use in cancer clients with uncontrolled pain include the following:*

A. Increase the daily dose of an oral preparation by no more than 33% every 24–48 hours.
B. Use sustained release preparations exclusively.
C. Nonpharmacological modalities should not be tried because they are not effective in these clients.
D. Start with the lowest effective dose.

18–70 *Some pharmacologic adjuncts to analgesics in clients with uncontrolled cancer pain include the following:*

A. anticonvulsants and tricyclic antidepressants.
B. anticonvulsants, tricyclic antidepressants, and corticosteroids.
C. selective serotonin receptor inhibitors.
D. benzodiazepines.

18–71 *Pernicious anemia is a result of:*

A. Not enough folic acid.
B. Not enough intrinsic factor.
C. Not enough vitamin D.
D. Not enough iron.

18–72 *The test in which a small, radioactive tracer dose of cyanocobalamin is given by mouth and then a 24-hour urine sample is collected and assayed for radioactivity is the:*

A. Coombs' test.
B. oligonucleotide probe test.
C. spherocytic test.
D. Schilling test.

18–73 *Sandra, age 19, is pregnant. She is complaining of breathlessness, tiredness, and weakness, and is* *pale. After diagnosing anemia, you order medication and tell her to take it:*

A. only with meals because it can be irritating to the stomach.
B. in the morning if she experiences morning sickness.
C. 1 hour before eating or between meals.
D. at bedtime.

18–74 *What is the mechanism of action of steroid hormones in cancer chemotherapy?*

A. They interfere with DNA or RNA synthesis.
B. They interfere with DNA replication by attacking DNA synthesis throughout the cell cycle.
C. They inhibit protein synthesis.
D. They alter the host environment for cell growth.

18–75 *Allie, age 5, is being treated with radiation for cancer. Her mother asks about the effect radiation will have on Allie's future growth. Although she knows that a specialist will be handling Allie's care, her mother asks for your opinion. How do you respond?*

A. "Let's worry about the cancer first, then see how her growth is affected."
B. "Chemotherapy may affect her future growth, but not radiation."
C. "She will probably have growth hormone problems, in which case she can then begin growth hormone therapy."
D. "That's the least of your worries now, everything will turn out OK."

18–76 *A platelet count less than 150,000/mm^3 may indicate:*

A. possible hemorrhage.
B. hypersplenism.
C. polycythemia vera.
D. malignancy.

18–77 *Macrocytic normochromic anemias are caused by:*

A. acute blood loss.
B. an infection or tumor.
C. a nutritional deficiency of iron.
D. a deficiency of folic acid.

18–78 *Thalassemia is caused by:*

A. blood loss.
B. impaired production of all blood-forming elements.
C. increased destruction of red blood cells.
D. autoimmune antibodies.

18–79 *Which type of leukemia produces symptoms with an insidious onset including weakness, fatigue, massive lymphadenopathy, pruritic vesicular skin lesions, anemia, and thrombocytopenia?*

A. Acute lymphocytic leukemia
B. Acute myelogenous leukemia
C. Chronic lymphocytic leukemia
D. Chronic myelogenous leukemia

18–80 *Physiological changes in the immune system of older adults include:*

A. an increase in immunoglobulin A and G antibodies.
B. a high rate of T-lymphocyte proliferation.
C. an increase in the number of cytotoxic T cells.
D. an increase in CD8, which affects regulation of the immune system.

18–81 *An increase of which immunoglobulin (Ig) signifies atopic disorders such as allergic rhinitis, allergic asthma, atopic dermatitis, and parasitic infestation?*

A. IgG
B. IgM
C. IgA
D. IgE

18–82 *Which hypersensitivity reaction results in a skin test that is erythematous with edema within 3–8 hours?*

A. Anaphylactic reaction
B. Cytotoxic reaction
C. Immune complex-mediated reaction
D. Delayed hypersensitivity reaction

18–83 *A fungal infection common in persons with acquired immunodeficiency syndrome that results in creamy patches surrounded by an erythematous base that can be wiped off, leaving a reddened or bleeding surface, is:*

A. candidiasis.
B. cryptococcosis.
C. onychomycosis.
D. histoplasmosis.

18–84 *Samuel, age 5, is receiving radiation therapy for his acute lymphocytic leukemia. He is at increased risk of developing which type of cancer as a secondary malignancy when he becomes an adult?*

A. Chronic lymphocytic leukemia
B. Brain tumor
C. Liver cancer
D. Esophageal cancer

18–85 *Robin has human immunodeficiency virus infection and is having a problem with massive diarrhea. You suspect the cause is:*

A. cryptococcosis.
B. toxoplasmosis.
C. cryptosporidiosis.
D. cytomegalovirus.

18–86 *What is the meaning of the term "shift to the left" or "left shift"?*

A. This indicates a rise in basophils.
B. This indicates a rise in monocytes.
C. This indicates a rise in neutrophils.
D. This indicates a rise in lymphocytes.

18–87 *Jill has just been given a diagnosis of human immunodeficiency virus infection and has a normal initial Pap test. When do the Centers for Disease Control and Prevention guidelines state that she should have a repeat Pap test?*

A. In 3 months
B. In 6 months
C. In 1 year
D. She should have a colposcopy every year rather than a Pap test.

18–88 *Maurice is an intravenous drug abuser with chronic hepatitis B (HBV). The development of which type of hepatitis poses the greatest risk to a client with HBV?*

A. Hepatitis A
B. Hepatitis C
C. Hepatitis D
D. Hepatitis E

18–89 *Sally has human immunodeficiency virus infection and asks which method of birth control, other than abstinence, would be best for her. You suggest:*

A. latex condoms.
B. the spermicide nonoxynol-9.
C. an intrauterine device (IUD).
D. an oral contraceptive.

18–90 *Prophylaxis for the first episode of* **Pneumocystis carinii** *pneumonia in an adult or adolescent client infected with human immunodeficiency virus is:*

A. isoniazid (Nydrazid) 300 mg PO and pyridoxine (vitamin B_6 [Beesix]) 50 mg PO qd for 12 days.
B. clarithromycin (Biaxin) 500 mg PO bid for 2 weeks.
C. rifampin (Rimactane) 600 mg PO qd for 12 months.
D. trimethoprim-sulfamethoxazole (TMP-SMZ) (Bactrim) DS 1 tablet PO qd for 10 days.

18–91 *Mandy's 16-year-old daughter has hepatitis A. Which of the following statements made by Mandy indicates that she understands the teaching you've just completed?*

A. "I guess she needs to be hospitalized until she's recovered."
B. "We'll keep her at home with strict isolation precautions."
C. "We'll stop at the store and buy plastic eating utensils."
D. "We'll stop at the drugstore and pick up prescription medications immediately."

18–92 *Julia asks how smoking increases the risk for folic acid deficiency. You respond that smoking:*

A. causes small-vessel disease and constricts all vessels that transport essential nutrients.
B. decreases vitamin C absorption.
C. affects the liver's ability to store folic acid.
D. causes nausea, thereby inhibiting the appetite and ingestion of folic-acid-rich foods.

18–93 *Which of the following is not an inherited condition that causes hemolytic anemia?*

A. Hereditary spherocytosis
B. Pernicious anemia
C. Glucose-6 phosphate dehydrogenase deficiency
D. Sickle cell anemia

18–94 *Caroline, an older adult, is homeless and has iron-deficiency anemia. She smokes and drinks when she can and has an ulcer. Which of the following is not one of the risk factors of iron-deficiency anemia?*

A. Smoking
B. Poverty
C. Ulcer disease
D. Age over 60

18–95 *Sheila, age 85, lives alone and has pernicious anemia. She has been coming into the clinic for weekly vitamin B_{12} injections, but finds this very inconvenient. What do you suggest?*

A. Have her come in every 2 weeks if her blood levels are stable.
B. Switch her to the nasal spray.
C. Switch her to oral vitamin B_{12}.
D. Forego the injections as long as she eats raw meat and raw liver.

18–96 *Which is the best serum test to perform to spot an iron-deficiency anemia early before it progresses to full-blown anemia?*

A. Hemoglobin
B. Hematocrit
C. Ferritin
D. Reticulocytes

18–97 *Which of the following laboratory studies is used to determine if a client has had hepatitis?*

A. Serum protein
B. Protein electrophoresis
C. Antibody testing
D. Globulin levels

18–98 *Under which of the following circumstances is the reticulocyte count elevated?*

A. Aplastic anemia.
B. Iron-deficiency anemias.
C. Poisonings.
D. Acute blood loss.

18–99 *The primary reason for newborn screening for sickle cell disease is to:*

A. present the parents with the option for genetic screening in the future.
B. test siblings if it is proven that the newborn has sickle cell disease.
C. allow for the prevention of septicemia with prophylactic medication.
D. prevent a sickle cell crisis.

18–100 *Samantha is being given platelets because of acute leukemia. One "pack" of platelets should raise her count by how much?*

A. 2000–4000 cu mm
B. 5000–8,000 cu mm
C. 9000–12,000 cu mm
D. About 15,000 cu mm

18–101 *How often should you order a complete blood count in your client?*

A. Routinely
B. Before dental work
C. In the case of infection
D. If she is pregnant

18–102 *Your client, Shirley, has an elevated MCV. What should you be considering in terms of diagnosis?*

A. Iron-deficiency anemia.
B. Hemolytic anemias.
C. Lead poisoning.
D. Liver disease.

18–103 *Sherri's blood work returns with a decreased mean cell volume (MCV) and a decreased mean cellular hemoglobin concentration (MCHC). What should you do next?*

A. Order a serum iron and total iron binding capacity (TIBC).
B. Order a serum ferritin.
C. Order a serum folate level.
D. Order a serum iron, TIBC, and serum ferritin level.

18–104 *Your 18-year-old client, Mandy, has infectious mononucleosis. What might you expect her blood work to reflect?*

A. Thrombocytopenia and elevated transaminase
B. Elevated white blood cells (WBCs)
C. Decreased WBCs
D. Decreased serum globulins

18–105 *Your client, Jackson, has decreased lymphocytes. You suspect:*

A. bacterial infection.
B. viral infection.
C. immunodeficiency.
D. parasitic infections.

18–106 *Your client, Ms. Jones, has an elevated platelet count. You suspect:*

A. systemic lupus erythematosus.
B. infectious mononucleosis.
C. disseminated intravascular coagulation (DIC).
D. Splenectomy.

Answers

18–1 Answer D

Mycobacterium tuberculosis, Neisseria gonorrhoeae, and *Streptococcus pneumoniae* are all multidrug-resistant, community-acquired bacterial pathogens that are causing major community healthcare concerns. Resistance is usually noted first among clients in the hospital, an environment characterized by heavy antimicrobial use and close proximity of clients, both factors that favor cross-contamination.

18–2 Answer A

Although certainly all of the answers listed may occur in clients with acquired immunodeficiency syndrome (AIDS), the key word is neurological. The neurological symptomatic triad that clients with AIDS typically experience consists of cognitive, motor, and behavioral changes. These changes are present to a greater or lesser degree in all clients with AIDS. Kaposi's sarcoma is not neurological; it is a multifocal neoplasm with vascular tumors in the skin and other organs.

18–3 Answer D

The spleen is not essential for life. When it is removed, the liver and bone marrow assume the spleen's functions. Although the bone marrow will produce and store hematopoietic stem cells, from which all cellular components of the blood are derived, it will not remove iron from old red blood cells for reuse.

18–4 Answer A

If your client has numerous petechiae, ask about the use of aspirin or aspirin compounds. Aspirin is a very effective antiplatelet agent. The recommended dosage for clients with chronic stable angina and certain other conditions is 325 mg (one tablet) per day. Many clients assume that if one tablet a day is good, two are better. Depending on the individual clotting time, even 325 mg per day may result in bleeding into the tissues. Antihypertensive agents, oral contraceptives, and anticonvulsants by themselves do not affect platelet activity.

18–5 Answer C

All infants should be screened for anemia using either hemoglobin or hematocrit testing at approximately 9 months of age. The cutoff points for a diagnosis of anemia at this age are a hemoglobin below 11 g/dL or a hematocrit below 33.0%. Cutoff points should be adjusted upward for children who live at high altitudes. You should consider repeat screening at age 3–4 years. Cutoff points for children this age are a hemoglobin of 11.2 g/dL or a hematocrit of 34.0%.

18–6 Answer A

Before acquired immunodeficiency syndrome (AIDS), *Pneumocystis carinii* pneumonia (PCP) was a rare disease that immunosuppressed persons and clients with leukemia sometimes developed. Today, PCP is usually the defining characteristic in clients with AIDS in both the United States and Europe. Cryptococcosis is a life-threatening systemic fungal infection that usually targets the central nervous system and the lungs, although it may attack anywhere. Cryptococcosis is a protozoal infection responsible for diarrhea in clients with AIDS. Candidiasis is the most common fungal infection, affecting 90% of all clients with AIDS, although it is common in the general population as well.

18–7 Answer C

Oral candidiasis (thrush) appears as white plaques that can be scraped off (removed), revealing an erythematous mucosal surface. Because of this, it is often referred to as a pseudomembranous lesion. Herpes simplex is an acute viral disease that causes small vesicles on the lip borders (cold sores). Leukoplakia is a disease of the mucous membranes of the cheeks, gums, or tongue with white thickened patches that may become malignant. Flat-topped papules with thin, bluish-white spiderweb lines are lesions of lichen planus, an inflammatory pruritic benign disease of the skin and mucous membranes.

18–8 Answer B

Tests for fecal occult blood in the stools should be done on all clients suspected of having iron-deficiency anemia. In the early stages of iron-deficiency anemia, both the hemoglobin and hematocrit measures are normal to slightly reduced. It is necessary to determine whether the iron deficiency is related solely to inadequate dietary intake, decreased absorption, or chronic blood loss.

18–9 Answer A

Clients with sickle cell anemia should have their hemoglobin and hematocrit levels maintained at a level slightly below normal because this is protective for some of the vaso-occlusive infarctive complications related to viscosity. When there is a painful sickle cell crisis, the client should be placed at rest, hydrated, given oral analgesics, and have the blood alkalinized mildly with an intravenous bicarbonate solution. Oxygen should be given to keep the hemoglobin well oxygenated and the amount of deoxyhemoglobin must be kept low.

18–10 Answer D

A metastatic tumor from below the diaphragm is suspected when you palpate Virchow's node in the left supraclavicular space. Virchow's node is an enlarged left supraclavicular node usually infiltrated with a metastatic tumor from below the diaphragm, especially of gastrointestinal origin. The other nodes listed do not exist. A wringer-type injury is seen in children who put their hands between the rollers of older washing machines still in use. Sims's is a side-lying position, and Wiscott-Aldrich syndrome is a childhood immunodeficiency disease.

18–11 Answer B

Glucose-6-phosphate dehydrogenase deficiency (G6PD) is an X-linked recessive disorder commonly seen in African-American men. It is an enzyme defect that causes episodic hemolytic anemia because of the decreased ability of red blood cells to deal with oxidative stresses. Sickle cell anemia is an autosomal recessive disorder in which an abnormal hemoglobin leads to chronic hemolytic anemia with a variety of severe clinical consequences. Pyruvate kinase deficiency is a rare autosomal recessive disorder that causes chronic hemolytic anemia, usually with the onset in childhood. Bernard-Soulier syndrome is a rare autosomal recessive intrinsic platelet disorder causing bleeding.

18–12 Answer C

Hemophilia is a classic example of an X-linked recessive disease, and as a rule only males are affected. In rare instances, female carriers are clinically affected if their normal X chromosomes are disproportionately inactivated. Women such as Judy may also become affected if they are the offspring of a father with hemophilia and a mother who is a carrier.

18–13 Answer B

The human immunodeficiency virus (HIV) viral load tests measure the amount of actively replicating HIV virus. They correlate with disease progression and response to antiretroviral drugs. Levels greater than 5,000–10,000 copies per milliliter indicate the need for treatment. The Western blot is a confirmatory test for HIV infection specificity when it is combined with the HIV enzyme-linked immunosorbent assay is greater than 99.9%. The absolute CD4 lymphocyte count is the most widely used predictor of the progression of HIV. The risk of progression to an acquired immunodeficiency syndrome opportunistic infection or malignancy is high if the CD4 count is less than 200 cells per microliter. The CD4 lymphocyte percentage is more reliable than the CD4 count.

18–14 Answer A

Also known as gamma globulin, immunoglobulin (Ig) G (IgG) is the most abundant Ig (75%) and is found in the blood, lymph, and intestines. IgG is active against bacteria, bacterial toxins, and viruses. IgA (10–15%) is found in the blood; lymph; saliva; tears; and bronchial, gastrointestinal (GI), prostatic, and vaginal secretions. IgA provides local protection on exposed mucous membrane surfaces and potent antiviral activity by preventing binding of the virus to cells of the respiratory and GI tracts. IgM (5–10%) is found in the blood and lymph and has high concentrations early in infection, decreasing within about a week. IgD (less than 1%) is found in the blood, lymph, and surfaces of B cells.

18–15 Answer B

Eosinophils are elevated in parasitic infections, hypersensitivity reactions, and autoimmune disorders. Neutrophils are increased in acute infections, the stress response, myelocytic leukemia, and inflammatory or metabolic disorders. Basophils are increased in hypersensitivity responses, chronic myelogenous leukemia, chickenpox or smallpox, after a splenectomy, and in hypothyroidism. Monocytes are increased in chronic inflammatory disorders, tuberculosis, viral infections, leukemia, Hodgkin's disease, and multiple myeloma.

18–16 Answer C

Lorie has the classic signs of iron-deficiency anemia: pale conjunctiva and nail beds, tachycardia, heart murmur, cheilosis (reddened lips with fissures at the angles), stomatitis, splenomegaly, koilonychia (thin and concave fingernails with raised edges), glossitis, esophageal webs (Plummer-Vinson syndrome), melena, and menorrhagia. Signs of vitamin B_{12} deficiency include weakness of the extremities, ataxia, pallor, loss of vibratory and position sense, memory loss, changes in mood, and hallucinations. Signs of a folate deficiency include weakness, pallor, and glossitis, with congestive heart failure occurring if the anemia is severe. A person with chronic fatigue syndrome might have a fever, a sore throat, muscle discomfort and myalgia, and generalized headaches.

18–17 Answer D

Acquired inhibitors of coagulation are found in women who are several weeks postpartum after a normal labor and delivery, clients with collagen vascular disease such as systemic lupus erythematosus, in older clients, and in clients with known inherited coagulation disorders, particularly factor VIII deficiency. There is no evidence that this is associated with mitral regurgitation, antibiotic usage, or as a sequela to a streptococcal infection.

18–18 Answer D

Skip has the characteristic symptoms of acute lymphoblastic leukemia. Diagnosis is made by the characteristic appearance found on a bone marrow smear. The enzyme-linked immunosorbent assay is the best test for rotavirus infection because it detects viral antigens. The monospot test is a latex agglutination test that measures production of heterophile antibodies during acute and recent episodes of Epstein-Barr virus infection. Its use is limited because of false-negative readings of 10–20%. A prothrombin time, partial thromboplastin time, bleeding time, complete blood count, and peripheral smear are included in an initial workup of bleeding disorders.

18–19 Answer C

When a neonate is initially protected against measles, mumps, and rubella (MMR) because the mother is immune, this is an example of natural passive immunity. This type of immunity is acquired by the transfer of maternal antibodies to the fetus or neonate via the placenta or breast milk. Chickenpox and hepatitis A are examples of natural active immunity, which is acquired by infection with an antigen, resulting in the production of antibodies. MMR, polio, diphtheria, pertussis, tetanus, and hepatitis B vaccines are examples of artificial active immunity, which is acquired by immunization with an antigen, such as attenuated live virus vaccine. A gamma globulin injection following hepatitis A exposure is an example of artificial passive immunity, which is acquired by administration of antibodies or antitoxins in the immune globulin.

18–20 Answer A

Systemic lupus erythematosus (SLE) is a multisystem autoimmune disease of unknown etiology. According to the American College of Rheumatology, 4 of 11 criteria must be present at some point through the course of the disease. These include positive antinuclear antibody; malar rash; photosensitivity; renal disease; neurological disorders, especially seizures and psychosis; oral or nasal ulcers; nonerosive arthritis with inflammation; pleuritis or pericarditis; hematologic disorder, specifically hemolytic anemia with reticulocytosis, leukopenia (WBC <4000 on two occasions), lymphopenia (<1500 on two occasions), or thrombocytopenia ($<100{,}000$ on two occasions); and immunologic disorder, specifically anti-DNA antibody, anti-Sm antibody, and antiphospholipid antibody, including false-positive syphilis. Weight loss and night sweats are not diagnostic for SLE.

18–21 Answer A

An isograft is a transplant in which the donor and recipient are identical twins. An autograft is a transplant of the client's own tissue, and is the most successful type of tissue transplant. An allograft is a graft between members of the same species, but who have different genotypes and, in the case of humans, human leukocyte antigens. A xenograft is a transplant from an animal species to a human, such as pigskin used as a temporary covering after a massive burn.

18–22 Answer A

Sjögren's syndrome is a multisystem autoimmune disease characterized by dysfunction of the exocrine glands, specifically notable for dry eyes and dry mouth. Thus, treatment is aimed at increasing comfort and lubrication. Artificial tears can be self-administered as needed; preservative-free products are usually better tolerated. For dry mouth, increasing hydration and chewing sugarless gum may be helpful; however, rinsing frequently with mouthwash, which contains alcohol, can prove more drying. Oral pilocarpine (Salagen), 5 mg qid, and cevimelene (Evoxac), 30 mg tid, have been shown to increase saliva production. Drinking milk is not recommended. Frequent removal of earwax is irrelevant to this problem.

18–23 Answer C

The first choice of therapy for a client who is positive for human immunodeficiency virus and has oral candidiasis would be clotrimazole troches (10 mg) 5 times daily or nystatin (Mycostatin) suspension 500,000–1,000,000 units 3–5 times daily. Because of common recurrence and increased rates of resistance, systemic fungicides should be reserved for severe cases, such as esophageal candidiasis and clients with dysphagia. Clotrimazole troches and nystatin suspension are the only nonsystemic medications listed.

18–24 Answer C

Regardless of whether the client is symptomatic or not, the Centers for Disease Control and Prevention standards call for therapy to be started when a client with human immunodeficiency virus infection has a CD4 count less than 500 and a HIV RNA level greater than 10,000.

18–25 Answer B

The most common signs and symptoms of primary human immunodeficiency virus (HIV) infection and their frequency are fever (95%), fatigue (90%), and pharyngitis (70%).

18–26 Answer C

The classic signs and symptoms of cytomegalovirus infection include cotton-wool spots ("cottage cheese and ketchup" appearance), hemorrhage, and exudates on fundoscopic exam. Decreased peripheral vision, blurriness, and partial blindness are other clinical manifestations. Referral to an ophthalmologist is imperative. Cryptococcosis is a systemic fungus infection that may involve any organ of the body, including lungs or skin, but has a marked predilection for the brain and its meninges. In the cerebral type, headache, dizziness, vertigo, and stiffness of the neck muscles are present. Toxoplasmosis produces symptoms that may be so mild as to be barely noticeable or may be more severe and include lymphadenopathy, malaise, muscle pain, or little, if any, fever. It may result in brain deterioration. Herpes simplex is characterized by thin-walled vesicles that tend to recur in the same area, usually at a site where the mucous membrane joins the skin; however, they may be limited to the gingiva, oropharynx, or conjunctiva.

18–27 Answer C

The "gold standard" for definitive diagnosis of sickle cell anemia is a hemoglobin electrophoresis, a test that determines the presence of hemoglobin S. The client with sickle cell anemia has a decreased hematocrit level as well as sickled cells on the smear. The baseline reticulocyte count is markedly elevated in sickle cell anemia and is not specific to that condition. The sickle cell test is a screening test. A peripheral blood smear is used for red cell morphology. Additional testing is always required to define the hemoglobin phenotype.

18–28 Answer C

At 6 months of age, Jimmy should be immunized with diphtheria, tetanus, and pertussis (DTP), *Haemophilus influenzae* type B (HIB), hepatitis B (HBV), and poliomyelitis vaccines. Children with sickle cell disease should receive all the standard well-baby care, but in addition to the standard immunizations, they should receive the pneumococcal vaccine at age 2 years. There is no cure for this disease. Children should be treated like other children and their activities should not be limited unless they are experiencing a painful sickle cell crisis.

18–29 Answer D

Genetic counseling, not early sterilization, is recommended for all clients with sickle cell disease; there is no routine risk in the use of oral contraceptives by women with the disease. Folic acid 1 mg PO each day should be given, as folic deficiency is common in these clients; 20% of these clients are iron deficient, so supplementation of iron is also often required. Adults should be immunized against *Streptococcus pneumoniae*, hepatitis B virus, and influenza. Hepatitis A vaccine is not routinely recommended; recommendation of this vaccine is limited to high-risk locales as determined by U.S. Centers for Disease Control and Prevention (CDC) guidelines.

18–30 Answer C

Certain precautions must be taken for infants with sickle cell disease to prevent vaso-occlusive crisis. Any activity or situation that would cause dehydration should be avoided. An example is sitting in a stroller in the heat for any length of time. Children with the disease should always have access to fluids. Exposure to cold temperatures slows the circulation and can cause sickling, as can any activity that can lead to hypoxia. Immunization for Hepatitis B should be done. The infant can be taken to visit relatives, although some care should be taken to avoid exposure to children and adults with URIs.

18–31 Answer A

The provider should always check a lead level before starting iron supplementation in children because an elevated lead level will cause anemia despite a normal iron level. Supplementation can cause iron overload. Regular milk (cow's milk) is often the cause of anemia in children; thus a thorough diet history must be obtained. Children under age 1 year are usually on iron-fortified infant formulas, and when they switch to cow's milk they do not receive sufficient iron.

18–32 Answer D

Parents often believe that milk is a good source of iron and vitamins for children. In the case of an iron-deficient child starting on iron supplementation, parents should know that milk, tea, and coffee inhibit iron absorption. They should be told that orange juice enhances the absorption of iron supplements. Iron, like all medications, should be kept out of the reach of children to prevent overdose.

18–33 Answer C

Abdominal pain, pallor, and tachycardia are all manifestations of splenic sequestration. Early recognition of splenic sequestration can be a life-saving skill. Parents can be taught to recognize signs of increasing anemia and enlarging spleen. Recognizing increasing abdominal girth or abdominal pain, as well as learning to palpate the spleen, is part of the educational plan. Vomiting and diarrhea do not necessarily accompany this complication, nor does a decrease in mental acuity.

18–34 Answer C

Kaposi's sarcoma in a client under age 60 is considered conclusive evidence of acquired immunodeficiency syndrome (AIDS) under the Centers for Disease Control and Prevention's definition. Other disorders, with or without laboratory evidence, of human immunodeficiency virus infections that also define AIDS include *Pneumocystis carinii* pneumonia; candidiasis of the esophagus, trachea, bronchi, or lungs; extrapulmonary cryptococcosis; cryptosporidiosis with persistent diarrhea; cytomegalovirus infection; herpes simplex virus infection with persistent skin lesions; *Mycobacterium avium* infection; progressive multifocal leukoencephalopathy; toxoplasmosis of the brain; and primary lymphoma of the brain in a client under age 60.

18–35 Answer C

The most significant increases in cancer death rates have been those seen with lung cancer in women. This is followed by melanomas of the skin, liver cancer, multiple myelomas, prostate cancer, non-Hodgkin's lymphoma, esophageal cancer, and cancer of the brain. The death rate from cancer of the cervix has declined over the past few years.

18–36 Answer D

A loss of DNA control over differentiation occurring in response to adverse conditions is referred to as dysplasia. Dysplastic cells show an abnormal degree of variation in size, shape, and appearance and a disturbance in the usual arrangement. An example of dysplasia is a change in the cervix in response to the human papillomavirus. Hyperplasia is an increase in the number or density of normal cells. Hyperplasia occurs in response to stress, increased metabolic demands, or elevated levels of hormones. An example of hyperplasia is the change in uterine cells in response to rising levels of estrogen during pregnancy. Metaplasia is a change in the normal pattern of differentiation such that dividing cells differentiate into cell types not normally found in that location in the body. An example of metaplasia is the replacement of normal columnar ciliated cells in the bronchial epithelium by stratified squamous cells in response to inhaled pollutants, primarily cigarette smoke. Anaplasia is the regression of a cell to an immature or undifferentiated cell type. Anaplastic cell division is no longer under DNA control. It usually occurs when a damaging or transforming event takes place inside the dividing, but still undifferentiated, cell. An example of anaplasia may be in response to an overwhelmingly destructive condition inside the cell or in the surrounding tissue.

18–37 Answer A

Burkitt's lymphoma is associated with Epstein-Barr virus. Kaposi's sarcoma is associated with human cytomegalovirus, a lymphoma with the human herpesvirus 6; and adult T-cell leukemia with human T-lymphotropic viruses.

18–38 Answer C

Prostate cancer is associated with the human cytomegalovirus. Carcinoma of the lip, cervical carcinoma, and Kaposi's sarcoma are all associated with herpes simplex virus types I and II; lymphoma with human herpesvirus 6; and adult T-cell leukemia and lymphoma, T-cell variant of hairy cell leukemia, and Kaposi's sarcoma with human T-lymphotropic viruses.

18–39 Answer B

Chemotherapy drugs are genotoxic carcinogens. Carcinogens can be classified in two groups: genotoxic and promotional carcinogens. Genotoxic carcinogens directly alter DNA and cause mutations. Other examples of genotoxic carcinogens include polycyclic hydrocarbons (smoke, soot, tobacco); arsenic; and methylaminobenzene. Promotional carcinogens cause other adverse biologic effects, such as hormonal imbalances, altered immunity, or chronic tissue damage. Examples include vinyl chloride polymers, asbestos, and wood and leather dust.

18–40 Answer D

Cervical cancer has not been linked to tobacco smoke. Individuals who smoke face an increased risk for pancreatic, bladder, and laryngeal cancer as well as oropharyngeal, esophageal, and gastric cancer. Persons who smoke pipes and cigars are especially susceptible to oropharyngeal and laryngeal cancers. Those who chew tobacco are especially susceptible to oral and esophageal cancers.

18–41 Answer D

Alcohol acts as a promoter by modifying the metabolism of carcinogens in the esophagus and liver, thereby increasing the effectiveness of the carcinogens in some tissues. Because Shelley smoked cigarettes and drank alcohol, she has an increased risk for oral, esophageal, and laryngeal cancers.

18–42 Answer C

Persons who are obese have an increased risk of hormone-dependent cancers because of their excessive body fat. Because sex hormones are synthesized from fat, these people have excessive amounts of the hormones that feed hormone-dependent malignancies such as cancer of the breast, bowel, ovary, endometrium, and prostate.

18–43 Answer B

Although anyone can get skin cancer, older adults have an increased risk because of decreased pigment in their skin. People of northern European ancestry with very fair skin, blue or green eyes, and light-colored hair seem to be the most vulnerable to skin cancer, but it is a problem for all people.

18–44 Answer A

A leiomyoma is a benign neoplasm of the smooth muscle. An osteosarcoma is a malignant neoplasm of the bone tissue, a glioma is a malignant neoplasm of the neuroglia cells, and a seminoma is a malignant tumor of the germ cells of the ectoderm and endoderm.

18–45 Answer C

Carcinoembryonic antigen is a tumor marker for adenocarcinomas of the colon, lung, breast, ovary, stomach, and pancreas. Prostate-specific antigen is the tumor marker for adenocarcinoma of the prostate; calcitonin is the tumor marker for a medullary cancer of the thyroid; and an immunoglobulin test will detect a multiple myeloma.

18–46 Answer C

Radiation therapy consists of delivering ionizing radiations of gamma and x rays in one of two ways. Brachytherapy is when radioactive material is placed directly into a tumor site and delivers a high dose to the tumor and a lower dose to the normal tissues. It is also referred to as internal, interstitial, or intracavitary radiation. Teletherapy is external radiation that involves placing the source of radiation at a distance from the client and delivering a relatively uniform dosage. Radiotherapy is another name for radiation therapy. Ionization involves the passage of radioactive particles.

18–47 Answer B

In the American Cancer Society's CAUTION model to help individuals be alert to many cancers, the N is for a nagging cough or hoarseness. The C is for change in bowel or bladder habits, the A for a sore that does not heal, the U for unusual bleeding or discharge, the T for thickening or lump in the breast or elsewhere, the I for indigestion or difficulty in swallowing, the O for obvious change in wart or mole, and the N for nagging cough or hoarseness.

18–48 Answer D

With the loss of a body part, there is an initial stage of shock and denial. It is a protective mechanism and should be neither challenged nor promoted. The best response to Nancy, who refuses to look at her mastectomy scar, would be to say: "You have to accept this eventually, just glance at it today." Then every day she could spend a little more time looking at it until she is able to care for the wound herself. Saying, "You'll look at it when you're ready" may mean that she'll never be ready. She should not be forced, but you should take a matter-of-fact approach with an empathetic attitude that will assist in her eventual acceptance of the change in body image. Practitioners should always avoid saying, "Everything's going to be OK," because sometimes it is not.

18–49 Answer D

Using an ice cap or a tight headband during chemotherapy helps to decrease the amount of drug that reaches the hair follicles. Although not 100% of clients receiving chemotherapy do lose their hair, you should prepare Trisha for that possibility. Suggesting that she buy a good wig while she still has hair enables the wig to be matched to her hair color and texture and minimizes obvious changes in appearance. Also suggest cheerful, brightly colored head wraps.

18–50 Answer C

The most significant reason why alcohol use is discouraged in persons with human immunodeficiency virus infection or acquired immunodeficiency syndrome is that alcohol decreases the ability of persons to adhere to a prescribed medical regimen. Current treatment regimens involve complex pharmacologic schedules with accurate dosing, strict compliance, and regular check-ups that are crucial to the success of the treatment and prevention of complications. Alcohol calories are empty and also fill up the person so that he or she may not eat important, essential food. If the client does have liver disease (which may have been caused by alcohol), it may be aggravated by the potentially hepatotoxic effects of various drugs that are commonly used.

18–51 Answer B

An endoscopic retrograde cholangiopancreatography uses an endoscope, which is inserted via the mouth and passed by the stomach and into the small intestine, where dye is injected into the pancreatic ducts and x rays are taken to determine if any obstruction is apparent. A percutaneous transhepatic cholangiography is a procedure in which a thin needle is put into the liver through the skin on the right side of the abdomen. Dye is injected into the bile ducts to visualize any blockages. An angiography is a procedure in which x rays are taken of the blood vessels after dye is injected. An upper gastrointestinal series is a series of x rays of the upper digestive system taken after barium is ingested. It shows the outline of the digestive organs. All four of these procedures are used to produce pictures of the pancreas and nearby organs to assist in the diagnosis of pancreatic cancer.

18–52 Answer C

Immunotherapy is also called biologic therapy. It is a form of treatment that uses the body's natural ability (immune system) to fight disease or to protect the body from adverse effects of treatment. Radiation therapy uses high-energy rays to damage cancer cells and prevent them from growing and dividing. Chemotherapy uses drugs to kill cancer cells.

18–53 Answer B

Although a high-carbohydrate diet and lack of activity may predispose one to obesity, which may lead to diabetes, this has not been documented as a risk factor for pancreatic cancer. Yo-yo dieting is not a documented risk factor. Smoking is a risk factor. Persons who smoke develop pancreatic cancer two to three times more often than nonsmokers. Diabetes is also a risk factor. Twice as many people with diabetes develop pancreatic cancer as opposed to people without diabetes. The risk of pancreatic cancer is also higher among people whose diet is high in fat and low in fruits and vegetables. Occupational exposure to petroleum and other chemicals also increases the risk of pancreatic cancer.

18–54 Answer D

Although drug trials and research and development with new drug products are important ways to work toward eradicating a disease, they do nothing for prevention. The three major approaches to cancer prevention are education, regulation, and host modification. Education reduces the cancer-causing behaviors of individuals, such as smoking. Regulations and guidelines help by prohibiting introduction of carcinogens and include methods such as encouraging nonsmoking areas, not selling cigarettes to minors, and workplace environmental guidelines. Host modification refers to increasing knowledge about cancer genetics. Healthcare providers are instrumental in educating the public and sharing decisions that may be made concerning the appropriate use of genetic testing. Colonoscopy is a screening measure aimed at detecting disease, not preventing it. The same is true of Pap smear.

18–55 Answer D

African Americans have the highest overall cancer incidence rate and the highest overall cancer mortality rate. Native Americans have the lowest overall cancer incidence and mortality rate of all of the populations in the United States. Asian and Pacific Islanders have a high rate of nasopharyngeal cancer. There is a high rate of gallbladder cancer among New Mexico Hispanics of Native American ancestry; liver cancer is more prevalent among Mexican-Americans; and cervical cancer is more prevalent among women from Central and South America.

18–56 Answer C

Lymphedema may occur many years after a radical mastectomy or radiation therapy on the affected side. Procedures such as venipuncture and blood pressure measurements should never be done on the affected arm because there is a greater risk for infection and compromised wound healing in that limb. About 15–20% of women develop lymphedema after treatment, some not until many years later. Several interventions have been tried with lymphadenopathy, ranging from nothing to aggressive surgical procedures, and have met with limited success. Most interventions include elevation, exercises, and pneumatic compression devices.

18–57 Answer A

It is important to maintain an adequate fluid intake to prevent dehydration, which may result in vomiting; therefore, decreasing the amount of liquids in the client's diet is not an effective strategy to prevent the nausea and vomiting associated with the effects of radiation and chemotherapy. Causes of nausea and vomiting include the effects of radiation and chemotherapy, obstruction of the gastrointestinal tract by tumor growth and metastasis, other metabolic abnormalities, and stress. Anticipatory nausea and vomiting should be expected and antiemetic therapy initiated before treatment and continued around the clock after starting the cancer treatment according to the anticipated length of symptoms. It can then be used on an as-needed basis. A soft, bland diet low in fat and sugar, as well as relaxation, distraction, and guided imagery, help to reduce the adverse effects of nausea and vomiting.

18–58 Answer B

Cervical cancer after a cone biopsy does not affect fertility; however, it does affect fertility after a hysterectomy or with radiation therapy. Fertility is affected by uterine cancer with surgery or radiation, Hodgkin's lymphoma (radiation to the pelvis affects the gonads by decreasing the number of sperm or ova), and prostate cancer.

18–59 Answer B

Mucosal erythroplasia (red inflammatory lesions) is the earliest visual sign of oral and pharyngeal squamous cell carcinomas. Leukoplakia (thickened whitish patches on the tongue or mucous membranes) is the most common premalignant lesion, but only about 30% of people with these lesions are later found to have malignancy. Other symptoms include pain in the face, jaw, or ear; bleeding; stuffy nose; sore throat; loss of sensation in the tongue; difficulty chewing or swallowing; or a feeling of a mass in the mouth or throat.

18–60 Answer C

Fecal occult blood testing (FOBT) is accurate in identifying 25–40% of colorectal cancers, specifically those in the sigmoid colon. It is less effective for identifying cancers of the right colon. It is not effective for identifying polyps. Persons over age 40 should have an annual stool examination performed, because this can help decrease colorectal cancer mortality rates by 33–57%. FOBT has a false-negative and a false-positive possibility. Certain medications such as aspirin and other nonsteroidal anti-inflammatory drugs, eating red meat or raw vegetables, or bleeding hemorrhoids may cause a false-positive reading. These medications and foods should be avoided for 3 days before the administration of the test. False-negative results may occur because of polyps or the fact that some cancers do not bleed or may bleed only occasionally.

18–61 Answer B

One of the most commonly used staging systems to label the extent of the cancer is the TNM staging system. The T is for primary tumor, N is for regional lymph nodes, and M is for distant metastasis. In an example of colorectal cancer, a person classified as T1N1M0 would have a tumor that invaded the submucosa, metastasis in one to three pericolic or perirectal lymph nodes, but no distant metastasis.

18–62 Answer D

There are no generally accepted guidelines for the prevention or early detection of bladder cancer. The first problem is usually gross hematuria, followed by dysuria, frequency, or urgency and symptoms of urethral obstruction. Bladder cancer comprises approximately 4–5% of all cancers in the United States. It is three times more common in men than women, and two times more common in whites than blacks. Smoking should be discouraged and exposure to certain chemicals used in the textile and rubber industries eliminated. There is no bladder tumor marker, and annual cystoscopies are not recommended.

18–63 Answer B

A chondrosarcoma arises from cartilage and is usually located in the pelvis, femur, proximal humerus, or ribs. It is the second most common bone malignancy, seen most frequently in men between ages 30 and 60. An osteosarcoma is the most common primary bone-forming tumor, usually affecting children and young adults. It arises from osteoblast cells that multiply rapidly during periods of skeletal growth. More common in men, osteosarcomas are usually located around the knee joint, with the proximal humerus also being a common site. Ewing's sarcoma is a marrow-originating tumor consisting of small round cells. It is seen primarily in male children and adolescents. It arises most commonly in the diaphysis of long bones and in flat bones. A fibrosarcoma is a rare type of bone tumor that consists of interlacing bundles of collagen cells. It is more common in men from age 20–60 and is commonly found in the femur and tibia.

18–64 Answer A

Alpha-fetoprotein levels may be elevated with embryonal cell tumors of the ovary or testis, hepatocellular carcinoma, and choriocarcinoma. Carcinoembryonic antigen detects colon, rectal, pancreatic, stomach, lung, breast, and ovarian tumors. Human chorionic gonadotropin detects choriocarcinoma, germ cell carcinoma, testicular teratoma, and hydatidiform moles. CA-125 is the tumor marker for epithelial ovarian neoplasms and breast and colorectal malignancies.

18–65 Answer B

The erythrocyte sedimentation rate (ESR) is a very nonspecific indicator of inflammation and is often elevated in inflammatory musculoskeletal conditions; it is not, however, diagnostic for rheumatoid arthritis. Additionally, anemia can cause an increased ESR. As people age, their "normal" sedimentation rate increases.

18–66 Answer C

Stage IV in the Rai classification system for chronic lymphatic leukemia (CLL) is the stage of thrombocytopenia where the life expectancy may be only 2 years. CLL is the only leukemia in which a staging system is commonly used because CLL has prognostic implications. A client with only an absolute lymphocytosis may live 7–10 years or more. In the Rai classification system, stage 0 indicates a lymphocyte count greater than 10,000 cu mm, stage I indicates enlarged lymph nodes, stage II indicates an enlarged liver and/or spleen, stage III indicates anemia, and stage IV indicates thrombocytopenia.

18–67 Answer C

Before initiating cancer therapy, the first crucial step is to confirm the diagnosis using tissue biopsy. This sounds simplistic, but some practitioners "diagnose" unconfirmed cancer that cannot then be effectively treated. The next step is to stage the disease using appropriate diagnostic means. The stage or the extent of the disease determines the prognosis and treatment. The third step is to define the goals of therapy—whether it is curative, adjuvant, or palliative—because that will influence the extent and aggressiveness of treatment. The last step before initiating therapy is to choose a treatment plan from the many therapeutic options, depending on many different client characteristics such as age, goals, wishes of the client and family, and extent of the cancer.

18–68 Answer D

Cancers with macroscopic disease that can be cured with chemotherapy include testicular and ovarian cancer and Hodgkin's disease. Bladder and breast cancers are cancers with microscopic disease that can be cured with adjuvant chemotherapy. A malignant melanoma has a low response rate or can be unresponsive to chemotherapy.

18–69 Answer D

When treating cancer clients who have uncontrolled, chronic pain with opioids, always start with the lowest effective dose; use around-the-clock dosing to avoid ups and downs; and use sustained-release preparations. Titrate dosage to provide adequate analgesia or avoid intolerable side effects. For uncontrolled pain you may increase the daily dose of oral preparations up to 50% every 24–48 hours. Always prescribe immediate-release formulations for breakthrough pain (use one-fourth to one-third of the total dose every 2–4 hours). Nonpharmacological modalities such as transcutaneous electrical nerve stimulation (TENS) and psychological therapies such as relaxation techniques may be used in addition to analgesics and may significantly improve control of chronic pain.

18–70 Answer B

Pain that is poorly controlled with opioids and NSAIDs is often neuropathic in nature, meaning that it is a result of direct nerve injury, such as nerve compression. This pain may be controlled with anticonvulsants, tricyclic antidepressants, and corticosteroids. Corticosteroids may also be effective for severe bone pain. SSRIs have not had the proven results with neuropathic pain that tricyclics have, although they may prove effective in clients with cancer in general. Benzodiazepines are not usually recommended because of their sedative-like effects. The goal with cancer clients who experience chronic pain is to provide adequate pain control while keeping the client awake and able to interact with those around them and maintain as normal a life as possible.

18–71 Answer B

Pernicious anemia is a macrocytic anemia marked by achlohydria. The parietal cells of the stomach fail to secrete enough intrinsic factor to ensure intestinal absorption of vitamin B_{12}, the extrinsic factor. This leads to a deficiency of B_{12}. Folic acid deficiency also causes a macrocytic anemia, but the B_{12} levels are normal and there are not the associated neurologic symptoms seen in pernicious anemia. Vitamin D is not essential for the absorption of vitamin B_{12}. A deficiency of iron results in iron deficiency anemia, a microcytic hypochromic anemia.

18–72 Answer D

The Schilling test is performed by giving a small, radioactive tracer dose of cyanocobalamin (about 0.5–2 mg) by mouth and then collecting and assaying a 24-hour urine sample for radioactivity. This is diagnostic of cobalamin deficiency (vitamin B_{12} deficiency). Coombs' tests ascertain the presence or absence of immunoglobulin and complement in the coating of red blood cells. The tests (direct and indirect) can differentiate between various types of hemolytic anemias; determine minor blood types, including the Rh factor; and test for erythroblastosis fetalis. The oligonucleotide probe test is a method used to diagnose antenatal thalassemia. Spherocytes are round rather than discoid cells.

18–73 Answer C

Sandra's symptoms indicate anemia, which is probably caused by a poor diet. She probably has an iron and folic acid deficiency. You should order iron, folic acid, and other supplements and tell her that for better absorption, she should take the iron supplement 1 hour before eating or between meals. You should also suggest that she eat foods high in vitamin C, such as citrus fruits and fresh, raw vegetables, because vitamin C makes iron absorption more efficient. Iron also will turn bowel movements black and often cause constipation, so you may want to discuss this with Sandra.

18–74 Answer D

Steroid hormones (androgens, such as fluoxymesterone [Halotestin]; estrogens, such as ethinyl estradiol [Estinyl]; and progestins, such as megestrol acetate [Megace]) are useful in cancer chemotherapy because they alter the host environment for cell growth. Antibiotics, such as doxorubicin (Adriamycin) and bleomycin (Blenoxane) interfere with DNA or RNA synthesis depending on the drug. Alkylating agents, such as chlorambucil (Leukeran) and melphalan (Alkeran), interfere with DNA replication by attacking DNA synthesis throughout the cell cycle. Other agents such as asparaginase (Elspar) and cisplatin (Platinol) inhibit protein synthesis.

18–75 Answer C

Growth complications depend on the direct damage to the endocrine tissue. Children with acute lymphocytic leukemia, brain tumors, nasopharyngeal cancers, and orbital tumors who have received radiation therapy are at the highest risk. Approximately 50–90% of these children will have some evidence of growth hormone deficiency. They may benefit from growth hormone therapy. Spinal radiation inhibits the vertebral body growth. Chemotherapy may result in a decrease in linear growth, but usually the child catches up when the chemotherapy is discontinued. Assuring the mother that "everything will be OK" is always a poor choice, as is negating her concern by saying "Let's worry about the cancer first, then see what happens."

18–76 Answer B

A platelet count less than 150,000/mm^3 may indicate hypersplenism as well as possible bone marrow failure or accelerated consumption of platelets. A count greater than 350,000/mm^3 may indicate possible hemorrhage, polycythemia vera, or malignancy.

18–77 Answer D

A folic acid and/or vitamin B_{12} deficiency causes macrocytic normochromic anemias in which the cell size is large and irregular. Acute blood loss and most hemolytic processes cause normocytic normochromic anemias in which the cell size is normal. Infections or tumor may cause an anemia of chronic disease that produces a normocytic red blood cell. Iron deficiency anemias are hypochromic microcytic and may result from dietary insufficiencies as well as acute blood loss.

18–78 Answer C

Thalassemia is caused by a decreased synthesis of hemoglobin and malformation of red blood cells (RBCs) that increases their hemolysis (increased destruction of RBCs). It is an inherited disorder that occurs primarily in Asians or persons of Mediterranean ancestry. Aplastic anemia is a depression or cessation of all blood-forming elements. An acquired hemolytic disorder is most often drug induced or autoimmune; in such cases antibodies are produced that cause premature destruction of the RBCs.

18–79 Answer C

Chronic lymphocytic leukemia (CLL) has an insidious onset with weakness, fatigue, massive lymphadenopathy, pruritic vesicular skin lesions, anemia, and thrombocytopenia. Acute lymphocytic leukemia (ALL) produces fever, respiratory infections, anemia, bleeding mucous membranes, lymphadenopathy, fatigue and weakness, and a tendency to infection. Acute myelogenous leukemia has the same symptoms as ALL but less lymphadenopathy. Chronic myelogenous leukemia produces weakness, fatigue, anorexia, weight loss, splenomegaly, anemia, thrombocytopenia, and fever, and can have a fulminant stage.

18–80 Answer A

Older adults have a change in their immunoglobulin (Ig) balance and a marked increase in IgA and IgG antibodies. Other physiologic changes in the immune systems of older adults include a low rate of T-lymphocyte proliferation in response to a stimulus, a decrease in the number of cytotoxic (killer) T cells, and a decrease in the relative production of CD4 (T4 or helper T cells) and CD8, affecting regulation of the immune system.

18–81 Answer D

An increase in immunoglobulin (Ig) E signifies atopic disorders such as allergic rhinitis, allergic asthma, atopic dermatitis, and parasitic infestation. An increase of IgG may signify bacterial infections, hepatitis A, glomerulonephritis, rheumatoid arthritis, systemic lupus erythematosus (SLE), and acquired immunodeficiency syndrome (AIDS). An increase in IgM would occur with hepatitis A and B infections, chronic infections, SLE, rheumatoid arthritis, Sjögren's syndrome, and AIDS. An increase in IgA would occur with SLE, rheumatoid arthritis, glomerulonephritis, and chronic liver disease.

18–82 Answer C

An immune complex-mediated hypersensitivity reaction may result from serum sickness, systemic lupus erythematosus, or rheumatoid arthritis. It results in a skin test that produces erythema and edema within 3–8 hours. An anaphylactic reaction may occur with allergic rhinitis or asthma. The mediator of injury is histamine and the skin test appears as a wheal and flare. A cytotoxic reaction, such as a transfusion reaction, does not produce any reaction from a skin test. A delayed hypersensitivity (cell-mediated) reaction, such as contact dermatitis or after a tuberculosis test, produces erythema and edema within 24–48 hours.

18–83 Answer A

Fungal infections are common in persons with acquired immunodeficiency syndrome. Candidiasis, cryptococcosis, and histoplasmosis are the most common types. Candidiasis produces the classic symptoms of creamy patches surrounded by an erythematous base that can be wiped off, leaving a reddened or bleeding surface. It can cause anorexia or dysphagia, because it is most common on the tongue or in the mouth, or it may result in a creamy vaginal discharge. Cryptococcosis may result in meningitis and produces symptoms such as fever, chills, fatigue, and night sweating. It may also produce a stiff neck, nausea and vomiting, and altered mentation. Onychomycosis is a fungal infection of the nails. Histoplasmosis results in pulmonary infections and disseminated disease with general symptoms of fever, weight loss, and fatigue. Enlargement of the liver and spleen is common, and may progress to respiratory failure.

18–84 Answer B

Children receiving radiation therapy for acute lymphocytic leukemia are at an increased risk for developing a brain tumor as a secondary malignancy. This has been seen more often in children who were treated with radiation at age 5 or less. In general, about 3–12% of children treated for cancer will develop a new cancer within 20 years of being treated for the primary cancer.

18–85 Answer C

When clients with human immunodeficiency virus infection have massive diarrhea, the protozoa C cryptosporidium is the most likely cause. The organism affects primarily the small intestine and produces massive diarrhea accompanied by nausea and fatigue. The diarrhea may exceed 4 L/day and can easily lead to dehydration and electrolyte imbalance if not treated promptly. Cryptococcosis is a fungal infection that usually appears as meningitis. Toxoplasmosis is a protozoal infection that causes encephalitis in persons with acquired immunodeficiency syndrome. Cytomegalovirus is a significant opportunistic infection of the herpesvirus family that can be acquired during the perinatal period, in the preschool years, or during the sexually active years.

18–86 Answer C

The term "shift to the left" or "left shift" indicates an elevated WBC count and a relative increase in segmented and band neutrophils. Usually seen in acute bacterial infections, it indicates clinically that the body is responding to an acute need before the neutrophils can fully mature in the bone marrow. The term originated from the Shilling hemogram which charted the maturation of the granulocytes from the least mature (blasts) on the left to most mature (segmented neutrophils) on the right. To represent the border between the bone marrow and the circulating blood a line was drawn between the band neutrophils and the segmented ones. When the body releases immature cells into the circulating blood, there is an increase in the cells in the circulating blood from the left of the line ("left shift"). Early hand devices for counting blood cells in a differential had the keys lined up in such a way that the technicians had to move their hand to the left to hit the keys for the more immature granulocytes.

18–87 Answer B

The Centers for Disease Control and Prevention guidelines state that if a woman infected with human immunodeficiency virus has a normal initial Pap test, then a second evaluation should be done in 6 months to reduce the likelihood of a false-negative initial test. If the initial two Pap smears are both negative, annual Pap smears are then adequate. If severe inflammation with reactive squamous cellular change is found, another Pap smear should be done within 3 months.

18–88 Answer C

Hepatitis D (delta) virus (HDV) poses the greatest risk to a client with chronic hepatitis B (chronic HBV). Chronic HBV carriers who acquire HDV infection have a much higher incidence of cirrhosis, approaching 70–80% compared with a 15–30% chance of liver cirrhosis with chronic HBV alone. Modes of transmission for HDV are similar to those of HBV.

18–89 Answer A

The latex condom, when used consistently and correctly, is the preferred contraceptive method for the client infected with human immunodeficiency virus (HIV) because it provides the most effective barrier between partners. The spermicide nonoxynol-9 has not been shown to prevent viral transmission in humans, especially when used alone. Because intrauterine devices increase menstrual blood flow, they expose a woman's partner to a greater viral load. Although the effect of oral contraceptive pills on HIV transmission is not known, the estrogen and progestin can promote HIV disease progression through opportunistic infections, as well as cervical neoplasia by their immunomodulating effects.

18–90 Answer D

Prophylaxis for the first episode of *Pneumocystis carinii* pneumonia in an adult or adolescent client infected with human immunodeficiency virus is trimethoprim-sulfamethoxazole (TMP-SMZ) (Bactrim) DS 1 tablet PO qd for 10 days. Clarithromycin (Biaxin) is the first choice for *Mycobacterium avium* complex infection; rifampin (Rimactane) is the first choice for combating isoniazid-resistant organisms; and isoniazid (Nydrazid) and pyridoxine (Beesix) are the first choice for combating *Mycobacterium tuberculosis* organisms.

18–91 Answer C

Clients with hepatitis A should have separate eating and drinking utensils or use disposable ones. Most clients can be cared for at home without undue risk;

strict isolation is not necessary. There is no specific medicine to treat hepatitis A.

18–92 Answer B

Smoking decreases vitamin C absorption, which is necessary for folic acid absorption. Smoking increases vitamin requirements. Clients with a folic acid deficiency should be encouraged to eat foods that are high in folic acid (asparagus spears, beef liver, broccoli, mushrooms, oatmeal, peanut butter, and red beans) daily because the liver can store folic acid for a limited time only.

18–93 Answer B

Pernicious anemia is caused by an inadequate absorption of vitamin B_{12}. The symptoms of pernicious anemia develop slowly and subtly and may not be recognized right away. Hemolytic anemias caused by the premature destruction of red blood cells (hemolysis) occur when the bone marrow cannot produce red blood cells fast enough to compensate for those being destroyed. These anemias can be acquired or congenital. Inherited conditions include hereditary spherocytosis, glucose-6-phosphate dehydrogenase deficiency, sickle cell anemia, and thalassemia.

18–94 Answer A

Smoking is not one of the risk factors for iron-deficiency anemia. The risk for iron-deficiency anemia increases in persons over age 60; those who live in poverty; and those with a recent illness, such as an ulcer, diverticulitis, colitis, hemorrhoids, or gastrointestinal tumors. Iron supplements should be taken.

18–95 Answer B

Cyanocobalamin 500 mg/0.1% intranasal spray (Nascobal) is indicated for maintenance of hematologic remission after intramuscular vitamin B_{12} therapy when vitamin B_{12} supplementation is still needed. Clients can administer this to themselves once per week with the same effect once they have been stabilized on the injections. The amount of vitamin B_{12} needed depends on the extent of the illness. The usual dosage is once a day by injection for 7 days, then one injection a week for 1 month, then possibly once a month for the rest of the client's life. Clients or significant others are usually taught how to give the injections because oral supplements are inadequate. Lifetime treatment is essential. Even with treatment, the ability to absorb vitamin B_{12} is not normal. Raw meat and raw liver are no longer prescribed.

18–96 Answer C

A serum measurement of ferritin, the body's iron-storing protein, can tell exactly how much iron is on hand in the body. It is the best way to spot an iron deficiency early before it progresses to full-blown anemia. If the ferritin level is borderline, a dietary and supplemental regimen of iron will rebuild the iron stores. Hemoglobin is the iron-containing pigment of the red blood cells that carries oxygen from the lungs to the tissues. Hematocrit is the volume of erythrocytes packed in a given volume of blood. The hemoglobin and hematocrit values give the values only at a given time, without regard for the body's stores. Reticulocytes are the last immature stage of red blood cells.

18–97 Answer C

Antibody testing may be ordered to determine whether a client has developed antibodies in response to an infection, such as hepatitis, or immunization. Antibody titers evaluate antibody-mediated responses. Serum protein is a measurement of the total protein in the blood. Albumin is a protein primarily responsible for the osmotic pressure of the blood. Globulins account for the majority of remaining serum protein. Globulins include all of the immunoglobulins and the antibodies they contain. Decreased globulin levels are noted with immunologic deficiencies. Protein electrophoresis further breaks down globulin into its specific components. Analysis of specific levels of each provides cues about the immune status of the client.

18–98 Answer D

The reticulocyte count indicates the percentage of newly maturing red blood cells released into the circulating blood from the bone marrow. As the red blood cell (RBC) matures, it loses its endothelial reticulum. The reticulocyte count is elevated in cases of blood loss, as the body tries to replace the loss; it might also be elevated during treatment of anemias (e.g., iron, folic acid, Vitamin B_{12}), and bone marrow disorders, when immature RBCs are displaced by other proliferating cells. It is decreased in aplastic anemia because the bone marrow has shut down all production of cells; it is also decreased in poisonings and disorders of red blood cell maturation such as iron-deficiency anemias.

18–99 Answer C

The primary reason for newborn screening for sickle cell disease is to allow the prevention of septicemia with prophylactic medication (penicillin) and prompt clinical intervention for infection and future crises. Early detection will not prevent future crises. Although the information obtained will allow the parents to make future decisions and have the benefit of possible genetic testing as well as testing siblings, this is not the primary reason for early screening.

18–100 Answer B

One "pack" of platelets should raise the count by 5000–8000 mm^3. One pack equals about 50 mL. A

"6-pack" refers to a pool of platelets from 6 units of blood. Platelets may be given for decreased production or destruction, such as aplastic anemia, acute leukemia, or after chemotherapy.

18–101 Answer C

Routine ordering of a complete blood count (CBC) is not indicated in asymptomatic adults; it should be ordered only when a specific condition is suspected, such as an infection or a hematologic disorder. Hemoglobin or hematocrit determination is recommended in pregnant women and high-risk infants, but not necessarily a CBC. There are no current recommendations for healthy adults to have a CBC as part of a routine, preadmission or preoperative physical exam if little or no blood loss is anticipated, as is the case in most dental procedures.

18–102 Answer D

MCV is an abbreviation for "mean cell volume," which indicates the average size of individual RBCs. Normal range, also referred to as normocytic, is 76–96 femtoliters. The MCV is increased (macrocytic) in megaloblastic anemias (Vitamin B_{12} deficiency, folate deficiency), liver disease (alcohol abuse), and some drugs (e.g., zidvudine). The MCV is decreased (microcytic) in iron-deficiency anemia, defects in porphyrin synthesis (lead poisoning), and hemolytic anemias.

18–103 Answer D

A decreased MCV and MCHC is indicative of a microcytic, hypochromic anemia. To make a more final diagnosis, you need to order both a serum iron and total iron binding capacity (TIBC) level and a serum ferritin level. You would order a folate level if you had an elevated MCV and a normal MCHC, indicative of macrocytic anemia.

18–104 Answer A

Infectious mononucleosis is a lymphocytic leukocytosis that may be confused with leukemia and other disorders. The presence of heterophile antibodies (monospot test) in the context of appropriate clinical and hematological findings is diagnostic; false-positive reactions are rare. Atypical lymphocytes usually account for more than 10% of the leukocytes in the peripheral blood smear. Detection of viral capsid antigen antibody IgM (elevated) is the most accurate test confirming acute infection. White blood count may be high, normal, or low; a relative and absolute neutropenia is present in many clients. Thrombocytopenia is common, and an elevated transaminase in most clients is related to hepatic involvement.

18–105 Answer C

A decrease in lymphocytes would be most consistent with immunodeficiency disorders, long-term corticosteroid therapy, or debilitating diseases such as Hodgkin's lymphoma or lupus erythematosus. Lymphocytes are increased primarily in viral infections (hepatitis, infectious mononucleosis, CMV, herpes zoster) and only occasionally in bacterial infections (pertussis, brucellosis). Eosinophils are elevated in parasitic infections such as malaria, trichinosis, and ascariasis).

18–106 Answer D

Platelets are decreased in coagulation disorders such as disseminated intravascular coagulation (DIC), septicemia, and eclampsia; increased destruction of platelets is seen in idiopathic thrombocytopenic purpura, systemic lupus erythematosus (SLE), and infectious mononucleosis; and decreased production of platelets is seen in aplastic anemia, most leukemias, and secondary to radiation and chemotherapy. Increased platelet count is seen in myeloproliferative leukemias, polycythemia vera, and status post-splenectomy.

References

Cheng, A, and Zaas, A: The Osler Medical Handbook. Mosby, Philadelphia, 2003.

Dambro, MR: Griffith's 5-Minute Consult. Lippincott Williams & Wilkins, Philadelphia, 2003.

Dunphy, LM, and Winland-Brown, JE (eds): Primary Care: The Art and Science of Advanced Practice Nursing. FA Davis, Philadelphia, 2001.

Gates, RA, and Fink, RM: Oncology Nursing Secrets. Hanley & Belfus, Philadelphia, 2002.

Goolsby, MJ: Nurse Practitioner Secrets. Hanley & Belfus, Philadelphia, 2002.

Hay, WW, et al: Current Pediatric Diagnosis and Treatment. Appleton & Lange, Stamford, CT, 2003.

Lin, TL, and Rypkema, SW: The Washington Manual of Ambulatory Therapeutics. Lippincott Williams & Wilkins, Philadelphia, 2002.

Rakel, RE: Textbook of Family Practice. WB Saunders, Philadelphia, 2001.

Speicher, CE: The Right Test: A Physician's Guide to Laboratory Medicine, ed 4. WB Saunders, Philadelphia, 2001.

Swartz, MN: Use of antimicrobial agents and drug resistance. N Engl J Med 337:7, 1997.

Tallia, AF, et al: Swanson's Family Practice Review, ed 4. Mosby, St. Louis, 2001.

Taylor, RB: Manual of Family Practice, ed 2. Little, Brown, Boston, 2002.

Tierney, L, et al: Current Medical Diagnosis and Treatment. Appleton & Lange, Stamford, CT, 2003.

Varricchio, C (ed): A Cancer Source Book for Nurses. American Cancer Society/Jones and Bartlett, Sudbury, MA, 2003.

HOW WELL DID YOU DO?

85% AND ABOVE CONGRATULATIONS! THIS SCORE SHOWS APPLICATION OF TEST-TAKING PRINCIPLES AND ADEQUATE CONTENT KNOWLEDGE.

75–85% KEEP WORKING! REVIEW TEST-TAKING PRINCIPLES AND TRY AGAIN.

65–75% HANG IN THERE! SPEND SOME TIME REVIEWING CONCEPTS AND TEST-TAKING PRINCIPLES AND TRY THE TEST AGAIN.

UNIT FOUR

ISSUES IN PRIMARY CARE

19

Issues in Primary Care

LYNNE M. DUNPHY
and
JILL E. WINLAND-BROWN

19–1 *The primary purpose of professional licensure is to:*

A. protect the public by ensuring a minimum standard for competency.
B. ensure high nursing care standards.
C. standardize nursing programs.
D. grant prescriptive privileges.

19–2 *The primary purpose of certification is to:*

A. document excellence and specialization.
B. regulate advanced practice nursing.
C. enable the practitioner to obtain third-party reimbursement.
D. assure the public that an individual has a special set of skills.

19–3 *Legal authority for advanced practice nursing rests with:*

A. the Health Care Financing Administration.
B. federal statutes.
C. state laws and regulations.
D. certifying bodies.

19–4 *Credentialing means that:*

A. an individual is permitted to practice advanced practice nursing.
B. the practitioner has met certain criteria through licensure, certification, and education.
C. an individual has completed a program of study.
D. an individual has prescriptive authority.

19–5 *What factors primarily determine the ability of an advanced practice registered nurse to obtain clinical privileges in an institution?*

A. The desires of the collaborating physician
B. Education, certification, and continuing education credits
C. Institutional policy, medical staff by-laws, state law, and Joint Commission on Accreditation of Healthcare Organizations (JCAHO) accreditation standards
D. Reimbursement and prescriptive privileges

19–6 *Goals and objectives for Healthy People 2010 include:*

A. improving access to healthcare for all Americans, increasing the life span for all Americans, and mandatory emergency care.
B. instituting a nationalized health insurance plan.
C. reducing disparities in healthcare, increasing healthy life span, and increasing access to healthcare for all Americans.
D. preserving choice of provider and healthcare plans for all Americans.

19–7 *"Indemnity insurer" refers to an insurer:*

A. in a health maintenance organization.
B. in a preferred provider organization.
C. that pays for the medical care of the insured, but does not provide that care.
D. that pays using a fee-for-service plan.

19–8 *"Usual and customary" refers to:*

A. an insurance term for how a charge compares to charges made to other persons receiving similar services and supplies.
B. how an insurer evaluates the need for an ordered diagnostic test.

C. a comparison of interventions across populations.
D. how much an insurer will charge to provide coverage.

19–9 *Most health maintenance organizations (HMOs) use a reimbursement mechanism called "capitation." This means that the:*

A. HMO reimburses the provider on a fee-for-service basis.
B. HMO reimburses the provider a set fee per client, per month, based on the client's age and sex.
C. fee paid to the provider fluctuates with the treatment.
D. provider is reimbursed by each individual client or family.

19–10 *When caring for a client who speaks a language different from yours, the ideal strategy is to:*

A. use gestures to convey the meaning of words and use a foreign-language dictionary of medical terms.
B. rely on family members to interpret.
C. review the case first with an interpreter before beginning the clinical visit.
D. use a pad and pencil to pass information back and forth with an interpreter.

19–11 *A good way to use an interpreter is to:*

A. try to use an interpreter who is of the same sex as and older than the client.
B. have the interpreter translate word for word so that you do not receive any misinformation.
C. use more than one interpreter if necessary.
D. attempt no communication with the client other than through the interpreter.

19–12 *The Agency for Healthcare Policy and Research, now renamed the Agency for Healthcare Research and Quality, was established to:*

A mandate treatment protocols.
B. dictate healthcare policy based on voluminous research.
C. promote outcome-based research.
D. develop cost-effective interventions.

19–13 *Which of the following statements is true regarding the consultative aspects of the advanced practice registered nurse (APRN) role?*

A. The APRN provides an ongoing supportive and educational relationship to a more junior clinician.
B. The problem is identified by the consultee, who calls on the consultant, a recognized expert, and a nonhierarchical relationship ensues or is established.
C. The APRN consultant assumes responsibility for the client once he or she is called into a clinical situation.
D. The consultee must take the recommendations of the APRN consultant.

19–14 *According to the Joint Commission on Accreditation of Healthcare Organizations, decisions regarding policy and client care should be made based on:*

A. experience.
B. clinical expertise.
C. consultation and collaboration.
D. research findings.

19–15 *Certain characteristics differentiate research from quality assurance. Which of the following is an example of research?*

A. Client satisfaction is evaluated relative to existing practice.
B. An intervention, well supported in the literature, is implemented and evaluated.
C. A standard assessment tool (e.g., risk assessment for falls) is implemented and evaluated.
D. A new intervention is implemented and compared with current practice to determine which is better.

19–16 *The primary purpose of an Institutional Review Board is to:*

A. protect human subjects.
B. evaluate the scientific merit of proposed research.
C. oversee and coordinate the research efforts of an institution.
D. oversee and coordinate the research efforts of an individual.

19–17 *Reviewing the literature refers to the ability to research existing literature about a specific problem, whether clinical or policy. The most important skill necessary to performing a thorough review of the literature is:*

A. talking with colleagues about the sources.
B. attending a research conference.
C. critiquing the findings and synthesizing the results.
D. reviewing clinical journals.

19–18 *Which of the following statements is true about case management?*

A. Case management oversees the client throughout acute-care hospitalization.
B. Case management is organized around a system of interdisciplinary resources and services.
C. Case management depends on physician-driven leadership to oversee the illness episode
D. Case management is applicable to the rehabilitative portion of the episode of the illness.

19–19 *Collaboration is best defined as:*

A. interdisciplinary teamwork.
B. a protocol arrangement with a physician.
C. case management.
D. cooperation with another to achieve mutual goals while not losing sight of one's own interests.

19–20 *The components that must all be present to establish malpractice include all of the following* ***except:***

A. harm (damages) to the client.
B. a duty to the client.
C. deviation (breach) from the standard of care.
D. negligence.

19–21 *You have seen a client who has tested positive for syphilis. You have treated the client, tested the client for other potential sexually transmitted diseases including human immunodeficiency virus (HIV) infection, counseled the client about safe sexual practices, and scheduled the client to return at 3 and 6 months for repeat serologic testing. The tests at those times demonstrated that no further syphilis was present. Should you have taken any other action?*

A. No, you have treated the client appropriately.
B. Yes, you must report the case to the local health authorities.
C. Yes, you need to notify all sexual contacts.
D. Yes, you must follow up on the client's HIV status.

19–22 *Sally, a nurse practitioner, sees Mr. Bell, who is suffering from congestive heart failure. She increases his diuretic, but makes no note of his potassium and orders no replacement potassium. Mr. Bell returns a week later for routine laboratory testing. His potassium level is found to be low; however, Mr. Bell has no complaints. Sally orders a potassium supplement to begin immediately and a follow-up potassium level measurement. Is Sally guilty of malpractice?*

A. Yes, because she breached the standard of care.
B. No, because no harm came to the client.
C. No, because she took remedial action.
D. Yes, because she was negligent.

19–23 *Which of the following nonverbal communication techniques are important to the establishment of rapport with the client?*

A. Taking notes only while the client is talking.
B. Making direct eye contact with the client with periodic breaks to check or take notes.
C. Having a desk between you and the client.
D. Wearing jeans in the clinical setting to ensure your comfort.

19–24 *The following verbal communication technique is helpful in establishing rapport with the client:*

A. Not calling the client by name because you do not want to appear intrusive.
B. Speaking directly to the client, introducing yourself by name, and establishing the purpose of the interaction.
C. Communicating slowly and quietly so as not to upset the client.
D. Very thoroughly discussing every detail of the client's history with the client.

19–25 *When caring for clients from a different culture, the following is an important piece of assessment data:*

A. Determining the ultimate decision maker.
B. Making decisions based on your general knowledge about the cultural background of the client.
C. Determining the family's perception of the client's problem.
D. Understanding that clients from other cultures expect their healthcare provider to be an authority figure.

19–26 *You are attempting to elicit a history from Mr. Barnes during his first visit to your office. He is becoming increasingly angry and belligerent. He says, "Can't you hurry up? Dr. Smith never takes this long! Why are all these questions necessary?" You respond:*

A. "I'm sorry, Mr. Barnes, but I need these questions answered."
B. "I want to provide the best possible care for you, Mr. Barnes."
C. "Perhaps your wife can assist with some of these questions."
D. "You seem very upset, Mr. Barnes. Could you share with me what is bothering you?"

19–27 *Medicare is divided into part A and part B.The difference between parts A and B is:*

A. Medicare part A provides coverage for hospital care and skilled nursing facility and home care; part B pays for outpatient fees at 80% of what Medicare determines to be reasonable.
B. Medicare part A covers healthcare expenses for individuals under age 65; part B pays for individuals over age 65.
C. Medicare part A covers disabled individuals under age 65, but they are not eligible for part B
D. Medicare A pays for outpatient fees including home care; part B provides coverage for hospital care only.

19–28 *Which of the following statements is true about Medicaid?*

A. Medicaid is a federal plan to provide care for all indigent persons.
B. Medicaid pays for family planning services, dental care, and eyeglasses.
C. Eligibility requirements for Medicaid are mandat ed by the Health Care Financing Administration.
D. Medicaid is a program for the indigent financed jointly by the federal and the state governments.

19–29 *All the following statements relate to the Medicare fee schedule called the resource-based relative value scale* ***except:***

A. It is a prospective payment system.
B. Geographic differences for rate of pay are factored into the formula.
C. It is a complex formula to quantify a healthcare encounter that includes the amount of time, the training required, the complexity of the decision making, and the risks associated with poor care, thus providing a rationale for reimbursement dollars.
D. It has been successful in controlling healthcare costs.

19–30 *The requirements for reportable communicable disease vary from state to state. Which of the following lists diseases that must be reported in every state?*

A. Syphilis, tuberculosis, and hepatitis
B. Human immunodeficiency virus (HIV) infection, *Chlamydia* infection, and syphilis
C. Gonorrhea, syphilis, and *Chlamydia* infection
D. Hepatitis, syphilis, and HIV

19–31 *Strategies for developing cultural competence include which of the following?*

A. Disregarding folk beliefs because they are not scientific
B. Learning basic words and sentences in the client's language
C. Explaining the pathophysiology of the disease process to the client so that he or she understands what is happening to him or her
D. Explaining your cultural beliefs to the client

19–32 *Which of the following is the best method for evaluating the efficacy of a new clinical intervention?*

A. A case report
B. A descriptive study
C. A randomized, controlled clinical trial
D. A correlational study

19–33 *Mr. Jones, age 44, is admitted to the emergency room (ER) complaining of chest pain. Which of the following actions would be the best way to establish a therapeutic relationship with Mr. Jones?*

A. Ask several quick and specific questions in rapid succession to establish the exact nature of this emergent clinical situation.
B. Ask open-ended questions to elicit pertinent clinical data.
C. Reassure the client that he is in good hands in a well-equipped ER and that all will be OK.
D. Ask the client about his anxiety level.

19–34 *According to the health belief model, motivation, or readiness to act, is determined by which of the following components?*

A. Perceived threat, efficacy, benefits of action, and perceived barriers to action
B. Education and positive reinforcement
C. Predisposing factors, reinforcing factors, and enabling factors
D. Self-efficacy theory and perceived ability to act

19–35 *Which of the following statements is accurate regarding primary care?*

A. The purpose of primary care is to provide and coordinate referrals.
B. Primary care provides integrated and accessible healthcare services.
C. Primary care uses a focus group methodology to assess community needs and plan care.
D. Primary care is only for those who cannot afford specialty care.

19–36 *There are a number of barriers to full implementation of an autonomous role for advanced-practice nurses (APNs) in primary care. Major barriers are:*

A. the need for medical specialists because of rapidly changing technologies.
B. the increasingly complex health problems of vulnerable populations.
C. prescriptive authority, scope of practice, and reimbursement.
D. managed care organizations' views of APNs.

19–37 *Health behaviors can be difficult to change. Which of the following is most important in influencing behavioral change?*

A. Motivation
B. Health beliefs
C. Cognitive knowledge
D. Social supports

19–38 *The marketing process is guided by a number of factors. These include:*

A. the prospective pool of clients.
B. your advertising budget and what you have to offer.
C. cost, benefit, and barriers.
D. product, price, place, and promotion.

19–39 *Your Native American client is convinced that her illness has been caused by the ill-will of a fellow tribeswoman. Her description of her illness is an example of her:*

A. explanatory reasoning.
B. lack of understanding of scientific medicine.
C. delusional ideation.
D. cultural bias.

19–40 *Which of the following statements related to statistical techniques and their usage in research is true?*

A. Statistical significance and clinical significance are the same.
B. If a journal article you are writing is required to be limited in length, you should delete the descriptive statistics and keep the inferential statistics.
C. Correlational coefficients infer causality.
D. To determine the appropriate statistical test to use, consider sample size, level of measurement, and data type.

19–41 *Multiple regression and analysis of variance and covariance are tests of:*

A. prediction.
B. statistical significance.
C. association.
D. correlation.

19–42 *Techniques used to enhance a client's adherence to a treatment plan include:*

A. stressing the dangers of missing medications.
B. giving clear written instructions and simplifying the drug regimen.
C. allowing plenty of time between follow up visits so that the client has time to adjust to the regimen.
D. explaining the importance of the regimen to the family.

19–43 *The best way to monitor compliance is to:*

A. obtain drug levels.
B. use clinical judgment.
C. ask the client.
D. monitor the responses to treatment.

19–44 *Strategies that can help to foster client compliance include*

A. in-depth client education.
B. frequency of medication dosing.
C. providing positive feedback and reinforcement.
D. performing serum drug levels to assess therapeutic range.

19–45 *Strategies effective in accomplishing behavioral change include all the following* ***except:***

A. consistency of the caretaker.
B. convenient, short, and frequent follow-up appointments to monitor progress and review expected outcomes.
C. positive reinforcement and individualization of the plan.
D. repeatedly stressing the importance of the need to change.

19–46 *All of the following are barriers to education and behavioral change* ***except:***

A. social issues.
B. psychologic issues.
C. social support.
D. physical issues.

19–47 *An effective method used to assess your client's retention and understanding of educational materials is:*

A. asking your client to restate what you have reviewed.
B. Providing pathophysiology book for your client to take home and read.
C. Repeating your explanations of disease pathology.
D. Objective testing.

19–48 *When teaching your client about medication that you are prescribing, the most important point(s) to discuss initially is (are):*

A. the action of the drug and its adverse effects.
B. whether to take the drug on a full or empty stomach.
C. what it is for, how much to take, and when to take it.
D. what to do if the client experiences any adverse effects.

19–49 *The maximum number of points you should attempt to make in one teaching session is (are):*

A. one.
B. two.
C. three to four.
D. as many as you need; there is no limit.

19–50 *Mr. Brill, age 50, is a house painter who has smoked 2 to 3 packs of cigarettes per day since he was 20 years old. He comes into the clinic complaining of a chronic cough. When you discuss his smoking behavior, he states, "I know I need to stop smoking, but I'm under too much stress right now." Mr. Brill is at which stage of learning?*

A. The precontemplative stage
B. The contemplative stage
C. The action stage
D. The maintenance stage

19–51 *To encourage reinforcement of client teaching, a useful strategy is to:*

A. be a role model.
B. have repeated discussions of the need for behavioral change.
C. provide additional written materials.
D. quiz the client periodically while monitoring the client's progress.

19–52 *Concrete strategies used to keep your client's attention as you institute client education include:*

A. providing the education session immediately after lunch.
B. going over the materials more than once.

C. translating theoretical information into practical terms.
D. using repetition.

19–53 *A plaintiff must prove which of the following in order to have a case of malpractice?*

A. Duty and breach of duty
B. Damage or injury
C. Causation
D. All of the above

19–54 *One theory regarding crisis postulates that there are three stages to a crisis: precrisis, crisis, and postcrisis. The crisis stage is defined as:*

A. stress.
B. an acute, temporary, self-limited state of disequilibrium.
C. an emergency.
D. the stage in which the individual is able to use previous coping mechanisms.

19–55 *The primary nursing responsibility during a crisis situation is to:*

A. provide for psychotherapeutic intervention.
B. refer.
C. establish a therapeutic relationship.
D. encourage hospitalization.

19–56 *The stages of grief include:*

A. shock, reality, and recovery.
B. awareness and resolution.
C. numbness, loss, and reawakening.
D. pain and loss.

19–57 *Some sources suggest that you create a marketing portfolio with documents that support what you have to offer as an advanced practice nurse or nurse practitioner. These documents include:*

A. your personal mission statement.
B. your scores on the certification exam or your college transcript.
C. the state nurse practice act and regulations, prescriptive authority legislation, third party reimbursement rules and regulations, and practice protocols.
D. letters of reference.

19–58 *Examples of abnormal and pathological grief responses include all the following* ***except:***

A. delayed grief.
B. catatonic grief.
C. exaggerated grief.
D. masked grief.

19–59 *Classic signs of normal grief include all of the following* ***except:***

A. loss of appetite and weight loss or gain.
B. manic episodes.
C. inability to concentrate or sleep.
D. inability to make decisions and carry out activities of daily living.

19–60 *The most common cause of litigation is:*

A. failure to provide services.
B. failure to diagnose breast cancer.
C. a medication error.
D. a surgical error.

19–61 *Factors that have led to the development of case management include all the following* ***except:***

A. Medicare and Medicaid.
B. the recent tobacco cases.
C. the Commission on Mental Retardation.
D. the Education for All Handicapped Children Act.

19–62 *The primary purpose of clinical paths is to:*

A. streamline healthcare services, contain costs, and improve or maintain quality of care.
B. make client care easier.
C. ensure that a client is discharged before money is lost by the institution.
D. increase client responsibility and self-care.

19–63 *A good resume can be crucial to your success in obtaining a job. It should include:*

A. religious activities.
B. community service.
C. demographic data, including marital status and age.
D. number of children.

19–64 *Sandy, age 16, is seen by you at the Women's Clinic. She asks you for information on birth control. Your course of action is to:*

A. provide her with birth control, because most states allow you to provide contraception to a 16-year-old without a parent being present.
B. not provide Sandy with any form of birth control because she is under legal age.
C. refer Sandy to the physician in control of the clinic.
D. determine if Sandy lives away from home and manages her own affairs. If she is an emancipated minor, you can supply her with birth control.

19–65 *Mr. Griffin, age 85, has been given a diagnosis of bowel cancer and surgery is indicated. He is mentally alert; however, he is refusing to give consent for the procedure. You respond by:*

A. ordering a psychiatric consultation.
B. having your collaborating physician talk with the client.
C. respecting his wishes.
D. talking with his family.

19–66 *Mrs. Smith, age 85, lost her husband 6 months ago. Since that time, she has been overwhelmed and has had difficulty coping. Today, she is in your office, tearful, weak, and discouraged. Her mobility has also been becoming increasingly limited because of her need for a hip replacement. She is indecisive, expresses fear about the surgery, and tells you that she does not want the surgery. Your action is to:*

A. treat the client's psychological problems and provide support.
B. respect the client's wishes.
C. consider placing the client in an assisted-living facility.
D. explain to the client that she is depressed and will feel better after the surgery.

19–67 *A situation in which medical information may be passed on without client consent is when:*

A. the client has a gunshot wound.
B. a potential employer asks for it.
C. certifying absence from work.
D. talking to another healthcare provider.

19–68 *In the outpatient office setting, the most common reason for a malpractice suit is failure to:*

A. properly refer.
B. diagnose correctly in a timely fashion.
C. obtain informed consent.
D. manage fractures and trauma correctly.

19–69 *As measured by the federal Health Care Financing Administration, national health expenditures are grouped into which two categories?*

A. Medicare A and B
B. Medicare and Medicaid
C. Research and medical facilities construction and payments for health services and supplies
D. Long-term care and medications

19–70 *APRNs are affected by laws and rules, although these vary from state to state. Some examples of these include:*

A. delegation of authority by physicians.
B. how many clients you must see every hour.
C. universal healthcare law.
D. making no more than five referrals for one client.

19–71 *The gerontological population is designated a vulnerable one when it comes to obtaining informed consent to serving as a research subject because of the potential for exploitation of older adults. Safeguards to follow when conducting research on a geriatric population include the following:*

A. Assess the competence of the individual before obtaining consent.
B. Obtain permission from the family or staff.
C. Stress how important the research is and why their participation and perspective, as an older adult, is important.
D. If the research is exempt, you do not need to obtain consent to participate.

19–72 *Elder abuse and neglect is an increasing concern, and it is estimated that 4–10% of older Americans are abused or neglected. What is the legal responsibility of the healthcare provider in reporting elder abuse and neglect?*

A. The healthcare provider should discuss the suspected abuse or neglect with the client.
B. The healthcare provider should discuss the suspected abuse or neglect with the client's family.
C. The healthcare provider must report the suspected abuse or neglect to the appropriate state protective agency.
D. The healthcare provider must confirm the suspected abuse or neglect before reporting it to the appropriate state protective agency.

19–73 *Mrs. Hernandez, age 79, is insisting on discharge from the skilled nursing facility where she is receiving rehabilitation after a left hip replacement. She lives alone and has very little support. You do not think that she is ready for discharge. Mrs. Hernandez's insistence on discharge is an example of your client exercising her right to:*

A. self-determination.
B. beneficence.
C. justice.
D. utilitarianism.

19–74 *The type of healthcare delivery system that allows the client the greatest freedom of choice is a:*

A. health maintenance organization.
B. preferred provider organization.
C. managed care plan.
D. fee-for-service plan.

19–75 *One way in which you, as an individual advanced practice registered nurse, can make a difference is by:*

A. reading about issues in the newspaper.
B. writing letters to the editor supporting APRNS.
C. thinking positively about the work that you do.
D. supporting a Democratic candidate.

19–76 *Prescriptive authority for advanced practice nurses:*

A. is permitted only under protocol.
B. is mandated by law in over 40 states.
C. varies from state to state.
D. includes the ability to prescribe controlled substances.

19–77 *Human research subjects are entitled to all of the following* ***except:***

A. the right to informed consent.
B. the right to compensation for their participation.
C. the right to withdraw from the research without being penalized.
D. the right to alternative treatments other than the experimental treatment.

19–78 *A number of factors are predicted to influence the mix of team providers for emerging primary-care systems. These include all of the following* ***except:***

A. the credentials of the providers.
B. the providers' skills and services and the target population.
C. the socio-economic status of the surrounding community.
D. the gender mix of the primary care providers.

19–79 *All of the following may contribute to the client's silence during the history taking and physical examination* ***except:***

A. a hearing impairment.
B. cultural barriers.
C. hostility toward the healthcare provider.
D. fear.

19–80 *It is important to word questions about sexual orientation in a nonjudgmental way. Which of the following is a good example of how to do this?*

A. "When did you begin abnormal sexual activity? This is important in addressing your risk factors. Please answer honestly. This behavior is not subject to judgment."
B. "Do you ever have sex in an abnormal way?"
C. "How many times do you permit penetration during intercourse?"
D. "Is your partner a man or a woman?"

19–81 *Advance directives, such as healthcare proxies and durable powers of attorney, are important for all clients to consider. In particular, persons who are unable to marry legally— for example, same-sex partners—and those who are single by choice or circumstance may preserve their healthcare wishes by:*

A. executing a durable power of attorney for healthcare.
B. drafting a letter stating that their next-of-kin is not the surrogate decision maker.
C. signing an institutional document stating that the healthcare provider is allowed to make all healthcare decisions for the client.
D. having one partner declared legally incompetent.

19–82 *Relapse is a common phenomenon seen during behavioral change. Useful strategies for the healthcare provider to institute to aid the client in a relapse situation include all of the following* ***except:***

A. using fear to reinforce the need to change.
B. telling the client that the relapse is a learning opportunity in preparation for the next action stage.
C. reminding the client that they must begin again as soon as possible.
D. expressing sincere disappointment so that the client senses your concern and caring.

19–83 *Research utilization is an important component of the advanced practice role. Literature has cited a number of barriers to the utilization of research. These include all of the following* ***except:***

A. self-image and lack of confidence.
B. lack of administrative support.
C. lack of knowledge and experience with research.
D. inadequate facilities and infrastructure for research.

19–84 *Do Not Resuscitate orders are decided by the:*

A. physician.
B. healthcare facility.
C. physician in consultation with the client, family, or surrogate decision maker.
D. interdisciplinary healthcare team.

19–85 *The majority of Medicaid enrollees are:*

A. young women and children.
B. unemployed, homeless clients.
C. older adults.
D. clients with a disability.

19–86 *The purpose of a block grant is to:*

A. provide more comprehensive services for Medicaid recipients.
B. encourage individuals to obtain their own health insurance and not need government assistance.
C. allow states to have greater flexibility in providing services to the poor.
D. decrease the proportion of state taxes that are allocated to paying for Medicare.

19–87 *"Direct costs" and "indirect costs" are terms used in drafting budgets. All the following statements are true regarding direct and indirect costs* ***except:***

A. Direct costs are incurred directly as a result of providing a specific service or operating a specific service-producing unit.
B. Indirect costs are incurred outside the service-producing unit.
C. From the standpoint of the organization as a whole, there are no indirect costs.
D. The market value of resources does not influence direct or indirect costs.

19–88 *Zero-base budgeting refers to a budgeting system that:*

A. accounts for unexpected budget variances.
B. accounts for expected budget variances only.
C. justifies each budget on its own merits, not on the basis of the previous era budget.
D. justifies each budget based on the previous period's budget.

19–89 *All of the following are examples of effective counseling techniques* ***except:***

A. providing reassurance.
B. beginning with the goal of helping.
C. recognizing limitations.
D. caring for self.

19–90 *The research function of the advanced practice nurse may be operationalized as both a consumer of research findings and a researcher. Being a consumer of research findings involves a number of activities, including:*

A. reading the literature, analyzing clinical applicability, and using new interventions.
B. organizing and conducting a research study.
C. collecting data.
D. ensuring protection of human subjects.

19–91 *What must you do as an advanced registered nurse practitioner before billing for visits?*

A. You must establish a collaborative agreement with a physician.
B. You must obtain a provider number and familiarize yourself with the rules and policies of the third-party payor.
C. You must provide evidence of continuing medical education.
D. You must have a Drug Enforcement Agency (DEA) number.

19–92 *What conditions must be met for you to bill "incident to" the physician, receiving 100% reimbursement from Medicare?*

A. You must initiate the plan of care for the client.
B. The physician must be on site and engaged in patient care.
C. You must be employed as an independent contractor.
D. You must be the main healthcare provider who sees the patient.

19–93 *What are important things to do before negotiating a contract?*

A. Do your homework.
B. Hire a lawyer.
C. Plan a signing-of-contract dinner.
D. Stand your ground.

19–94 *If conflict should arise during a job negotiation, you should consider:*

A. separating the issue from the person.
B. always standing your ground.
C. getting a legal opinion.
D. basing your actions on the contract a friend of yours has secured in a local practice.

19–95 *What is the difference between a referral and a consultation?*

A. A consultation is officially telephoned in by your office and implies continued treatment.
B. A referral is a request that another provider accept ongoing treatment responsibility.
C. A consultation may occur informally.
D. In a consultation, the patient is sent to another healthcare provider for a more in-depth evaluation.

19–96 *What is the responsibility of the primary care provider?*

A. The primary care provider is the coordinator of the patient's healthcare.
B. Once the patient is referred to another provider for ongoing treatment, the responsibility of the primary healthcare provider is relieved.
C. The primary care provider should dictate all aspects of the client's plan of care.
D. The primary care provider turns over care of the client to the specialist.

Answers

19–1 Answer A

The primary purpose of professional licensure is to protect the public from unsafe practitioners by ensuring a minimum standard for competency. Licensure is a legal status granted by a regulating authority (in the case of nursing, by individual state boards of nursing). In nursing, this is accomplished by mandating passage of the National Council Licensure Exam (NCLEX-RN) by an individual before state licensure. Licensure does not ensure high nursing standards; passage of the NCLEX is designed to assess minimum competency to practice safely. The curriculum of a nursing program, although providing a foundation of nursing knowledge that will graduate a safe and competent practitioner, is not specifically geared to the NCLEX exam. Nursing programs retain autonomy over their own curricula. Although the licensing statutes may spell out prescriptive privileges for advanced practice nurses, they do not necessarily do that, nor is that the primary purpose of professional licensure.

19–2 Answer A

The primary purpose of certification is to document excellence and specialization. Certification is a voluntary process by which a nongovernmental agency or association certifies that an individual has met certain predetermined standards for competency and specialization in a particular area. Although some states mandate that an advanced practice nurse pass a national certification exam before granting licensure to practice at an advanced level, this is not the case in all states. National certification may be necessary to obtain third-party reimbursement; however, that is not the primary purpose of certification, either. Although certification at the national level does provide the public with information about the skills of the practitioner, that is the realm of licensure, not the primary purpose of certification.

19–3 Answer C

Legal authority for all nursing practice, including advanced practice nursing, rests with the individual state boards of nursing who administer the legal statutes that define nursing practice in their state. The Health Care Financing Administration oversees the administration of federal Medicare and Medicaid funds. Legal authority for professional practice was delegated to the states and territories by the Constitution and is not regulated by federal statutes. Certification by certifying bodies is a voluntary process with no legal significance.

19–4 Answer B

Credentialing means that the practitioner has met certain criteria through licensure, education, and certification. The criteria for credentialing vary depending upon the credentialing body. Hospitals, for example, may use credentialing to grant hospital privileges. An individual is permitted to practice basic or advanced practice nursing by licensure. An academic degree is awarded when one has completed a program of study. Prescriptive authority is mandated by state statutes.

19–5 Answer C

Although the desires of the collaborating physician; education, certification, and continuing education credits; and reimbursement and prescriptive privileges may influence institutional policy and medical staff by-laws, the factors that primarily determine the ability of an advanced practice nurse to obtain clinical privileges in an institution are institutional policy, medical staff by-laws, state law, and the Joint Commission on Accreditation of Healthcare Organizations accreditation standards.

19–6 Answer C

The goals and objectives contained in Healthy People 2010 include reducing disparities in healthcare, increasing healthy life span, and increasing accessibility to healthcare for all Americans. They do not include mandatory provision of emergency care. Healthy People 2010 does not advocate instituting a nationalized health insurance plan. Preserving choice of provider for all Americans is not one of the goals and objectives of Healthy People 2000.

19–7 Answer C

"Indemnity insurer" refers to an insurer that pays for the medical care of the insured, but does not provide that care. A health maintenance organization provides the medical care as well as the insurance of the insurer. A preferred provider organization is a network of healthcare providers linked together through similar reimbursement mechanisms. A fee-for-service plan refers to reimbursement for healthcare services under a fee schedule.

19–8 Answer A

The term "usual and customary" refers to comparing charges made to other like charges for services and supplies received in the immediate vicinity as well as in a broader geographic area. It does not refer to the "usual and customary" charge to obtain insurance, but rather how much the insurer will reimburse for a service. Whether to order a diagnostic test is up to the provider's discretion, although the payor may hold the provider to the standard of care. "Usual and customary" is not a term used to compare interventions across populations.

19–9 Answer B

The reimbursement mechanism called "capitation" that some health maintenance organizations (HMOs) use is one in which the HMO reimburses the provider a set fee per client, per month, based on the client's age and sex. HMOs are prepaid, comprehensive systems of health benefits that combine both financing and delivery of services to subscribers. They may pay providers on a capitated or fee-for-service basis. Capitation is a set fee that does not fluctuate. The provider is reimbursed by the HMO and not the client. Most plans require clients to make a copayment at the time of the visit. Capitated fees for primary care range from $5.00 to $35.00 per month depending on the client's age and sex and, thus, relative risk. Fee for service refers to reimbursement for healthcare services under a fee schedule that is based on a complex variety of factors. These include the number and type of services provided, the current procedural terminology, International Classification of Disease (ICD-9) codes, the geographic area (the "usual and customary" fee), and certain office and training expenses of the provider.

19–10 Answer C

Reviewing the case with an interpreter before seeing the client is a useful strategy that can help enhance cross-cultural communication. Information about the reason for the visit and the purpose of the healthcare encounter can be exchanged beforehand, potentially enhancing communications. It is helpful for the practitioner to face the interpreter and the client together, thus maintaining eye contact and the ability to assess nonverbal cues as well as maintaining close contact with the interpreter. It may be necessary to rely on family members to translate, but it is not a good strategy. For example, it is often the school-age child who has the best grasp of English; however, relying on the child to interpret reverses parent-child roles and places unnecessary and sometimes inappropriate burdens on the child. It also lessens the client's sense of authority and privacy. A trained interpreter is usually best. Gesturing and relying on a dictionary may be necessary but distracts from the general flow of communication and slows the speed and comprehension of the communication.

19–11 Answer A

The role of an interpreter in a healthcare setting is often one of cultural broker, to act not just as a translator of words, but also of cultural concepts and beliefs. Additionally, cultural values may make it more difficult for the client to discuss certain issues in the presence of an interpreter. Using a trained same-sex interpreter, preferably one older than the client, has been found to work best. The client also needs to be reassured about the confidentiality of the information shared. For this reason, it is best to use only one interpreter and for the provider to establish rapport with the client in any way possible.

19–12 Answer C

The Agency for Healthcare Policy and Research (AHCPR) was established to promote outcome-based (medical effectiveness) research as well as to develop databases for research, develop clinical guidelines, and disseminate research findings and clinical guidelines for care. The AHCPR routinely publishes reviews of studies on clinical problems with summaries of treatment protocols and effectiveness. It does not mandate these in practice, although the provider may be held to these as a standard of care. It also does not dictate healthcare policy or develop cost-effective interventions, although it does do cost-benefit analysis of the interventions.

19–13 Answer B

Principles of consultation include the identification of a problem by a consultee who calls in a consultant with documented expertise in a given area; the consultant making recommendations based on his or her assessment of the situation; and the consultee remaining free to accept or reject these recommendations and retaining responsibility for the outcome of care. (Likewise, the consultee is free to disregard the advanced practice nurse [APN] consultant.) Classically, there is a nonhierarchical relationship between the consultant and consultee. APNs working in the same organization as the consultee often have a higher degree of accountability in relation to client care; however, the issue of responsibility for outcome of care is what should separate collaboration from consultation. A situation where a senior clinician provides a supportive and educative relationship with a junior clinician is defined as "clinical supervision" and implies that responsibility for the outcome of care remains in the hands of the senior clinician.

19–14 Answer D

According to the Joint Commission on Accreditation of Healthcare Organizations (JCAHO), decisions regarding policy and client care should be based on research findings. The JCAHO mandates that decisions be based on research and rooted in and supported by scientific literature. Experience, clinical expertise, and consultation and collaboration are no longer solely acceptable as the rationale for policy and client-care decisions.

19–15 Answer D

One characteristic that differentiates research from quality assurance is that research compares a new intervention with current practice to determine which is better. Research asks a new question that will improve or expand new knowledge with some degree of generalizability. Additionally, there may be a risk implied to a human subject. Clients receiving the new and untested interventions may be at risk. With quality assurance, client satisfaction may be evaluated relative to existing practice or when an intervention that is well supported in the literature is implemented and evaluated. It is not new knowledge, but evaluation of existing knowledge. Similarly, with the implementation and evaluation of a standardized assessment tool, new knowledge is not gained.

19–16 Answer A

The purpose of an Institutional Review Board (IRB) is to protect human subjects. The primary purpose of the IRB is ethical; it does not evaluate the scientific merit of proposed research, nor does it oversee and coordinate the research efforts of an institution or an individual. These functions are usually performed by the institution's research committee. It is your obligation as a researcher to obtain some form of IRB approval any time you are conducting research on human subjects. If you are planning a research project in a private practice setting, approval should be obtained from the IRB of some affiliating institution such as a hospital where you are credentialed and permitted to admit clients.

19–17 Answer C

Although talking with colleagues, attending a research conference, and reviewing your own clinical journals may all help identify relevant databases, the most important skill necessary to performing a thorough review of the literature is critiquing the findings and synthesizing the results.

19–18 Answer B

Case management is organized around a system of interdisciplinary resources and services; the clinical and financial aspects of care are overseen by a case manager who has a financial incentive to manage risk and maximize the quality of care. It is not physician driven. Case management is applicable to the entire episode of the illness, not just the client's acute care, hospitalization, or rehabilitative care.

19–19 Answer D

Collaboration is best defined as cooperation with another to achieve mutual goals while not losing sight of one's own interests. True collaboration combines the activities of cooperation or concern for another's interests with assertiveness. The interest considered most important in nurse-physician collaboration is the professionals' concern for the care of the client rather than the provider's personal agenda. Collaboration is essential in interdisciplinary teamwork, but is not the definition of collaboration. Collaboration may include a protocol arrangement with a physician, but is not solely defined that way. Case management is defined as managing an entire episode of illness from the standpoint of coordination of resources and services. This will involve collaboration, but is a different concept.

19–20 Answer D

The components that must all be present to establish malpractice are a duty to the client, a deviation (breach) from the standard of care, and harm (damages) to the client that occurs because of the breach of duty and the deviation from the standard of care (causation).

19–21 Answer B

The practitioner is also responsible for reporting the case of syphilis to the local health authorities. All sexual partners of the client should be contacted; however, it is the health department that has trained staff who will perform the investigation of contacts and follow-up. Syphilis is easily treated and controllable if its presence is reported. It is not necessary to retest the client's human immunodeficiency virus status unless there is a new clinical reason on subsequent visits.

19–22 Answer B

Sally is not guilty of malpractice because no harm came to Mr. Bell as a result of her actions. For malpractice to occur, the provider must have a duty to the client (which Sally had), a standard of care must have been breached (which Sally did), and harm or damages must occur as a result of the duty and the breach of the standard of care (which did not occur). Because all of the components were not met, malpractice has not been established.

19–23 Answer B

Nonverbal communication techniques important to the establishment of rapport with the client include making direct eye contact with the client, with periodic breaks to check or take notes; avoiding having a desk between you and the client; and having personal grooming appropriate to the setting. Taking notes only while the client is talking does not help establish rapport with the client, because making direct eye contact with the client aids in establishing trust. A break in eye contact, however, is important because some cultures view staring as disrespectful. Other nonverbal communication techniques that help establish rapport include sitting while interviewing the client rather than standing; standing or sitting near the client, but not invading the client's personal comfort zone; and maintaining a friendly, helpful expression.

19–24 Answer B

Verbal communication techniques helpful in establishing rapport with the client include verifying the name of the client and using it throughout the conversation; speaking directly to the client, introducing yourself by name, and establishing the purpose of the interaction; and communicating in a tone of voice, speed, and choice of words that are similar to the client's. Very thoroughly discussing every detail of the client's history with the client, unless absolutely necessary, can be disturbing to the client. It is important to take cues from the client. Some areas of the history will be much more important than others. You must be astute and attuned to the client without missing important information.

19–25 Answer A

When caring for clients from a different culture, important pieces of assessment data include determining the ultimate decision maker (it may be someone else, for example, the male patriarch of the family); determining the client's perception of the cause of his or her problem (e.g., some clients may view it as fate or a curse); and ascertaining the client's, not the family's, expectations of the provider. Making decisions based on your general knowledge about the cultural background of the client is not appropriate. Assuming the client expects an authoritarian healthcare provider is cultural stereotyping. The practitioner should not fall into this common trap. Each clinical visit needs to be evaluated in the light of the general cultural background of the client as well as the specific reasons for the visit.

19–26 Answer D

The most important aspect of communicating with clients is acknowledging their feelings. By responding, "You seem very upset, Mr. Barnes. Could you share with me what is bothering you?" you acknowledge Mr. Barnes's discomfort by reflecting back his feelings, and you offer to assist him. If you respond by saying: "I'm sorry, Mr. Barnes, but I need these questions answered" or "I want to provide the best possible care for you, Mr. Barnes," you have not acknowledged Mr. Barnes's feelings. If you respond by saying: "Perhaps your wife can assist with some of these questions," you violate Mr. Barnes's autonomy and right to self-determination.

19–27 Answer A

Medicare part A provides coverage for inpatient care, including hospital care, skilled nursing facility care, and home healthcare; part B pays for outpatient fees at 80% of what Medicare determines to be reasonable. Disabled individuals under age 65 are eligible for Medicare A and B.

19–28 Answer D

Financed jointly by the federal and state governments, Medicaid is a program to pay for healthcare services for the indigent. Each state defines income eligibility and the benefit structure. Minimally, Medicaid must provide inpatient, skilled nursing facility, and home care; physician services; outpatient care; family planning services; and periodic screening, detection, and treatment care of children under age 12. As for services such as dental care, eyeglasses, and prescription drugs, each state makes its own decisions concerning payment.

19–29 Answer D

Although a complex formula, the resource-based relative value scale (RBRVS) is a prospective payment system. It calculates a standard fee schedule for physician services in advance. Patterns of geographic variation are built into the conversion formulas. The purpose of the RBRVS is to control escalating medical costs, but it has not yet proven effective in doing this. Some commercial insurers are instituting similar programs to control costs and convert from the fee-for-service reimbursement mechanisms that have previously existed.

19–30 Answer A

Of the lists presented, the communicable diseases that must be reported in every state include syphilis, tuberculosis, and hepatitis. The diseases that are notifiable by law vary by state and over time. Criteria for determining notifiable diseases have generally been based on the potential for control or prevention of additional cases of the disease. Practitioners should be familiar with what diseases need to be reported in their state; for example, invasive *Haemophilus influenzae* infection, meningitis, encephalitis, giardiasis, measles, and Reye's syndrome are reportable in over 40 states.

19–31 Answer B

Strategies for developing cultural competence include learning basic words and sentences in the client's language, attending special cultural events and celebrations, and relating a client's belief to your own even if it is different. It is important to recognize that clients who have English as a second language may regress back to their first language under the stress of an illness. Learning a few key phrases in the client's native language and knowing how to address the client properly can go a long way in establishing rapport and trust. Disregarding folk beliefs because they are not scientific is not a strategy to develop cultural competence. Folk beliefs must be taken into consideration because they can profoundly affect the course of the client's illness. If the client believes his or her illness is the result of a "curse," you may need to strategize ways to "undo" the curse.

19–32 Answer C

The best method for evaluating the efficacy of a new clinical intervention is a randomized controlled clinical trial. Case reports, descriptive studies, and correlational studies are methodological approaches that are less reliable in establishing causal relationships, and thus the attribution of an effect to the new clinical intervention would be less clear. The effect might be attributable to other confounding variables.

19–33 Answer B

Asking open-ended questions is essential to establishing a therapeutic relationship, even in an emergency situation, and is a good interviewing technique. Asking several questions in rapid succession may help establish the nature of the clinical situation, but it will not facilitate a therapeutic relationship or communication. To reassure the client may be unrealistic. False reassurance is considered a block to therapeutic communication. Asking the client about his anxiety level will probably only increase the client's anxiety. It is also an irrelevant question because the client would most certainly be anxious.

19–34 Answer A

An underlying assumption of the health belief model (HBM) is that behavior is determined more by a person's perceived reality than by environmental factors. Components include perceived threat, efficacy, benefits of action, and perceived barriers to action. People take actions to change their lifestyle to prevent a disease only to the extent that the disease exists in their perception. They must also perceive the benefits of action as well as feel the confidence (often referred to as efficacy) to act. These benefits must outweigh the barriers to action. Benefits and barriers are people's beliefs rather than objective facts about the effectiveness of action. Education and positive reinforcement are not concepts associated with the HBM. Predisposing factors, reinforcing factors, and enabling factors are concepts from the precede-proceed model, which is used for comprehensive planning in health education and health promotion with individuals and communities. Self-efficacy theory and the perceived ability to act are one and the same and form only part of the HBM.

19–35 Answer B

According to the 1996 revised Institute of Medicine report, primary care addresses a large majority of personal healthcare needs, provides integrated and accessible healthcare services, sustains a partnership with clients, and is practiced in the context of the family and community. Public healthcare commonly uses focus-group methodology to assess community needs and design a plan of care for a community. It is not meant solely to provide a source of referrals, nor is it only for those who cannot afford specialty care.

19–36 Answer C

The limitation on prescriptive authority and the scope of practice and reimbursement issues are major barriers, as cited by Safriet, to full implementation for an autonomous role for advance practice nurses (APNs) in primary care. Research by entities such as the Pew Commission has shown that the need for medical specialists is not increasing—there are more than enough such physicians available. The complex health problems of vulnerable populations are frequently rooted in lifestyle issues such as poverty, violence, and poor housing. These social problems are often more amenable to traditional nursing-based approaches. Managed care organizations' views are shifting and variable at the present time. In some settings it is one barrier; in other settings it is something else.

19–37 Answer A

Motivation is the most important factor influencing behavioral change. Health beliefs and self-efficacy may underlie motivation for change, but it is motivation that is most strongly correlated with actual behavioral change. Cognitive knowledge and social supports have some relationships to the concept of self-efficacy, but not directly to motivation.

19–38 Answer D

The marketing process is guided by a number of factors including product, price, place, and promotion. Referred to by Burke and Bair as the "4 P's of the marketing process," "product" stands for the service you offer; "price" is identification of the right cost for the service; "place" refers to where the services are delivered or the demands of the market where the service will be offered; and "promotion" is your ability to increase your market's awareness of what you have to offer. The prospective pool of clients, your advertising budget, and what you have to offer are only portions of a marketing plan. Cost, benefit, and barriers do not describe the marketing process in a meaningful or coherent way.

19–39 Answer A

Explanatory reasoning—reasoning which explains, in the client's view, the cause of the client's illness—has been labeled by Kleinman the "explanatory model." The client may have a cognitive understanding of scientific medicine, but reject it. The client's view, in this situation, is not necessarily delusional or a cultural bias.

19–40 Answer D

The statement related to statistical techniques and their usage in research that is true is: to determine the appropriate statistical test to use, consider sample size, level of measurement, and data type, as well as other factors. Statistical significance and clinical significance are not the same. If a journal article you are writing is limited in length, you should not delete the descriptive statistics and keep the inferential statistics. You must describe your sample and possibly a number of other things before explaining your inferences. Correlational coefficients measure the strength of the relationship between variables; correlation does not infer causality, nor can you make firm predictions based on these data.

19–41 Answer A

Multiple regression and analysis of variance and covariance are tests of prediction. They are statistical techniques of inferences and imply causality, not just correlation. Statistical significance is a level set by the researcher to establish when results are sufficient to make inferences. A test of association does not exist.

19–42 Answer B

Techniques used to enhance a client's adherence to the treatment plan include giving clear written instructions, simplifying the drug regimen (such as once-a-day dosing), and having the client be an active participant (the factor most highly correlated to adherence). Negative statements that generate fear, such as stressing the dangers of missing medications, have not been found to be conducive to adherence. Positive reinforcement is best. Frequent and convenient appointments have also been correlated with higher levels of adherence. You must deal directly with the client to increase adherence, not the family.

19–43 Answer C

Although obtaining drug levels, using clinical judgment, and monitoring the responses to treatment will all assist you in assessing the degree of the client's compliance, the best way to monitor compliance is to ask the client. Most clients will be truthful.

19–44 Answer C

Strategies that help to avoid client noncompliance include providing positive feedback and reinforcement and performing careful follow-up on canceled and missed appointments. In-depth client education does not help avoid client noncompliance. Instead, client education that is short, uses multiple ways of learning, and is meaningful to the client's situation is usually more effective. Likewise, frequency of medication dosing not foster compliance, but rather leads to a greater likelihood that the client will miss the medication. Monitoring blood levels to assess therapeutic efficacy does not involve the client as a partner in their healthcare.

19–45 Answer D

Strategies effective in accomplishing behavioral change are those including personal involvement and positive reinforcement, such as the consistency of the caretaker; use of convenient, short, and frequent follow-up appointments to monitor progress and review expected outcomes; and positive reinforcement and individualization of the plan formulated and negotiated with the client. Repeatedly stressing the importance of the need to change (negative reinforcement) is not effective in accomplishing behavioral change.

19–46 Answer C

Social support is not a barrier to education and behavioral change; rather, it is a positive force in instituting behavioral change and compliance with the plan of care. Setting concrete, achievable goals for change is also an effective strategy for behavioral change. Barriers to education and behavioral change include social issues, such as cost, inconvenience, cultural and language differences, and family stressors; psychologic issues, such as depression, anxiety, insomnia, and cognitive difficulties such as the ability to read; and physical issues, such as poor vision or hearing, adverse effects of medications, and certain diseases or conditions.

19–47 Answer A

Methods used to assess your client's retention and understanding of educational materials include asking your client to restate or do a return demonstration of what you have reviewed, having your client keep a diary or record of his or her behaviors, and reviewing written materials with your client. Providing a pathophysiology book to your client does not help assess your client's retention and understanding of educational material. Repeated explanations of pathophysiology of disease will most likely not increase your client's retention, nor will objective testing.

19–48 Answer C

It can be difficult to find time to do client teaching; therefore, apply the 3 S rule: short, specific, and simple. The most important points you need initially to teach your client about a new drug are what the medication is for, how much to take, and when to take it. The specifics of taking the medication and what to do if there are adverse effects are also important, but should be explained after the other information. Discussing the action and adverse effects of the drug might distract the client from what he or she really needs to know initially.

19–49 Answer C

The maximum number of points you should attempt to make in one teaching session are three to four. The average adult can only remember five to seven points at a time. Therefore, to enhance your client's recall, limit your instructions to three to four major points in any one teaching session. Teaching more points may overwhelm even the most advanced learner. Additionally, healthcare situations are often charged with anxiety, which can further interfere with learning. Be specific about what you want the client to know, and use simple, everyday language.

19–50 Answer A

To assess Mr. Brill's readiness to learn, ask: "What do you think you should do about your smoking?" If Mr. Brill had said, "I have no problem," he would be in the precontemplative stage of learning. You would focus your teaching on increasing his awareness of his condition. Mr. Brill's response indicates that he is in the contemplative stage of learning. He is considering change, but has not taken any action. You would focus your teaching on reinforcing his understanding of the need to change, teaching him the skills needed to make the change, pointing out the positive aspects of making the change, and stressing his ability to do so. If the client had already begun to change his behavior, he would be in the action stage. You would focus your teaching on reinforcing his behavior with modeling and reward. This is a crucial stage because you do not want the client to stop the behavioral change. You must support his actions in every way possible. A client in the maintenance stage is practicing the behavior regularly. Your intervention is to continue to reinforce the new behavior and the need to maintain the change.

19–51 Answer A

To encourage reinforcement of client teaching, a useful strategy is to model the healthy behaviors. Role modeling is a very successful reinforcement strategy. Many people learn best by imitating the behavior of others. For example, if you are teaching your client exercises, demonstrate them, then have the client practice them. Videos or pictures of others performing the exercises can also be helpful. Repeated discussions of the need for behavioral change are not often effective. Although providing some written materials is helpful, providing them without behavioral support may not add to the client's motivation. Likewise, although quizzing the client may provide information about his or her knowledge base, it does not positively reinforce behavior or lead to positive behavioral change.

19–52 Answer C

Concrete strategies used to keep your client's attention as you institute client education include making your point clear from the start; varying your tone of voice (speaking in a monotone may communicate a lack of interest); using various teaching methods (visual aids work best); and translating theoretical information into practical terms. Repetition is usually not an effective strategy for keeping your client's attention. Providing an educational session immediately after eating lunch is also not necessarily conducive to learning.

19–53 Answer D

A plaintiff must prove all of the following elements in order to have a case of malpractice: duty, breach of the duty, damages or injuries, and causation. Duty means that a relationship has been established between the defendant and the plaintiff. Breach of the duty is the failure to do what a reasonable and prudent practitioner would have done in the same or similar circumstances. Damages or injuries include medical expenses; pain and suffering, both physical and mental; lost wages and lost earning capacity; loss of companionship, society, affection, and sexual relations; hedonic damages; and punitive or exemplary damages. Causation means that the plaintiff must prove a direct causal connection between the act of negligence and the alleged injuries.

19–54 Answer B

The crisis stage is defined as an acute, temporary, self-limited state of disequilibrium from which a previously intact individual may emerge even stronger. A crisis may offer an opportunity for renewal and growth. An individual in the crisis state is temporarily unable to cope with or adapt to the stressor by using previous coping mechanisms. Stress refers to pressure and tension, not a crisis. An emergency is a situation that demands immediate action to ensure survival. This is not necessarily the case during crisis.

19–55 Answer C

The primary nursing responsibility during a crisis situation is to establish a therapeutic relationship. Other nursing responsibilities include providing education regarding the recovery process, stress management and reduction, and integration of the crisis experience. The establishment of support mechanism and the development of coping mechanisms frequently enable the client to mobilize effectively and move beyond the crisis stage. Occasionally hospitalization may be necessary during an acute crisis and psychotherapy may be a useful intervention.

19–56 Answer A

The stages of grief include shock, reality, and recovery. The shock stage is characterized as numbness, the reality stage as deep pain, and the recovery stage as beginning to live again. Numbness, pain, loss, and resolution are all components of the process of grief. A grieving person shares many behavioral similarities with a depressed individual; however, grieving is a natural and not a pathologic process and is usually time-limited.

19–57 Answer C

A marketing portfolio that will support what you have to offer as an advanced practice nurse or nurse practitioner should include the state nurse practice act and regulations, prescriptive authority legislation, third-party reimbursement rules and regulations, and practice protocols. This type of information provides concrete data to potential employers and reimbursers concerning the range of services you can offer. Your personal mission statement should be used to help you personally focus your job search and options. Your scores on the certification exam and the specifics of your transcript are usually not relevant. Letters of reference should be provided only when requested.

19–58 Answer B

Examples of abnormal and more pathologic grief responses include delayed, exaggerated, and masked grief. Catatonic grief is not a grief response. Abnormal grief situations are thought to occur particularly in situations where the client had ambivalent feelings toward the person and unresolved emotional issues in the relationship. Sudden death may also precipitate abnormal grief responses.

19–59 Answer B

Classic signs of normal grief include loss of appetite, weight loss or gain, inability to concentrate or sleep, and the inability to make decisions and carry out activities of daily living. Manic episodes are not typically a component of the normal grief response.

19–60 Answer B

From the listing provided, the most common cause of litigation is failure to diagnose breast cancer.

19–61 Answer B

Legislation in the 1960s affected the development of case management, specifically Medicare and Medicaid. The 1962 Commission on Mental Retardation recommended, among other things, the use of a "program coordinator" for managing and facilitating the care of the mentally disturbed. The 1975 Education for All Handicapped Children Act recommended case management of children in schools. Additionally, the Older Americans Act of 1973 authorized the creation of Area Agencies on Aging to develop community-based networks for the delivery of coordinated services for older adults in the community. Prospective payment systems in the 1980s and managed care's dominance in the 1990s have also supported the increased usage of case managers. The recent tobacco cases, although bringing revenue in the form of punitive settlements to some states, have not necessarily had any effect on case managers.

19–62 Answer A

The primary purposes of clinical paths are to streamline healthcare services, contain costs, and improve or maintain the quality of care. Clinical paths are not designed to make client care easier. The use of clinical paths has facilitated earlier discharge of clients, but this again is not the only focus of the path. Likewise, client responsibility and self-care are often increased, but that is not the primary purpose of the path.

19–63 Answer B

A good resume should include name, address, telephone and fax numbers, e-mail address, educational background and degrees, professional employment, community service, research interests, grants written, publications, speaking engagements, consulting activities, honors and awards, professional memberships, and military history. Religious and demographic data, including number of children, should not be included to avoid being ruled out by any of these noncontributing factors.

19–64 Answer A

State laws vary on issues related to minors and you should be knowledgeable about the laws in your state. Most states consider a teenager capable of receiving birth control information and devices without the presence or consent of a parent. In the case of a teenager seeking abortion, this is not as clear. You are freer not to seek parental approval or consent when a teenager is living on his or her own and managing his or her own affairs because the emancipated minor concept is recognized in most jurisdictions. You should not need to refer Sandy to the clinic physician.

19–65 Answer C

Respecting the client's wishes is the most correct response to this situation. You may want to consider a psychological overlay, such as depression, and be sure this is not a driving component of the client's behavior. If the client appears to be of sound mind, his wishes should be respected. Ordering a psychiatric consult or having your collaborating physician talk with the client is not necessary. Talking to his family interferes with the client's autonomy, a primary value of care.

19–66 Answer A

Your action is to treat the client's psychological problems and provide support. With Mrs. Smith, there are enough symptoms to warrant evaluation and possible intervention for psychological problems, most likely depression. Then it would be appropriate to support the client's decision. There is not enough data to evaluate the need for placement in an assisted living facility at this point. To try to convince the client that she is in need of surgery would be coercive and would violate the client's autonomy.

19–67 Answer A

One situation in which medical information may be passed on without client consent is when the client has a gunshot wound. Other situations include when the client has a sexually transmitted or communicable disease. All other situations need the client's consent for release of medical records and information.

19–68 Answer B

In the outpatient office setting, the most common reason for a malpractice suit is failure to diagnose correctly. Approximately one-third of malpractice cases brought against general practitioners involve cases of failure to diagnose in a timely manner. These cases usually involve cancer, particularly cancer of the breast (failure to diagnose promptly accounts for the highest number of liability cases), lung, colon, or testes. Failure to refer and failure to manage fractures and trauma are among the top seven allegations in malpractice cases. Failure to obtain informed consent accounts for approximately 10% of the cases.

19–69 Answer C

As measured by the federal Health Care Financing Administration, national health expenditures are grouped into two categories: research and medical facilities construction and payments for health services and supplies. Medicare and Medicaid account for more than 76% of personal healthcare services. Long-term care and medications are subsumed under the other categories. Public spending for research and facilities construction totals approximately $17 billion, only a small fraction of the approximately $900 billion spent on all healthcare in recent years. Of that, more than 75% was dedicated to research paid for at the federal level.

19–70 Answer A

Advanced-practice registered nurses are overseen by laws and rules such as scope of practice, reimbursement for healthcare services, delegation of authority by physicians, quality of care, and requirements for collaboration. However, the number of clients seen per hour is not regulated by law, nor are universal health coverage nor number of referrals.

19–71 Answer A

Safeguards to follow when conducting research on a geriatric population include assessing the competence of the individual before obtaining consent, making sure the consent form is in understandable language, and obtaining verbal consent (in some situations, verbal consent is all that is required). Permission must be obtained from the client. Obtaining permission from the family or staff is usually not acceptable because it may interfere with client autonomy. Additionally, stressing the importance of the research to encourage participation is coercive. Research deemed exempt does not negate the necessity of consent to participate.

19–72 Answer C

If a healthcare provider suspects elder abuse or neglect, the provider, in most states, must report the suspected abuse or neglect to the appropriate state protective agency. Most states have laws mandating reporting of elder and dependent-adult abuse. The goals of intervention are to protect the client and prevent further injury. Although data regarding the abuse may have come from the client, depending on the situation, it is not always advisable to confront the client or the family directly. Most state laws mandate reporting of suspected abuse or neglect, not just confirmed abuse or neglect. Trained investigators can then be called in to make a more detailed assessment. Healthcare providers should be involved in educating the public about the problems of elder abuse and neglect and should be aware of community resources and supports that might help the client and their family.

19–73 Answer A

Mrs. Hernandez's insistence on discharge is an example of her exercising her right to self-determination or autonomy. The principle of beneficence implies doing the greatest good for the client and preventing harm; justice implies treating individuals fairly; and utilitarianism implies doing the greatest good for the greatest number of individuals.

19–74 Answer D

The type of healthcare delivery system that allows the client the greatest freedom of choice is a fee-for-service plan. A health maintenance organization, a preferred provider organization, and a managed care plan all have greater restrictions.

19–75 Answer B

As an individual advanced practice registered nurse, you can make a difference in advancing the role of all APRNs by writing letters to the editor on healthcare issues that outline the positive impact of advanced practice registered nurses. Reading the newspapers, although it keeps you well informed, is not enough to affect others unless you also speak out in a knowledgeable fashion. Likewise, thinking positive thoughts about your role may help you communicate a positive attitude, but the communication element is essential if you are to affect others. Supporting a Democratic candidate may or may not help advance the cause of advanced practice nursing. The stances of candidates of both parties need to be researched to ascertain each one's personal stance on this issue. There is no one "party line" on this issue.

19–76 Answer C

Prescriptive authority for advanced practice nurses varies from state to state. Some states mandate the filing of a protocol that documents physician oversight, but other states do not. It is not mandated by law in more than 40 states. The ability to prescribe controlled substances varies from state to state.

19–77 Answer B

Human research subjects are entitled to the right to informed consent, the right to withdraw from the research without being penalized, and the right to treatments other than the experimental treatment. Subjects are not guaranteed any compensation for participation, although some research studies do provide compensation.

19–78 Answer A

A number of factors are predicted to influence the mix of team providers for emerging primary-care systems. These include the provider's skills and services, the target population, and incentives for interdisciplinary teamwork. The specifics of the credentials of a provider are usually not relevant, and the socio-economic structure of the surrounding community is just one variable in taking into account the target population. Likewise, the gender mix of the primary care providers should not make a difference.

19–79 Answer C

Hostility toward the healthcare provider is not a likely cause of silence; a hearing impairment, cultural barriers, and fear are. If you suspect hearing impairment, try the whisper test. If you suspect cultural barriers, ascertain that the client can understand English. Obtain an interpreter if necessary. Fear may be caused by several different factors—it may have to do with fear of the practitioner's authority—so a gentle demeanor may help in this situation. If the client is fearful of being told bad news, reassure the client that the practitioner will be there to help, regardless of the outcome. Pointing out the problem, such as by saying "You are being very quiet," may also help to clarify the situation. Explain the need for collaboration—in some cultures this is not an acceptable model.

19–80 Answer D

Asking a question such as "Do you ever have sex in an abnormal way?" is a judgmental way of requesting information about sexual activity, even if you state that no judgment will be made. Asking questions such as the number of times penetration occurs during intercourse is invasive and, in almost all cases, irrelevant. Asking "Is your partner a man or a woman?" conveys greater tact in gathering sexual history information.

19–81 Answer A

A durable power of attorney for healthcare (DPAHC) authorizes another person or agent to make medical decisions on behalf of an individual if and when that client becomes unable or unwilling to make those decisions. It is a version of the power of attorney used in commercial transactions. In the absence of such a document, in most cases, the client's next of kin (typically a spouse, parent or child, depending on individual circumstances) is legally mandated to assume that role. Unlike the "living will," which is used for end-of-life decisions, a DPAHC is used to make decisions when the client is incapacitated.

19–82 Answer B.

Useful strategies for the healthcare provider to institute to aid the client in a relapse situation include telling the client that the relapse is a learning opportunity in preparation for the next action stage (positive reframing). Expressing disappointment, even if in a sincere and caring manner, will only increase the client's guilt. Likewise, stressing that the client must begin again as soon as possible with whatever phase of the recovery process will take away autonomy from the client. Using fear to reinforce the need to change usually does not work for behavioral issues.

19–83 Answer C

Although self-image and lack of confidence may be present and interfere with integration of research into daily practice, nurses are actually very well versed in problem-solving methods. In reality, they collect data every day, make hypotheses on the outcomes of care, and evaluate and document clinical judgments, as well as discussing their observations with others in clinical conferences. Therefore, lack of knowledge and experience with research is usually not a barrier to the utilization of research. Lack of administrative support and inadequate facilities, as well as lack of a proper infrastructure (such as library and computer support) are well-documented barriers to lack of utilization of research findings in advanced nursing practice.

19–84 Answer C

Do Not Resuscitate (DNR) orders are decided by the physician in consultation with the client, family, or surrogate decision maker. Advanced directives may help clarify end-of-life decisions, but the lack of a documented DNR order in the chart presumes that the client desires full intervention and holds healthcare providers legally responsible to initiate life-sustaining treatment. A DNR order, written by the physician, relieves the healthcare providers of that responsibility. The individual decision is never made by the healthcare facility, although the facility may draft generic guidelines to assist procedurally in end-of-life situations.

19–85 Answer A

The majority of Medicaid enrollees are young women and children. The majority of Medicaid funds, however, go to long-term care services for older adults and clients with disabilities.

19–86 Answer C

The purpose of a block grant is to allow states to have greater flexibility in providing services to the poor. Accelerating costs of the Medicaid program have prompted state-based initiatives for reform of the program. The federal government has considered converting Medicaid funds to block grants to allow states greater flexibility in providing Medicaid services.

19–87 Answer D

The market value of resources does influence direct and indirect costs. That direct costs are incurred directly as a result of providing a specific service or operating a specific service-producing unit; indirect costs are incurred outside the service-producing unit; and, from the standpoint of the organization as a whole, there are no indirect costs, are all true statements.

19–88 Answer C

Zero-based budgeting refers to a budgeting system that justifies each budget on its own merits, not on the basis of the previous period's budget. It is a process in which the budgets for succeeding budget periods are unrelated to those of earlier budget periods, but rather are justified on their own merits, as if no previous budgets had ever been prepared.

19–89 Answer A

Effective counseling techniques include beginning with the goal of helping, recognizing limitations, and caring for self. Providing reassurance is not an effective counseling technique, because reassurance may be false and does not build trust. Other effective counseling techniques include confidentiality, recognizing the effect of one's own interpersonal responses on the counseling situation, understanding the application of theory to specific and practical situations, understanding cultural differences, having flexible responses to a wide variety of situations, and acknowledging human dignity in all situations.

19–90 Answer A

A consumer of research findings engages in a number of activities that include reading the literature, analyzing clinical applicability, and using new interventions. Organizing and conducting research study, as well as ensuring the protection of human subjects, are tasks of the researcher. Collecting data may be done by anyone trained to do it and does not necessarily require advanced knowledge of the research process. Research utilization, on the other hand, involves reading the current literature; critically evaluating the study, including its methods and conclusions, to evaluate applicability to practice; introducing relevant findings into clinical practice; evaluating the results of the new treatments on clients; and disseminating those results in clinical practice.

19–91 Answer B

To bill your clients for services, you must obtain a provider or panel membership as necessary and familiarize yourself with the rules and policies of each payor. Some but not all states require a collaborative agreement with a physician for you to practice; some states require national certification to practice, but not all do. In some states you are able to provide controlled substances, and this will require that you have a DEA number; other states do not allow you to prescribe controlled-substances. There is not at present a requirement that you have a specific number of continuing medical education credits in order to bill for services provided.

19–92 Answer B

The term "incident to" implies that your services as an Advanced Registered Nurse Practitioner (ANP) are performed in connection with a physician. The reimbursement rate for Medicare billing "incident to" a physician is 100%. The physician must be on site when the care is provided, and must be providing medical services as opposed to performing administrative work. The physician must have previously seen the client and initiated the plan of care; and the physician must see the client frequently enough to provide ongoing input into the care of the client.

19–93 Answer A

You need to do your homework. This means being prepared to present the facts clearly and succinctly. Talk with your colleagues by networking with other nurse practitioners in your area. Write down an optimal salary and benefits as well as your required bottom-line salary and benefits to help establish a reasonable range. You do not necessarily need to hire a lawyer; you can handle most or all of this process yourself with proper preparation. It is premature, and is not your best use of time, to plan a signing dinner. Standing your ground is important but not if it means being unreasonable. Negotiate for agreement, not for winning or losing.

19–94 Answer A

Seeking a legal opinion might be prudent but is usually not necessary and can set up additional roadblocks in some situations. You should not base your actions or decisions on a similar situation that someone you know may have experienced. Although the experiences of others may be useful sources of comparisons, your decisions should be based on your own analysis of your own situation. Standing your ground, again, is important, but not if it means being unreasonable. During the process of negotiation an honest difference of opinion can arise. Resolving the issue is wise and prudent behavior. Always separate the issue from the person. It is about achieving a mutually satisfying outcome—a win-win situation. Clarifying misconceptions and focusing on what has been achieved thus far can be an effective strategy. You want to leave the process with positive feelings even if a work agreement is not achieved.

19–95 Answer B

A consultation implies a more informal arrangement and may occur formally or informally. It is a request for direction or guidance on diagnosis or treatment from another provider. A referral, on the other hand, is a request for another provider to accept the ongoing treatment of a patient, at least in regard to one specific health problem. A consultation does not imply the continued treatment that is part and parcel of a referral.

19–96 Answer A

The primary care provider is the coordinator of all care that the client receives. The primary care provider does not necessarily dictate all aspects of the client's care—for example, the cardiologist may decide on the antihypertensive regimen, and the primary care provider may continue to monitor the client's response. But neither does the primary care provider turn over all aspects of the care to the specialist.

Bibliography

American Association of Colleges of Nursing: The Essentials of Master's Education for Advance Practice Nursing. American Association of Colleges of Nursing, Washington, DC, 1996.

American Nurses Association: Nursing Social Policy Statement. American Nurses Association, Washington, DC, 1995.

Buppert, CK: Justifying nurse practitioner existence: Hard facts to hard figures. Nurse Pract 20:43, 1995.

Buppert, CE: Nurse Practitioner's Business Practice and Legal Guide. Aspen, Gaithersburg, MD, 1999.

Burke, CE, and Bair, JP: Marketing the role. In Sheehy, CM, and McCarthy, M. Advanced Practice Nursing: Emphasizing Common Roles. FA Davis, Philadelphia, 1998.

Cronenweit, L: Molding the future of advance practice nursing. Nurs Outlook 43:13, 1995.

Dunphy, LM, and Winland-Brown, JE (eds): Primary Care: The Art and Science of Advanced Practice Nursing. FA Davis, Philadelphia, 2001.

Goolsby, Mary Jo: Nurse Practitioner Secrets. Hanley & Belfus, Philadelphia, 2002.

Harrington, C, and Estes, CL (eds): Health Policy and Nursing. Jones and Bartlett, Boston, 2002.

Hickey, JV, et al (eds): Advance Practice Nursing. Lippincott-Raven, Philadelphia, 2000.

Katz, JR: Back to basics: Providing effective patient teaching. Am J Nurs 97:5, 1997.

King, CS: Second licensure. Adv Pract Nurs Q 1:1, 1995.

Kovner, A (ed): Health Care Delivery in the United States, ed 5. Springer, New York, 2002.

Larrabee, JH, et al: Patient satisfaction with nurse practitioner care in primary care. J Nurs Care Quality 11:5, 1997.

Mahoney, DF: Employer resistance to state authorized prescriptive authority for nurse practitioners. Nurse Pract 20:58, 1995.

National Organization of Nurse Practitioner Faculties: Curriculum Guidelines and Program Standards for Nurse Practitioner Education. National Organization of Nurse Practitioner Faculties, Washington, DC, 1995.

Nobel, J: Primary Care Medicine. Mosby, St. Louis, 2002.

Parr, MBE: The changing role of advance practice nursing in a managed care environment. AACN Clin Issues 7:300, 1996.

Pearson, LJ: Annual update of how each state stands on legislative issues affecting advance nursing practice. Nurse Pract 23:11, 2003.

Pew Health Professions Commission: Interdisciplinary Collaborative Teams in Primary Care: A Model Curriculum and Resource Guide. The University of California, San Francisco Center for the Health Professions, San Francisco, 1995.

Pew Health Professions Commission: Nurse Practitioners: Doubling Graduates by the Year 2000. In Commission Policy Papers. Pew Health Professions Commission, San Francisco, 1994.

Rakel, R: Textbook of Family Medicine. WB Saunders, Philadelphia, 2002.

Rustia, J, and Bartek, JK. Managed care credentialing of APNs. Nurse Pract 22:9, 1997.

Schaffner, J, et al: Utilization of advance practice nurses in health care systems and multispecialty group practice. J Nurs Admin 25:12, 1995.

Sheehy, CM, and McCarthy, M. Advanced Practice Nursing: Emphasizing Common Roles. FA Davis, Philadelphia, 1998.

Snyder, M, and Mirr, MP: Advanced Practice Nursing: A Guide to Professional Development. Springer, New York, 2000.

HOW WELL DID YOU DO?

85% AND ABOVE CONGRATULATIONS! THIS SCORE SHOWS APPLICATION OF TEST-TAKING PRINCIPLES AND ADEQUATE CONTENT KNOWLEDGE.

75–85% KEEP WORKING! REVIEW TEST-TAKING PRINCIPLES AND TRY AGAIN.

65–75% HANG IN THERE! SPEND SOME TIME REVIEWING CONCEPTS AND TEST-TAKING PRINCIPLES AND TRY THE TEST AGAIN.

UNIT FIVE

PRACTICE EXAMINATIONS

Examination 1

JILL E. WINLAND-BROWN
and
LYNNE M. DUNPHY

1 *Which of the following symptoms is not typical in fibromyalgia?*

A. Widespread pain at multiple sites
B. Poor sleep
C. Afternoon fatigue
D. Difficulty with memory

2 *According to the American Nurses Association's Social Policy Statement, the authority for the practice of nursing is based on:*

A. a social contract that acknowledges professional rights and responsibilities as well as being a mechanism for public accountability.
B. the values and assumptions of nursing theorists, with the society as a sounding board.
C. state regulatory laws and legislation.
D. legislation set by the state boards of medicine.

3 *Jenny is a primigravida. You talk to her about "quickening" and tell her to expect it at about:*

A. 12–14 weeks' gestation.
B. 14–16 weeks' gestation.
C. 18–20 weeks' gestation.
D. 22–24 weeks' gestation.

4 *Collaboration, as described in the American Nurses Association's Social Policy Statement, is defined as all of the following* ***except:***

A. the exchange of ideas and knowledge.
B. the recognition of expertise of others within and outside of one's expertise.
C. shared functions and a common focus on the same mission.
D. a group of people following the leader's direction.

5 *Liability insurance that covers claims made against the practitioner only while the policy is in force is referred to as:*

A. an "occurrence" policy.
B. an annual aggregate policy.
C. a "claims made" policy.
D. a functional policy.

6 *You are examining a pregnant woman. Measuring from the symphysis pubis, you find that the fundal height is palpable at the umbilicus. As a rule of thumb, you would estimate this woman to be at:*

A. 12 weeks' gestation.
B. 16 weeks' gestation.
C. 20 weeks' gestation
D. 24 weeks' gestation.

7 *Damages covered by the "personal injury" clause in a practitioner's liability insurance might include:*

A. the practitioner's dog biting the physician.
B. false arrest, detention, or imprisonment.
C. a visitor tripping over the practitioner's child's toy.
D. clients not being able to get an appointment within 24 hours.

8 *Healthy People 2010 is about improving the health of individuals, communities, and the nation. Which one of the following is not one of Healthy People 2010's overarching goals for the nation?*

A. Increase quality and years of healthy life
B. Provide health care to all Americans
C. Eliminate health disparities

9 *Which person or group stated that health reflects a philosophic ideal, encompassing optimal mental, physical, and emotional well-being, and not merely the absence of disease?*

A. Nola Pender
B. The World Health Organization
C. Betty Newman
D. The American Nurses Association

10 *Educating the public and industry to use healthy rehabilitated persons to the fullest extent possible is an example of:*

A. primary prevention.
B. secondary prevention.
C. tertiary prevention.
D. general prevention.

11 *Which document "drives" the health-care agenda for the nation?*

A. The Pew Health Professions Commission Report
B. The World Health Organization report
C. Healthy People 2010
D. The ANA Social Policy Statement

12 *The process of enabling people to increase control over and to improve their health is referred to as:*

A. primary care.
B. health promotion.
C. primary prevention.
D. collaborative care.

13 *An ultrasound is often the most reliable way of ascertaining the estimated date of confinement (EDC) because a woman's memory regarding the date of her last menstrual period is often unreliable. When performed during the first trimester, ultrasound is able to predict the EDC to within 7–10 days using which measurement?*

A. Biparietal diameter
B. Femur length
C. Skull width
D. Crown-rump length

14 *Which legislation is the basis for the federal Medicare program?*

A. Title XVIII of the amendments to the Social Security Act
B. The original Social Security Act
C. The Health Insurance Association of America Act
D. Title XIX of the amendments to the Social Security Act

15 *Home health services are provided under which part of Medicare?*

A. Part A.
B. Part B.
C. Parts A and B.
D. Home health services are not covered under Medicare.

16 *Which type of communication tends to be misunderstood the most?*

A. Verbal
B. Nonverbal
C. Written
D. Telephone

17 *The study of proxemics has identified that personal space is appropriate for close relationships in which touching may be involved and good visualization is desired. Personal space is defined as a distance of:*

A. up to 18 inches.
B. 18 inches to 4 feet.
C. 4–9 feet.
D. 9 feet and over.

18 *The use of silence when communicating:*

A. is never appropriate.
B. implies that the interviewer is unsure.
C. reduces pressure on the interviewee.
D. forces the interviewee to speak.

19 *Ethel, age 72, lives by herself quite capably. Her daughter feels that she is sometimes forgetful and needs to move in with her. She calls Ethel's physician to try and convince him that he should persuade Ethel to move in with her. This is:*

A. a violation of Ethel's personal autonomy.
B. evidence of a thoughtful daughter.
C. evidence of a daughter who feels ethically obliged to take care of her mother.
D. not the daughter's decision; the physician should decide Ethel's competency.

20 *All of the following statements about adults in the United States are true* ***except:***

A. Over 75% of clients visit a physician's office at least once per year.
B. The average client visits a physician about three times a year.
C. Older adults visit their physicians about twice as often as other clients.
D. Five percent of all physician visits require hospital admissions.

21 *All of these women are currently pregnant and are at high risk, warranting a referral,* ***except:***

A. Sandra, age 29, who is expecting twins.
B. Marcie, age 35, whose son was delivered by C-section.

C. Georgia, age 24, who has a history of deep venous thrombosis.
D. Maxine, age 38, whose daughter was born at 35 weeks' gestation.

22 *Which of the following is the best statement regarding blood pressure in pregnancy?*

A. The blood pressure is lower during the second trimester and higher in the third.
B. The blood pressure tends to be somewhat higher during the second and third trimester.
C. The blood pressure tends to be somewhat lower during the second and third trimesters.
D. The blood pressure is higher during the second trimester because of weight gain, and lower during the third.

23 *Susan is 36 weeks pregnant, and during a routine exam you test her urine and note a 3+ proteinuria. Her blood pressure is normal. Your next step is to:*

A. refer her to an obstetrician.
B. monitor her blood pressure and urine 2 days later.
C. obtain a clean-catch midstream urine specimen for culture and sensitivity.
D. have her drink several glasses of water and test a second urine specimen.

24 *All of the following features at an initial prenatal assessment suggest that a woman is at higher risk for the development of gestational diabetes* ***except:***

A. previous stillbirth.
B. glucosuria.
C. yeast infection.
D. macrosomia.

25 *Gestational diabetes occurs in what percentage of all pregnancies?*

A. 0.5%
B. 1–2%
C. 5%
D. 7%

26 *The TNM staging system for cancer assists in guiding therapeutic choices. The T in TNM stands for:*

A. the type of tumor.
B. the extent of the primary tumor.
C. the length of time the tumor has been in existence.
D. how solid the tumor feels to touch.

27 *Which of the following indicates an impending complication of influenza?*

A. Myalgia and headache
B. Diffuse crackles in the lungs
C. Sore throat and productive cough
D. Fever of 100.4° F with chills

28 *When performing a respiratory assessment on a client with pneumococcal pneumonia, you would expect to find:*

A. increased vocal fremitus.
B. fine crackles.
C. hyperresonance.
D. asymmetric chest expansion.

29 *What assessment finding indicates sarcoidosis?*

A. Use of accessory muscles
B. Increased resistance to airflow into the lungs
C. Decreased lung compliance
D. Increased vital capacity and total lung capacity

30 *A client has a diagnosis of bronchiectasis. When he asks what caused this, the nurse practitioner tells him that the structural changes in the bronchi are usually associated with:*

A. chronic bronchitis.
B. lung tumors.
C. bacterial infections.
D. congenital defects.

31 *A positive Phalen's sign indicates:*

A. splenomegaly.
B. carpal tunnel syndrome.
C. a fractured hip.
D. rheumatoid arthritis.

32 *The majority of ovarian malignancies are caused by:*

A. granulosa stromal cell tumors.
B. germ cell tumors.
C. undifferentiated tumors.
D. epithelial tumors.

33 *Which test differentiates iron deficiency anemia from the anemia of chronic disease in clients with normal or low mean corpuscular volume values?*

A. Ferritin
B. Total iron-binding capacity
C. Folate
D. Erythrocyte sedimentation rate

34 *A class III PAP test result indicates:*

A. a normal Pap test.
B. carcinoma in situ.
C. adenocarcinoma.
D. mild dysplasia.

35 *In which age group does the highest incidence of rape and other sexual assault occur?*

A. Age less than 10 years
B. Ages 14–19

C. Young and middle-aged adults
D. Older adults

36 *Risk factors for the development of cervical cancer include:*

A. a postmenopausal state.
B. nulliparity.
C. a history of endometrial, breast, or colon cancer.
D. a history of exposure to diethylstilbestrol and smoking.

37 *Mary is at risk for endometrial cancer because she:*

A. is between 40 and 50 years of age.
B. is underweight.
C. has a history of hypertension, diabetes, and endometrial hyperplasia.
D. has a family history of ovarian and breast cancer.

38 *June is at risk for ovarian cancer because she:*

A. has been exposed to talc and asbestos.
B. is postmenopausal.
C. had twins.
D. has had an abnormal Pap smear.

39 *Pain or discomfort during or after intercourse is termed:*

A. metrorrhagia.
B. dyspareunia.
C. dysmenorrhea.
D. dysphagia.

40 *Ben, age 72, is complaining of insomnia and asks your advice. You recommend that he:*

A. take alprazolam (Xanax) at bedtime.
B. go for a walk before bedtime.
C. eat a large meal before bedtime for relaxation.
D. refrain from napping during the day.

41 *John, age 46, has acquired immunodeficiency syndrome. He comes to the office with white lesions in his oropharynx. What do you suspect?*

A. Kaposi's sarcoma
B. Herpes simplex virus
C. Thrush or oral hairy leukoplakia
D. Gingivitis

42 *How often should a CD4 count be evaluated in a client with acquired immunodeficiency syndrome if the client's previous levels have been greater than 500?*

A. Every month
B. At every visit
C. Every 6 months
D. Annually

43 *Martha is experiencing an acute clinical syndrome characterized by fever, night sweats, lethargy and malaise, myalgias, arthralgias, general lymphadenopathy, pharyngitis, maculopapular rash, and a headache. You suspect this to be an acute primary infection that usually follows exposure to the human immunodeficiency virus (HIV). How many weeks ago do you think she was exposed to HIV?*

A. 1 week
B. 2–4 weeks
C. 1–2 months
D. 2–4 months

44 *Erythropoietin replacement therapy is indicated in:*

A. chronic renal failure.
B. thalassemia minor.
C. sickle cell disorders.
D. aplastic anemia.

45 *Mrs. Jay has just been placed on warfarin (Coumadin) therapy. To maintain adequate anticoagulation to reduce the risk of recurrent thrombosis as well as the potential for hemorrhage, the goal is a(n):*

A. partial thromboplastin time (PT) of 55–80 seconds.
B. prothrombin time ratio of 2.0–2.5 times the control.
C. PT of 17–19.
D. international normalized ratio of 2.0–3.0.

46 *When should all pregnant women first be screened for gestational diabetes?*

A. Between 16 and 20 weeks' gestation.
B. Between 20 and 24 weeks' gestation.
C. Between 24 and 28 weeks' gestation.
D. Between 30 and 32 weeks' gestation.

47 *Lymphedema may be differentiated from venous edema by:*

A. being a soft pitting edema with skin of normal texture.
B. affecting the foot but not the toes.
C. being a firm edema that pits poorly, with thickened skin.
D. an increase in the superficial venous pattern.

48 *Fundamental concepts involved with the pathophysiology of heart failure include all the following* ***except:***

A. preload.
B. contractility.
C. first-degree atrioventricular block.
D. afterload.

49 *Congestive heart failure results from a reduced output of the heart as a result of increased hemodynamic burden or coronary insufficiency. It is the* *result of adaptive mechanisms to preserve function. These adaptive mechanisms can result in all* ***except:***

A. systolic dysfunction (impaired contraction).
B. diastolic dysfunction (impaired ventricular filling).
C. remodeling that causes structural changes in the myocardium.
D. decreased heart size as a result of decreased volume output.

50 *The most common clinical manifestation of heart failure is:*

A. tachycardia.
B. syncope.
C. dyspnea.
D. peripheral edema.

51 *Clinical symptoms of congestive heart failure noted on physical exam may include:*

A. collapsed neck veins.
B. splenomegaly.
C. hepatomegaly and tenderness.
D. hyperactive bowel sounds and diarrhea.

52 *Auscultation of the chest of a client with congestive heart failure typically reveals:*

A. an S3 gallop.
B. a pericardial rub.
C. bronchial vesicular breath sounds.
D. S4 sounds.

53 *Pharmacological approaches for the client with chronic systolic dysfunction include the use of:*

A. angiotensin-converting enzyme inhibitors.
B. diuretics as monotherapy.
C. vasoconstrictive agents.
D. digoxin as monotherapy.

54 *The purpose of administering a vasodilating drug to a client in heart failure is to:*

A. reduce contractility.
B. increase preload.
C. increase afterload.
D. reduce afterload.

55 *In examining a child with possible rheumatic fever, you may note:*

A. a murmur consistent with valvular sufficiency.
B. subcutaneous nodules on the extensor surfaces of the lower extremities.
C. an erythematous rash over the trunk and proximal part of the limbs.
D. confusion caused by low fevers.

56 *Which type of skin cancer is most common in adults?*

A. Basal cell
B. Squamous cell
C. Melanoma
D. Actinic keratosis

57 *When assessing abdominal pain, determine the severity of the pain by asking the client:*

A. "Is it the worst pain you've ever experienced?"
B. "Do you feel at the 'end of your rope'?"
C. "How would you rate it on a scale of 1–10?"
D. "Please describe it for me."

58 *Constipation in older adults is commonly caused by all of the following* ***except:***

A. a low-fiber diet.
B. an inadequate fluid intake.
C. chronic laxative use.
D. caffeine intake.

59 *At which disc levels of the lumbar spine do most herniations occur?*

A. L1–L3.
B. L2–L4.
C. L3–L5.
D. L4–S1.

60 *Which nerve root is responsible for the patellar reflex?*

A. L2
B. L3
C. L4
D. L5

61 *Which nerve root is responsible for the Achilles reflex?*

A. L4
B. L5
C. S1
D. S2

62 *Which of the following is not an indication for a lumbar discectomy?*

A. Severe, intractable pain
B. Sciatica
C. A progressive neurological deficit
D. Cauda equina syndrome

63 *You are wondering whether to order a magnetic resonance imaging (MRI) scan for your client with a herniated nucleus pulposus (HNP). When is an MRI not indicated to rule out an HNP?*

A. When the client has acute low back pain
B. When the client experiences a loss of bowel and bladder function
C. When there is no improvement after 2 months
D. When the client is complaining of severe, intractable low back pain

64 *What is the most common presentation of a client with a sprained ankle?*

A. Point tenderness over a ligament, ecchymoses, edema, and pain
B. General achiness, reddened skin, and no edema
C. Bony deformity, no edema, and cool skin
D. Crepitus, ecchymoses, severe pain, and no point tenderness

65 *All of the following can trigger lesions in the client with psoriasis* ***except:***

A. tobacco.
B. alcohol.
C. infection.
D. salt water.

66 *Classic psoriasis lesions exhibit:*

A. diffuse macules over the torso.
B. sharply marginated plaques and papules with marked silvery-white scales.
C. ulcerations on flexor surfaces of the extremities.
D. transient thin-roofed vesicles with honey-colored crusts.

67 *Signs of elder mistreatment may include:*

A. minimal visits from family members at a nursing home.
B. polypharmacy.
C. clean dry skin
D. decubiti

68 *All of the following statements regarding visual acuity screening are true* ***except:***

A. Screening should be performed with a standard Snellen wall chart at a distance of 20 feet.
B. A tumbling "E" chart may be used for clients who are not familiar with the western alphabet.
C. Corrective lenses should not be worn during screening.
D. Each eye should be tested separately.

69 *Martin is coming in for his exam directly after a dental appointment at which he was told he had gingival overgrowth. What medication do you think he must be on?*

A. Phenytoin (Dilantin)
B. Methyldopa (Aldomet)
C. Prednisone (Deltasone)
D. Sertraline (Zoloft)

70 *Which positive sign on physical examination is indicative that the client may have appendicitis?*

A. McBurney's
B. Rovsing's
C. Psoas
D. Obturator

71 *Mr. Forrest has a positive purified protein derivative (PPD) result of 7 mm. Preventive therapy for tuberculosis should be administered for at least:*

A. 10 weeks.
B. 12 weeks.
C. 10 months.
D. 12 months.

72 *The most significant factor in a client developing recurrent urinary tract infections is the:*

A. type of bacteria present.
B. presence of a urinary obstruction.
C. type of antibiotic taken.
D. lack of hydration.

73 *You are using a penlight to attempt to transilluminate Tommy's left testicle, which on physical exam revealed a scrotal mass, as well as being swollen and reddened. Which finding will be translucent?*

A. A testicular tumor
B. A hematocele
C. A hydrocele
D. A varicocele

74 *Separation anxiety and stranger anxiety occur around age:*

A. 5–6 months.
B. 7–8 months.
C. 8–9 months.
D. 10–11 months.

75 *The cremasteric reflex can be avoided by using all of the following techniques* ***except:***

A. warming the hands and examining the client in a warm environment.
B. having the client bear down.
C. placing the thumb and index finger of one hand over the inguinal canal at the upper part of the scrotal sac before palpating the scrotum.
D. using gentle touch.

76 *Your client with a colostomy seems to have excessive flatus. What would you not suggest when advising him or her?*

A. "Do not smoke or chew gum."
B. "Do not drink beer."
C. "Avoid broccoli, brussels sprouts, cabbage, cauliflower, cucumbers, mushrooms, and peas."
D. "Poke multiple holes in the bottom of the bag to let the air out."

77 *Jennifer, age 36, has systemic lupus erythematosus. She exhibits erythematous raised patches with adherent keratotic scaling and follicular plugging. This is characteristic of:*

A. a malar rash.
B. a discoid rash.
C. photosensitivity.
D. an oral ulcer.

78 *The system that affects about 75% of all clients with systemic lupus erythematosus and has one of the most serious systemic sequelae, leading to significant morbidity and mortality, is the:*

A. renal system.
B. cardiovascular system.
C. neuromuscular system.
D. integumentary system.

79 *Sue, age 53, comes to your office for a routine exam. In passing, she mentions that she has Sjögren's syndrome. What do you think is her major complaint related to this syndrome?*

A. Fatigue
B. Diarrhea
C. Constipation
D. A dry, gritty sensation in her eyes

80 *Joan, age 24, has chronic fatigue syndrome. She is so frustrated with her family and friends thinking that it is all in her head that she tells you that she has actually thought about suicide. Knowing which of the following would be most helpful in assessing Joan's suicidal risk?*

A. If there is a history of suicide in the family
B. If Joan lives alone
C. If Joan uses any alcohol or recreational drugs
D. If Joan has developed a plan for the suicide

81 *Marnie comes to the clinic with multiple bruises and complaining of low back pain. She answers all questions with monosyllabic answers and averts your gaze. What should be your first response?*

A. "Don't worry, we'll take care of everything."
B. "Is someone hurting you at home?"
C. "Are your children bruised also?"
D. "What happened to you?"

82 *All of the following are common changes in the head and neck of older adults* ***except:***

A. more prominent facial bones and orbits.
B. sagging facial skin.
C. decreased subcutaneous fat.
D. increased skin moisture.

83 *A benign heart murmur, previously undocumented and discovered after an episode of pharyngitis, may be a clue to the diagnosis of:*

A. scarlet fever.
B. Reye's syndrome.
C. rheumatic fever.
D. diphtheria.

84 *Monique has insulin-dependent diabetes and states that she always has a blood sugar level of 230 mg/dL before breakfast. Your action is to:*

A. increase her neutral protamine Hagedorn (NPH) insulin dosage at bedtime.
B. start her on metformin (Glucophage) 500 mg bid.
C. have her test her blood sugar at 3 AM.
D. ask when she last changed the batteries in her home glucose monitoring kit.

85 *Junior can say approximately 900 words and speaks intelligible 4-word phrases. How old do you think he is?*

A. 2 years old
B. 3 years old
C. 4 years old
D. 5 years old

86 *A man who is inadequately treated for gonorrhea may develop:*

A. a reinfection.
B. an immunity to the microorganism.
C. ureteritis, pyelonephritis, and nephritis.
D. prostatitis, epididymitis, and orchitis.

87 *You suspect that Marcia has an eating disorder because she is 5 feet 6 inches tall, weighs 110 lb, and seems disgusted with herself when you weigh her. During your examination, you suspect bulimia rather than anorexia because of her:*

A. sensitivity to cold.
B. hair loss.
C. swollen salivary glands.
D. statement regarding irregular menstruation.

88 *Alexandra, age 48, has a bad complexion and has been treated for acne unsuccessfully. You suspect rosacea rather than acne because rosacea:*

A. appears as blackheads and whiteheads.
B. causes the skin to become oily.
C. appears primarily around the nose and cheeks.
D. appears red and waxy.

89 *Which of the following is a "trigger" that may aggravate rosacea?*

A. Nonalcoholic beer
B. Salt
C. Mild exercise
D. Caffeine

90 *The most common ocular manifestation with rosacea is:*

A. blepharitis.
B. conjunctivitis.
C. hordeolum.
D. tearing.

91 *Samantha, age 35, states that she wants to be tested for "thyroid disease" because it runs in her family. Her thyroid-stimulating hormone level comes back mildly high and she has normal T^3 and T^4 levels. What is the diagnosis?*

A. Primary hypothyroidism
B. Subclinical hypothyroidism
C. Primary hyperthyroidism
D. Subclinical hyperthyroidism

92 *Marta, age 52, is scheduled for sclerotherapy. She asks you what to expect during her recovery. You tell her that she will:*

A. be able to walk out of the office wearing shorts and looking great.
B. have to go home and put her feet up (either in bed or in a lounge chair) for several days.
C. be in the hospital for several days.
D. have her legs wrapped afterward with graduated compression stockings.

93 *Which of the following foods, which has the highest amount of calcium, should be recommended to your client with osteoporosis?*

A. Swiss cheese
B. Cottage cheese
C. Eggs
D. Yogurt

94 *Which of the following exercises would you recommend as being the best for your client with osteoporosis?*

A. Swimming
B. Walking
C. Chair aerobics
D. None of the above because the client should avoid any exercise that might cause an injury.

95 *Mason has chronic nonbacterial prostatitis. He is predisposed to develop:*

A. infertility.
B. decreased fertility.
C. benign prostatic hypertrophy.
D. prostate cancer.

96 *The antibiotic of choice for all forms of prostatitis is:*

A. trimethoprim-sulfamethoxazole (Bactrim).
B. tetracycline (Achromycin).
C. doxycycline (Vibramycin).
D. erythromycin (E-Mycin).

97 *Jeff, a nurse practitioner, is pressing down on the client's prostate with his index finger, moving from the base to the distal end of the gland. He is sweeping the gland's entire surface in a series of longitudinal strokes. What is he doing?*

A. A digital rectal exam
B. Checking for induration of the prostate
C. Assessing for benign prostatic hypertrophy
D. Prostatic massage

98 *Sam has prostate cancer and tells you that the surgeon wants to remove his testes. All of the following statements are true* ***except:***

A. Normal circulating testosterone levels influence the growth and spread of prostate cancer.
B. Radiation therapy is just as effective as radical surgery in eliminating the cancer.
C. A bilateral orchiectomy is the most efficient way to reduce the circulating testosterone.
D. A bilateral orchiectomy does not necessarily lead to impotence.

99 *Marie has a 9-month-old daughter whose first tooth has not erupted yet. She asks you when she should take her daughter to the dentist. You tell her:*

A. "She should go to the dentist now."
B. "Wait until her first tooth erupts."
C. "She should go at 1 year of age even if her first tooth has not come in or as soon as it does."
D. "When she's 1 1/2 years old and ready to brush her teeth, she should go to the dentist."

100 *Lynne asks you about the site selection for a blood specimen on her newborn. You tell her that the best site is:*

A. the most lateral surface of the plantar aspect of the infant's heel.
B. the central area of the newborn's foot.
C. the newborn's finger.
D. a previous puncture site.

101 *All of the following place a person at risk for gastric malignancy* ***except:***

A. smoking.
B. female gender.
C. age over 65.
D. presence of a hiatal hernia.

102 *Your client brings her daughter to the clinic with her. She says three words over and over again. About what age do you think she is?*

A. 10 months
B. 13 months
C. 15 months
D. 18 months

103 *In the screening portion of a routine physical, you ask a child to copy a cross after observing you; to stand on 1 leg for at least 10 seconds; to hand you 2 sticks from a pile of 4 tongue depressors; and to draw a man (expecting a head, 2 appendages, and possibly 2 eyes, but probably not a torso). What age would you expect the child to be?*

A. 2–3 years
B. 3–4 years
C. 4–5 years
D. 5–6 years

104 *All of the following statements are true about cluster headaches* ***except:***

A. They predominantly affect middle-aged men.
B. There is often no family history of headache or migraine.
C. The episodes usually awaken the client at night and then last for about 4 hours.
D. Alcohol may trigger an attack.

105 *Saul comes today with a history of a sudden headache that started yesterday with a severity never experienced previously. It was followed by nausea and vomiting and a transient loss of consciousness. When he awakened, he was slightly confused and irritable. He exhibits nuchal rigidity. What do you suspect?*

A. Subarachnoid hemorrhage
B. Intracranial aneurysm
C. Intracerebral hemorrhage
D. Cerebral infarction

106 *Which is the most effective method of preventing the accelerated phase of bone mass loss after menopause?*

A. Calcium supplementation
B. Regular weight-bearing exercise
C. Estrogen replacement therapy
D. Vitamin D supplementation

107 *Which type of cancer has the highest mortality rate of all cancers and yet is one of the most preventable?*

A. Cervical cancer
B. Bladder cancer
C. Breast cancer
D. Lung cancer

108 *A rule of thumb for the growth guideline of children is that their birth weight triples by age:*

A. 6 months.
B. 9 months.
C. 12 months.
D. 15 months.

109 *Permanent teeth begin erupting around age:*

A. 3 years.
B. 4–5 years.
C. 6–7 years.
D. 7–8 years.

110 *You suspect that a pregnant client with a diagnosis of anemia practices pica. What makes you suspect this?*

A. She smokes when no one is looking.
B. She keeps boxes of starch under her bed.
C. Her breath smells like alcohol.
D. There are many empty vitamin bottles in the trash.

111 *A child with slanted eyes with inner epicanthal folds; a short, flat nose; and a thick, protruding tongue probably has:*

A. Down syndrome.
B. hypertelorism.
C. craniosynostosis.
D. Marfan's syndrome.

112 *The expected change in weight in the neonate, physiologic weight loss, is the result of a loss of:*

A. intracellular fluid.
B. extracellular fluid and meconium.
C. loss of blood through the umbilical cord.
D. blood, fluid, and meconium.

113 *In which Tanner developmental stage is Josh, whose pubic hair is becoming darker and coarser, slightly curled, and spreads over his symphysis; whose penis is starting to lengthen; and whose scrotum shows a little increase in size?*

A. Tanner stage 1
B. Tanner stage 2
C. Tanner stage 3
D. Tanner stage 4

114 *The most common cause of erectile dysfunction is:*

A. prostate surgery.
B. generalized atherosclerosis.
C. drug use (antihypertensives, antidepressants).
D. diabetes.

115 *Maura, age 36, has just been given a diagnosis of Bell's palsy and asks you about her chances for a complete recovery. How do you respond?*

A. "Don't worry; I'm sure you'll have a complete recovery."
B. "You have about a 50–50 chance of complete recovery; otherwise you may have some minor problems."
C. "About 80% of clients have a complete recovery within 2 months."
D. "Although you won't recover completely, the residual effects are minor."

116 *George, age 62, just had a carotid Doppler scan done to determine what type of cerebrovascular accident (CVA) he had suffered. If the results show an occlusion of the carotid artery, which type of CVA is suspected?*

A. Transient ischemic attack
B. Ischemic CVA
C. Embolic CVA
D. Hemorrhagic CVA

117 *Sandy, age 9, has seizures with brief, jerking contractions of her arms, legs, and trunk. Which seizure type is this?*

A. Myoclonic
B. Clonic
C. Tonic
D. Tonic-clonic

118 *Mavis, age 76, comes to the office with a unilateral throbbing headache in the periorbital region. She states that the pain has been gradually increasing over the past several hours and when she went out into the cold weather, the pain was extremely bad. What do you suspect?*

A. Trigeminal neuralgia
B. A migraine
C. Giant-cell arteritis
D. A transient ischemic attack

119 *Susan, age 46, states that she has a slowly developing, painless, hard mass on her right eye. Physical examination with eversion of the eyelid reveals a red, elevated mass that is quite large on the meibomian gland pressing against the eye, causing nystagmus. What is your diagnosis?*

A. Hordeolum
B. Blepharitis
C. Sebaceous cell carcinoma
D. Chalazion

120 *Sally, age 8, has frequent episodes of epistaxis. What prevention strategy do you suggest to her mother?*

A. Vigorously blow her nose before going to bed to ensure a patent airway.
B. Start low-dose daily aspirin therapy.
C. Humidify the bedroom.
D. Tilt her head back and pinch her nose.

121 *A classic symptom of carpal tunnel syndrome is acroparesthesia, which is:*

A. the relief of tingling and numbness of the fingers by shaking or rubbing the hands.
B. awaking at night with numbness and burning pain in the fingers.
C. wrist pain with repetitive motions.
D. pain on percussion of the median nerve.

122 *Which of the following is an important step to be taken before assisting with a lumbar puncture?*

A. Obtain a complete blood count.
B. Assess the fundi for papilledema.
C. Obtain other diagnostic tests that might preclude the need for a lumbar puncture.
D. Have a cerebrospinal-fluid-pressure-reading device readily available.

123 *Which of the following topical preparations should not be used in intertriginous areas or in the perineum because they increase maceration?*

A. Gel solutions
B. Ointments
C. Emollient creams
D. Powders

124 *Which skin disorder in newborns occurs when the infant is placed on one side and the dependent half develops an erythematous flush while the upper half of the body becomes pale?*

A. Sebaceous gland hyperplasia
B. Erythema toxicum
C. Erythema toxicum neonatorum
D. Harlequin color change

125 *Which bacterial infection in children appears as a firm, dry crust, surrounded by erythema, that exudes purulent material?*

A. Ecthyma
B. Impetigo
C. Bullous impetigo
D. Cellulitis

126 *The most common pathogen for bronchiolitis in children under age 2 is:*

A. parainfluenza.
B. influenza.
C. respiratory syncytial virus.
D. adenovirus.

127 *Marsha is taking her healthy 8-lb newborn home and has been reading many conflicting statements regarding positioning and sudden infant death syndrome. What position do you recommend that she not place the baby in when putting her down for sleep?*

A. Supine
B. Sidelying
C. Prone
D. Semi-Fowler

128 *Matthew, age 3, is rushed into the office with an upper airway obstruction as a result of foreign body aspiration. A partial obstruction is present. What is your next step?*

A. Place him face down over your arm and give him five measured back blows.
B. Use the Heimlich maneuver.
C. Allow him to use his own cough reflex to extrude the foreign body.
D. Blindly probe his airway to dislodge the foreign body.

129 *Jill's son, Nathan, has asthma, and she can not decide whether he should play Little League baseball or not. She asks for your advice. What do you tell her?*

A. "Exercise should be encouraged rather than restricted."
B. "Sports are recommended unless exercise-induced bronchospasm occurs."

C. "He should find some other type of recreational activity."
D. "If he has a nebulization treatment before playing, he should do fine."

130 *Johnny, age 2, is brought in by his mother with painless rectal bleeding with dark red and black stools. You suspect:*

A. Hirschsprung's disease.
B. chylous ascites.
C. duplications of the gastrointestinal tract.
D. Meckel's diverticulum.

131 *Jason, age 14 months, is carried into the exam room screaming and drawing up his knees. His abdomen is tender and distended. You palpate a sausage-shaped mass in the upper midabdomen. Your next step is to order:*

A. stools for guaiac times 3.
B. an ultrasound.
C. a barium enema.
D. a computed tomography scan.

132 *Which laboratory finding would be indicative of celiac disease?*

A. Excessive fecal fat
B. Hyperproteinemia
C. Many villi apparent in the jejunal mucosa on intestinal biopsy
D. A normal carbohydrate metabolism

133 *Your client of many years calls you for advice because she states that her obstetrician just told her that her newborn has breast milk jaundice. She wants to know if she has to stop breast-feeding. What do you tell her?*

A. "Yes, you should start the infant on a bottle."
B. "You should stop breast-feeding for a week, pump your breasts, then resume feedings when the jaundice clears up."
C. "The jaundice clears before 3 months in almost all infants, even when breast-feeding is continued."
D. "You need to stop breastfeeding for at least 1 month, but may resume after that."

134 *The presence of which type of cast in the urine is not indicative of renal disease?*

A. Red cell casts
B. Hyaline casts
C. Renal tubular cell casts
D. White cell casts

135 *Judy has been on hemodialysis for several years and wants to try continuous ambulatory peritoneal dialysis (CAPD). In teaching her about this, you tell her that the major complication is:*

A. dehydration.
B. hemorrhage.
C. peritonitis.
D. electrolyte imbalance.

136 *Goodpasture's syndrome includes a triad of all of the following conditions* ***except:***

A. acute renal failure.
B. pulmonary hemorrhage.
C. iron-deficiency anemia.
D. glomerulonephritis.

137 *You suspect a bladder neck or prostatic urethral problem with Bob because he is complaining of:*

A. initial hematuria.
B. terminal hematuria.
C. total hematuria.
D. "spotty" hematuria.

138 *Chronic urinary retention may result in:*

A. total incontinence.
B. stress incontinence.
C. urge incontinence.
D. overflow incontinence.

139 *Jacob, age 56, is started on finasteride (Proscar) to improve his benign prostatic hyperplasia symptoms by reducing the size of his prostate. Which of the following statements is true regarding finasteride?*

A. Liver function tests should be done every 3–6 months to assess for potential liver damage.
B. The dose should be started low initially, then titrated upward.
C. For a complete therapeutic trial, the medication should be continued for a full 12 months.
D. If not effective by 6 months, the drug should be discontinued.

140 *Joe has had several kidney stones over the past year. They have been analyzed and been determined to be calcium stones. What question might you ask him to help determine prevention recommendations?*

A. "Do you use vitamin D supplements?"
B. "Are you on any antidepressants?"
C. "Do you take excessive amounts of vitamin C?"
D. "Do you have a history of frequent urinary tract infections?"

141 *In trying to determine which type of urinary incontinence Mona, age 56, has, you order a postvoid residual urine. The results come back with a low reading. Which type of incontinence would this indicate?*

A. Hypoactive bladder (neurogenic bladder).
B. Outlet incompetence (stress incontinence).

C. Outlet obstruction (overflow incontinence).
D. All types of incontinence result in a high level (amount) of postvoid residual urine.

142 *Marian has newly diagnosed diabetes, and diet modification has failed. You decide to try sulfonylurea therapy and tell her that it:*

A. acts as an insulin sensitizer.
B. acts as an antihyperglycemic agent.
C. augments pancreatic insulin secretion.
D. interferes with digestion and absorption of dietary carbohydrate.

143 *Barbara has type II diabetes and now has dyslipidemia. Which drug should be added to her regimen to lower the triglycerides into an acceptable range?*

A. Gemfibrozil (Lopid)
B. Nicotinic acid (Niacin)
C. Cholestyramine (Questran)
D. Bile acid sequestrant (Colestid)

144 *Jack, age 42, has diabetes, and now has a diagnosis of hypertension. You may decide to start him on any of the following antihypertensive agents* ***except:***

A. enalapril (Vasotec).
B. amlodipine (Norvasc).
C. atenolol (Tenormin).
D. doxazocin (Cardura)

145 *Joyce is hypothyroid and has been taking levothyroxine (Synthroid) 112 mcg for 6 months. You order a thyroid-stimulating hormone (TSH) test and the results come back at 0.3 mL U/L. You change her levothyroxine dosage to:*

A. 88 mcg.
B. 100 mcg.
C. 125 mcg.
D. 150 mcg.

146 *Ginger says she was taught that because she has diabetes, she should carry sweets with her in case she has a hypoglycemic episode. However, she is unsure of how much to take. How much rapidly absorbable carbohydrate do you tell her to take to abort a hypoglycemia episode?*

A. 5–10 g
B. 10–15 g
C. 15–20 g
D. 20–25 g

147 *Which of the following statements is not true regarding eye disease and persons with diabetes?*

A. Cataracts are more common in people with diabetes than in those without diabetes.
B. Open-angle glaucoma is more common in people with diabetes.
C. Eye surgery must be approached with caution in people with diabetes because of poor healing.
D. Cataracts occur at a younger age and progress more rapidly in people with diabetes.

148 *Mindy is taking levothyroxine (Synthroid) for her hypothyroidism, along with several other medications. She asks if she needs to stop taking any of her medications when she comes in for blood work because she has heard that many drugs affect thyroid function test results. You tell her that all of the following drugs affect the results* ***except:***

A. corticosteroids.
B. cough medications.
C. estrogens.
D. antibiotics.

149 *Lorie has been given a diagnosis of Cushing's disease. You tell her that 80% of all cases are cured by:*

A. subtotal transsphenoidal hypophysectomy.
B. irradiation.
C. adrenal enzyme inhibitors.
D. adrenalectomy.

150 *Which type of pharyngitis do you suspect when a client has a sore throat with dysphagia and thin, white nonvesicular diffuse exudative ulcers on the mucosa?*

A. Allergic pharyngitis
B. Streptococcal pharyngitis
C. Mononucleosis
D. *Candida* infection

Answers

1 Answer C

Content area: Female Genitourinary Problems (Chap. 15)

2 Answer A

Content area: Issues in Primary Care (Chap. 19)

3 Answer C

Content area: Care of the Emerging Family (Chap. 4)

4 Answer D

Content area: Issues in Primary Care (Chap. 19)

5 Answer C

Content area: Issues in Primary Care (Chap. 19)

6 Answer C

Content area: Care of the Emerging Family (Chap. 4)

7 Answer B
Content area: Issues in Primary Care (Chap. 19)

8 Answer B
Content area: Health Promotion (Chap. 3)

9 Answer B
Content area: Health Promotion (Chap. 3)

10 Answer C
Content area: Health Promotion (Chap. 3)

11 Answer C
Content area: Issues in Primary Care (Chap. 19)

12 Answer B
Content area: Health Promotion (Chap. 3)

13 Answer D
Content area: Care of the Emerging Family (Chap. 4)

14 Answer A
Content area: Issues in Primary Care (Chap. 19)

15 Answer C
Content area: Issues in Primary Care (Chap. 19)

16 Answer B
Content area: Health Counseling (Chap. 6)

17 Answer B
Content area: Health Counseling (Chap. 6)

18 Answer C
Content area: Health Counseling (Chap. 6)

19 Answer A
Content area: Issues in Primary Care (Chap. 19)

20 Answer D
Content area: Health Promotion (Chap. 3)

21 Answer B
Content area: Care of the Emerging Family (Chap. 4)

22 Answer A
Content area: Care of the Emerging Family (Chap. 4)

23 Answer C
Content area: Care of the Emerging Family (Chap. 4)

24 Answer C
Content area: Care of the Emerging Family (Chap. 4)

25 Answer B
Content area: Care of the Emerging Family (Chap. 4)

26 Answer B
Content area: Hematologic and Immune Problems (Chap. 18)

27 Answer B
Content area: Respiratory Problems (Chap. 10)

28 Answer A
Content area: Respiratory Problems (Chap. 10)

29 Answer C
Content area: Respiratory Problems (Chap. 10)

30 Answer C
Content area: Respiratory Problems (Chap. 10)

31 Answer B
Content area: Musculoskeletal Problems (Chap. 16)

32 Answer D
Content area: Female Genitourinary Problems (Chap. 15)

33 Answer A
Content area: Hematologic and Immune Problems (Chap. 18)

34 Answer D
Content area: Female Genitourinary Problems (Chap. 15)

35 Answer B
Content area: Female Genitourinary Problems (Chap. 15)

36 Answer D
Content area: Female Genitourinary Problems (Chap. 15)

37 Answer C
Content area: Female Genitourinary Problems (Chap. 15)

38 Answer A
Content area: Female Genitourinary Problems (Chap. 15)

39 Answer B

Content area: Female Genitourinary Problems (Chap. 15)

40 Answer D

Content area: Health Counseling (Chap. 6)

41 Answer C

Content area: Hematologic and Immune Problems (Chap. 18)

42 Answer C

Content area: Hematologic and Immune Problems (Chap. 18)

43 Answer B

Content area: Hematologic and Immune Problems (Chap. 18)

44 Answer A

Content area: Hematologic and Immune Problems (Chap. 18)

45 Answer D

Content area: Cardiovascular Problems (Chap. 11)

46 Answer C

Content area: Care of the Emerging Family (Chap. 4)

47 Answer C

Content area: Hematologic and Immune Problems (Chap. 18)

48 Answer C

Content area: Cardiovascular Problems (Chap. 11)

49 Answer D

Content area: Cardiovascular Problems (Chap. 11)

50 Answer C

Content area: Cardiovascular Problems (Chap. 11)

51 Answer C

Content area: Cardiovascular Problems (Chap. 11)

52 Answer A

Content area: Cardiovascular Problems (Chap. 11)

53 Answer A

Content area: Cardiovascular Problems (Chap. 11)

54 Answer D

Content area: Cardiovascular Problems (Chap. 11)

55 Answer C

Content area: Cardiovascular Problems (Chap. 11)

56 Answer A

Content area: Integumentary Problems (Chap. 8)

57 Answer C

Content area: Abdominal Problems (Chap. 12)

58 Answer D

Content area: Abdominal Problems (Chap. 12)

59 Answer D

Content area: Musculoskeletal Problems (Chap. 16)

60 Answer C

Content area: Musculoskeletal Problems (Chap. 16)

61 Answer C

Content area: Musculoskeletal Problems (Chap. 16)

62 Answer B

Content area: Musculoskeletal Problems (Chap. 16)

63 Answer A

Content area: Musculoskeletal Problems (Chap. 16)

64 Answer A

Content area: Musculoskeletal Problems (Chap. 16)

65 Answer D

Content area: Integumentary Problems (Chap. 8)

66 Answer B

Content area: Integumentary Problems (Chap. 8)

67 Answer D

Content area: Health Promotion (Chap. 3)

68 Answer C

Content area: Head and Neck Problems (Chap. 9)

69 Answer A

Content area: Head and Neck Problems (Chap. 9)

70 Answer A

Content area: Abdominal Problems (Chap. 12)

71 Answer D
Content area: Respiratory Problems (Chap. 10)

72 Answer B
Content area: Renal Problems (Chap. 13)

73 Answer C
Content area: Male Genitourinary Problems (Chap. 14)

74 Answer C
Content area: Growth and Development (Chap. 5)

75 Answer B
Content area: Male Genitourinary Problems (Chap. 14)

76 Answer D
Content area: Abdominal Problems (Chap. 12)

77 Answer B
Content area: Hematologic and Immune Problems (Chap. 18)

78 Answer A
Content area: Hematologic and Immune Problems (Chap. 18)

79 Answer D
Content area: Musculoskeletal Problems (Chap. 16)

80 Answer D
Content area: Neurological Problems (Chap. 7)

81 Answer B
Content area: Health Counseling (Chap. 6)

82 Answer D
Content area: Head and Neck Problems (Chap. 9)

83 Answer C
Content area: Head and Neck Problems (Chap. 9)

84 Answer C
Content area: Endocrine and Metabolic Problems (Chap. 17)

85 Answer B
Content area: Growth and Development (Chap. 5)

86 Answer D
Content area: Male Genitourinary Problems (Chap. 14)

87 Answer C
Content area: Neurological Problems (Chap. 7)

88 Answer C
Content area: Integumentary Problems (Chap. 8)

89 Answer D
Content area: Integumentary Problems (Chap. 8)

90 Answer A
Content area: Integumentary Problems (Chap. 8)

91 Answer B
Content area: Head and Neck Problems (Chap. 9)

92 Answer D
Content area: Health Counseling (Chap. 6)

93 Answer D
Content area: Health Promotion (Chap. 3)

94 Answer B
Content area: Health Promotion (Chap. 3)

95 Answer B
Content area: Male Genitourinary Problems (Chap. 14)

96 Answer A
Content area: Male Genitourinary Problems (Chap. 14)

97 Answer D
Content area: Male Genitourinary Problems (Chap. 14)

98 Answer B
Content area: Male Genitourinary Problems (Chap. 14)

99 Answer C
Content area: Health Counseling (Chap. 6)

100 Answer A
Content area: Health Counseling (Chap. 6)

101 Answer B
Content area: Abdominal Problems (Chap. 12)

102 Answer B
Content area: Growth and Development (Chap. 5)

103 Answer C
Content area: Growth and Development (Chap. 5)

104 Answer C
Content area: Neurological Problems (Chap. 7)

105 Answer A
Content area: Neurological Problems (Chap. 7)

106 Answer C
Content area: Health Promotion (Chap. 3)

107 Answer D
Content area: Health Promotion (Chap. 3)

108 Answer C
Content area: Growth and Development (Chap. 5)

109 Answer C
Content area: Growth and Development (Chap. 5)

110 Answer B
Content area: Health Counseling (Chap. 6)

111 Answer A
Content area: Growth and Development (Chap. 5)

112 Answer B
Content area: Growth and Development (Chap. 5)

113 Answer C
Content area: Growth and Development (Chap. 5)

114 Answer B
Content area: Male Genitourinary Problems (Chap. 14)

115 Answer C
Content area: Neurological Problems (Chap. 7)

116 Answer B
Content area: Neurological Problems (Chap. 7)

117 Answer A
Content area: Neurological Problems (Chap. 7)

118 Answer C
Content area: Neurological Problems (Chap. 7)

119 Answer D
Content area: Head and Neck Problems (Chap. 9)

120 Answer C
Content area: Head and Neck Problems (Chap. 9)

121 Answer B
Content area: Musculoskeletal Problems (Chap. 16)

122 Answer B
Content area: Neurological Problems (Chap. 7)

123 Answer B
Content area: Integumentary Problems (Chap. 8)

124. Answer D
Content area: Integumentary Problems (Chap. 8)

125 Answer A
Content area: Integumentary Problems (Chap. 8)

126 Answer C
Content area: Respiratory Problems (Chap. 10)

127 Answer C
Content area: Respiratory Problems (Chap. 10)

128 Answer C
Content area: Respiratory Problems (Chap. 10)

129 Answer A
Content area: Respiratory Problems (Chap. 10)

130 Answer D
Content area: Abdominal Problems (Chap. 12)

131 Answer C
Content area: Abdominal Problems (Chap. 12)

132 Answer A
Content area: Abdominal Problems (Chap. 12)

133 Answer C

Content area: Abdominal Problems (Chap. 12)

134 Answer B

Content area: Renal Problems (Chap. 13)

135 Answer C

Content area: Renal Problems (Chap. 13)

136 Answer A

Content area: Renal Problems (Chap. 13)

137 Answer B

Content area: Renal Problems (Chap. 13)

138 Answer D

Content area: Renal Problems (Chap. 13)

139 Answer C

Content area: Renal Problems (Chap. 13)

140 Answer A

Content area: Renal Problems (Chap. 13)

141 Answer B

Content area: Renal Problems (Chap. 13)

142 Answer C

Content area: Endocrine and Metabolic Problems (Chap. 17)

143 Answer A

Content area: Endocrine and Metabolic Problems (Chap. 17)

144 Answer C

Content area: Endocrine and Metabolic Problems (Chap. 17)

145 Answer C

Content area: Endocrine and Metabolic Problems (Chap. 17)

146 Answer B

Content area: Endocrine and Metabolic Problems (Chap. 17)

147 Answer C

Content area: Endocrine and Metabolic Problems (Chap. 17)

148 Answer D

Content area: Endocrine and Metabolic Problems (Chap. 17)

149 Answer A

Content area: Endocrine and Metabolic Problems (Chap. 17)

150 Answer D

Content area: Head and Neck Problems (Chap. 9)

GOOD LUCK ON YOUR CERTIFICATION EXAMINATION!

Examination 2

LYNNE M. DUNPHY
and
JILL E. WINLAND-BROWN

1 *The intended purpose of national certification is to:*

A. ensure quality beyond the basic registered nurse license.
B. assist the nurse in obtaining a higher salary.
C. identify nurses who may be eligible for direct reimbursement for services.
D. assist the nurse in job promotion.

2 *One disadvantage of the "claims-made" type of policy for liability insurance is that the coverage:*

A. must have a high liability limit.
B. does not cover personal acts of negligence.
C. must be continued indefinitely.
D. There are no disadvantages.

3 *Which organization is a delivery method in the private sector that gives the sponsoring organization discounts from their usual charges?*

A. Health maintenance organization
B. Preferred provider organization
C. Gatekeeper organization
D. Fee-for-service organization

4 *Countries that have socialized medicine have more cost-effective healthcare systems than the United States, partly because:*

A. they have fewer nurses.
B. they have more primary-care physicians than consultants.
C. they have a lower cost of living.
D. they have no health maintenance organizations.

5 *The most important activity that the care provider performs is:*

A. taking the history.
B. the ordering of appropriate tests.
C. disease follow-through.
D. the ordering of appropriate medications.

6 *Sam just left your office with a diagnosis of prostate cancer after an extensive workup. His wife is on the phone demanding to know what his problem turned out to be. How do you respond?*

A. "Don't worry, everything will be okay after we send Sam to a specialist."
B. "You'll have to ask Sam; I can't tell you."
C. "He has prostate cancer, but you'll have to talk to Sam about what his choices are."
D. You refuse to take the call.

7 *David, age 19, has end-stage renal disease and needs to continue on dialysis, which he started 2 years ago. He is on a waiting list for a kidney transplant, but his chance to receive one is slim because of his rare blood type. He has made the choice to stop dialysis. How do you respond?*

A. "You're crazy, any life is better than no life at all."
B. "You don't have the right to make that decision, I'm your healthcare provider."
C. "Let me talk to your parents about this."
D. "Let's discuss the risks and consequences."

8 *By the time a child reaches 7 years old, how many doses of oral polio vaccine (OPV) should have been administered?*

A. 1 dose.
B. 2 doses.
C. 3 doses.
D. 4 doses.

9 *The most common risk factors for thromboembolism include:*

A. fractures and prolonged immobilization.
B. myocardial infarction and atrial fibrillation.
C. cardiomyopathy and pregnancy.
D. abnormal fibrinolysis and congestive heart failure.

10 *Which valve is most affected in rheumatic heart disease?*

A. Aortic
B. Tricuspid
C. Mitral
D. Pulmonary

11 *You suspect that Marvin has digitalis toxicity. What is the most dangerous manifestation that you will be on the alert for?*

A. Seizures
B. Diarrhea
C. Delirium
D. Arrhythmias

12 *Sara, age 57, comes in with a complaint of pain and swelling in her right lower leg. The pain is worse if she tries to walk or stand on the leg. She smokes a half pack of cigarettes a day and takes a hormone replacement pill every night. She states that she returned from Tokyo 3 days ago and still feels jet lagged. Her vital signs are normal. Her physical exam reveals a warm and slightly reddened right lower leg with marked edema extending from the knee to the foot; intact popliteal, dorsalis pedis, and posterior tibial pulses; and an unremarkable Homan's sign. You suspect:*

A. edema from increased salt intake from the foods she had been eating while in Tokyo.
B. acute arterial occlusion.
C. deep venous thrombosis.
D. dependent edema from sitting for long periods of time during her flight home.

13 *The initial diagnostic procedure for evaluation of a deep venous thrombosis is:*

A. a contrast venography.
B. a duplex ultrasound.
C. an arteriogram.
D. an MRI of the affected limb.

14 *Rose, age 66, comes in with an intractable headache accompanied by weakness, difficulty chewing, and visual changes. You note some swelling and tenderness on her left forehead. What do you suspect?*

A. A migraine headache
B. Temporal arteritis
C. A cluster headache
D. A cerebral aneurysm

15 *Anne has a history of hyperlipidemia, and today you note a soft, yellowish, raised, waxy lesion beneath her right eyelid. You diagnose this as a:*

A. xanthelasma.
B. hordeolum.
C. chalazion.
D. lagophthalmos.

16 *When performing an ophthalmoscopic exam, you note retinal hemorrhages and narrowing, obliteration, dilation, and tortuousness of the retinal vessels. You diagnose this as:*

A. macular degeneration.
B. hypertensive retinopathy.
C. diabetic retinopathy.
D. a cataract.

17 *Ginny, age 62, comes to the office with a sudden onset of severe, throbbing eye pain and unilateral vision loss. Even before you examine her, you suspect:*

A. a unilateral cataract.
B. iritis.
C. a detached retina.
D. acute angle-closure glaucoma.

18 *Mark has a diagnosis of bullous myringitis. What might you expect to see during an otoscopic exam?*

A. Bulging of the tympanic membrane (TM)
B. Serous amber fluid and air behind the TM
C. Vesicles on the TM
D. Perforation of the TM

19 *When examining a client's chest wall, you note crepitus. What condition might you suspect?*

A. Emphysema
B. Pleuritis
C. Pulmonary edema
D. Pneumonia

20 *When auscultating Marie's heart sounds in the left semilateral position, you hear an atrial gallop. When documenting this sound, you refer to it as:*

A. S1.
B. S2.
C. S3.
D. S4.

21 *Of the abnormalities that might show up on an ultrasound during pregnancy, all of the following warrant a referral* ***except:***

A. hydramnios.
B. placenta previa (after 28 weeks).
C. breech position at 28 weeks.
D. oligohydramnios.

22 *Betsy, age 23, is 38 weeks pregnant and has a urinary tract infection. Which drug is the best choice for treatment?*

A. Cefprozil (Cefzil)
B. Tetracycline (Achromycin)
C. Nitrofurantoin (Furadantin)
D. Amoxicillin (Amoxil)

23 *All of the following are common discomforts of pregnancy* ***except:***

A. leg cramps.
B. edema of the face and fingers.
C. varicosities.
D. urinary frequency.

24 *Janice is 28 weeks pregnant and makes an emergency visit complaining of painful vaginal bleeding. You palpate a tender, boardlike uterus. What is this most indicative of?*

A. Placenta previa
B. Abruptio placentae
C. Gestational trophoblastic disease
D. Emboli

25 *Pregnancy-induced hypertension occurs in what percentage of pregnant clients?*

A. Less than 3%
B. 3–5%
C. 5–7%
D. 7–10%

26 *Your client has no signs or symptoms other than a fever and coarse crackles. What must you assess for further?*

A. Congestive heart failure
B. Pneumonia
C. Bronchitis
D. Pulmonary fibrosis

27 *The most common cause of a chronic cough that is more severe early in the morning and produces a yellowish-brown mucus is:*

A. cigarette smoking.
B. asthma.
C. bronchogenic carcinoma.
D. angiotensin-converting enzyme inhibitor use.

28 *Sol, age 46, is overweight and comes in with dyspnea. He also has peripheral edema, ascites, and neck vein distention. What do you further evaluate him for?*

A. Anemia
B. Pulmonary hypertension
C. Pleural effusion
D. Central nervous system lesion

29 *A complication of emphysema may be:*

A. polycythemia.
B. ascites.
C. pain.
D. elevated LDL.

30 *George has ischemic changes and gangrene of the hands and fingers. This may be a result of:*

A. Raynaud's disease.
B. Buerger's disease.
C. Allen's disease.
D. Hodgkin's disease.

31 *All of the following systemic diseases may lead to pruritus* ***except:***

A. liver disease.
B. diabetes mellitus.
C. Parkinson's disease.
D. thyroid disorders.

32 *A "liver flap," associated with hepatic encephalopathy, uremia, and respiratory acidosis, refers to:*

A. nonrhythmic flapping of the wrists and hands.
B. a palpable liver that "flaps" against the palpating hand.
C. a jaundiced color of the skin.
D. urine that is the color of liver.

33 *When palpating lymph nodes, it is essential to also palpate the supraclavicular nodes located:*

A. along the chest wall, high in the axilla.
B. superficially on the medial side of the elbow.
C. hidden behind the sternocleidomastoid muscle's clavicular head.
D. directly in the axillary region.

34 *Abnormal bony growths on the distal and proximal interphalangeal joints are associated with:*

A. rheumatoid arthritis.
B. osteoarthritis.
C. scleroderma.
D. Lyme disease.

35 *Abnormal bony growths on the proximal interphalangeal joints are referred to as:*

A. Heberden's nodes.
B. Bouchard's nodes.
C. subcutaneous nodules.
D. tophi.

36 *Marsha, age 36, comes for a physical. Her chart mentions a swan-neck deformity. You will be sure to assess her:*

A. hands.
B. neck.
C. shoulders.
D. ankles.

37 *You are assessing the direction of Jim's abdominal venous blood flow and note a centrifugal venous return radiating outward from his umbilicus. This may be a sign of:*

A. inferior vena cava obstruction.
B. normal blood flow.
C. portal hypertension.
D. an abdominal aortic aneurysm.

38 *Karen, age 43, was recently in a car accident but is now up and about. She comes into the office with vague complaints of being tired. You assess Cullen's sign and Grey Turner's sign. You assume therefore that she has:*

A. anemia.
B. retroperitoneal bleeding.
C. portal hypertension.
D. liver dysfunction.

39 *Timmy, age 5, comes for a preschool physical. You note that his urethral meatus opens on the ventral surface of the penis and document this as:*

A. epispadias.
B. paraphimosis.
C. phimosis.
D. hypospadias.

40 *When doing a pelvic exam on Tara, age 19, you note painful, raised, reddened lesions filled with fluid around the labia. You diagnose these as:*

A. lesions associated with syphilis.
B. a vaginal infection.
C. condyloma.
D. herpetic vesicles.

41 *When auscultating bowel sounds, you note high-pitched tinkling sounds. What might this indicate?*

A. Peritonitis
B. Progressive bowel obstruction
C. Paralytic ileus
D. Gastric outflow obstruction

42 *Marge comes for a pelvic exam complaining of vaginal burning and itching and painful intercourse. You note strawberry spots on her cervix, along with a greenish-yellow, frothy, foul-smelling vaginal discharge. What is your diagnosis?*

A. *Candida albicans* infection
B. *Gardnerella vaginalis* infection
C. *Trichomonas vaginalis* infection
D. Atrophic vaginitis

43 *When performing sensory testing on the lower extremities, vibration is the first sense to be lost in the client with:*

A. peripheral vascular disease.
B. alcoholism.
C. vitamin B_6 deficiency.
D. TIA.

44 *Melissa has multiple sclerosis and has reached the point at which she needs to use a wheelchair. She anticipates that soon she will not be able to do anything for herself and has decided that, when that time comes, she is going to take an overdose of sleeping pills. If her husband supports her decision, which ethical principle is he using?*

A. Beneficence
B. Veracity
C. Autonomy
D. Justice

45 *Which would be the best question or statement to use to facilitate open communication between yourself and a morbidly obese woman?*

A. "Don't you want to live to dance at your daughter's wedding?"
B. "It took you a long time to get like this; it will take a while to get the weight off."
C. "What steps have you taken to change your patterns of eating and exercising?"
D. "I'm going to come up with some goals that I think you can live with."

46 *The leading cause(s) of death in all age groups under age 44 is (are):*

A. accidents.
B. heart disease.
C. malignant neoplasms.
D. human immunodeficiency virus infection.

47 *Judy has come to have an influenza immunization today. Which of the following would be a contraindication for her to receive the injection?*

A. She is pregnant.
B. She has a temperature of 102°F (38.8°C).
C. She has a history of neurological reaction.
D. She had a previous anaphylactic reaction to neomycin and streptomycin.

48 *A good technique for assessment of the supraclavicular nodes is:*

A. Have the client sit up and perform the Valsalva's maneuver.
B. Use the diaphragm of the stethoscope.
C. Palpate the axilla.
D. Use the bell of the stethoscope.

49 *Most persons who are advised to perform monthly self-examinations do not do so. Which of the following statements is true regarding self-examination?*

A. Women perform a monthly breast self-exam 50–60% of the time.
B. Adults perform a routine self-examination 20% of the time.
C. Men perform a testicular self-examination 10–15% of the time.
D. Adults check their skin on a routine basis.

50 *Many Americans have their urine tested for illegal drugs for different purposes. At about what percentage is there a likelihood of false-positive results?*

A. Less than 10%
B. 10–30%
C. 30–60%
D. More than 60%

51 *Mr. Smith, age 68, comes to the primary care office complaining of inability to sleep, fatigue, and lack of concentration. As you talk with him, you discover that his wife died less than a year ago. You note that he has lost over 15 lb since his last visit 6 months ago. Although he is taking enalapril (Vasotec) 5 mg PO qd, you measure his blood pressure to be 154/94 mm Hg. An immediate priority would be to:*

A. adjust his antihypertensive medication regimen.
B. assess him for suicidal ideation.
C. discuss beginning antidepressant therapy.
D. refer him to a counselor and suggest a grief support group.

52 *Mrs. Jones, age 58, comes to your primary care office complaining of dull, left-sided chest pain that increases somewhat on inspiration. This has been going on since the previous day and has no relation to movement or exercise. The pain intensifies when she lies down, and she obtains some relief sitting up and leaning slightly forward. On auscultation, you hear a pericardial friction rub. Her electrocardiogram shows ST-segment elevation, a T-wave inversion, and PR-segment depression. The ST elevations are diffuse and across leads. You suspect:*

A. an evolving myocardial infarction.
B. angina.
C. pericarditis.
D. costochondritis.

53 *Angie, age 17, is complaining of nasal congestion, sneezing, and itchiness of the eyes that worsens when she does yard work. She has been self-medicating with an over-the-counter nasal decongestant spray. Although this has been temporarily helpful, she reports that her symptoms are now worsening. You should:*

A. counsel her to avoid yard work.
B. advise her of the rebound effect of the nasal spray.
C. order a nonsedating antihistamine and a corticosteroid nasal spray.
D. advise a combination nonsedating antihistamine and decongestant tablet.

54 *The term "sensitivity" is most accurately defined as:*

A. the percentage of clients with a positive test result who actually have the disease.
B. the percentage of clients with the disease in whom the test is positive.
C. the percentage of clients with a negative test result who really do not have the disease.
D. a true positive result.

55 *John, age 18, has a seizure disorder. He has been taking a combination of phenytoin (Dilantin) and phenobarbital (Luminal) to treat his seizures. He reports a new rash. You know that:*

A. the phenobarbital should be discontinued.
B. the phenytoin should be discontinued.
C. either of these drugs could cause a rash.
D. you must begin John on an entirely new drug regimen.

56 *Mrs. Dorman, age 65, is complaining of a sharp, tingling sensation and itchiness on the right side of her back below the scapula that radiates around her ribcage. Careful examination of this area reveals clear, unbroken skin. She is also complaining of feeling tired and achy. One of your differential diagnoses is herpes zoster. You know all the following to be true* ***except:***

A. 90% of the adult population harbors latent herpes zoster infection that can reactivate at any time.
B. This type of pain could recur for months, or even years, after reactivation of the virus and an outbreak of shingles.
C. This type of pain can signal a new outbreak of herpes zoster.
D. You should begin this client on antiviral therapy immediately.

57 *Marty, age 7, was brought to your primary care office with dog bites on his right hand and arm. You would send him home on:*

A. amoxicillin and clavulanate (Augmentin).
B. penicillin (Pentids).
C. amoxicillin (Amoxil).
D. clarithromycin (Biaxin).

58 *In assessing the susceptibility of Frank having been exposed to rabies after a dog bite, you should evaluate all of the following* ***except:***

A. whether Frank provoked the dog.
B. whether Frank knew the dog.
C. the immunization status of the dog.
D. whether the wound was cleaned out thoroughly.

59 *What is the correct procedure for assessing for arterial bruits?*

A. Auscultate at a point 2.5 cm above and lateral to the umbilicus.
B. Palpate the epigastric region with light pressure.

C. Position the bell of the stethoscope over the right lateral abdominal area.
D. Position the diaphragm of the stethoscope over the abdominal aorta and apply moderate pressure.

60 *You have just seen Mrs. Hill with her 4-month-old infant boy for a well-baby visit. You would schedule the next appointment in:*

A. 1 month.
B. 2 months.
C. 3 months.
D. 4 months.

61 *On Mrs. Hill's well-baby visit with her 4-month-old infant son, the following immunizations would be given:*

A. diphtheria, tetanus, pertussis (DTP); measles, mumps, rubella (MMR); and hepatitis B vaccine (HBV).
B. DTP, HBV, and *Haemophilus influenzae* type B vaccine (Hib).
C. HBV, Hib, DTP, and oral poliovirus (live) (OPV).
D. DTP, MMR, HBV, and Hib.

62 *Mrs. Hill's 4-month-old infant son is formula fed. An infant that age should have approximately how much formula per day?*

A. 8–9 oz given in 4 feedings per day
B. 6–7 oz given in 4–5 feedings per day
C. 5–6 oz given in 6 feedings per day
D. 5 oz given in 7 feedings per day

63 *Mrs. Hill wonders when she should start her 4-month-old infant on solid foods. You advise her that:*

A. solid foods may be added to liquid formula in formula-fed infants whenever they are unable to be satisfied with formula alone.
B. formula-fed infants should not begin on solid foods until they are over 6 months of age.
C. solid foods may be begun safely in formula-fed infants between 4 and 6 months of age.
D. solid foods may be begun safely in formula-fed infants between 6 and 8 months of age.

64 *Mr. Hughes is a 41-year-old African-American man who is in your primary care office for a physical exam. You recommend the following screening for prostate cancer:*

A. a digital rectal exam (DRE).
B. none; there is no need for screening until age 50 and older.
C. a DRE and prostate-specific antigen (PSA) level test.
D. a PSA test.

65 *Mr. Brown is 50 years old. His prostate-specific antigen (PSA) level the year before was 2.8 ng/mL. His PSA this year is 4.3 ng/mL. Your first course of action would be to:*

A. refer him for possible biopsy.
B. wait for 2 weeks, then repeat the test.
C. prescribe sulfamethoxazole and trimethoprim (Bactrim) PO bid or doxycycline (Vibramycin) 100 mg PO bid for 4 weeks and repeat the PSA 1 week after completion of the medication.
D. refer him for transrectal ultrasound.

66 *Andrea, age 16, is seen in your office for an injury to her eye. You remove a small foreign body from her cornea. There is no rust ring. In preparation for discharge, you would:*

A. patch her eye.
B. prescribe anesthetic eye drops.
C. prescribe steroid eye drops.
D. tell her that she may return to normal activity and take a nonsteroidal anti-inflammatory drug for pain if needed.

67 *Ms. Clancy, age 28, is complaining of a "cold that won't go away." She "thinks" that she has had a fever (she is afebrile in your office) and reports a nasal discharge that has become greenish in color. She also reports a cough. You decide that she has an acute, uncomplicated sinusitis and order:*

A. amoxicillin (Amoxil) 500 mg PO tid for 14–21 days.
B. sulfamethoxazole and trimethoprim (Bactrim) 1 DS tab PO bid for 7–10 days.
C. amoxicillin (Amoxil) 500 mg PO bid for 3–4 weeks.
D. ciprofloxin (Cipro) 500 mg bid for 14 days.

68 *Ms. Stanley is in your primary care office today complaining of burning on urination that has persisted for 3 days. She has no fever and no flank pain. This is the second urinary tract infection that she reports this year, and she thinks that the infections are related to increased sexual activity. She does not use a diaphragm for contraception and has tried drinking cranberry juice to offset this problem, something she read about in a women's magazine. You order:*

A. sulfamethoxazole and trimethoprim (TMP-SMZ) (Septra or Bactrim) 1 DS tab PO bid for 3 days.
B. TMP/SMZ 1 DS tab PO bid for 7–14 days.
C. TMP/SMZ 1 DS tab PO bid for 3 weeks.
D. a single dose of TMP/SMZ 1 DS tab PO.

69 *The most common cause of disability in clients under age 45 is:*

A. stress-related psychological disturbances.
B. low back pain.
C. severe migraine headaches.
D. alcohol and drug-related problems.

70 *The single most reliable indicator of readiness to return to work after an episode of back pain is:*

A. cessation of pain.
B. full mobility.
C. work satisfaction.
D. personal motivation.

71 *All of the following are clear indications for surgical intervention for the treatment of low back pain **except:***

A. progressive neurological deficit.
B. evidence of a bulging disc or protrusion on the computed tomography scan or magnetic resonance imaging.
C. incapacitating leg pain with demonstrated neural compromise.
D. failure of conservative therapy.

72 *Ms. Clayton, a 32-year-old office worker, comes to your ambulatory care setting complaining of paresthesias and burning in the fingers of her right hand, specifically the thumb, index, and middle fingers. She reports that these symptoms wake her up at night and are relieved by shaking or rubbing her hand. She has noted increasing weakness of her right hand and is concerned. You suspect carpal tunnel syndrome. Some other differential diagnoses that you must rule out include all the following **except:***

A. rotator cuff syndrome.
B. general peripheral neuropathy.
C. vascular insufficiency.
D. thoracic outlet obstruction.

73 *There are a number of parameters that allow you to distinguish between physiological and nonphysiological jaundice in the newborn. These include all of the following **except:***

A. Jaundice in the first 24 hours of life falls into the category of nonphysiological jaundice.
B. Physiological jaundice that arises by the third day of life and resolves by the tenth day is physiological.
C. Any jaundice after 10 days in a full-term infant is considered physiological.
D. Total bilirubin of more than 12 mg/dL in a full-term infant indicates nonphysiological jaundice.

74 *The treatment of choice for an adult with a diagnosis of group A beta-hemolytic streptococcal pharyngitis is:*

A. ofloxacin (Floxin) 500 mg PO bid for 5 days.
B. sulfamethoxazole and trimethoprim (Bactrim) DS 1 tab PO bid for 10 days.
C. penicillin V (PenVee K) 500 mg PO bid for 10 days.
D. cefaclor (Ceclor) 500 mg PO for 7 days.

75 *Mrs. Moore brings her 3-year-old son to your primary care office for evaluation. She is very upset and reports that, after eating dinner last evening, her son seemed to lose consciousness for a brief period. She states that he was sitting up, but that his head drooped and he did not respond to calls from her. She could not recall exactly how long this episode lasted, but reports that he returned to normal as the evening progressed and is also acting normally today. You suspect that the child had a(n):*

A. absence seizure.
B. tonic-clonic seizure.
C. myoclonic seizure.
D. atonic seizure.

76 *When diagnosing seizures in a child, despite an appropriate workup, the etiology remains undetermined 50% of the time. Differential diagnoses for seizure disorders in a child include the following:*

A. autism.
B. benign paroxysmal vertigo.
C. drug reaction.
D. labyrinthitis.

77 *The proper technique for measuring the fundal height in a pregnant client is to have the client:*

A. empty her bladder, then lie supine with legs flexed.
B. empty her bladder, then lie supine with legs extended.
C. empty her bladder, then assume a semi-Fowler's position with legs flexed.
D. lie in a completely flat position with legs extended.

78 *Postcoital contraception, or disruption of fertilization or of implantation of the egg within 72 hours after unprotected intercourse, is based on all of the following theoretical premises **except:***

A. Progestational agents change or interfere with sperm migration or the capacity of a sperm to penetrate the egg.
B. Progestational agents are thought to inhibit motility of the fallopian tubes.
C. Testosterone probably causes atrophy of the endometrium and prohibits implantation.
D. Estrogen increases the plasma level of progesterone, which assists in preventing ovulation.

79 *The serum albumin level gives a variety of valuable clinical information. All of the following are true regarding albumin **except:***

A. The albumin to total protein ratio should be greater than 1:2.
B. A low albumin level always indicates liver disease.
C. Along with the prothrombin time, albumin is a good, although indirect, indicator of the body's ability to synthesize proteins
D. Trauma, sepsis, or severe burns may all rapidly lower the albumin level as a result of fluid shifts.

80 *When a client comes in with hematuria, it is important to assess whether it is accompanied by pain or is painless. Etiologies of painful hematuria include all of the following* ***except:***

A. bladder tumor.
B. endometriosis.
C. glomerulonephritis.
D. papillary necrosis.

81 *Marcus, age 60, has just been given a diagnosis of urologic cancer. He asks what the risk factors are. You tell him that they include age older than 40 as well as:*

A. tobacco and alcohol use.
B. tobacco use and analgesic abuse.
C. exposure to aniline dyes and a low-fiber diet.
D. a diet high in fat and nitrates.

82 *A variety of different drugs may lead to hematuria. These include all of the following* ***except:***

A. nonsteroidal anti-inflammatory drugs.
B. penicillin (Pen-Vee K).
C. allopurinol (Zyloprim).
D. warfarin (Coumadin).

83 *The primary screening test for thyroid abnormalities is:*

A. thyroid-stimulating hormone level.
B. thyroxine (T_4)
C. free thyroxine index.
D. thyrotropin-releasing factor.

84 *Thyroxine (T_4) level may be influenced by a number of factors, thus giving an inaccurate result. These factors include:*

A. pregnancy, malnutrition, and alcohol use.
B. pregnancy, birth control pills, and malnutrition.
C. birth control pills, alcohol use, and use of opiates.
D. physical activity level, malnutrition, and alteration in liver function.

85 *Dementia is often acute and reversible. Reversible causes of dementia include:*

A. depression, deafness, and use of nitrates.
B. psychosis, vitamin B_{12} deficiency, and migraine headache.
C. sepsis, syphilis, and use of warfarin (Coumadin).
D. subdural hematoma, depression, and use of anticholinergics.

86 *You suspect that Bill, age 44, is abusing alcohol. There are several effective ways of eliciting sensitive information from such a client. Which of the following is most effective?*

A. Ask Bill directly, "How much do you drink?"
B. Ask Bill if he has had a drink in the last 24 hours.
C. Ask Bill if he has ever tried to cut down on his drinking.
D. Ask Bill if he has ever had health, legal, or personal problems as a result of alcohol and if the response is yes, ask him "When was the last time you had a drink?"

87 *Immunizations in adults age 65 and older should include:*

A. diphtheria, tetanus, and pertussis every 5 years and pneumococcal vaccine every 6 years starting at age 65.
B. pneumococcal vaccine at age 65 and tetanus and diphtheria every 10 years.
C. diphtheria, tetanus, and acellular pertussis every 10 years; and pneumococcal vaccine at age 65.
D. influenza immunization every fall, tetanus and diphtheria every 10 years, and pneumococcal vaccine at age 65.

88 *According to Erikson's 8 Stages of Man schemata for life span development, the chief psychosocial task for children ages 6–12 is:*

A. initiative vs. guilt.
B. productivity vs. stagnation.
C. generativity vs. boredom.
D. identity vs. confusion.

89 *An 18-month-old child is able to demonstrate the following competencies and characteristics:*

A. walks up steps, puts two words together, and performs simple tasks.
B. walks down steps, puts two words together, and has stranger anxiety.
C. throws overhand, zips and unzips, and points to and vocalizes wants.
D. kicks ball, puts four to six words together, and turns doorknob.

90 *Mrs. Greene scheduled an appointment for her 50-year-old husband for a routine check of his blood pressure. He is currently taking enalapril (Vasotec) 5 mg PO qd. She tells the receptionist that she would really like the nurse practitioner to talk with her husband about his alcohol use and smoking. When you press Mr. Greene for details about his alcohol and tobacco use during his visit, he becomes irritated and defensive. What stage of change is Mr. Greene exhibiting regarding the possibility of behavioral change?*

A. Contemplation
B. Precontemplation
C. Resistance
D. Prepreparation

91 *When you are counseling clients about behavioral change, there are many useful strategies. As the client is preparing and strengthening his or her determination to change, the nurse practitioner should do all of the following* ***except:***

A. Encourage the client to set a "start" date for action and note this in the chart.
B. Chart the specific actions in the plan, such as "will begin walking 30 minutes a day 3 times a week," in plain view of the client.
C. Generate much enthusiasm and demonstrate complete confidence in the client's ability to change.
D. Follow up with a phone call, note, or postcard.

92 *Often clients do not freely admit their difficulties in adhering to a treatment plan. Signs that the client may not be following the treatment plan include:*

A. active involvement, asking many questions; inconsistent response to treatment.
B. obedient and passive attitude; inconsistent response to treatment.
C. dissatisfaction with recommendations; attempts at negotiation.
D. consistent and measurable response to treatment.

93 *Research has demonstrated essential elements in achieving client adherence. These include all of the following* ***except:***

A. Developing a specific plan for implementation and clearly communicate this to the client.
B. Being empathic regarding the client's point of view.
C. Not hesitating to ask openly about the client's adherence.
D. Altering the plan to suit the client.

94 *Mrs. Garvey brings her 10-year-old son, Steve, to your primary care office. He has a 3-inch laceration on his leg that occurred over 24 hours before this visit. He did not tell his mother about this injury when it happened and the bleeding has stopped. No special efforts had been taken to cleanse the wound until the evening, when his mother discovered it. The wound edges are in close approximation. You should:*

A. cleanse, suture, and dress the wound, then have Steve return in 5 days for suture removal.
B. cleanse the wound and apply Steri-Strips.
C. cleanse and dress the wound, then have the client return in 3–5 days.
D. irrigate and cleanse the wound with antiseptic agents.

95 *An area of deep abrasion, including a "road burn," on the left forearm is best treated by doing all of the following:*

A. icing the wound after irrigation.
B. cleansing it several times a day and leaving it open to air.
C. prescribing prophylactic antibiotic therapy.
D. removing ground-in dirt using forceps.

96 *You, the nurse practitioner, have come down with a mild upper respiratory infection. You should take all of the following steps to prevent transmitting the infection:*

A. Begin treatment with antibiotics to minimize secondary bacterial infection.
B. Stay home until symptoms subside.
C. Take medications to reduce respiratory secretions.
D. Go in to work, but do not see clients—catch up on charts, follow up phone calls and the like.

97 *Clients with respiratory infections frequently call the office. You usually must make the decision regarding whether to treat over the phone or have the client come in to be seen. Some general parameters for this situation include all of the following* ***except:***

A. Being aware of the prevalent conditions in your community.
B. If a client has what sounds like a typical "cold," telephoning reassurance is all that is needed.
C. Calling in an antibiotic prescription if the client is insistent or has severe symptoms.
D. Advising decongestants, rest, fluid, and acetaminophen (Tylenol).

98 *Certain "red flags" signal the presentation of a true abdominal emergency. The nurse practitioner should be alert for all of the following conditions* ***except:***

A. light-headedness on standing and a history of alternating between constipation and diarrhea.
B. decreased urine output, light-headedness on standing, and a normal blood pressure.
C. increasing abdominal distention.
D. acute onset of abdominal pain.

99 *The Miller Assessment for Preschoolers screens all the following domains* ***except:***

A. sensory.
B. motor.
C. language.
D. cognitive.

100 *Jean wonders whether her 2-year-old son is developing normally. She is concerned because he seems to have a lot of temper tantrums. About what percentage of all children between the ages of 2–3 have a daily temper tantrum?*

A. 10%
B. 20%
C. 50%
D. 70%

101 *Tommy, age 5, wants to go to his grandfather's funeral, but his parents have conflicting opinions. They ask you for advice. What do you say?*

A. "Children under age 7 should not be exposed to funerals."
B. "He should go, but have him sit in the back and do not allow him to view the corpse."

C. "Let him attend, participate as much as he seems to want, and have someone willing to leave with him when he's ready."
D. "All children at this age should be encouraged to view the corpse to say their final good-byes."

102 *As a school-age child, Joshua, age 10, should master all of the following principal developmental tasks* ***except:***

A. winning approval from peers and adults.
B. obtaining a place in a peer group.
C. developing analytic thinking.
D. adopting moral standards for behavior.

103 *Sandy says that her baby can now roll from side to side and from back to front. How old do you suspect her baby to be?*

A. 3 months
B. 4 months
C. 5 months
D. 6 months

104 *Julie says that her doctor told her to participate in 20–30 minutes of vigorous activity at least three times per week and asks you to qualify "vigorous." How do you respond?*

A. "Exercise that makes you sweat is vigorous, as long as you sweat for the entire 20–30 minutes."
B. "It's vigorous if the heart rate is elevated to at least 60% of maximum for your age with the maximum heart rate calculated as 220 minus your age."
C. "If your heart rate is increased to 1 1/2 times your walking rate, the exercise is vigorous."
D. "If your heart rate is increased to twice your resting rate and is no more than 160, the exercise is vigorous."

105 *Curt's teenage daughter has a congenital heart problem and the doctor told her that she could participate only in nonstrenuous sports activities. These would include all the following* ***except:***

A. archery.
B. table tennis.
C. golf.
D. riflery.

106 *Martina has several young children and says that the information regarding safety seats is so confusing. You tell her that safety seats should:*

A. be used until the child weighs at least 50 lb.
B. face backwards until the infant weighs 15 lb.
C. be in the middle of the rear seat.
D. be used all the time even though they are not required in all states.

107 *In teaching your client about birth control, you tell her that the highest failure rate is with which birth control method?*

A. Spermicide
B. Withdrawal
C. Cervical cap
D. Condoms

108 *Jill is perimenopausal and asks you about the relationship between exercise and preventing osteoporosis. You tell her that:*

A. exercise has no effect; she should take calcium supplements.
B. weight-bearing exercise prevents bone mass loss.
C. all types of exercise assist in preventing osteoporosis.
D. after one has exercised regularly for 5 years, even after stopping, bone mass decreases slowly.

109 *Which type of stroke has a gradual onset and results in a pure motor or pure sensory stroke?*

A. Thrombotic
B. Embolic
C. Hemorrhagic
D. Lacunar

110 *Which type of tremor is goal-directed, more prominent with willful action, and may be located in proximal as well as distal extremities?*

A. Cerebellar
B. Physiologic
C. Parkinsonian
D. Essential

111 *Sigrid, age 78, is given a diagnosis of bacterial meningitis. What is the most probable offending pathogen?*

A. *Neisseria meningitides*
B. Staphylococci
C. *Streptococcus pneumoniae*
D. Gram-negative bacilli

112 *Beulah, age 86, has stasis dermatitis of her left lower leg. Her ankle is edematous and there is a rusty, brownish discoloration of the skin. What is your diagnosis?*

A. Arterial valvular insufficiency
B. Venous valvular insufficiency
C. Cellulitis
D. Diabetic nephropathy

113 *Jane, age 74, is incontinent of urine about 50% of the time. Which of the following is the absolute last resort in management of incontinence?*

A. Incontinence pads
B. Intermittent catheterization
C. A bladder training program (because of her age)
D. Indwelling catheterization

114 *Your neighbor calls you and states that her doctor told her that her mother developed septicemia as* *a result of zoonoses. She asks you what that is. You tell her that:*

A. Zoonosis is a cross-contamination type of disease between animals and humans.
B. She must have misunderstood the doctor; there is no such thing.
C. Zoonosis is a disease communicable from lower animals to humans under natural conditions.
D. He must have said xanthosis.

115 *Early descriptions of this disease were centered on the cutaneous manifestations. In fact, the word means "wolf" and was used to describe the destructive eating away of the skin that was a result of the rash. Which disease is this?*

A. Systemic lupus erythematosus
B. Herpes zoster (shingles)
C. Malaria
D. Rubeola

116 *The major cause of chronic renal failure is:*

A. hypertension.
B. glomerulonephritis.
C. diabetes mellitus.
D. obstructive uropathy.

117 *Maurice has gynecomastia. His evaluation should include:*

A. measuring testosterone level.
B. an evaluation of the adequacy of his liver function.
C. ordering a bilateral mammogram stat.
D. reassuring him that this is nothing and will pass.

118 *A condition with the symptoms of prostatitis but without infection is:*

A. prostatodynia.
B. acute nonbacterial prostatitis.
C. epididymitis.
D. chemical prostatitis.

119 *Jack had a routine screening and was found to have proteinuria. Your next action would be to:*

A. schedule a renal ultrasound.
B. refer him to a urologist.
C. ask the physician to schedule a renal biopsy.
D. collect a 24-hour urine for quantification.

120 *The major risk of a red blood cell transfusion is:*

A. cytomegalovirus infection.
B. hepatitis B infection.
C. human immunodeficiency virus infection.
D. a hemolytic transfusion reaction.

121 *Margaret thinks that her husband has toxoplasmosis and asks you about the symptoms. You tell her that the most common symptom is:*

A. confusion.
B. a fever.
C. a headache.
D. lethargy.

122 *Which glomerular disease occurs 10–14 days after an acute illness (commonly streptococcal in children) and is characterized by tea-colored urine, mild to severe renal insufficiency, and edema?*

A. Henoch-Schönlein purpura glomerulonephritis
B. Glomerulonephritis of systemic lupus erythematosus
C. Postinfection glomerulonephritis
D. Immunoglobulin A nephropathy

123 *About what percentage of children have congenital anomalies of the genitourinary tract, with severity ranging from abnormalities that remain asymptomatic through adulthood to malformations incompatible with life?*

A. Less than 3%
B. 5%
C. 10%
D. More than 10%

124 *Sadie, age 26, complains of a headache, backache, edema, breast tenderness, abdominal bloating, and lethargy for 3 days before each menstrual period. You diagnose premenstrual syndrome. You might suggest that Sadie try all of the following* ***except:***

A. evening primrose oil 2 caps bid.
B. vitamin E 66 mg daily.
C. prostaglandin inhibitors taken during the first half of the menstrual cycle.
D. vitamin B^6 (pyridoxine) 150–200 mg total daily dose initially.

125 *Marjorie has a Bartholin's cyst. What is the most common offending pathogen?*

A. Gonococcus
B. *Staphylococcus aureus*
C. *Streptococcus faecalis*
D. *Escherichia coli*

126 *Scott, age 22, has cryptorchidism and was never treated. To what is he more susceptible than men who do not have this?*

A. Malignant neoplasm of the testes
B. Epididymitis
C. Prostate cancer
D. Diverticular disease

127 *James is a high-school senior and cannot understand why you will not prescribe testosterone for him. He states that all of his bodybuilding friends take anabolic androgenic steroids to increase their muscle mass. You tell him that you have seen it ordered:*

A. for weight loss.
B. for decreased immune function

C. for fibrocystic breast disease.
D. to increase energy and appetite in older adults.

128 *In a 4-year-old child, the ideal glucose level after 2 or more hours of fasting should be:*

A. 80–180 mg/dL.
B. 100–200 mg/dL.
C. 70–150 mg/dL.
D. 120–220 mg/dL.

129 *Good diabetes management calls for a urine microalbumin level to be done:*

A. annually after the condition is first diagnosed.
B. every 2 years.
C. annually after the client has had diabetes for 5 years.
D. every 6 months.

130 *Betty states that she is infertile because of polycystic ovary syndrome. She asks you what causes the symptoms of amenorrhea, hirsutism, acne, and obesity. You tell her they are related to:*

A. androgen excess.
B. estrogen deficiency.
C. inadequate gonadotropin stimulation.
D. excessive adrenocorticotropic hormone.

131 *Prophylaxis for the first episode of* Pneumocystis carinii *pneumonia, an opportunistic disease in human immunodeficient virus-infected adults and adolescents, is:*

A. rifampin (Rimactane) 600 mg PO qd.
B. isoniazid (Nitrazid) 300 mg PO plus pyridoxine (Beesix) 50 mg PO qd.
C. trimethoprim-sulfamethoxazole (TMP-SMZ) (Bactrim) 1 DS PO qd.
D. clarithromycin (Biaxin) 500 mg PO bid.

132 *Marissa is going to have a splenectomy for her idiopathic thrombocytopenic purpura (ITP). The following is true about this:*

A. splenectomy produces permanent remission in 70–90% of children with ITP.
B. splenectomy is a first-line therapy.
C. vitamin B-12 supplementation is essential.
D. anticoagulant therapy is indicated postoperatively when the platelet count rises.

133 *Shelley, age 21, a single woman, comes to your primary care office for birth control. You are considering placing Shelley on birth control pills. The following are contraindications to placing Shelley on birth control pills:*

A. use of carbamazepine (Tegretol).
B. dysmenorrhea.
C. endometriosis.
D. need for contraception.

134 *Mrs. Graves, age 38, has been on birth control pills for approximately 15 years. She is a smoker, has a blood pressure of 110/70 mm Hg, and has lipid levels within normal limits. You advise that she should:*

A. discontinue the birth control pills because of her smoking.
B. remain on the pill because her blood pressure and lipids are within normal limits.
C. remain on the pill until her follicle-stimulating hormone level is greater than 30.
D. discontinue the pill because of her age.

135 *Goals for management of the client with diabetes mellitus include all of the following:*

A. maintaining blood glucose near normal (100–150 mg/dL); achieving normal weight; and eating a low-carbohydrate, high-protein diet.
B. exercising 20–30 minutes 3 times a week; maintaining a glycosylated hemoglobin (HgbA1C) greater than 12%.
C. maintaining a HgbA1C between 8 and 10%; minimizing complications; avoid hypoglycemia; and maintaining a normal lifestyle.
D. achieving a weight of 10% less than normal; exercising vigorously 60 minutes a day, 5 times a week; and minimizing complications.

136 *Diabetic clients who are most at risk for hypoglycemic episodes include the following:*

A. older adults, alcohol abusers, and those with hepatic and/or renal dysfunction.
B. clients with insulin pumps.
C. clients who are taking certain antifungal agents concurrently with oral hypoglycemic drugs and eating a diet of complex carbohydrates.
D. clients who exercise regularly or take birth control pills.

137 *Retinopathy is the leading cause of new blindness in the United States. Given this fact, you should recommend the following ophthalmologic exams to your clients with diabetes:*

A. Clients with insulin-dependent diabetes mellitus (type 1) should have their first ophthalmologic exam within first 5 years of diagnosis and then yearly exams thereafter; clients with non-insulin–dependent diabetes mellitus (type 2) should have their first ophthalmologic exam immediately on diagnosis and then yearly exams thereafter.
B. Clients with type 2 diabetes should be referred to an ophthalmologist within 5 years of diagnosis and have yearly exams thereafter; clients with type 1 diabetes should be referred immediately on diagnosis and then every 3 years.
C. Clients with either type 1 or type 2 diabetes should be referred immediately on diagnosis and then yearly thereafter.
D. Clients with either type 1 or type 2 diabetes should be referred on diagnosis and then followed up every other year depending on age.

138 *You should be suspicious of the accuracy of the results of a positive protein dipstick test that you have done in the office under which of the following circumstances?*

A. The urine concentration is very diluted.
B. The urine is very concentrated.
C. The urine has a very high sugar content.
D. The urine has blood in it.

139 *Urinary incontinence in older adults is widely underreported. It affects the following percentage of older adults:*

A. 15–30% of those living in the community and as high as 50% of those in institutional settings.
B. 10–15% of all those living in the community and 35% of those in institutional settings.
C. 40% of those living in the community and 60% of those in institutional settings.
D. 7–10% of those living in the community and 40% of those in institutional settings.

140 *Food sources rich in iron include:*

A. potatoes, bananas, and green, leafy vegetables.
B. enriched grain cereals, cabbage, and sweet potatoes.
C. liver, red meats, prunes, apples, and raisins.
D. enriched grain cereals, strawberries, watermelon, and honeydew melons.

141 *Menstruating women lose approximately how much iron per day?*

A. 5 mg
B. 10 mg
C. 0.1–1.6 mg
D. 2 mg

142 *Previous full-term pregnancies, even if uncomplicated, may cause a woman to lose approximately how much iron?*

A. 1500–1700 mg
B. 500–1000 mg
C. 250–500 mg
D. 1200–1500 mg

143 *The term "pica" refers to:*

A. an insatiable craving for such substances as laundry starch, clay, and ice, and is thought to suggest iron deficiency.
B. poverty and violence.
C. mental retardation in children.
D. a folic acid deficiency.

144 *Clients with refractive asthma should be evaluated along a number of parameters. These include:*

A. continued exposure to known causes, evaluation of compliance with treatment, examination of behavioral aspects, and evaluation of possible other causes of airway obstruction.
B. underlying, unresolved infectious processes; behavioral aspects of the disease; and compliance with treatment.
C. environmental aspects, family support systems, and socioeconomic status.
D. compliance with treatment, an evaluation of underlying nutritional status, family structure, and behavioral aspects of the disease.

145 *Your client, Mr. Lane, who suffers from chronic obstructive pulmonary disease, calls to say that, while visiting his daughter, he was exposed to influenza. He had received a flu shot in your office less than a week ago. He is calling because he is concerned that it is not working as yet. You tell him that:*

A. the flu shot will be sufficient to protect him.
B. because the flu shot will not be fully effective for several weeks, he should wash his hands frequently and get adequate rest.
C. he should start amantadine (Symmetrel) because it has been less than 48 hours since exposure to the infected person.
D. he should start amantadine (Symmetrel) immediately because the time since exposure has been over 72 hours.

146 *Your client, Mr. Lane, who has chronic obstructive pulmonary disease (COPD), reports a worsening of his respiratory symptoms. You review his entire medication list, noting that he is taking a beta blocker for his hypertension and nitrates for his angina in addition to the theophylline that he takes daily for his COPD. You decide to:*

A. switch him to a different bronchodilator.
B. discontinue the beta blocker.
C. switch his beta blocker to a calcium channel blocker.
D. discontinue his nitrates.

147 *Constipation is a frequent and common problem in older adults. Principles of treatment include:*

A. beginning supplemental bulk agents and encouraging exercise.
B. suggesting a combination of applesauce, bran, and prunes to be eaten every morning.
C. establishing a routine for early morning defecation and teaching clients not to ignore the urge to defecate.
D. encouraging adequate hydration and exercise and providing client education regarding a high-fiber diet and stopping laxatives.

148 *Inflammatory bowel disease is commonly seen in the primary care setting. It affects what percentage of all clients?*

A. 10%
B. 15%
C. 20%
D. 30%

149 *The majority of clients affected with inflammatory bowel disease are:*

A. older adults, with men and women equally affected.
B. young adults, with men and women equally affected.
C. older adults, with women affected twice as frequently as men.
D. young adults, with women affected twice as frequently as men.

150 *A variety of drugs have been implicated in erectile dysfunction. These include but are not limited to:*

A. diuretics, beta blockers, and angiotensin-converting enzyme (ACE) inhibitors.
B. vasodilators, anticholinergic agents, and antihistamines.
C. cimetidine (Tagamet), beta blockers, and diuretics.
D. ACE inhibitors, calcium channel blockers, estrogens, and digoxin.

Answers

1 Answer A

Content area: Issues in Primary Care (Chap. 19)

2 Answer C

Content area: Issues in Primary Care (Chap. 19)

3 Answer B

Content area: Issues in Primary Care (Chap. 19)

4 Answer B

Content area: Issues in Primary Care (Chap. 19)

5 Answer A

Content area: Issues in Primary Care (Chap. 19)

6 Answer B

Content area: Issues in Primary Care (Chap. 19)

7 Answer D

Content area: Issues in Primary Care (Chap. 19)

8 Answer D

Content area: Cardiovascular Problems (Chap. 11)

9 Answer B

Content area: Cardiovascular Problems (Chap. 11)

10 Answer C

Content area: Cardiovascular Problems (Chap. 11)

11 Answer D

Content area: Cardiovascular Problems (Chap. 11)

12 Answer C

Content area: Cardiovascular Problems (Chap. 11)

13 Answer B

Content area: Cardiovascular Problems (Chap. 11)

14 Answer B

Content area: Neurological Problems (Chap. 7)

15 Answer A

Content area: Head and Neck Problems (Chap. 9)

16 Answer C

Content area: Head and Neck Problems (Chap. 9)

17 Answer D

Content area: Head and Neck Problems (Chap. 9)

18 Answer C

Content area: Head and Neck Problems (Chap. 9)

19 Answer A

Content area: Cardiovascular Problems (Chap. 11)

20 Answer D

Content area: Cardiovascular Problems (Chap. 11)

21 Answer C

Content area: Care of the Emerging Family (Chap. 4)

22 Answer D

Content area: Care of the Emerging Family (Chap. 4)

23 Answer B

Content area: Care of the Emerging Family (Chap. 4)

24 Answer B

Content area: Care of the Emerging Family (Chap. 4)

25 Answer C

Content area: Care of the Emerging Family (Chap. 4)

26 Answer C
Content area: Respiratory Problems (Chap. 10)

27 Answer A
Content area: Respiratory Problems (Chap. 10)

28 Answer B
Content area: Respiratory Problems (Chap. 10)

29 Answer D
Content area: Respiratory Problems (Chap. 10)

30 Answer B
Content area: Musculoskeletal Problems (Chap. 16)

31 Answer C
Content area: Integumentary Problems (Chap. 8)

32 Answer A
Content area: Abdominal Problems (Chap. 12)

33 Answer C
Content area: Integumentary Problems (Chap. 8)

34 Answer B
Content area: Musculoskeletal Problems (Chap. 16)

35 Answer B
Content area: Musculoskeletal Problems (Chap. 16)

36 Answer A
Content area: Musculoskeletal Problems (Chap. 16)

37 Answer C
Content area: Abdominal Problems (Chap. 12)

38 Answer B
Content area: Abdominal Problems (Chap. 12)

39 Answer D
Content area: Male Genitourinary Problems (Chap. 14)

40 Answer D
Content area: Female Genitourinary Problems (Chap. 15)

41 Answer B
Content area: Abdominal Problems (Chap. 12)

42 Answer C
Content area: Female Genitourinary Problems (Chap. 15)

43 Answer D
Content area: Musculoskeletal Problems (Chap. 16)

44 Answer C
Content area: Issues in Primary Care (Chap. 19)

45 Answer C
Content area: Health Promotion (Chap. 3)

46 Answer A
Content area: Health Promotion (Chap. 3)

47 Answer B
Content area: Health Promotion (Chap. 3)

48 Answer A
Content area: Hematologic and Immune Problems (Chap. 18)

49 Answer B
Content area: Health Promotion (Chap. 3)

50 Answer C
Content area: Health Promotion (Chap. 3)

51 Answer B
Content area: Neurological Problems (Chap. 7)

52 Answer C
Content area: Cardiovascular Problems (Chap. 11)

53 Answer D
Content area: Head and Neck Problems (Chap. 9)

54 Answer B
Content area: Health Promotion (Chap. 3)

55 Answer C
Content area: Neurological Problems (Chap. 7)

56 Answer D
Content area: Integumentary Problems (Chap. 8)

57 Answer A
Content area: Integumentary Problems (Chap. 8)

58 Answer D
Content area: Integumentary Problems (Chap. 8)

59 Answer D
Content area: Health Promotion (Chap. 3)

60 Answer B
Content area: Care of the Emerging Family (Chap. 4)

61 Answer C
Content area: Care of the Emerging Family (Chap. 4)

62 Answer B
Content area: Care of the Emerging Family (Chap. 4)

63 Answer C
Content area: Care of the Emerging Family (Chap. 4)

64 Answer C
Content area: Male Genitourinary Problems (Chap. 14)

65 Answer C
Content area: Male Genitourinary Problems (Chap. 14)

66 Answer D
Content area: Head and Neck Problems (Chap. 9)

67 Answer A
Content area: Head and Neck Problems (Chap. 9)

68 Answer A
Content area: Female Genitourinary Problems (Chap. 15)

69 Answer B
Content area: Musculoskeletal Problems (Chap. 16)

70 Answer C
Content area: Musculoskeletal Problems (Chap. 16)

71 Answer B
Content area: Musculoskeletal Problems (Chap. 16)

72 Answer A
Content area: Musculoskeletal Problems (Chap. 16)

73 Answer C
Content area: Growth and Development (Chap. 5)

74 Answer C
Content area: Head and Neck Problems (Chap. 9)

75 Answer A
Content area: Neurological Problems (Chap. 7)

76 Answer D
Content area: Neurological Problems (Chap. 7)

77 Answer B
Content area: Growth and Development (Chap. 5)

78 Answer D
Content area: Female Genitourinary Problems (Chap. 15)

79 Answer B
Content area: Abdominal Problems (Chap. 12)

80 Answer A
Content area: Renal Problems (Chap. 13)

81 Answer B
Content area: Male Genitourinary Problems (Chap. 14)

82 Answer C
Content area: Renal Problems (Chap. 13)

83 Answer A
Content area: Endocrine and Metabolic Problems (Chap. 17)

84 Answer B
Content area: Endocrine and Metabolic Problems (Chap. 17)

85 Answer D
Content area: Neurological Problems (Chap. 7)

86 Answer D
Content area: Health Promotion (Chap. 3)

87 Answer D
Content area: Health Promotion (Chap. 3)

88 Answer A
Content area: Growth and Development (Chap. 5)

89 Answer A
Content area: Growth and Development (Chap. 5)

90 Answer B
Content area: Health Counseling (Chap. 6)

91 Answer C
Content area: Health Counseling (Chap. 6)

92 Answer B
Content area: Health Counseling (Chap. 6)

93 Answer A
Content area: Health Counseling (Chap. 6)

94 Answer C
Content area: Integumentary Problems (Chap. 8)

95 Answer C
Content area: Integumentary Problems (Chap. 8)

96 Answer A
Content area: Respiratory Problems (Chap. 10)

97 Answer B
Content area: Respiratory Problems (Chap. 10)

98 Answer A
Content area: Abdominal Problems (Chap. 12)

99 Answer C
Content area: Growth and Development (Chap. 5)

100 Answer B
Content area: Growth and Development (Chap. 5)

101 Answer C
Content area: Growth and Development (Chap. 5)

102 Answer C
Content area: Growth and Development (Chap. 5)

103 Answer C
Content area: Growth and Development (Chap. 5)

104 Answer B
Content area: Health Counseling (Chap. 6)

105 Answer B
Content area: Health Counseling (Chap. 6)

106 Answer C
Content area: Health Counseling (Chap. 6)

107 Answer C
Content area: Health Counseling (Chap. 6)

108 Answer B
Content area: Health Promotion (Chap. 3)

109 Answer D
Content area: Neurological Problems (Chap. 7)

110 Answer A
Content area: Neurological Problems (Chap. 7)

111 Answer C
Content area: Neurological Problems (Chap. 7)

112 Answer B
Content area: Integumentary Problems (Chap. 8)

113 Answer D
Content area: Renal Problems (Chap. 13)

114 Answer C
Content area: Hematologic and Immune Problems (Chap. 18)

115 Answer A
Content area: Integumentary Problems (Chap. 8)

116 Answer C
Content area: Renal Problems (Chap. 13)

117 Answer D
Content area: Endocrine and Metabolic Problems (Chap. 17)

118 Answer A
Content area: Male Genitourinary Problems (Chap. 14)

119 Answer D
Content area: Renal Problems (Chap. 13)

120 Answer A
Content area: Hematologic and Immune Problems (Chap. 18)

121 Answer C
Content area: Hematologic and Immune Problems (Chap. 18)

122 Answer C

Content area: Renal Problems (Chap. 13)

123 Answer C

Content area: Renal Problems (Chap. 13)

124 Answer C

Content area: Female Genitourinary Problems (Chap. 15)

125 Answer A

Content area: Female Genitourinary Problems (Chap. 15)

126 Answer A

Content area: Male Genitourinary Problems (Chap. 14)

127 Answer D

Content area: Male Genitourinary Problems (Chap. 14)

128 Answer B

Content area: Endocrine and Metabolic Problems (Chap. 17)

129 Answer C

Content area: Endocrine and Metabolic Problems (Chap. 17)

130 Answer A

Content area: Endocrine and Metabolic Problems (Chap. 17)

131 Answer C

Content area: Hematologic and Immune Problems (Chap. 18)

132 Answer D

Content area: Hematologic and Immune Problems (Chap. 18)

133 Answer C

Content area: Female Genitourinary Problems (Chap. 15)

134 Answer A

Content area: Female Genitourinary Problems (Chap. 15)

135 Answer C

Content area: Endocrine and Metabolic Problems (Chap. 17)

136 Answer A

Content area: Endocrine and Metabolic Problems (Chap. 17)

137 Answer A

Content area: Endocrine and Metabolic Problems (Chap. 17)

138 Answer B

Content area: Renal Problems (Chap. 13)

139 Answer A

Content area: Renal Problems (Chap. 13)

140 Answer C

Content area: Hematologic and Immune Problems (Chap. 18)

141 Answer D

Content area: Hematologic and Immune Problems (Chap. 18)

142 Answer B

Content area: Hematologic and Immune Problems (Chap. 18)

143 Answer A

Content area: Hematologic and Immune Problems (Chap. 18)

144 Answer A

Content area: Respiratory Problems (Chap. 10)

145 Answer C

Content area: Respiratory Problems (Chap. 10)

146 Answer C

Content area: Respiratory Problems (Chap. 10)

147 Answer D

Content area: Abdominal Problems (Chap. 12)

148 Answer B

Content area: Abdominal Problems (Chap. 12)

149 Answer D

Content area: Abdominal Problems (Chap. 12)

150 Answer C

Content area: Male Genitourinary Problems (Chap. 14)

GOOD LUCK ON YOUR CERTIFICATION EXAMINATION!